E·S·S·E·N·T·I·A·L·S   O·F

DENTAL
ASSISTING

E·S·S·E·N·T·I·A·L·S   O·F

DENTAL ASSISTING

Ann Ehrlich, CDA, MA

Hazel O. Torres, CDA, RDA, RDAEF, MA

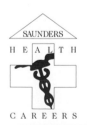

W. B. Saunders Company
Harcourt Brace Jovanovich, Inc.
Philadelphia   London   Toronto   Montreal   Sydney   Tokyo

W. B. Saunders Company
Harcourt Brace Jovanovich, Inc.

The Curtis Center
Independence Square West
Philadelphia, Pennsylvania 19106

Library of Congress Cataloging-in-Publication Data

Ehrlich, Ann B. (Ann Beard)
    Essentials of dental assisting / Ann Ehrlich, Hazel O. Torres.
        p.   cm.
    Includes bibliographical references and index.
    ISBN 0-7216-3262-9
    1. Dental assistants.   2. Dentistry.   I. Torres, Hazel O.
II. Title.
    [DNLM: 1. Dental Assistants.   2. Dental Care-methods.   WU 90 E33e]
RK60.5.E37   1992
617.6'0233—dc20
DNLM/DLC   92-9660

Editor: Margaret M. Biblis
Developmental Editor: Shirley Kuhn
Designer: W. B. Saunders Staff
Production Manager: Linda R. Garber
Manuscript Editor: W. B. Saunders Staff
Illustration Specialist: Peg Shaw
Indexer: Mary Chris Lindsay

Essentials of Dental Assisting   ISBN 0-7216-3262-9

Printed in the United States of America

Last digit is the print number: 9   8   7   6   5   4   3   2   1

Preface

Essentials of Dental Assisting is an exciting new undertaking for us. In this combination text and workbook, our primary goal is to present the basic *what* and *how-to-do-it* information that an entry-level dental assistant needs to know to get started on the job.

Our secondary goal is to present this information in simple, easy to follow steps, with generous illustrations. We believe that this book meets this challenge and can be used effectively by

▼ Students in entry-level dental assistant training programs.

▼ Dental assistants who are receiving on-the-job-training in a dental office or clinic.

▼ Dental assistants who want current information about topics such as disease transmission, universal precautions (infection control), the handling of hazardous substances in the dental office, and dental radiography.

The dental assistant who understands the what, why, and how of dental procedures is better able to effectively assist the dentist and to be a valued member of the dental health team. Therefore, we are optimistic that students using this book as a primary text will seek continuing education so that they will also learn *why* things are done in a certain manner.

The use of the pronouns "he" and "she" in this text is made necessary by the limitations of the English language. We do not mean to indicate that any sex limitations exist with regard to the qualifications for a position as part of the dental health team.

Many people have contributed to making *Essentials of Dental Assisting* possible, and we wish to express special thanks to

▼ Margaret Hooper, Lynn Strickland, and Linda Stewart of the Dental Assisting Program of Alamance Community College, Haw River, NC.

▼ Arnold Eilers, Wayne Feamster, and Steve Rizzuto for their photographic and artistic contributions to this book.

▼ Kimball C. Kaufman, DDS, San Rafael, CA, and Alonso D. Chattan, BA, Kentfield, CA.

▼ Barbara Cancilla, CDA, MA, RDAEF, and the students of the Registered Dental Assisting Program, College of Marin, Kentfield, CA.

▼ Michael Danford, DDS, and Robert Espino, University of California School of Dentistry, San Francisco.

We also wish to express thanks to the editorial staff of W. B. Saunders Company for their continued support and sincere interest in the concept of this text. Without the support and interest of all these individuals, this text might not have been realized.

ANN EHRLICH
HAZEL O. TORRES

Contents

1 Orientation to Dentistry

▼ LEARNING OBJECTIVES

The student will be able to:

1. Describe the functions of the reception area, business office, and dental laboratory.
2. Discuss the educational and licensure requirements of the dentist and the registered dental hygienist.
3. List and describe briefly the eight dental specialties.
4. Describe the role of the dental assistant as an administrative assistant, as a chairside assistant in four-handed dentistry, as a coordinating assistant in six-handed dentistry, and as an extended function dental assistant.
5. Identify the roles of the dental laboratory technician and the other members of the dental health team.
6. Discuss the assistant's responsibilities to the dentist, to the patients, and to the other members of the dental health team.
7. Demonstrate greeting patients in a professional manner.

OVERVIEW OF THE DENTAL OFFICE

The majority of dentists are in a "solo" or private practice in which one or two dentists work with their staff members. These dentists may be generalists, who provide all dental services, or specialists, who limit their practice to one area of dentistry.

Dental practices also range in size and variety all the way to very large group practices that include many general dentists and specialists plus a large staff of dental auxiliaries.

Although the size and type of practices vary greatly, there are certain areas found in every dental office.

The Reception Area

All persons coming to the dental office are always treated with courtesy and respect.

The reception area is where patients are received, greeted, and made to feel welcome. This should not be a "waiting area," for with proper scheduling patients can be seen on time for their appointments.

Patients often judge the quality of their care by the appearance of the office; therefore, this and all areas of the dental office must be kept neat and clean at all times.

Upon arrival the patient is greeted promptly, pleasantly, and by name. Adults are always greeted

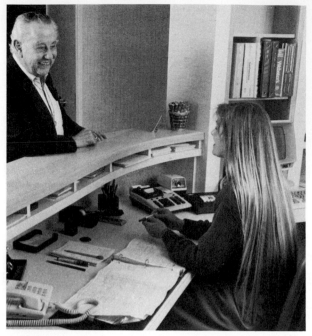

▼ **Figure 1–1**

The patient is greeted promptly and pleasantly upon his arrival at the dental office. (Torres HO, Ehrlich A: Modern Dental Assisting, 4th Ed. Philadelphia, WB Saunders, 1990, p 258.)

using the appropriate title such as Mr., Mrs., Miss, or Ms. (Fig. 1–1). Children may be greeted with their first name or nickname.

The Business Office

This area is the hub for the management of the business side of the practice, including:

▼ Appropriate patient flow, which is controlled through effective scheduling. *Unless patients have been properly scheduled, there are no patients to be treated.*

▼ Management of accounts receivable (money owed to the practice) and accounts payable (money owed by the practice). *Unless the dentist makes a profit from the practice, he or she cannot afford to stay in practice.*

▼ Records management and protection to safeguard patient and practice records. *These records are important legal documents, which must be protected against damage or loss.*

▼ Many other activities that are necessary for the smooth operation of the practice. *This enables the dentist to concentrate on providing quality patient care.*

The Treatment Area

The treatment area consists of several identically equipped "operatories." It is here that most patient care is provided. These operatories are described in Chapter 10, "The Dental Operatory."

The Central Sterilization and Supply Area

The sterilization and supply area is centrally located to provide easy access from the operatories and other office areas. The use of this area is discussed further in Chapters 7, "Infection Control," and 11, "Dental Hand Instruments."

The Dental Laboratory

The dental laboratory is where basic dental laboratory procedures are performed. In most practices, unless a certified dental technician is employed, more complex cases are sent to a commercial laboratory (Fig. 1–2).

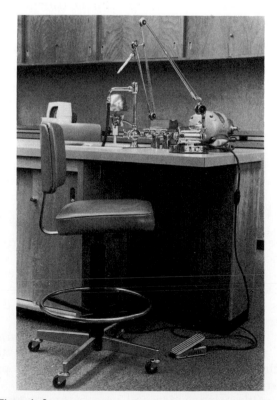

▼ **Figure 1–2**

Basic dental laboratory equipment. (Torres HO, Ehrlich A: Modern Dental Assisting, 4th Ed. Philadelphia, WB Saunders, 1990, p 345.)

Basic dental laboratory equipment includes:

▼ Well-lighted workbenches.

▼ Laboratory handpieces, burs, and rheostat.

▼ A model trimmer.

▼ Vibrator.

▼ Bench lathe.

▼ Vacuum spatulator for mixing stone.

▼ Plaster or investment material.

▼ A vacuum unit for the construction of custom trays and mouth guards.

After each use, the laboratory work surfaces and equipment must be cleaned and returned to their appropriate places.

Other Office Areas

Private Office. Each dentist usually maintains a private office for his or her personal use. Other staff members must respect the privacy of this area.

Consultation Room. This room is equipped with a table, comfortable chairs, and good lighting. Here the dentist "presents the case" and discusses the proposed treatment plan with the patient.

If there is no consultation room, the dentist's private office may be used for this purpose.

Darkroom. If radiographs are processed manually, a dark room is maintained for this purpose. (See Chapter 16, "Dental Radiography: Paralleling Techniques," for a further explanation.)

Staff Lounge. Some practices maintain a separate area for use as a lounge where staff members may change into their uniforms, eat lunch, and hold meetings.

Staff members are responsible for keeping this area neat and clean at all times.

MEMBERS OF THE DENTAL HEALTH TEAM

The Dentist

The educational requirements for the dentist within the United States include undergraduate college plus graduation from a dental school that has been accredited by the Commission on Dental Accreditation of the American Dental Association (Fig. 1-3).

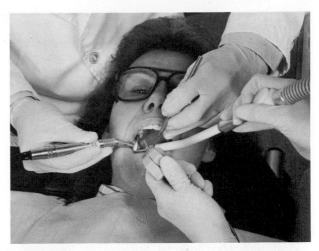

▼ Figure 1-3

In four-handed dentistry, the assistant works in close cooperation with the dentist. (Torres HO, Ehrlich A: Modern Dental Assisting, 4th Ed. Philadelphia, WB Saunders, 1990, p 12.)

The degree granted usually is the DDS (Doctor of Dental Surgery) or the DMD (Doctor of Medical Dentistry). Most dentists are members of their professional organizations, the American Dental Association (ADA) or the National Dental Association.

Prior to beginning to practice dentistry in a state, the dentist must pass both written and clinical examinations in order to be licensed by that state.

The Dental Specialties

Training for dental specialists includes an additional 2 years of postgraduate and graduate education in the area of specialization in a program approved by the Commission on Dental Accreditation of the American Dental Association.

The dental specialties officially recognized by the American Dental Association's Commission on Dental Accreditation are outlined in the chart on page 4.

The Dental Hygienist

The hygienist uses the title Registered Dental Hygienist (RDH) and is an important member of the dental health team, particularly in the area of preventive dentistry (Fig. 1-4). The hygienist is trained to:

▼ Scale and polish the teeth.

▼ Record case histories and chart conditions of the oral cavity.

▼ The Dental Specialties

Dental Public Health is concerned with preventing and controlling dental diseases, preventing the spread of communicable diseases, and promoting dental health through organized community efforts.

Endodontics is concerned with the etiology, diagnosis, prevention, and treatment of diseases and injuries of the dental pulp and associated periradicular tissues.

Oral Pathology is concerned with the etiology and the nature of the diseases affecting the oral structures and adjacent regions. (**Etiology** is the study of the cause of diseases.)

Oral and Maxillofacial Surgery is concerned with the diagnosis and surgical and adjunctive treatment of diseases, injuries, and defects involving both the functional and the esthetic aspects of the hard and soft tissues of the oral and maxillofacial regions.

Orthodontics is concerned with the supervision, guidance, and correction of all forms of malocclusion of the growing or mature dentofacial structures.

Pediatric Dentistry is concerned with the preventive and therapeutic oral health care of children from birth through adolescence. It also includes care for special patients beyond adolescence who demonstrate mental, physical, and/or emotional problems.

Periodontics is concerned with the diagnosis and treatment of disease of the supporting and surrounding tissues of the teeth.

Prosthodontics is concerned with the restoration and maintenance of oral functions by the restoration of natural teeth and/or the replacement of missing teeth and contiguous oral and maxillofacial tissues with prostheses (artificial substitutes).

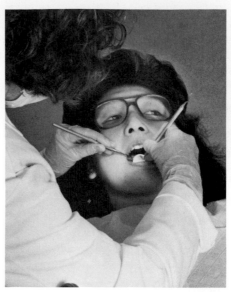

▼ Figure 1-4

A dental hygienist is licensed by the state in which he or she works to scale and polish teeth. (Torres HO, Ehrlich A: Modern Dental Assisting, 4th Ed. Philadelphia, WB Saunders, 1990, p 11.)

academic years of college study in a dental hygiene program that has been accredited by the Commission on Dental Accreditation of the American Dental Association.

Dental hygiene education is also offered in bachelor's and master's degree programs.

The hygienist must pass both a written and a clinical state or regional examination in order to be licensed by the state in which he or she plans to practice. The hygienist is then governed by the dental practice act of that state.

The Dental Assistant

Educational programs for dental assistants vary considerably in length. An "accredited dental assisting program" is one that has been evaluated and approved by the Commission on Dental Accreditation of the American Dental Association.

Dental assistants fill many roles in the dental practice, and the importance of these roles is discussed further in Chapter 2, "The Professional Dental Assistant."

The Generalist

Working as a generalist is a challenging but increasingly rare role. In a "one-employee" practice this dental assistant divides her time between the business office, treatment areas, dental laboratory, and darkroom.

▼ Expose, process, and evaluate the quality of radiographs.

▼ Polish restorations.

▼ Apply topical fluoride treatments.

▼ Instruct the patient in preventive dentistry and nutrition.

▼ Administer local anesthetic materials and nitrous oxide-oxygen.

The hygienist is also permitted to perform the tasks of a chairside assistant and, in some states, has been assigned additional extended responsibilities.

In the majority of states, the minimal education required for dental hygiene licensure is 2

A more common situation is one in which several assistants are employed, each of whom is a "specialist" in her own area. However, each assistant has basic knowledge of other areas and is able to substitute or help out as necessary.

The Administrative Assistant

The administrative assistant, also known as the *secretarial assistant* or *receptionist,* is primarily responsible for the smooth and efficient operation of the business office (Fig. 1–5). These duties include:

▼ Patient reception and answering the telephone.

▼ Appointment control.

▼ Records management.

▼ Accounts receivable and accounts payable bookkeeping.

▼ Handling of all correspondence and management of the recall and inventory control systems.

The Chairside Assistant

The term **four-handed dentistry** describes the seated dentist and chairside assistant working smoothly as a team to provide quality dental care with a minimum of time, motion, and stress.

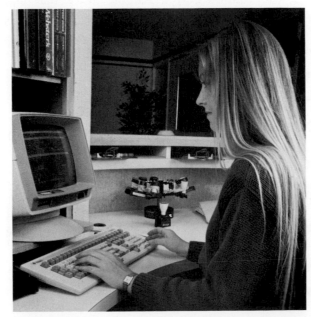

▼ Figure 1–5

The administrative assistant is primarily responsible for the smooth functioning of the business office. (Torres HO, Ehrlich A: Modern Dental Assisting, 4th Ed. Philadelphia, WB Saunders, 1990, p 904.)

The chairside assistant is responsible for working directly with the dentist in the treatment area. Responsibilities here may include:

▼ Patient seating and preparation.

▼ Instrument and operatory care.

▼ Oral evacuation.

▼ Tongue and tissue retraction.

▼ Instrument exchange.

▼ The preparation and storage of materials and supplies.

▼ Some radiography and patient education.

In a practice where there *is* a coordinating assistant, the chairside assistant's duties are usually modified so that more time may be spent "chairside" working directly with the dentist.

The Coordinating Assistant

The term **six-handed dentistry** describes the use of an additional assistant, usually the coordinating assistant, who "serves as an extra pair of hands where needed" throughout the dental treatment (Fig. 1–6).

In six-handed dentistry, the coordinating assistant also has specific responsibilities of her own. These may include:

▼ Exposing, processing, and mounting radiographs.

▼ Patient seating and dismissal.

▼ Mixing and passing materials to the chairside assistant or dentist.

▼ Operatory and instrument care and preparation.

▼ Patient education.

▼ Limited laboratory procedures and control of cases to and from the dental laboratory.

Very often a new assistant is assigned to work as a coordinating assistant until she becomes familiar with all aspects of the practice.

The Extended Functions Dental Assistant (EFDA)

Under the State Dental Practice Act, "extended functions" are those duties that may legally be assigned to qualified dental auxiliaries functioning in that state (Fig. 1–7).

An assistant who is qualified and registered to perform these duties is known as an extended function dental auxiliary (EFDA). (See Chapter 2,

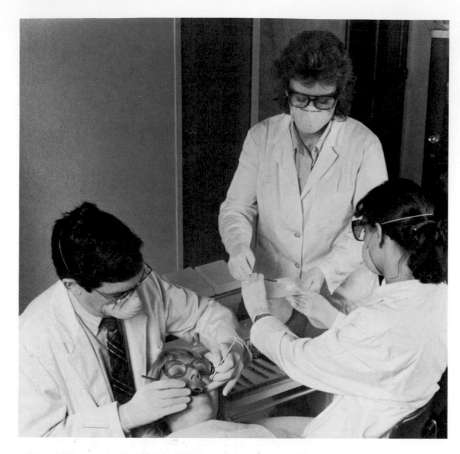

▼ Figure 1-6

In six-handed dentistry, the coordinating assistant serves "as an extra pair of hands where needed" throughout treatment. (Torres HO, Ehrlich A: Modern Dental Assisting, 4th Ed. Philadelphia, WB Saunders, 1990, p 335.)

"The Professional Dental Assistant," for more details on the legal regulations that control these activities.)

The following is a list of duties that may *potentially* be allowed for performance by an extended functions registered dental assistant:

▼ Making radiographic exposures.

▼ Taking impressions for opposing study casts.

▼ Taking a bite registration.

▼ Retracting gingivae prior to impression procedures.

▼ Taking impressions for cast restorations.

▼ Taking impressions for space maintainers, orthodontic appliances, and occlusal guards.

▼ Determining root length and endodontic file length.

▼ Fitting trial endodontic filling points.

▼ Placing and removing periodontal and surgical dressings.

▼ Removing sutures.

▼ Applying topical anesthetics.

▼ Assisting in the administration of nitrous oxide–oxygen analgesia or sedation.

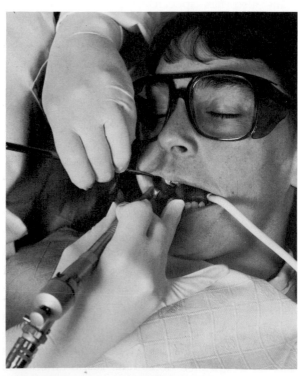

▼ Figure 1-7

The extended functions dental assistant (EFDA) performs direct patient functions in keeping with the state's dental practice act and his or her educational qualifications. (Torres HO, Ehrlich A: Modern Dental Assisting, 4th Ed. Philadelphia, WB Saunders, 1990, p 904.)

▼ Performing preliminary oral examinations.

▼ Polishing coronal surfaces of teeth.

▼ Providing oral health instruction.

▼ Applying anticariogenic agents topically.

▼ Placing and removing rubber dams.

▼ Placing and removing wedges and matrices.

▼ Placing and removing sedative or temporary restorations and crowns.

▼ Placing, carving, and finishing amalgam restorations.

▼ Placing and finishing composite restorations.

▼ Removing excess cement from coronal surfaces of teeth.

▼ Preparing teeth for bonding by etching.

▼ Applying pit and fissure sealants.

▼ Applying cavity liners and bases.

▼ Performing additional functions that may be delegated within specialties for the state in which the auxiliary is employed.

The Dental Laboratory Technician

The dental laboratory technician may legally fabricate and repair dental prostheses (such as cast restorations and removable dentures), as specified by the *written* prescription of the dentist (Fig. 1–8).

Most dental laboratory technicians are employed by large commercial laboratories; however, some are employed by individual dentists and the military services. Others maintain their own laboratories.

Other Members of the Dental Health Team

Dental Supply Salesperson

A dental supply salesperson is a representative from a dental supply house who routinely calls at the dental office. His or her services include taking orders for supplies, providing new product information, and helping to arrange for equipment service and repairs.

Detail Person

A detail person is a representative of a specific company, usually a drug or dental product manu-

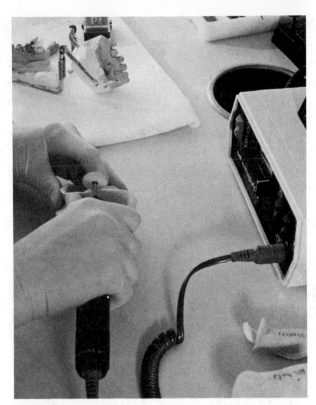

▼ **Figure 1–8**

A dental laboratory technician fabricates prosthetic devices based on the written prescription of the dentist. (Torres HO, Ehrlich A: Modern Dental Assisting, 4th Ed. Philadelphia, WB Saunders, 1990, p 13.)

facturer, who visits dental offices for the purpose of providing the doctor with information concerning his or her company's products.

Dental Equipment Technician

A dental equipment technician is a specialist who installs and provides service and repairs of dental equipment. This service may be provided under a maintenance contract or on an "as needed" basis.

THE DENTAL HEALTH TEAM

Although the individual members of the dental health team have specific duties and areas of responsibility, they are *all* working together toward the shared goal of providing the best possible care for their patients.

The dentist is the leader of this team. He or she is in charge and must retain responsibility for the well-being of the patients and the actions of the employees.

All members of the team must give their complete support and loyalty to the dentist who is the leader of their team. They must also be able to work together in close harmony and be willing to help each other at all times.

The Role of the Assistant as a Team Member

As a member of the dental health team, the assistant has very definite obligations and responsibilities to the dentist, the patients, and the other team members.

The Assistant's Responsibilities to the Dentist

1. The assistant must give complete and loyal support to the dentist and must at all times treat the dentist with dignity and respect.
2. The assistant must be able to accept the dentist's method of practice and share his or her belief in the value of preventive dental care.
3. The assistant must hold in strict confidence all things seen or heard in the dental office pertaining to the dentist, the patients, and the other team members.
4. The assistant must perform only those duties delegated by the dentist and that can be performed in keeping with the assistant's educational qualifications and the state dental practice act.
5. The assistant must at all times carefully follow the instructions given, and work to the best of his or her ability.
6. The assistant must conduct himself or herself in such a professional manner as to reflect favorably on the dentist, the dental health team, and the dental profession.
7. The assistant must maintain positive mental attitudes in working relationships and not convey personal problems in professional activities.
8. The assistant who is not able to accept these responsibilities should give due notice to the employer and seek employment elsewhere.

The Assistant's Responsibilities to the Patient

1. The assistant must always perform all duties to the very best of his or her ability, for performance that is less than 100 percent could have disastrous effects for the patient.
2. The assistant must recognize that all persons have a basic need for approval and respect, and that this need is exaggerated in times of stress, such as the dental situation.

3. The assistant must make every effort to understand the patient's needs and be willing to help the patient meet these needs, in an acceptable manner.
4. The assistant should work toward personal development and maturity, which will enable him or her to:

   Recognize that the patient may be motivated by factors totally unknown to the assistant.

   Accept the patient as he or she is.

   Be tolerant of behavior that is not readily understood.

   Be willing to make the extra effort to be pleasant and understanding, although the patient may be irritable and demanding.

5. The assistant must take necessary steps to protect the health of the patient, herself, and co-workers by carefully following the procedures necessary for maintaining asepsis. Also, if the assistant is ill, she must take precautions to prevent the spread of her disease to patients or co-workers.
6. The assistant must be neat, clean, properly attired, and professional in appearance, for this creates a favorable impression and helps inspire patient confidence.
7. The assistant must try to educate the patient in the values of modern preventive dental care. By personal example and enthusiasm, the assistant demonstrates his or her belief in these values.
8. The assistant must try to be a good representative of the dental profession.

The Assistant's Responsibilities to the Other Dental Health Team Members

1. The assistant must treat all team members with respect and work with them in a spirit of cooperation.
2. The assistant must carefully perform his or her duties and responsibilities and not try to shift these duties onto someone else.
3. The assistant must help others when not occupied with his or her own duties.
4. The assistant must be prepared to interrupt those duties in order to help other team members in an emergency.
5. The assistant must make every effort to arrive at work on time and to be on duty at all assigned times. (This includes guarding his or her health because any absence may cause an unfair hardship to the other team members.)
6. If, for any reason, the assistant must be absent

from work, advance arrangements should be made to ensure that his or her position is covered.

7. The assistant must realize that supervision, criticism, and change are occasionally necessary and should accept these in the constructive manner in which they are offered.

8. The assistant must at all times maintain current skills and knowledge through active participation in continuing education programs.

9. The assistant must handle grievances through the accepted office procedure, such as the staff conference, before they become major in nature.

10. If unable to work harmoniously with other team members, the assistant should give notice and seek employment elsewhere.

▶ EXERCISES

1. The assistant must perform only those duties that are _a b c_
   _____.

   a. delegated by the dentist
   b. in keeping with the assistant's educational qualifications
   c. permitted by the state dental practice act
   d. a, b, and c

2. The educational requirements for a dentist include ___D. D. S___
   _D M D_.

   a. graduation from a dental school accredited by the Commission on Dental Accreditation of the American Dental Association
   b. membership in the American Dental Association
   c. undergraduate college
   d. a and c

3. A/An ___d_____ is a specialist who fits and designs bridge-work and dentures to replace teeth.

   a. exodontist
   b. orthodontist
   c. periodontist
   d. prosthodontist

4. The assistant must ___d_____.

   a. be able to accept the dentist's method of practice
   b. give complete and loyal support to the dentist
   c. hold in strict confidence all things seen or heard in the dental office
   d. a, b, and c

5. A ___d_____ is trained to scale and polish the teeth and is licensed by the state in which he or she is employed.

   a. certified dental assistant
   b. certified dental hygienist
   c. registered dental assistant
   d. registered dental hygienist

6. In _(b) Four handed___ dentistry, the coordinating assistant serves as *an extra pair of hands* where needed.

   a. extended function
   b. four-handed
   c. seated
   d. six-handed

7. ___D. P. H (a)_____ is the specialty concerned with preventing and controlling dental diseases and promoting dental health through organized community efforts.

   a. Dental public health
   b. Oral pathology
   c. The dental hygienist
   d. The state board of dentistry

8. The assignment of extended functions to qualified dental auxiliaries is controlled by the _____.

   a. American Dental Assistants Association
   b. American Dental Association
   c. Dental Assisting National Board
   d. State Dental Practice Act

9. The degree DDS stands for _____.

   a. Doctor of Dental Science
   b. Doctor of Dental Specialties
   c. Doctor of Dental Surgery
   d. none of the above

10. A proposed treatment plan is presented to the patient in the _____.

    a. business office
    b. consultation room
    c. staff lounge
    d. treatment area

11. A _____ generalist _____ works in a "one-employee" practice.

    a. chairside assistant
    b. coordinating assistant
    c. generalist
    d. receptionist

12. _____ N_2O-O_2 Analgesia _____ is/are functions which may be assigned to an EFDA.

    a. Preparing a tooth for an amalgam restoration
    b. Administering nitrous oxide–oxygen analgesia
    c. Fitting a full or partial denture
    d. None of the above

13. An assistant who is unable to work harmoniously with other team members should _____ (b) _____.

    a. complain to the dentist
    b. give notice and seek employment elsewhere
    c. report the situation to the state dental board
    d. a and c

14. A _____ (a) _____ is a specialist who installs and provides service and repairs of dental equipment.

    a. dental equipment technician
    b. dental laboratory technician
    c. dental supply salesperson
    d. detail person

15. A/An _____ c _____ is concerned with the diagnosis and treatment of diseases of the supporting and surrounding tissues of the teeth.

    a. endodontist
    b. oral pathologist
    c. periodontist
    d. prosthodontist

16. It is the role of the _____(a)_____ to make and repair dental prostheses as specified by the written prescription of the dentist.

    a. dental laboratory technician
    b. detail person
    c. extended function dental assistant
    d. registered dental hygienist

17. When not occupied with his or her own duties, the assistant should _____(d)_____.

    a. notify the receptionist
    b. report immediately to the dentist
    c. retire quietly to the staff lounge
    d. try to help others

18. All persons have a basic need for approval and respect. In times of stress, such as the dental situation, this need is _____c._____.

    a. diminished
    b. exaggerated
    c. minimized
    d. sublimated

19. In the majority of states, the minimal education requirement for dental hygiene licensure is _____c._____ in a dental hygiene program accredited by the Commission on Dental Accreditation of the American Dental Association.

    a. a master's degree
    b. 4 academic years of college study
    c. 2 academic years of college study
    d. a or b

20. Prior to beginning to practice in a state, the _____dentist_____ must pass both written and clinical examinations to become licensed by that state.

    a. dental assistant
    b. dental laboratory technician
    c. dentist
    d. a, b, and c

21. Training for dental specialists includes at least _____2_____ years of postgraduate and graduate education in an approved program in the area of specialization.

    a. 1
    b. 2
    c. 3
    d. 4

22. The _____reception_____ is where patients are received, greeted, and made to feel welcome in the dental office.

    a. business office
    b. consultation room
    c. private office
    d. reception area

23. _____c._____ is the specialty concerned with the preventive and therapeutic oral health care of children from birth through adolescence.

    a. Dental public health
    b. Orthodontics
    c. Pediatric dentistry
    d. Periodontics

24. The assistant should handle grievances _c._ _____.

    a. by discussing them with co-workers
    b. by reporting them immediately to the dentist
    c. through the accepted office procedure
    d. a and b

25. The duties of the _____ include patient reception and answering the telephone, appointment control, and records management.

    a. administrative assistant
    b. coordinating assistant
    c. registered dental hygienist
    d. a or b

▼ Criterion Sheet 1–1

Student's Name _____

Procedure: *GREETING DENTAL PATIENTS*

Performance Objective:

In a classroom simulation, the student will greet an arriving patient and ask him to accompany her to the treatment area.

Another student will play the role of the patient *Randolph Patterson*. He is hard of hearing, but does not wear a hearing aid. Mr. Patterson is very irritable and nervous about coming to the dentist.

SE = Student evaluation IE = Instructor evaluation	C = Criterion met X = Criterion not met	SE	IE
Instrumentation: None			
1. Greeted the patient pleasantly and by name.			
2. Politely asked the patient to accompany her to the operatory.			
3. Recognized the patient's difficulty and repeated the request.			
4. Dealt appropriately with the patient's irritability.			
Comments:			

2 The Professional Dental Assistant

▼ LEARNING OBJECTIVES

The student will be able to:

1. Identify at least three benefits of being a member of the American Dental Assistants Association (ADAA).
2. Discuss the role of certification, and state where information may be gathered concerning becoming a certified dental assistant (CDA).
3. Describe the role of the State Dental Practice Act, the State Board of Dentistry, licensure, and registration in regulating dentistry within the state.
4. Describe the requirements for renewal for the certified and/or registered dental assistant.
5. List three places where a dental assistant may find information regarding potential employment opportunities.
6. Describe the responsibilities of both the employer and the employee in maintaining employment.
7. Demonstrate preparing a personal résumé.
8. Demonstrate preparing a letter of application.

OVERVIEW OF THE PROFESSIONAL DENTAL ASSISTANT

Assistants fill many interesting, important, and varied roles in the dental office. Each assistant must fulfill the role to the best of her ability and training. It is also essential that the assistant perform *only* those duties that may legally be assigned to her under the laws of the state in which she is employed.

AMERICAN DENTAL ASSISTANTS ASSOCIATION

The American Dental Assistants Association (ADAA) is the professional organization of dental assistants, with local and state components and a national office maintained in Chicago. The "American Dental Assistants Association Principles of Ethics" is shown in the chart on page 16.

Membership in the ADAA gives the assistant representation and a voice in national affairs, with a far-reaching effect on the career and future of all dental assistants.

The ADAA also provides journals, continuing education opportunities, and group and professional liability insurance plus local, state, and national meetings.

CERTIFICATION

Certification carries with it the prestige of knowledge and the ability to apply it properly; however, it is in no sense a degree, nor does it hold any legal status except in those states recognizing it under their dental practice acts.

Upon satisfactory completion of an accredited training program, or having met the work experience requirements, and holding current cardiopulmonary resuscitation (CPR) certification, the assistant is eligible to sit for the certification examination given by the Dental Assisting National Board, Inc. (DANB).

More specific information concerning the certification program may be obtained from the Chicago office of the DANB.

The examination for a certified dental assistant (CDA) covers primarily chairside duties plus dental radiation health and safety. Certification is also awarded in the following specialty areas:

▼ Certified Orthodontic Assistant (COA).

▼ Certified Oral and Maxillofacial Surgery Assistant (COMSA).

▼ Certified Dental Practice Management Assistant (CDPMA).

The Certified Dental Assistant (CDA) must earn a certain number of continuing education credits each year in order to renew certification. Assistants who do not meet these requirements are no longer permitted to use the title Certified Dental Assistant.

It is also expected that the assistant will maintain *current* certification in basic first aid and cardiopulmonary resuscitation (CPR).

THE EXTENDED FUNCTION DENTAL AUXILIARY (EFDA)

The EFDA performs reversible dental procedures in compliance with the state's dental practice act, his or her educational qualifications, and that state's registration requirements.

Although assistants may be trained to perform all of these functions, legally they may perform only those functions that have been officially delegated to auxiliaries under the dental practice act of their state.

Direct Supervision

In most states, when the practice act assigns extended functions to the auxiliary, it specifies that these functions be performed under the direct supervision of the dentist. Compliance with this requirement is important.

Direct supervision means that the dentist:

▼ Is in the dental office or treatment facility.

▼ Personally authorizes the procedures.

▼ Remains in the office while the procedures are being performed by the auxiliary.

▼ Evaluates the performance of the dental auxiliary before the patient is dismissed.

General Supervision

The dental practice act may stipulate general supervision for the delegation of certain functions by qualified personnel.

In most states, general supervision means that the dentist is responsible for the actions of the auxiliary; however, that procedure may legally be performed without the dentist being present in the treatment facility.

THE STATE DENTAL PRACTICE ACT

The state dental practice act contains the legal restrictions, responsibilities, and controls on the dentist, the dental auxiliaries, and the practice of dentistry within that state.

The educationally qualified assistant is able to relieve the dentist of those activities that do not require the dentist's professional skill and judgment. However, the responsibilities assigned to the assistant are limited by the regulations of the dental practice act of the state in which the dentist and assistant are working.

Licensure

The State Board of Dental Examiners is responsible for supervising and regulating the practice of dentistry within the state.

Licensure is one means of supervising and regulating those practicing dentistry within the state. It is a means of establishing and enforcing standards to protect the interests and well-being of the general public.

The dentist and the dental hygienist must be licensed by the State Board of Dental Examiners in order to practice within that state.

Dental assistants are not licensed to perform their routine functions; however, in some states a registered dental assistant, who is assigned specific extended functions, may be licensed at that level.

Engaging in the unlicensed practice of dentistry is a criminal act. This includes performing functions that are assigned to the dentist—but not those assigned to the auxiliary.

Ignorance of the dental practice act, licensure, or the rules and regulations interpreting the act is no excuse for illegally practicing dentistry.

Registration

Although dental assistants are not licensed, some states do require registration for those assistants who expose radiographs and/or perform extended functions (Fig. 2–1).

Some states require that the assistant pass a state examination or meet specific educational requirements. Other states grant registration to those assistants who have passed the DANB certification examination.

Having met these requirements, the assistant is known as a Registered Dental Assistant (RDA) or Registered Dental Assistant in Extended Functions (RDAEF).

The states that require registration may also require periodic (annual or biannual) renewal of that registration. Practicing without a current (renewed) registration or license is illegal.

If you work in a state that requires registration of any sort for dental assistants, contact your state board of dentistry for information regarding these requirements.

▼ The Illegal Practice of Dentistry

The assistant who performs "extended functions" that are not legal in his or her state is guilty of the unlicensed practice of dentistry and is committing a criminal act.

Also, if the function is legal *but* the assistant is not qualified by education and appropriate certification or registration, he or she is guilty of the unlicensed practice of dentistry.

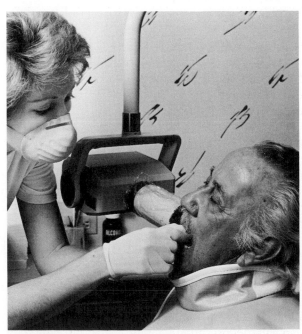

▼ Figure 2–1

Some states require registration for any assistant who exposes radiographs and/or performs extended functions. (Torres HO, Ehrlich A: Modern Dental Assisting, 4th Ed. Philadelphia, WB Saunders, 1990, p 904.)

Continuing Education

In some states, the dentist, hygienist, and registered dental assistant are required by law to have completed a number of hours of continuing education each year or biannually before their license or registration can be renewed.

Even when continuing education is not required, the assistant should voluntarily attend continuing education programs that will update and improve her professional skills.

EMPLOYMENT

Locating Employment Opportunities

Information about employment opportunities may come from many sources, including the following.

Newspaper Classified Advertising

Newspaper classified advertising is an excellent source. It is not uncommon for a dentist to place an advertisement describing the position open and listing a box number rather than a telephone number.

This is done for two reasons: First, to protect the office routine from being disrupted by phone calls of inquiry; second, to give the dentist an opportunity to screen the letters of application before calling any of the applicants for an interview.

Placement Service

If you are attending a dental assisting training program, the school probably will have at least an informal placement service, since area dentists frequently call the school first when they need an assistant.

Even after you have graduated, it is usually possible for you to continue to use the school placement service.

Dental Supply Representative

The sales representative who calls on dental offices in the area frequently knows when a dentist is looking for an assistant. When you are seeking employment, let the salesman know that you are looking and the type of employment you prefer.

Professional Organizations

Your local dental assistants' society and the local dental society frequently serve as informal employment information centers.

Many local dental societies publish monthly news bulletins in which it may be possible to place a classified ad at very little cost.

Employment Agencies

Federal and state governments provide Human Resources Development services and information without charge.

A private employment agency charges a fee if it finds you a position. You are responsible for paying this fee unless, by special prearrangement, your new employer agrees to pay it.

First Contacts

Telephone

If the advertisement you are answering includes a telephone number, your first contact will be by telephone. When you call, identify yourself and your reasons for calling.

The first impression via the telephone is an all-important one, for if you do not make a good impression here, you may not get a chance to "prove yourself" in an interview.

It is unlikely that you will be able to speak to the dentist at this time; however, the administrative assistant or someone else in the office will be able to handle calls of inquiry and to set up an interview appointment.

Letter of Application

Most frequently, initial contact is made through a letter of application, and the appearance and contents of your letter create that all-important first impression of you (Fig. 2–2).

Your letter should be brief, business-like, well written, and neatly typed on white stationery or typing paper. Do not include personal information in the letter since that should be contained in your résumé, which should be enclosed with your letter of application.

However, you may want to include in the letter just enough information to create interest—for example, that you are a certified dental assistant.

Mary Jones, CDA
212 Pleasant Drive
Midville, US 27740

June 16, 19XX

Box 782
Area Tribune
Midville, US 27740

Dear Doctor:

In response to your advertisement in the June 15th Area Tribune, I am applying for the position of chairside assistant in your practice.

I am a Certified Dental Assistant and a graduate of the Accredited School of Dental Assisting. Enclosed is my résumé which will provide you with additional information as to my background and experience.

I would appreciate the opportunity to interview with you. I may be reached at 965-1255 any day after 5 P.M.

Sincerely,

Mary Jones

Mary Jones, CDA

enclosure

▼ Figure 2–2

A neatly typed letter of application helps to make a good "first impression." (Torres HO, Ehrlich A: Modern Dental Assisting, 4th Ed. Philadelphia, WB Saunders, 1990, p 908.)

Résumé

A résumé is a neatly organized statement of your applicable personal information. A good résumé goes a long way toward helping you make a good impression.

A sloppy résumé, with careless erasures and misspelled words, is inexcusable and may cost you a good chance at a position.

A copy of your résumé should be enclosed with your letter of application. If you do not send a letter of application, take a copy of your résumé with you to the interview and leave it with the interviewer.

Your résumé should be typed and well organized to create an impression of neatness and orderliness. Space can be used to isolate important points to which you want to draw attention. Also, sufficient spacing between all elements helps to create a clean, inviting impression (Fig. 2-3).

Information to be included is as follows:

Your Personal Directory. This is a simple listing of your name, address, and telephone number.

Objective. State clearly your job objective—for example, to work as a chairside assistant in either a general dentistry or a pediatric dentistry practice. It is important that you be clear regarding the kind of job you want; however, a too narrowly stated objective may limit your job opportunities.

Work Experience. Dates should be given along with the company address and a brief description of your work. Your job listing should be in reverse order, beginning with the last job you held.

Education. Usually only schools from which you have graduated and dates of graduation are listed; for example, high school and dental assisting school. However, if you took special courses that may be of interest to your potential employer, you may want to make note of them.

Other Activities, Special Honors. If you are active in organizations or have received special honors that may relate to your potential as an employee, you may include them in a special category, or you may list them with the appropriate groups. For example, school honors could be listed with education.

Personal Data. This section *may* include date of birth, number of children, sex (if name is ambiguous), and state of health. Health is usually listed as "excellent" or "good."

Under **Federal Equal Employment Opportunity (EEO) regulations,** employers may *not* ask questions regarding race, color, religion, sex, national origin, marital status, and child care arrangements, unless they relate to **bona fide occupational qualifications** (BFOQ). If you are under 19, age may be a BFOQ question. Although you are not required to supply this information, you may do so voluntarily if you so choose.

Omit References. Instead of listing references, note that references and further data are available "on request." You should be prepared to supply these to an interested employer at the time of your interview. Relatives are never used as references.

References related to your work experience are preferred to those of social acquaintances. A former employer and/or an instructor from your dental assisting program may be included if he or she knows you well. It is courteous to receive a person's permission before using his or her name as a reference.

The Employment Application

Prior to your interview, you may be asked to complete an application form. This serves as the initial basis of your conversation with the interviewer.

In completing this form, be sure that you *follow directions exactly* and that the information you give is accurate and complete.

The Interview

The employment interview is an important exchange of information and impressions. During the interview you will gather information to help you determine if you would be happy working for this dentist, with this staff, and in this practice. At the same time, the dentist is trying to determine if you are the right employee for this position.

Your appearance is all-important. In selecting your clothes, remember that you are looking for employment, not going to a ball game or a party.

You want your appearance to reflect the fact that you are a neat, well-organized, and competent professional. However, it is not appropriate to wear your dental assisting uniform to an interview.

Try to answer the interviewer's questions courteously, completely, and honestly. Remember, your attitude during the interview is an important

Mary Jones, CDA
212 Pleasant Drive
Midville, US 27740

(912) 965-1255

Objective:

- Chairside assistant in either pediatric or general dentistry practice.

Work Experience:

- Student intern in the practice of Dr. Janis Davison. I also worked as a part-time chairside assistant for Dr. Davison from March 19XX to the present.

- Circulating assistant in the practice of Dr. Harry Randolph during the summer of 19XX.

Education:

- Accredited School of Dental Assisting, Sept 19XX - June 19XX. Graduated with honors in pediatric dentistry.

- Midville High School, 19XX - 19XX.

Other Activities:

- I have applied to be a Registered Dental Assistant in our state.

Personal Data:

- Excellent health.

References:

- References and additional information available on request.

▼ Figure 2–3

Sample résumé. (Torres HO, Ehrlich A: Modern Dental Assisting, 4th Ed. Philadelphia, WB Saunders, 1990, p 909.)

determining factor. You want to convey a positive attitude without overselling yourself.

You must also be prepared for surprise questions such as, "What can I do for you?" or "Tell me about yourself."

You too will have questions to ask. Feel free to question and, if it seems to be a convenient time, ask to be shown around the office and to meet the other staff members.

Salary Negotiations

Although salary should *not* be the first question in your mind, it is an important factor and should be discussed openly.

The interviewer may ask, "What do you expect in terms of salary?" If you have a definite and realistic idea, by all means state it.

However, if you are uncertain, you may phrase your response along the lines of, "To be fair to everybody, it is open to negotiation," and then wait to see what sort of offer is made.

The Employment Agreement

Before you accept a position, there are several topics that you and the dentist, or office manager, need to explore. These should be organized into a written employment agreement (Fig. 2–4).

An employment agreement is a written document, prepared in duplicate and signed by both employer and employee. One copy is retained in the personnel file, and the other is given to the employee for her records.

Reaching a clear understanding of the following topics is important, for it can prevent later misunderstandings.

Duties and Responsibilities. You need to know exactly what your duties will be. The dentist should have developed a written job description that includes a list of the specific responsibilities of your job.

Working Hours. What hours and days of the week will you routinely be expected to work? How far in advance are these scheduled, and how is overtime handled?

Salary and Benefits. Although salary should have already been discussed, you also need to know what provisions are made for increases and benefits.

Uniform Requirements. If there are uniform requirements, you need to know who is responsible for supplying and maintaining uniforms and whether there is a uniform allowance.

Conditional Period of Employment. Most employers routinely consider the first several weeks as a conditional period during which either party may terminate the relationship without notice.

Continuing Education. Determine what continuing education is provided and who is expected to pay for it.

Periodic Performance Review. At specified intervals, usually on an annual basis, the employee is provided with a formal evaluation or performance review. This may include a discussion of the employee's job skills, ability to get along with patients, and interactions with other employees. Performance reviews are often tied to salary increases.

Termination. You should be aware of how much notice you are expected to give, or to receive, should you or the dentist terminate your employment after the conditional period.

MAINTAINING EMPLOYMENT

Maintaining employment is a two-sided situation. There are responsibilities on the part of the assistant and other auxiliaries as employees. There are also responsibilities on the part of the dentist as the employer.

Before accepting employment, try to determine, through observation and by talking to other employees, if the dentist does indeed carry out the responsibilities of a good employer.

If it is apparent that the dentist does not, perhaps you should consider employment elsewhere.

The Employee's Responsibilities in Maintaining Employment

1. To be a willing, punctual, cooperative, and responsible worker who performs her regularly assigned duties cheerfully and competently and helps others as needed.
2. To be always neat and appropriately uniformed during working hours.
3. To be pleasant, respectful, and cooperative, yet professional, with *all* patients.

EMPLOYMENT AGREEMENT

(Complete in duplicate. One copy to employee, one for personnel records.)

NAME _____Mary Jones_____ DATE _9/10/19xx_

JOB TITLE _Chairside Assistant_ FULL TIME/PART TIME _full time_

DUTIES AND RESPONSIBILITIES (check appropriate space)

___XX___ Listed on reverse side. _____ Copy of job description attached.

WORKING HOURS

Usual working hours are from _8:30_ to _5:30_ ; lunch _1 hr._ ; breaks _____ .

Days per week: S _____ M _X_ T _X_ W _1/2_ Th _X_ F _X_ S _1/2_

When working hours vary, you will be notified in the following manner:

_____Schedule is posted in the staff lounge._____

_____

_____

_____

SALARY AND BENEFITS

Starting rate: _$XX per hour_____

Provisions for increases: _Review at end of conditional employment._

_____Thereafter, annual review in October._____

Paid: Vacation days _5_ ; Sick days _3_ ; Personal time _2_ ;

Other benefits _Employer paid health insurance._

_____After 3 years, participation in pension plan._

_____

_____

UNIFORM REQUIREMENTS (if applicable)

_____Clinical personnel wear white slacks, white shoes._

_____Uniform top to be light color with short sleeves._

CONDITIONAL PERIOD OF EMPLOYMENT

For each new employee the first __6__ weeks of employment are considered a conditional or probationary period. During this time the employee may leave, or be dismissed, with 24 hours' notice.

TERMINATION

The employee is expected to give __2__ weeks' notice.

If dismissed, the employee will receive __2__ weeks' notice or the equivalent in severance pay. In the event of fraud, theft or unprofessional conduct, the employee may be dismissed without notice or severance pay.

Mary Jones CDA _Roger Walters_ DDS
Employee's signature Employer's signature

Form 9876 Colwell Co., Champaign, Illinois

▼ **Figure 2–4**

Sample employment agreement form. (Courtesy of Colwell Systems, Inc., Champaign, IL.)

4. To be able to accept and act upon constructive criticism and continually to upgrade and update her professional skills and knowledge through continuing education.
5. To maintain high personal, professional, and ethical standards.

The Employer's Responsibilities in Maintaining Employment

1. To establish and maintain fair employee policies and practices.
2. To treat all employees with professional and personal dignity and respect.
3. To organize and maintain the practice so that it provides safe, pleasant working conditions for all.
4. To encourage employees to their best performances through praise, encouragement, and other more tangible indications that their efforts have been noticed and appreciated.

Physical Well-Being

Physical well-being is an important part of maintaining employment, for you must be healthy so that you can work to the best of your ability.

You need that glow of healthy well-being that comes from proper nutrition, regular exercise, sufficient rest, and a zest for living.

General Health

Good nutrition, which involves eating the proper food in the proper quantities, is the basis of good general health.

Exercise, relaxation, and weight control are important keys to physical and mental well-being. Although you are active at work, you should also engage regularly in a pleasurable form of general exercise such as walking, yoga, jogging, or swimming.

Fatigue and lack of sufficient rest are hazards to good health and attractive appearance. The start of every health program is to get *sufficient* sleep on a *regular* basis. For most people this means getting 8 hours of sleep every night. You should take all the necessary preventive care steps to preserve your physical well-being. These include:

▼ As an assistant you are exposed to a wide variety of communicable diseases. Keeping your immunizations up to date is important for yourself and your patients.

▼ Every woman should have a Papanicolaou (Pap) test at least once a year.

▼ An annual eye examination is also important because faulty vision may affect your appearance, your health, and your work.

Dental Health

Your dental health is important. You must believe in, and carry through, a good program of preventive dental care, which includes having regular dental examinations and completion of any necessary treatment.

Complexion Care and Makeup

A clear, bright, and healthy complexion can be one of your greatest assets, and a good program of skin care is an important part of being healthy.

Your diet affects your skin, and fresh air and exercise provide the natural stimulation to the bloodstream that your complexion needs.

Obvious or excessive makeup is never appropriate in the professional office. The desired effect is to achieve a natural glowing and healthy look. This look is achieved through good health plus careful makeup selection and application. The makeup selected should be quietly flattering and appropriate for daytime wear, natural looking, and never harsh in appearance.

Hairstyles

Well-groomed hair is an important part of your professional appearance. A suitable hairstyle is one that is neat, clean, easily controlled, and not falling over the face (either yours or the patient's).

It is impossible to maintain a clean or clear operating field if the chairside assistant must keep fussing with her hair. Therefore, a hairstyle must also be manageable. This means that it does not require constant fussing, touching, or pushing back into place. If the chairside assistant's hair is long, it must be secured effectively throughout the hours of employment.

Care of the Hands and Nails

Fingernails must be kept short and clean. Dark or bright red nail polish is not appropriate for the dental office. However, clear protective polish or a soft natural color is acceptable. If worn, nail polish should be maintained in excellent repair at all times. No polish is preferable to chipped polish.

The assistant should take good preventive care

of her hands to minimize damage caused by frequent contact with soap, water, and gloves. Any cut or damage to the skin is an invitation to infection.

Lotions are available for use before hands are placed in water whose effect should last through several washings. Also, a wide range of lotions is available for use after the hands have been washed. Use such a lotion as often as practical; however, avoid selecting one that is either extremely sticky or highly perfumed.

Rings

Because rings may tear gloves and/or accumulate debris, jewelry should not be worn on the hands during working hours.

Professional Uniforms and Appearance

The uniform should not be worn out of the office and in public places. Change into and out of your uniform at the office.

The dentist should make the final recommendation in uniform selection for the staff; however, there are certain basic rules that the assistant should apply to all uniform selections.

No matter what the current fashions, a uniform should be selected that will always present a pleasing professional appearance. This means one that is:

▼ Appropriate for the work situation.

▼ Well fitted and flattering.

▼ Neat.

▼ Capable of maintaining its fresh look throughout the day.

The uniform selected should be comfortable and easy to wear without being baggy or sloppy. It should not be too tight, too short, or of a revealing nature or require constant adjustments.

Uniforms must fit properly at all times. If weight is gained, the uniform size must be adjusted accordingly. The promise of tomorrow's diet does nothing to correct the problem of today's appearance.

Sloppy appearance does not create a positive image of the dental assistant or of the dentist who is her employer. Therefore, uniforms must be kept clean and in good repair at all times.

This means a clean uniform daily and, if necessary, wearing a cover-up while doing messy jobs. A spare uniform should be kept at the office for use in case of emergency.

Also, a neatly uniformed appearance does not include jewelry or colored hair bows. Jewelry should be limited to the association pin, a name pin, and a watch with a second hand.

Another important aspect of neat appearance is the selection of undergarments. These should be well fitted, adequate, modest, in good repair, and clean daily. Colored undergarments that show through the uniform or hems that show below are neither attractive nor professional in appearance.

A dental assistant spends a lot of time on her feet, and well-fitted shoes and stockings are essential. A good duty shoe should offer adequate support and be well fitted. These shoes must be kept in good repair, clean and well polished, with clean laces at all times.

Stockings should be of an appropriate shade and style. They should also be well fitted, comfortable, and free of runs. Because of the amount of "leg work" done by the assistant each day, many find that a lightweight support hose is helpful in preventing aching legs.

TERMINATION

If the dental assitant decides to terminate employment, she should abide by the terms of the employment agreement. Always give the employer adequate notice. If the assistant is leaving under friendly conditions, she may be asked to help select and train a replacement.

If the dental assistant is leaving under other circumstances, it is best that she leave quickly and quietly. She may be given severance pay and asked to leave immediately.

Summary Dismissal

Summary dismissal is termination without notice or severance pay. The causes for summary dismissal include stealing, use of drugs, and any other form of unprofessional behavior.

▼ EXERCISES

1. Sources of information concerning employment opportunities include ____
   _____ .

   a. dental supply representatives
   b. placement services
   c. professional organizations
   d. a, b, and c

2. Most employers routinely consider the first several weeks of employment to
   be a _____ period.

   a. conditional
   b. temporary
   c. trial
   d. training

3. Before being eligible to sit for the certification examination, the dental
   assistant must _____ .

   a. hold a current cardiopulmonary resuscitation (CPR) certificate
   b. hold an associate degree in dental assisting
   c. pass a state licensure examination
   d. b and c

4. During the interview, the employer _____ legally ask
   questions regarding race, color, religion, sex, and national origin.

   a. may
   b. may not

5. In most states, a dental assistant must be _____ in order
   to expose radiographs.

   a. certified
   b. licensed
   c. registered
   d. a or c

6. A member in the ADAA receives _____ .

   a. a voice in national affairs
   b. continuing education opportunities
   c. journals
   d. a, b, and c

7. If terminating employment under less than favorable conditions, it is best to
   _____ .

   a. give 2 week's notice
   b. insist upon training your replacement
   c. leave as quickly as possible
   d. a and b

8. In is *not* proper to list _____ as references.

   a. friends
   b. relatives
   c. teachers
   d. a and b

9. When telephoning a dental office in response to a newspaper advertisement, you should expect to _____.

   a. be told the amount of the salary being offered
   b. make an appointment for an interview
   c. speak to the dentist
   d. a and b

10. The dental assistant's uniform should be worn _____.

    a. only in the office
    b. to and from work
    c. to the job interview
    d. b and c

11. It _____ appropriate for the dental assistant to wear bright red nail polish at work.

    a. is
    b. is not

12. Stealing, the illegal use of drugs, or any other form of unprofessional behavior is considered cause for _____.

    a. conditional dismissal
    b. salary reduction
    c. suspension
    d. summary dismissal

13. In a résumé, your personal directory is a listing of your _____.

    a. education and experience
    b. name, address, and telephone number
    c. name, age, and health
    d. school activities and honors

14. The responsibilities for maintaining employment lie with the _____.

    a. dental assistant
    b. dentist
    c. a and b

15. The _____ must be licensed by the State Board of Dental Examiners in order to practice within that state.

    a. dental assistant
    b. dentist
    c. registered dental hygienist
    d. b and c

16. References _____ be included as part of your résumé.

    a. should
    b. should not

17. _____ supervision means that the dentist is in the dental office or treatment facility and personally authorizes the procedure.

    a. Clinical
    b. Direct
    c. General
    d. Legal

18. Unless you have made a previous special arrangement, a _____ _____ employment agency charges a fee if it finds you a position.

    a. federal
    b. private
    c. state
    d. a, b, and c

19. A/an _____ is a written document that clarifies the terms of employment.

    a. contract
    b. employment agreement
    c. job description
    d. office procedures manual

20. The assistant who performs extended functions that are not legal in his or her state is guilty of committing a _____ act.

    a. criminal
    b. felonious
    c. negligent
    d. a and b

21. It _____ appropriate to openly discuss salary during a job interview.

    a. is
    b. is not

22. _____ is one means of supervising and regulating those practicing dentistry within the state.

    a. Certification
    b. Continuing education
    c. Licensure
    d. Supervision

23. The certification examination for dental assistants is given by the _____ .

    a. Certifying Board of the ADA
    b. Certifying Board of the ADAA
    c. Dental Assisting National Board
    d. National Board of the American Dental Association

24. During the interview, it _____ appropriate to ask the interviewer questions.

    a. is
    b. is not

25. Each year the Certified Dental Assistant must _____ .

    a. earn continuing education credits
    b. pass a renewal examination
    c. renew certification
    d. a and c

▼ Criterion Sheet 2–1

Student's Name _____

Procedure: *PREPARING A RÉSUMÉ*

Performance Objective:

The student will prepare a personal résumé for use in seeking employment.

SE = Student evaluation **C** = Criterion met **IE** = Instructor evaluation **X** = Criterion not met	**SE**	**IE**
Instrumentation: Plain paper, typewriter, word processor or pen.		
1. Prepared a résumé including the following parts: _____ Personal directory _____ Objective _____ Work experience _____ Education _____ Other activities _____ Personal data		
2. The résumé was neat and professional in appearance.		
3. The résumé was free of grammatical errors and misspelled words.		
Comments:		

▼ Criterion Sheet 2–2

Student's Name _____

Procedure: *WRITING A LETTER OF APPLICATION*

Performance Objective:

The student will write a letter of application, to accompany the résumé. The letter is being sent in response to a classified advertisement in the *Daily Times* newspaper.

SE = Student evaluation **C** = Criterion met **IE** = Instructor evaluation **X** = Criterion not met	**SE**	**IE**
Instrumentation: Plain paper, typewriter, word processor or pen.		
1. The letter contained appropriate information.		
2. The letter was free of misspelled words.		
3. The letter was free of grammatical errors.		
4. The letter was neat and concise.		
Comments:		

3 Structures of the Head and Neck

▼ LEARNING OBJECTIVES

The student will be able to:

1. State at least two reasons why it is important for the assistant to have a basic understanding of the structures of the head and neck.
2. Identify the major anatomic landmarks of the face and skull.
3. Describe the glide and hinge action of the temporomandibular joint (TMJ).
4. Describe the major muscles of mastication and facial expression.
5. Name the three pairs of salivary glands and the major ducts for each.
6. Describe the major landmarks of the hard palate, soft palate, and oral mucosa.
7. Describe the characteristics of healthy gingiva.
8. Demonstrate identification of major bones and landmarks of the face.

OVERVIEW OF THE STRUCTURES OF THE HEAD AND NECK

There are many reasons why a dental assistant must have at least a basic understanding of the structures of the head and neck. One reason is that the differences in bone structure affect how the local anesthetic solution is administered. However, the most important reason is so that the assistant can carry out her duties without risking injury to the hard and soft tissues of the oral cavity or harm to the patient. The more the assistant understands about these structures, the more effective she can be in performing her duties.

THE STRUCTURE OF BONE

Bone is the hard connective tissue that makes up most of the human skeleton. There are two types of bone: compact bone and cancellous bone (Fig. 3–1).

Compact bone, also known as **cortical bone**, is hard, dense, and very strong. It forms the outer layer of bones, where it is needed for strength.

Cancellous bone, also known as **spongy bone**, is lighter in weight but not as strong as compact bone. It is found in the interior of bones.

The **periosteum** is the specialized connective tissue covering all bones of the body.

BONES AND ANATOMIC LANDMARKS OF THE SKULL

The skull is made up of the bones of the cranium and the face. (The **cranium** forms the bony protection for the brain.) These bones are summarized in Table 3–1.

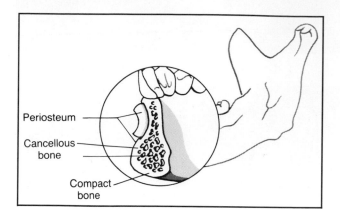

▼ **Figure 3-1**

The structure of bone. A cross section of the mandible is shown with a portion of the periosteum reflected. (Torres HO, Ehrlich A: Modern Dental Assisting, 4th Ed. Philadelphia, WB Saunders, 1990, p 21.)

There are many anatomic landmarks of the skull that are important in dentistry. These are included in the illustrations of the bones of the skull (Figs. 3–2 through 3–9).

Table 3-1. BONES OF THE SKULL

Cranium	Face
1 Frontal	2 Zygomatic
2 Parietal	2 Maxillary
1 Occipital	2 Palatine
2 Temporal	2 Nasal
1 Sphenoid	2 Lacrimal
1 Ethmoid	1 Vomer
6 Auditory ossicles	2 Inferior conchae

(Torres HO, Ehrlich A: Modern Dental Assisting, 4th Ed. Philadelphia, WB Saunders, 1990, p 26.)

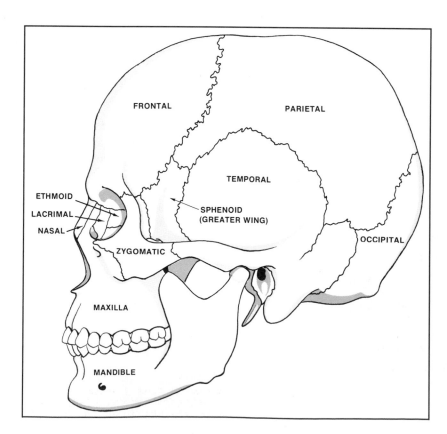

▼ **Figure 3-2**

Bones of the skull (lateral view). (Torres HO, Ehrlich A: Modern Dental Assisting, 4th Ed. Philadelphia, WB Saunders, 1990, p 24.)

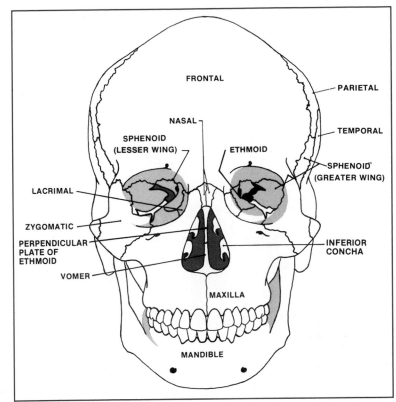

▼ Figure 3-3

Bones of the skull (frontal view). (Torres HO, Ehrlich A: Modern Dental Assisting, 4th Ed. Philadelphia, WB Saunders, 1990, p 25.)

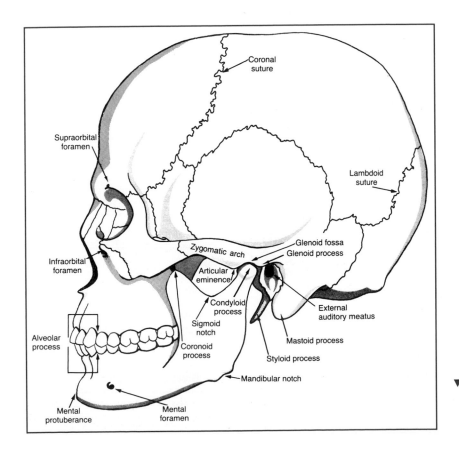

▼ Figure 3-4

Anatomic landmarks of the skull (lateral view). (Torres HO, Ehrlich A: Modern Dental Assisting, 4th Ed. Philadelphia, WB Saunders, 1990, p 27.)

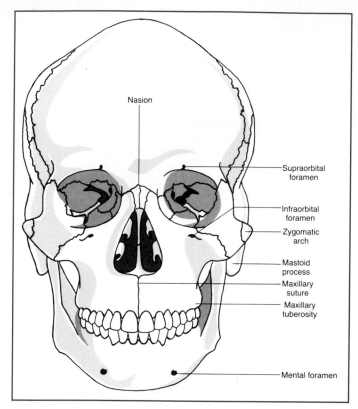

Nasion

Supraorbital
foramen

Infraorbital
foramen

Zygomatic
arch

Mastoid
process

Maxillary
suture

Maxillary
tuberosity

Mental foramen

▼ Figure 3–5

Anatomic landmarks of the skull (frontal view). (Torres HO, Ehrlich A: Modern Dental Assisting, 4th Ed. Philadelphia, WB Saunders, 1990, p 28.)

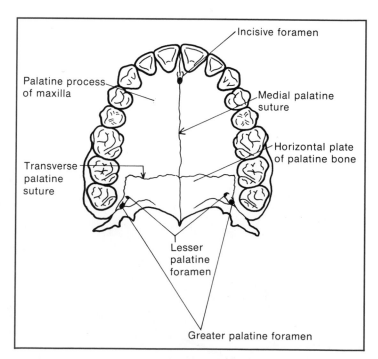

Incisive foramen

Palatine process
of maxilla

Medial palatine
suture

Horizontal plate
of palatine bone

Transverse
palatine
suture

Lesser
palatine
foramen

Greater palatine foramen

▼ Figure 3–6

Bones and landmarks of the hard palate. (Torres HO, Ehrlich A: Modern Dental Assisting, 4th Ed. Philadelphia, WB Saunders, 1990, p 29.)

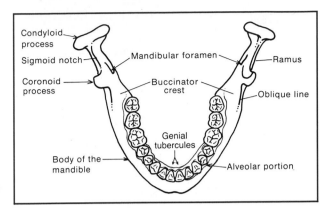

▼ **Figure 3-7**

Topical view of the mandible. (Torres HO, Ehrlich A: Modern Dental Assisting, 4th Ed. Philadelphia, WB Saunders, 1990, p 29.)

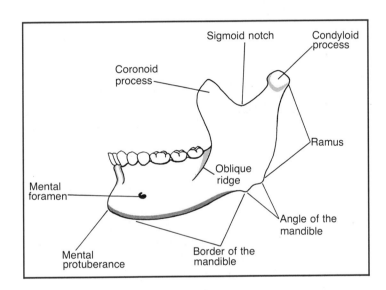

▼ **Figure 3-8**

Anatomic landmarks of the mandible (lateral view). (Torres HO, Ehrlich A: Modern Dental Assisting, 4th Ed. Philadelphia, WB Saunders, 1990, p 29.)

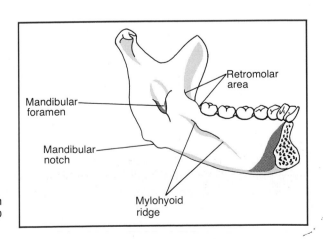

▼ **Figure 3-9**

Anatomic landmarks of the mandible (medial view). (Torres HO, Ehrlich A: Modern Dental Assisting, 4th Ed. Philadelphia, WB Saunders, 1990, p 30.)

Paranasal Sinuses

The paranasal sinuses are air-containing spaces within the bones of the skull that communicate with the nasal cavity (Fig. 3–10). One of their functions is to make the cranium lighter. These sinuses are named for the bones in which they are located.

The **maxillary sinuses,** located in the maxillary bones, are the largest of the paranasal sinuses.

The **frontal sinuses,** located in the frontal bone, are located within the forehead, just above the eyes.

The **ethmoid sinuses,** located in the ethmoid bones, are irregularly shaped air cells, separated from the orbital cavity by a very thin layer of bone.

The **sphenoid sinuses,** located in the sphenoid bone, are close to the optic nerves, and an infection here may damage vision and/or cause brain damage.

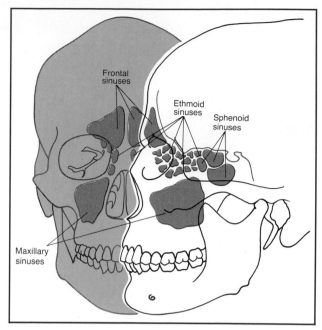

▼ **Figure 3–10**

The paranasal sinuses. (Torres HO, Ehrlich A: Modern Dental Assisting, 4th Ed. Philadelphia, WB Saunders, 1990, p 51.)

THE TEMPOROMANDIBULAR JOINT

The temporomandibular joint (TMJ) is located where the temporal bone and the mandible articulate. (**Articulate** means to come together.)

Components of the Temporomandibular Joint

Bony Components

The temporomandibular joint is made up of three bony parts (Fig. 3–11):

1. The **glenoid fossa** is an oval depression in the temporal bone just anterior to the external auditory meatus.
2. The **articular eminence** is a raised portion of the temporal bone just anterior to the glenoid fossa.
3. The **condyloid process** of the mandible lies in the glenoid fossa.

Meniscus

The meniscus, also known as the **articular disc,** is a cushion of tough, somewhat elastic, specialized connective tissue.

The meniscus divides the articular space between the glenoid fossa and the condyle into upper and lower compartments.

Capsular Ligament

The ligaments of the temporomandibular joint attach the mandible to the cranium.

The capsular ligament is a dense fibrous capsule that completely surrounds the temporomandibular joint. It is attached to the neck of the condyle of the mandible and to the nearby surfaces of the temporal bone.

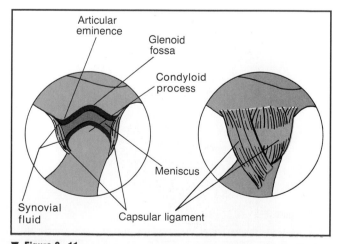

▼ **Figure 3–11**

The parts of the temporomandibular joint. (Torres HO, Ehrlich A: Modern Dental Assisting, 4th Ed. Philadelphia, WB Saunders, 1990, p 32.)

Movements of the Temporomandibular Joint

The left and right temporomandibular joints function in unison. Their structure permits specialized hinge and glide movements and different degrees of mouth opening and closing (Fig. 3–12).

Hinge Action

The hinge action is the first phase in mouth opening, and only the lower compartment of the joint is used.

During hinge action, the condyle head rotates around a point on the undersurface of the menis- cus, and the body of the mandible drops almost passively downward and backward.

The jaw is opened by the combined actions of the external pterygoid, digastric, mylohyoid, and geniohyoid muscles.

The jaw is closed and **retracted** (pulled backward) by the action of the temporal, masseter, and internal pterygoid muscles.

Gliding Action

The gliding action is the second phase in mouth opening and movement. It involves both the lower and the upper compartments of the joint.

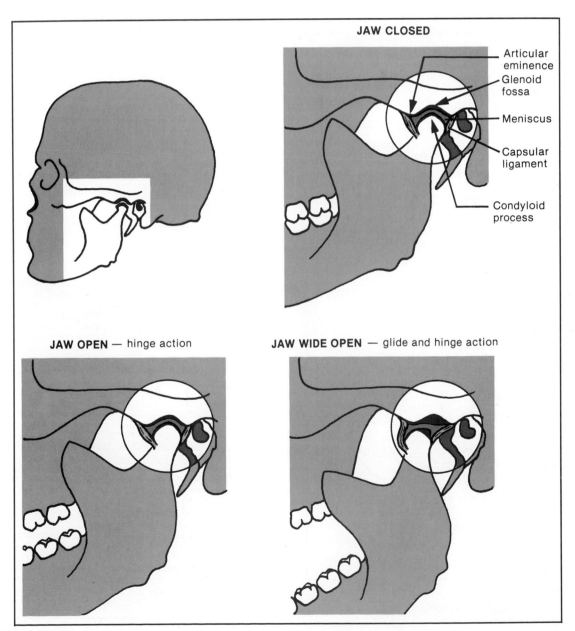

▼ Figure 3–12

Hinge and glide action of the temporomandibular joint. (Torres HO, Ehrlich A: Modern Dental Assisting, 4th Ed. Philadelphia, WB Saunders, 1990, p 33.)

The phase consists of a gliding movement by the condyle and meniscus forward and downward along the articular eminence.

This occurs only during protrusion and lateral movements of the mandible and in combination with the hinge action during the wider opening of the mouth.

Protrusion is the forward movement of the mandible. This happens when the internal and external pterygoid muscles on both sides contract together.

Lateral movement (sideways) of the mandible occurs when the internal and external pterygoid muscles on the same side contract together.

Side-to-side lateral **grinding movements** are brought about by alternating contractions of the internal and external pterygoid muscles, first on one side and then on the other.

THE MAJOR MUSCLES OF MASTICATION AND FACIAL EXPRESSION

The major muscles of mastication and facial expression are shown in Figures 3–13 and 3–14 and function as follows:

▼ **Buccinator.** Serves to compress the cheeks and hold food in contact with the teeth. Also retracts the angles of the mouth.

▼ **External (lateral) pterygoid.** Depresses, protrudes, and moves the mandible from side to side.

▼ **Internal (medial) pterygoid.** Closes jaw.

▼ **Masseter.** Acts to raise the mandible, close the jaws, and occlude the teeth

▼ **Mentalis.** Raises and wrinkles the skin of the chin and pushes up the lower lip.

▼ **Orbicularis oris.** Closes and puckers the lips. Also aids in chewing and speaking by pressing the lips against the teeth.

▼ **Temporal.** Acts to raise the mandible, close the jaws, and occlude the teeth. The posterior fibers of the muscle draw the protruding mandible backward.

▼ **Zygomatic major.** Draws the angles of the mouth upward and backward, as in laughing.

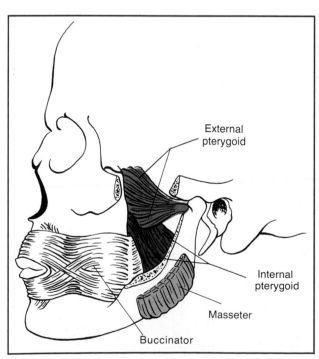

▼ **Figure 3–13**

Muscles of mastication and facial expression (internal view). (Torres HO, Ehrlich A: Modern Dental Assisting, 4th Ed. Philadelphia, WB Saunders, 1990, p 36.)

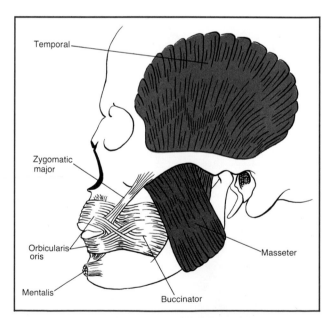

▼ **Figure 3–14**

Muscles of mastication and facial expression (internal view). (Torres HO, Ehrlich A: Modern Dental Assisting, 4th Ed. Philadelphia, WB Saunders, 1990, p 36.)

BLOOD SUPPLY TO THE FACE AND ORAL CAVITY

Arteries carry oxygenated blood away from the heart to all parts of the body with a pulsing motion. The **major arteries of the face and mouth** are shown in Figure 3–15 and Table 3–2.

Veins carry blood back to the heart. The **major veins of the face and mouth** are shown in Figure 3–16.

Lymph Nodes

Lymph nodes are small round or oval structures located in lymph vessels. In acute infections, the lymph nodes become swollen and tender. The lymph nodes of the face and neck are shown in Figure 3–17.

INNERVATION OF THE ORAL CAVITY

The **trigeminal nerve** is the primary source of innervation for the oral cavity. At the **semilunar ganglion,** the trigeminal nerve subdivides into three main branches: the ophthalmic, the maxillary, and the mandibular. The branches of the

Table 3–2. MAJOR ARTERIES TO THE FACE AND MOUTH

Structure	Blood Supply
Muscles of facial expression	Branches and arterioles from maxillary, facial, and ophthalmic arteries
Maxilla	Anterior, middle, and posterior alveolar arteries
Maxillary teeth	Anterior, middle, and posterior alveolar arteries
Mandible	Inferior alveolar arteries
Mandibular teeth	Inferior alveolar arteries
Tongue	Lingual artery
Muscles of mastication	Facial arteries

(Torres HO, Ehrlich A: Modern Dental Assisting, 4th Ed. Philadelphia, WB Saunders, 1990, p 43.)

nerve serving the oral cavity are shown in Figures 3–18 through 3–21.

Maxillary Innervation

The maxillary division of the trigeminal nerve supplies the maxillary teeth, periosteum, mucous membrane, maxillary sinuses, and soft palate.

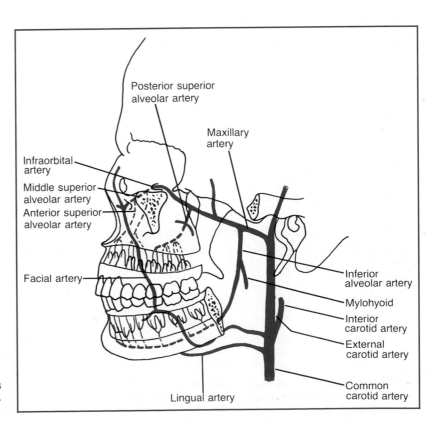

▼ Figure 3–15

Major arteries of the face and mouth. (Torres HO, Ehrlich A: Modern Dental Assisting, 4th Ed. Philadelphia, WB Saunders, 1990, p 43.)

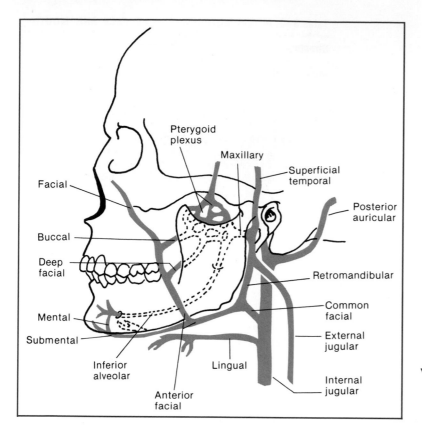

▼ Figure 3-16

Major veins of the face and mouth. (Torres HO, Ehrlich A: Modern Dental Assisting, 4th Ed. Philadelphia, WB Saunders, 1990, p 44.)

The maxillary division subdivides to provide the following innervation:

▼ The **nasopalatine nerve,** which passes through the incisive foramen, supplies the tissues palatal to the maxillary anterior teeth. (A **foramen** is

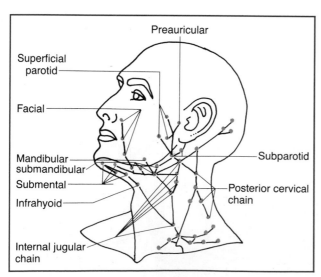

▼ Figure 3-17

Major lymph nodes of the face and neck. (Torres HO, Ehrlich A: Modern Dental Assisting, 4th Ed. Philadelphia, WB Saunders, 1990, p 45.)

an opening in a bone through which blood vessels, nerves, and ligaments pass.)

▼ The **anterior palatine nerve,** which passes through the posterior palatine foramen and forward over the palate, supplies the mucoperiosteum. (**Mucoperiosteum** is periosteum having a mucous membrane surface.)

▼ The **anterior superior alveolar nerve** supplies the maxillary central, lateral, and cuspid teeth, plus their periodontal membrane and gingiva. This nerve also supplies the maxillary sinus.

▼ The **middle superior alveolar nerve** supplies the maxillary first and second premolars, the mesiobuccal root of the maxillary first molar, and the maxillary sinus.

▼ The **posterior superior alveolar nerve** supplies the other roots of the maxillary first molar and the maxillary second and third molars. It also branches forward to serve the lateral wall of the maxillary sinus.

▼ The **buccal nerve** supplies branches to the buccal mucous membrane and to the mucoperiosteum of the maxillary and mandibular molar teeth.

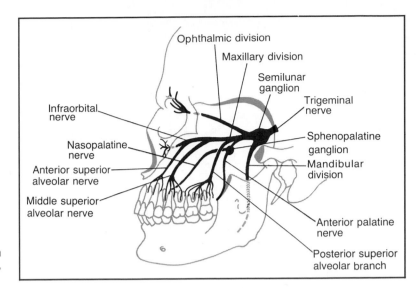

▼ **Figure 3-18**

Maxillary innervation. (Torres HO, Ehrlich A: Modern Dental Assisting, 4th Ed. Philadelphia, WB Saunders, 1990, p 49.)

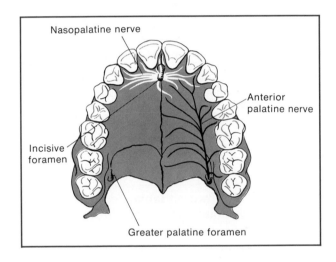

▼ **Figure 3-19**

Palatal innervation. (Torres HO, Ehrlich A: Modern Dental Assisting, 4th Ed. Philadelphia, WB Saunders, 1990, p 50.)

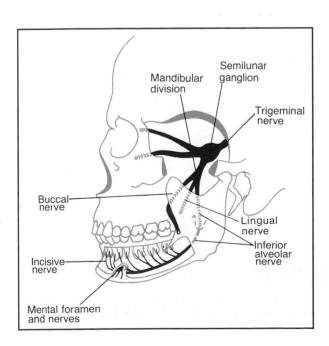

▼ **Figure 3-20**

Mandibular innervation. (Torres HO, Ehrlich A: Modern Dental Assisting, 4th Ed. Philadelphia, WB Saunders, 1990, p 50.)

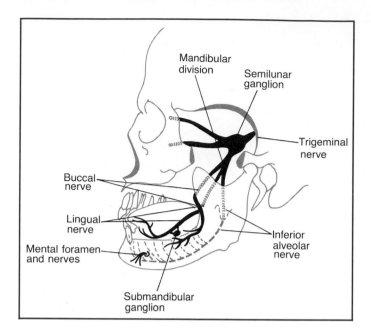

▼ Figure 3-21

Lingual and buccal innervation. (Torres HO, Ehrlich A: Modern Dental Assisting, 4th Ed. Philadelphia, WB Saunders, 1990, p 51.)

Mandibular Innervation

The mandibular division of the trigeminal nerve subdivides into the (1) buccal, (2) lingual, and (3) inferior alveolar nerves.

The **buccal nerve** supplies branches to the buccal mucous membrane and to the mucoperiosteum of the maxillary and mandibular molar teeth.

The **lingual nerve** supplies the anterior two thirds of the tongue and gives off branches to supply the lingual mucous membrane and mucoperiosteum.

The **inferior alveolar nerve** subdivides into the following:

1. The **mylohyoid nerve** supplies the mylohyoid muscles and the anterior belly of the digastric muscle.
2. The **small dental nerves** supply the molar and premolar teeth, alveolar process, and periosteum of the mandible.
3. The **mental nerve** moves outward through the mental foramen and supplies the chin and mucous membrane of the lower lip.
4. The **incisive nerve** continues anteriorly and gives off small branches to supply the cuspid, lateral, and central teeth.

STRUCTURES OF THE FACE AND ORAL CAVITY (Figs. 3-22 through 3-28)

Landmarks of the Face

The ala of the nose is the wing-like tip of outer side of each nostril.

The outer canthus of the eye is the fold of tissue at the outer corner of the eyelids.

The inner canthus of the eye is the fold of tissue at the inner corner of the eyelids.

The tragus of the ear is the cartilage projection anterior to the external opening of the ear.

The Lips

The lips, also known as **labia,** form the anterior border of the mouth. They are formed externally by the skin and internally by mucous membrane. (**Labial** means of, or pertaining to, the lip.)

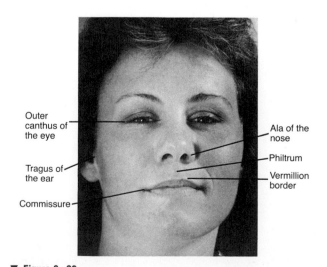

▼ Figure 3-22

Landmarks of the face.

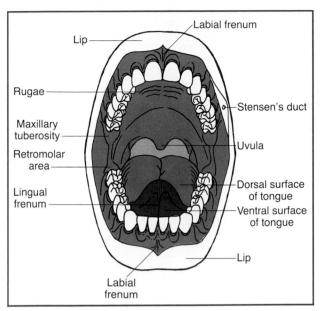

▼ **Figure 3-23**

Structures of the oral cavity. (Torres HO, Ehrlich A: Modern Dental Assisting, 4th Ed. Philadelphia, WB Saunders, 1990, p 53.)

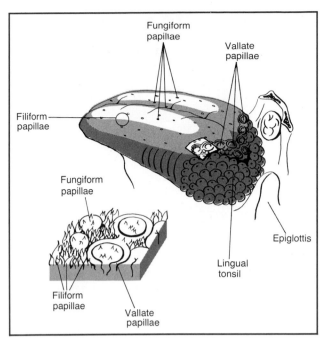

▼ **Figure 3-25**

The dorsal (top) surface of the tongue showing the locations of the taste buds. (Torres HO, Ehrlich A: Modern Dental Assisting, 4th Ed. Philadelphia, WB Saunders, 1990, p 48.)

The red free margins of the lips, where the skin of the face joins the mucous membrane of the lips, is known as the **vermilion border.** The corners of the lips are called the **commissures.**

The **philtrum** is the soft vertical groove running from under the nose to the midline of the upper lip.

The Cheeks

The cheeks form the side walls of the oral cavity. The **buccal vestibule** is the area between the cheeks and the teeth or alveolar ridge. (**Buccal** means pertaining to, or directed toward, the cheek.)

The **labial vestibule** is the area between the lips and the teeth or alveolar ridge.

Frenum

A frenum is a narrow band of tissue that connects two structures. (The term *frenum* is singular; the plural is *frena*.)

▼ The **upper labial frenum** passes from the midline of the gingiva of the outer surface of the mucosa of the maxillary arch to the midline of the inner surface of the upper lip.

▼ The **lower labial frenum** passes from the midline of the gingiva of the outer surface of the mucosa of the mandibular arch to the midline of the inner surface of the lower lip.

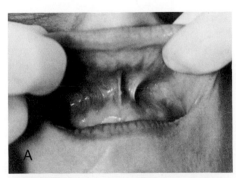

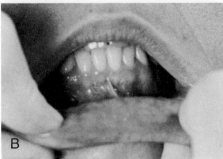

▼ **Figure 3-24**

The labial vestibule, upper and lower labial frena. *A.* The maxillary labial mucosa and frenum attachments. *B.* The mandibular labial mucosa and frenum attachments. (Torres HO, Ehrlich A: Modern Dental Assisting, 4th Ed. Philadelphia, WB Saunders, 1990, p 459.)

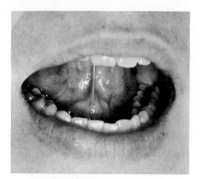

▼ Figure 3-26

The ventral (under) surface of the tongue and the floor of the mouth. (Torres HO, Ehrlich A: Modern Dental Assisting, 4th Ed. Philadelphia, WB Saunders, 1990, p 461.)

▼ The **lingual frenum** passes from the floor of the mouth to the midline of the undersurface of the mucosa of the tongue.

▼ The **buccal frenum** is located in the area of the first maxillary permanent molar. It passes from the gingiva of the outer surface of the maxillary arch to the inner surface of the cheek.

The Tongue

The tongue, which is attached only at the posterior end, consists of a very flexible group of muscles that are arranged to enable it to change size, shape, and position quickly.

The **dorsal** (top) surface, or *dorsum,* of the tongue is covered by a thick and highly specialized epithelium. The taste buds are contained on the posterior portion of the dorsum of the tongue.

The **ventral** (underside) surface of the tongue and the floor of the mouth are covered with lining mucosa. These delicate tissues are highly vascular and easily injured.

The Salivary Glands

There are three pairs of salivary glands: The **parotid, sublingual,** and **submandibular glands.** These are shown in Figures 3-27 and 3-28.

Parotid Glands

The parotid glands are the largest of the salivary glands. One lies subcutaneously just in front of and below each ear.

Saliva from the parotid gland is conveyed to the mouth via **Stensen's duct** (also known as the **parotid duct).** This duct opens into the mouth from the cheek opposite the maxillary second molar.

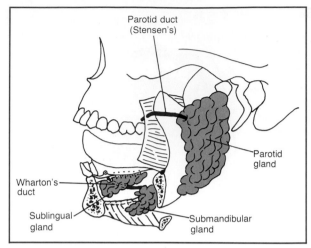

▼ Figure 3-27

Diagram of the salivary glands and ducts. (Torres HO, Ehrlich A: Modern Dental Assisting, 4th Ed. Philadelphia, WB Saunders, 1990, p 54.)

Sublingual Glands

The sublingual glands are the smallest of the salivary glands. They are located one on either side underneath the tongue.

Saliva from these glands is conveyed into the mouth through **Wharton's duct** along with the **ducts of Rivinus,** which lie parallel to the lingual frenum and open under the tongue.

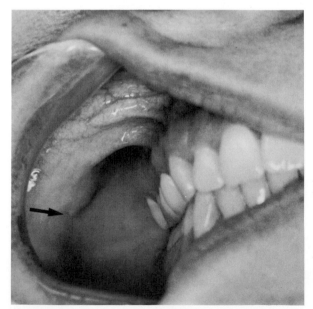

▼ Figure 3-28

The buccal frenum attachment and the opening of Stenson's duct (arrow). (Torres HO, Ehrlich A: Modern Dental Assisting, 4th Ed. Philadelphia, WB Saunders, 1990, p 460.)

Submandibular Glands

The submandibular glands are about the size of a walnut and lie on the floor of the mouth beneath the posterior portion of the mandible.

Saliva from these glands is conveyed to the mouth by **Wharton's duct,** which opens through the floor of the mouth just lingual to the lower incisors.

The Hard Palate (Fig. 3–29)

The palate serves as the roof of the mouth and separates it from the nasal cavity. The hard palate is the bony anterior portion.

It is formed by the inferior surfaces of the palatine processes of the maxillae and the horizontal plates of the palatine bones.

The hard palate is covered with masticatory mucosa. The **palatine rugae** are irregular ridges or folds in this mucous membrane that are located on the anterior portion of the hard palate just behind the maxillary incisors.

The **palatine raphe** is a narrow whitish streak in the midline of the palate.

The **incisive papilla** is a pear-shaped or oval structure formed on dense connective tissue. It is located directly posterior to the maxillary central incisors.

The Soft Palate

The soft palate forms the flexible posterior portion of the palate. The **uvula** hangs from the free edge of the soft palate (Fig. 3–30).

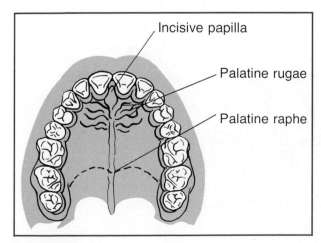

▼ **Figure 3–29**

Tissues of the hard palate. (Torres HO, Ehrlich A: Modern Dental Assisting, 4th Ed. Philadelphia, WB Saunders, 1990, p 88.)

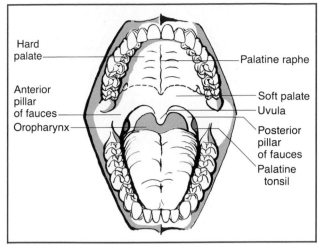

▼ **Figure 3–30**

The pillars of fauces. (Torres HO, Ehrlich A: Modern Dental Assisting, 4th Ed. Philadelphia, WB Saunders, 1990, p 38.)

The soft palate can be lifted upward and back to meet the posterior pharyngeal wall. This blocks the entrance to the nasopharynx during swallowing and speech.

The Pillars of Fauces

The two arches at the sides and back of the mouth are called the pillars of fauces (see Fig. 3–30). These are the **anterior pillar of fauces** and the **posterior pillar of fauces**.

The opening between the two arches is called the **isthmus of fauces** and contains the palatine tonsil.

The posterior opening of the mouth is into the **oropharynx**.

The Gag Reflex (Fig. 3–31)

The gag reflex is a protective mechanism located in the posterior region of the mouth. This very sensitive area includes the soft palate, the uvula, the fauces, and the posterior portion of the tongue.

Contact of a foreign body with the membranes of this area causes gagging, retching, or vomiting.

The Alveolar Process

The alveolar process is the extension of the bone of the body of the mandible and the maxilla. It supports the teeth in their functional positions in the jaws (Fig. 3–32).

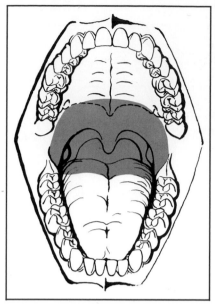

▼ **Figure 3–31**

Sensitive tissues of the oropharynx or tissues that react in a gag reflex when touched. (Torres HO, Ehrlich A: Modern Dental Assisting, 4th Ed. Philadelphia, WB Saunders, 1990, p 54.)

Cortical Plate

The dense outer cortical plate of bone covering the alveolar process provides strength and protection.

The cortical plate of the mandible is denser than that of the maxilla and has fewer openings

for the passage of nerves and vessels. This difference in structure affects the technique of injection for local anesthetic.

Alveolar Crest

The alveolar bone joins with the cortical plates on the facial and lingual sides of the crest of the alveolar process.

This alveolar crest is the highest point of the alveolar ridge. In a healthy mouth, the distance between the cementoenamel junction of the teeth and the alveolar crest is fairly constant.

Trabeculae

The central part of the alveolar process consists of trabeculae, which are bony spicules in cancellous bone (singular, *trabecula*).

In a radiograph, this trabecular bone has a web-like appearance and is known as **trabeculation**.

Alveolar Socket

The alveolar socket, or *alveolus,* is the cavity within the alveolar process in which the root of a tooth is held by the periodontal ligament.

The bony projection separating one socket from another is called the **interdental septum**.

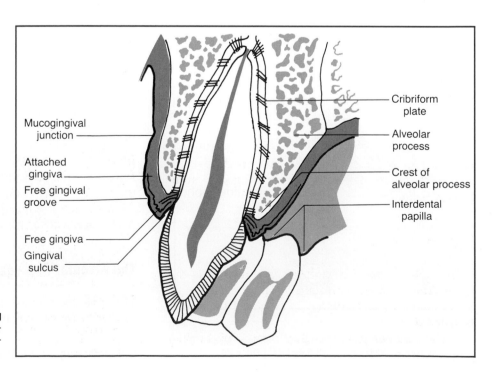

▼ **Figure 3–32**

The anterior teeth and supporting tissues. (Torres HO, Ehrlich A: Modern Dental Assisting, 4th Ed. Philadelphia, WB Saunders, 1990, p 87.)

Mucogingival junction

Attached gingiva

Free gingival groove

Free gingiva

Gingival sulcus

Cribriform plate

Alveolar process

Crest of alveolar process

Interdental papilla

The bone separating the roots of a multirooted tooth is called the **interradicular septum**.

Lamina Dura

The lamina dura, also known as the **cribriform plate**, is thin compact bone that lines the alveolar socket. Because of its structure, the lamina dura appears opaque on a radiograph.

THE TEETH

The teeth are discussed in Chapter 4, "Dental Anatomy and Tooth Morphology."

THE ORAL MUCOSA

The entire oral cavity is lined with mucous membrane. This tissue is specialized and adapted to meet the needs of the area it covers.

Lining Mucosa

The lining mucosa covers the inside of the cheeks, vestibule, lips, ventral surface of the tongue, and soft palate.

This delicate tissue is thin, moves freely, and injures easily. Beneath the lining mucosa is the **submucosa,** which contains the larger blood vessels and nerves.

Masticatory Mucosa

Masticatory mucosa covers the gingiva, the hard palate, and the dorsum of the tongue. There is no submucosa beneath the masticatory mucosa, and it is firmly affixed to the bone.

Masticatory mucosa is a very dense, tough covering in the mouth that is designed to withstand the vigorous activity of chewing and swallowing food.

The Gingiva

The gingiva, a form of masticatory mucosa, is the tissue immediately surrounding the teeth (Figs. 3–33 and 3–34.) (*Gingiva* is singular; the plural is *gingivae*.)

The following are characteristics of healthy gingival tissue:

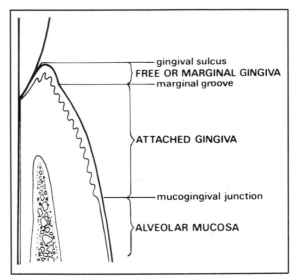

▼ Figure 3–33

Diagram showing anatomic landmarks of the gingiva. (Carranza FA Jr: Glickmann's Clinical Periodontology, 7th Ed. Philadelphia, WB Saunders, 1990, p 15.)

1. It surrounds the tooth in collar-like fashion.
2. It is self-cleansing in form.
3. It is firm and resistant.
4. It is tightly adapted to the tooth and bone.
5. The surfaces of the attached gingiva and interdental papillae are firm and stippled and are similar in appearance to the skin of an orange.

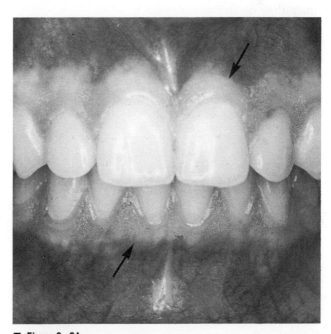

▼ Figure 3–34

Clinically normal gingiva in a young adult. Arrows indicate the mucogingival line between the light color of the attached gingiva and the darker alveolar mucosa. (Carranza, FA Jr: Glickmann's Clinical Periodontology, 7th Ed. Philadelphia, WB Saunders, 1990, p 15.)

6. In Caucasians, the surface is coral or salmon-pink in color; in other races, it is usually darker.

Epithelial Attachment

Healthy gingiva covers the alveolar bone and attaches to the teeth on the enamel surface just above the cervical line of the tooth. This is known as the epithelial attachment.

Free Gingiva

The free gingiva is that part of the gingiva that is higher than the epithelial attachment.

It is made up of the tissues from the gingival margin to the base of the gingival sulcus and is normally light pink or coral in color.

Gingival Sulcus

The gingival sulcus is the space between the free gingiva and the tooth. A normal, healthy gingival sulcus is 3 mm or less in depth.

Gingival Margin

The gingival margin is the upper edge of the gingiva. Its shape follows the curvatures of the cervical line of the tooth.

Free Gingival Groove

The free gingival groove is a shallow groove that runs parallel to the margin of the gingiva.

Interdental Papilla

The interdental papilla fills the interproximal embrasure between two adjacent teeth. It is usually triangular or conical in shape. It may also be referred to as the *gingival papilla.*

Attached Gingiva

Attached gingiva extends from the base of the sulcus to the **mucogingival junction.** It is a stippled, dense tissue, self-protecting in form, and is firmly bound and resilient.

Alveolar Mucosa

The alveolar mucosa, located below the mucogingival junction, is movable and darker in color due to additional pigment and blood supply.

▼ **EXERCISES**

1. The _____ salivary glands lie just in front of, and below, each ear.

   a. frontal
   b. parotid
   c. sublingual
   d. submandibular

2. The _____ is the cartilage projection anterior to the external opening of the ear.

   a. ala
   b. outer canthus
   c. philtrum
   d. tragus

3. The _____ is the space between the free gingiva and the tooth. When healthy, it rarely exceeds 3 mm in depth.

   a. epithelial attachment
   b. free gingiva
   c. gingival margin
   d. gingival sulcus

4. The term _____ means pertaining to, or directed toward, the cheek.

   a. buccal
   b. labial
   c. lingual
   d. a or b

5. The maxillary anterior teeth are innervated by the _____ nerve.

   a. anterior superior alveolar
   b. inferior alveolar
   c. incisive
   d. nasopalatine

6. _____ duct carries saliva from the parotid gland to the mouth.

   a. Hansen's
   b. Stensen's
   c. The Rivinus
   d. Wharton's

7. The _____ is compact bone that lines the tooth socket.

   a. alveolar crest
   b. cortical plate
   c. lamina dura
   d. trabecula

8. The area of the lips where the skin joins the mucous membrane is called the
   _____.

   a. frenum
   b. labial vestibule
   c. philtrum
   d. vermilion border

9. The underside of the tongue is referred to as the _____ surface.

   a. dorsal
   b. ventral

10. _____ mucosa is thin, freely movable tissue that tears and injures easily.

    a. Attached gingival
    b. Free gingival
    c. Lining
    d. Masticatory

11. The _____ muscle closes the jaw.

    a. external pterygoid
    b. internal pterygoid
    c. masseter
    d. mylohyoid

12. In the temporomandibular joint, the _____ action is the second phase in mouth opening and movement.

    a. gliding
    b. hinge

13. The _____ sinuses are located within the forehead just above the eyes.

    a. ethmoid
    b. frontal
    c. maxillary
    d. sphenoid

14. The _____ muscle serves to compress the cheeks, hold food in contact with the teeth, and retract the angles of the mouth.

    a. buccinator
    b. masseter
    c. orbicularis oris
    d. temporal

15. _____ extends from the base of the sulcus to the mucogingival junction.

    a. Alveolar mucosa
    b. Attached gingiva
    c. Free gingiva
    d. Lining mucosa

16. The major blood supply to the mandibular teeth is from the _____ _____.

    a. anterior artery
    b. inferior alveolar arteries
    c. lingual artery
    d. a and c

17. The two arches at the back of the mouth, which form the opening into the throat, are called the _____.

    a. alveolar crest
    b. oropharynx
    c. pillars of fauces
    d. uvula

18. The _____ are irregular ridges or folds in the mucous membrane that are located on the anterior portion of the hard palate just behind the maxillary incisors.

    a. fauces
    b. frena
    c. rugae
    d. symphysis

19. The _____ is the bony projection separating one alveolar socket from another.

    a. interdental septum
    b. interradicular septum
    c. lamina dura
    d. trabeculation

20. _____ bone is hard, dense, and strong.

    a. Cancellous
    b. Compact
    c. Cortical
    d. b and c

21. _____ is the forward movement of the mandible.

    a. Excursion
    b. Mastication
    c. Protrusion
    d. Retraction

22. A _____ is a narrow fold of mucous membrane passing from a more fixed to a movable part.

    a. fauce
    b. frenum
    c. philtrum
    d. vestibule

23. The _____ is a pear-shaped structure of dense connective tissue that is located immediately posterior to the maxillary anterior centrals.

    a. incisive papilla
    b. palatine rugae
    c. palatine raphe
    d. pillar of fauces

24. The _____, which consists of dense fibrous tissue, surrounds the temporomandibular joint.

    a. articular eminence
    b. capsular ligament
    c. meniscus
    d. periosteum

25. The _____ is the opening located on the lingual surface of each ramus of the mandible.

    a. genial tubercle
    b. mandibular foramen
    c. mandibular notch
    d. oblique ridge

Criterion Sheet 3-1

Student's Name _____

Procedure: *IDENTIFY MAJOR BONES AND LANDMARKS OF THE FACE*

Performance Objective:

Given a drawing or the replica of a skull, the student will identify the bones and landmarks of the face listed below.

	SE	IE
SE = Student evaluation **C** = Criterion met **IE** = Instructor evaluation **X** = Criterion not met		
Instrumentation: Unlabeled drawing or skull replica		
1. Identified the temporal bone.		
2. Identified the mandible.		
3. Identified the maxilla.		
4. Identified the mental foramen.		
5. Identified the condyloid process.		
Comments:		

Criterion Sheet 3-2

Student's Name _____

Procedure: *IDENTIFY MAJOR LANDMARKS OF THE FACE*

Performance Objective:

Using a mouth mirror and working with another student, the student will identify the landmarks of the face listed below.

	SE	IE
SE = Student evaluation **C** = Criterion met **IE** = Instructor evaluation **X** = Criterion not met		
Instrumentation: Mirror and another student		
1. Identified the inner and outer canthus of the eye.		
2. Identified ala of the nose.		
3. Identified commissure of the lips.		
4. Identified tragus of the ear.		
5. Identified the philtrum.		
Comments:		

Dental Anatomy and Tooth Morphology

The student will be able to:

1. Name and describe the parts and tissues of the teeth.

2. List and describe the teeth of the primary and permanent dentition.

3. Name the types of teeth and describe the principal characteristics of each.

4. Describe the dental arches, quadrants, surfaces of the teeth, and the Universal Numbering system.

5. Define overbite and overjet, line and point angles, contours, contacts, embrasures, and antagonists.

6. Describe normal occlusion and Angle's classification of occlusion and malocclusion.

7. Demonstrate identification of the permanent teeth by type and differentiate between anterior and posterior teeth.

OVERVIEW OF DENTAL ANATOMY AND TOOTH MORPHOLOGY

Anatomy is the study of the structures of the body. **Morphology** is the study of the form of these structures.

The dental assistant must understand the structure and form of the teeth and the tissues that surround and support the teeth, so that she may perform her duties effectively without accidentally injuring these delicate tissues.

This knowledge also helps the assistant understand how the teeth and tissues function together and why it is so important to maintain the oral tissues in healthy condition.

PARTS AND TISSUES OF THE TOOTH (Fig. 4–1)

Each tooth consists of a crown and one or more roots. The size and shape of the crown and the size and number of roots are determined by the function of the tooth.

The Crown

The **anatomic crown** of the tooth is that portion covered with enamel and extending from the incisal edge or occlusal surface to the cementoenamel junction. The anatomic crown remains constant throughout the life of the tooth.

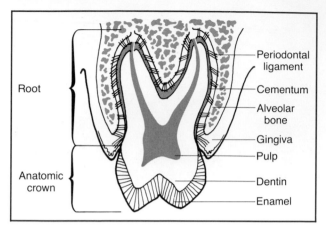

▼ **Figure 4 – 1**

Parts of the tooth and surrounding tissues in cross section. (Torres HO, Ehrlich A: Modern Dental Assisting, 4th Ed. Philadelphia, WB Saunders, 1990, p 78.)

The **clinical crown** is that portion which is visible in the mouth. The clinical crown may vary during the life cycle of the tooth as the tooth erupts into position, is worn away through attrition, and as the surrounding tissues recede.

The Root

The root of the tooth is that portion normally embedded in the alveolar process and covered with cementum.

The root portion of the tooth may be single, as found in a normal anterior tooth, or multiple, with a **bifurcation** (division into two roots) or a **trifurcation** (division into three roots). The tapered end of each root tip is known as the **apex**.

The Cervix

The constricted area where the anatomic crown and the root meet is called the cervix, or *neck,* of the tooth.

The **cementoenamel junction** is a line formed by the junction of the enamel of the crown and the cementum of the root and is also referred to as the *cervical line.*

Enamel

Enamel, which makes up the anatomic crown of the tooth, is the cap that covers and protects the underlying tissues of the tooth.

Enamel is translucent and ranges in color from yellowish to grayish white. The variation in color may be caused by differences in the thickness and in the translucent qualities of the enamel.

Enamel is the hardest, most dense, calcified tissue of the body and is able to withstand crushing stresses to about 100,000 pounds per square inch during mastication (chewing).

Although it is strong, enamel is also brittle. Unless it has sufficient bulk or is properly supported, enamel is prone to splitting and chipping. Unlike other body tissues, enamel is not capable of repairing itself.

The cushioning effect of the underlying dentin and the suspensory action of the periodontium, combined with the hardness of the enamel, enable it to withstand the pressures brought against it.

Structurally, enamel is composed of millions of calcified **enamel rods**, or *prisms,* which originate at the dentinoenamel junction and extend the width of the enamel to the surface. The diameter of the rods averages 4 microns.

Each rod appears to be encased in a *rod sheath,* and the sheathed rods seem to be cemented together by an *interrod substance.*

Of these three structures, the rods are the most highly calcified; however, all three are extremely hard. This difference is an important factor in the "acid etch" technique of bonding materials directly to the enamel surface.

Dentin

Dentin constitutes the main portion of the tooth structure and extends almost the entire length of the tooth. It is covered by enamel on the crown and by cementum on the root.

The internal surface of the dentin forms the walls of the pulp cavity. This internal wall closely follows the outline of the external surface of the dentin.

In the permanent teeth, dentin is pale yellow in color and somewhat transparent. The color in primary teeth is paler.

The hardness of dentin is less than that of enamel but is greater than that of either bone or cementum. Although dentin is considered a hard structure, it has elastic properties that are important for the support of the brittle enamel of the tooth. Because it is less calcified than enamel, dentin is more radiolucent.

Dentin is very porous tissue. It is penetrated through its entire thickness by many microscopic canals called **dentinal tubules**. Each tubule contains a **dentinal fiber**.

Dentin, an excellent thermal conductor, also transmits pain stimuli by way of the dentinal fibers. In addition, when not protected by enamel, the dentinal tubules form a passage for invading bacteria to reach the pulp.

Each dentinal fiber is an extension from one of the odontoblasts in the pulp chamber. Because of these fibers, dentin is considered to be a living tissue. As a living tissue, it is capable of limited repair and continued growth.

However, because dentin is living tissue, it must be protected from dehydration and thermal shock during operative procedures.

Secondary dentin, which is formed later in the life of the tooth, is a somewhat uniform layer of dentin around the pulp chamber that is laid down routinely throughout the life of the tooth.

Reparative dentin is formed in response to irritation. During operative procedures, lining materials are used to encourage the formation of reparative dentin.

Cementum

Cementum is the root covering of the tooth. It overlies the dentin and joins the enamel at the cementoenamel junction. Cementum is not quite as hard as dentin; however, in structure and appearance, it is much like bone.

Cementum is light yellow and is easily distinguishable from enamel by its lack of luster and its darker hue. It is somewhat lighter in color than dentin.

The **cementodentinal junction**, which is the attachment of the cementum to the dentin, is almost impossible to distinguish, even with the electron microscope.

Cementum functions as an attachment to anchor the tooth to the bony socket by means of attachment fibers within the periodontium.

The Pulp

The inner aspect of the dentin forms the boundaries of the **pulp chamber**. The surface of the pulp chamber more or less follows the contours of the exterior surface of the tooth.

At the time of eruption, the pulp chamber is large, but because of continuous deposition of dentin it becomes smaller with age.

The pulp contains blood vessels, connective tissue, and an extensive nerve supply that receives and transmits pain stimuli.

The part of the pulp that lies within the crown portion of the tooth is called the **coronal pulp**. This includes the **pulp horns**, which are extensions of the pulp that project toward the cusp tips and incisal edges (Fig. 4–2).

The other portion of the pulp is more apically

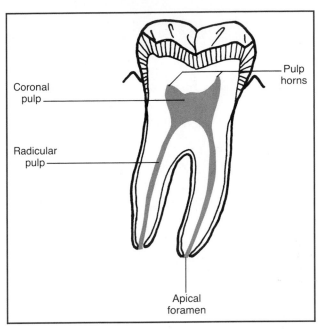

▼ **Figure 4–2**

The dental pulp. Mandibular first molar in cross section. (Torres HO, Ehrlich A: Modern Dental Assisting, 4th Ed. Philadelphia, WB Saunders, 1990, p 83.)

located and is referred to as the **radicular** or **root pulp**. The radicular pulp is continuous with the tissues of the periapical area via an **apical foramen**.

This foramen provides a channel through which blood and lymph vessels, nerves, and connective tissue elements gain access to the interior regions of the tooth.

In relatively young teeth, the apical foramen is not yet fully formed and the apical orifice is rather wide. However, with increasing age and exposure of the tooth to functional stress, secondary dentin decreases the diameter of the pulp chamber and the apical foramen.

The Periodontal Ligament

The periodontal ligament is not part of the tooth; however, it plays an important role in supporting the the tooth within its bony socket. (The bony support for a tooth is described in Chapter 3.)

The periodontal ligament, which is a series of fiber groups, holds the tooth suspended in its socket. This cushioning makes it possible for the tooth to withstand the pressures and forces of mastication (Fig. 4–3).

Because of its structure, the periodontal ligament appears translucent on a radiograph.

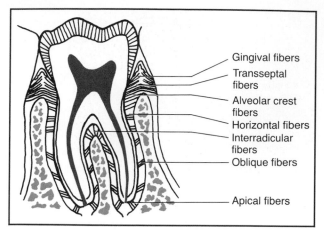

▼ **Figure 4-3**

Periodontal ligament fiber groups. (Torres HO, Ehrlich A: Modern Dental Assisting, 4th Ed. Philadelphia, WB Saunders, 1990, p 85.)

THE DENTITION

Primary Dentition

The 20 teeth of the primary dentition are also referred to as the *deciduous, baby,* or *milk teeth.* As the term *primary* implies, these teeth are shed to make way for their permanent successors, which are known as **succedaneous teeth.**

All the primary teeth should be in normal alignment and occlusion shortly after the age of 2 years. The roots should be fully formed by the time the child is 3 years old.

Figure 4-4 shows the eruption and shedding dates for the primary dentition.

Mixed Dentition Stage

During the mixed dentition stage, the child has some permanent and some primary teeth in position. Figure 4-5 is a radiographic view of the normally developing mixed dentition in a 7-year-old child.

Between the ages of 4 and 5, as the result of jaw growth, the anterior teeth begin to separate to make room for the larger permanent teeth that will follow.

During this phase, the occlusion is supported and made more efficient by the eruption of the first permanent molars immediately in back of the primary second molars.

The exfoliation of the primary teeth takes place between the fifth and twelfth years. (**Exfoliation** is the normal process by which primary teeth are shed.)

Permanent Dentition

The permanent dentition consists of 32 teeth. As the name implies, these teeth are designed to last a lifetime. Figure 4-6 shows the eruption dates of the permanent dentition.

Figures 4-7 and 4-8 detail the names of the cusps and roots of the teeth in the permanent dentition.

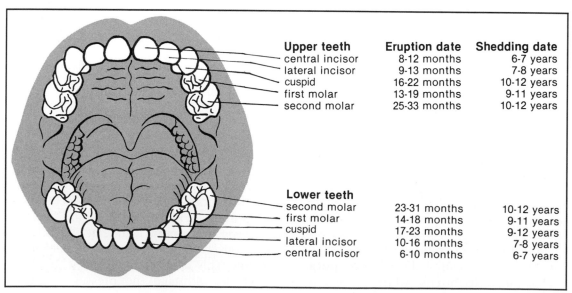

Upper teeth	Eruption date	Shedding date
central incisor	8-12 months	6-7 years
lateral incisor	9-13 months	7-8 years
cuspid	16-22 months	10-12 years
first molar	13-19 months	9-11 years
second molar	25-33 months	10-12 years
Lower teeth		
second molar	23-31 months	10-12 years
first molar	14-18 months	9-11 years
cuspid	17-23 months	9-12 years
lateral incisor	10-16 months	7-8 years
central incisor	6-10 months	6-7 years

▼ **Figure 4-4**

Normal eruption and shedding ages for the primary teeth. (Torres HO, Ehrlich A: Modern Dental Assisting, 4th Ed. Philadelphia, WB Saunders, 1990, p 74.)

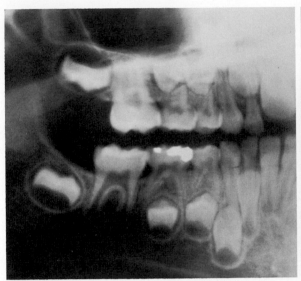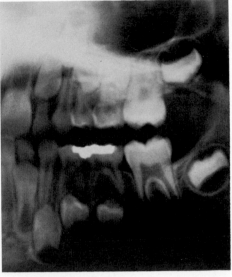

▼ Figure 4-5

Panoramic radiograph showing the mixed dentition stage of a 7-year-old boy. (Courtesy of Dr. E. Howden.)

THE TYPES OF TEETH

On the basis of form and function, the human teeth of the permanent dentition are divided into four types or classes: incisors, cuspids, premolars, and molars.

Incisors

The incisors are single-rooted teeth with a relatively sharp and thin edge (Fig. 4-9). They are designed for cutting food without the application of heavy forces.

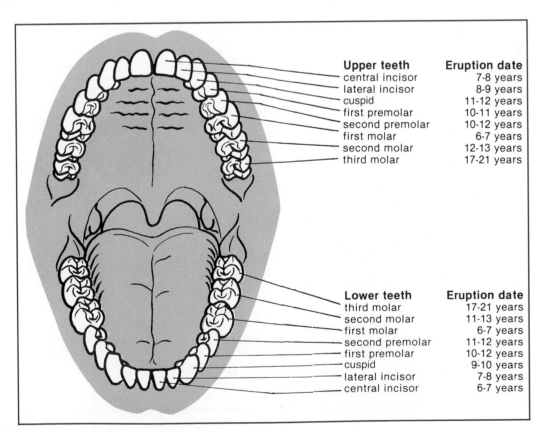

Upper teeth	Eruption date
central incisor	7-8 years
lateral incisor	8-9 years
cuspid	11-12 years
first premolar	10-11 years
second premolar	10-12 years
first molar	6-7 years
second molar	12-13 years
third molar	17-21 years

Lower teeth	Eruption date
third molar	17-21 years
second molar	11-13 years
first molar	6-7 years
second premolar	11-12 years
first premolar	10-12 years
cuspid	9-10 years
lateral incisor	7-8 years
central incisor	6-7 years

▼ Figure 4-6

Normal eruption ages for the permanent teeth. (Torres HO, Ehrlich A: Modern Dental Assisting, 4th Ed. Philadelphia, WB Saunders, 1990, p 74.)

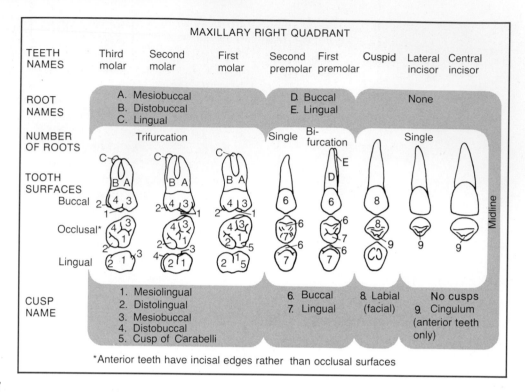

▼ Figure 4–7

Names of the cusps and roots of the teeth of the maxillary right quadrant (permanent dentition). (Torres HO, Ehrlich A: Modern Dental Assisting, 4th Ed. Philadelphia, WB Saunders, 1990, p 109.)

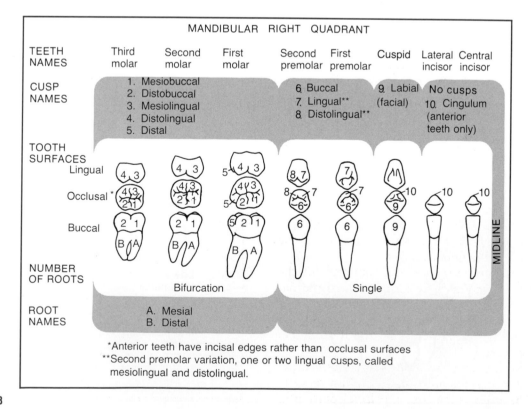

▼ Figure 4–8

Names of the cusps and roots of the teeth of the mandibular right quadrant (permanent dentition). (Torres HO, Ehrlich A: Modern Dental Assisting, 4th Ed. Philadelphia, WB Saunders, 1990, p 109.)

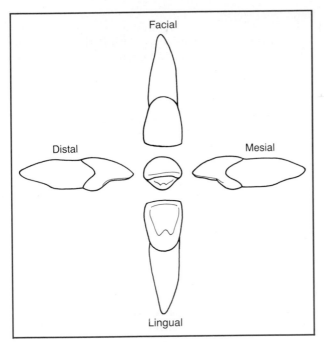

▼ **Figure 4-9**

Permanent maxillary right central incisor.

There is a central incisor and a lateral incisor in each quadrant of the primary and permanent dentition.

The **incisal edges** of these teeth are formed at the labioincisal line angle and do not exist until an edge has been created by wear. The incisal edge is also known as the *incisal surface* or *incisal plane.*

Cuspids

The cuspids are located between the lateral incisors and the first premolar at the "corners" of the mouth (Fig. 4–10). Because of their strength and location, these teeth are often referred to as the cornerstones of the dental arches.

There is one cuspid in each quadrant of the primary and permanent dentition. Each cuspid has a single pointed cusp and a single well-developed root. The cuspid is the longest rooted tooth in the dentition and is well designed for the functions of cutting and tearing.

Because they are the most stable teeth in the dentition, the cuspids are usually the last teeth to be lost. The bony ridge over the facial portion of the root of the cuspid is known as the **canine eminence.**

Premolars

The premolars, or *bicuspids,* are like the cuspids in that they have points and cusps for grasping and tearing (Fig. 4–11). They also have a somewhat broader working surface for chewing food. The premolars are located posterior to the cuspids and immediately anterior to the molars.

There are two premolars in each quadrant of the permanent dentition. There are no premolars in the primary dentition.

The **maxillary first premolar** has two cusps and two roots. The **maxillary second premolar** has two cusps and one root.

The **mandibular first** and **second premolars** each have two cusps and a single-root.

Molars

There are two molars in each quadrant of the primary dentition. There are three molars in each quadrant of the permanent dentition.

The molars have more cusps and multiple roots to support the broad occlusal surface that is necessary to withstand the application of heavy forces that are required in chewing food (Fig. 4–12).

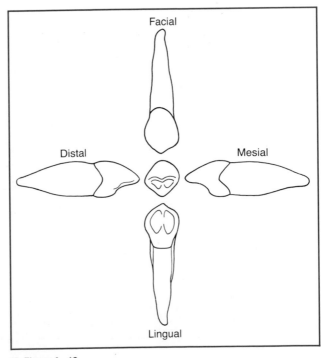

▼ **Figure 4-10**

Permanent maxillary right cuspid.

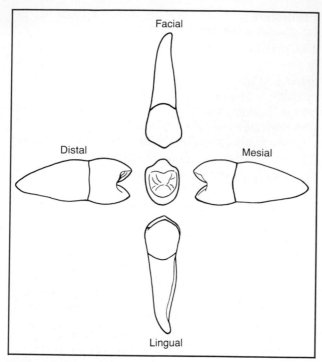

▼ **Figure 4–11**

Permanent maxillary right second premolar.

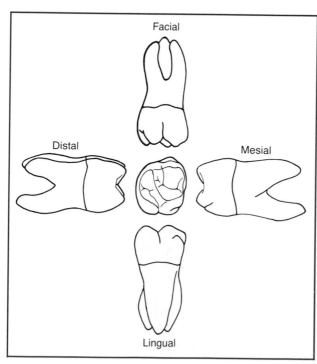

▼ **Figure 4–12**

Permanent maxillary right first molar.

Permanent Molars

The **maxillary permanent molars** each have three trifurcated roots. (**Trifurcated** means divided into three.) The three roots are located one on the lingual area and two on the buccal (facial) area.

The **mandibular permanent molars** each have two bifurcated roots. (**Bifurcated** means divided into two.) These two roots are located one on the mesial area and one on the distal area.

The **maxillary permanent first molar** is normally the largest tooth in the maxillary arch. It has four well-developed functioning cusps and frequently one supplemental cusp.

This fifth cusp is called the **cusp of Carabelli.** This cusp is found lingual to the mesiolingual cusp and often is so poorly developed that it is scarcely distinguishable.

The **maxillary second molar** has four cusps. The **maxillary third molar** often differs considerably in size, contour, number or roots, and relative position from the other teeth.

The **mandibular first molar** normally is the largest tooth in the mandibular arch. It has five well-developed cusps and two well-developed roots.

The **mandibular second molar** has four cusps. The **mandibular third molar** presents many developmental irregularities in form, in number of roots, and in position.

THE DENTAL ARCHES

The teeth are aligned into two dental arches, the **maxillary** and the **mandibular**, each of which contains the same number and types of teeth (Fig. 4–13).

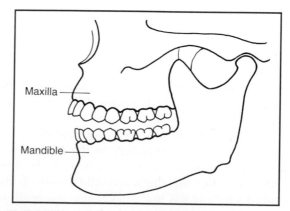

▼ **Figure 4–13**

The dental arches. (Torres HO, Ehrlich A: Modern Dental Assisting, 4th Ed. Philadelphia, WB Saunders, 1990, p 91.)

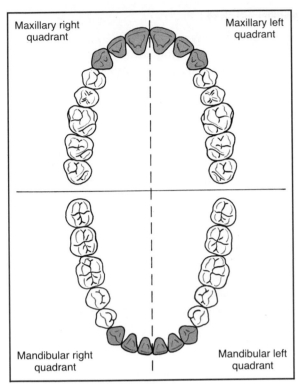

▼ **Figure 4-14**

Occlusal view of the dental arches divided into quadrants. The anterior teeth are shaded. The posterior teeth are not shaded. (Torres HO, Ehrlich A: Modern Dental Assisting, 4th Ed. Philadelphia, WB Saunders, 1990, p 92.)

As the arches function, the *movable* mandibular arch brings the primary forces of occlusion to bear against the *immovable* maxillary arch.

Through normal development and proper positioning of all of its parts, the dental arch is designed to be an efficient unit, and stability is ensured as long as the normal arrangement is maintained.

However, malocclusion and/or the premature loss of teeth greatly reduces the functioning, efficiency, and stability of the dentition.

Anterior and Posterior Teeth

As an aid in describing their location within the arches, teeth are classified as anterior or posterior (Fig. 4-14).

The **anterior teeth** are the incisors and cuspids. These teeth are aligned so as to form a smooth, curving arc from the distal of the cuspid on one side of the arch to the distal of the cuspid on the opposite side.

The **posterior teeth** of the permanent dentition are the premolars and molars. There is little or no lateral curvature in the posterior portion of

the dental arch; hence, the teeth appear to be almost in a straight line.

Quadrants

An imaginary midline divides each arch into mirror halves. The two arches, each divided into halves, create four sections, or quarters, which are called quadrants (see Fig. 4-14). These are:

▼ The maxillary right quadrant.

▼ The maxillary left quadrant.

▼ The mandibular left quadrant.

▼ The mandibular right quadrant.

In the primary dentition, each quadrant contains the central incisor, lateral incisor, cuspid, first molar, and second molar (there are no premolars in the primary dentition).

The permanent dentition has in each quadrant the central incisor, lateral incisor, cuspid, first premolar, second premolar, first molar, second molar, and third molar.

Surfaces of the Teeth

Axial Surfaces (Figs. 4-15 and 4-16)

Each tooth has four **axial surfaces.** *Axial* refers to the long axis, which is an imaginary line passing longitudinally through the center of a tooth.

Thus, an axial surface is a longitudinal surface of the tooth from the occlusal surface (or incisal edge) through the apex of the root. However, not all tooth surfaces are axial.

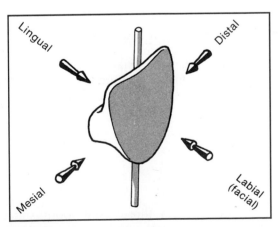

▼ **Figure 4-15**

Axial surfaces of an anterior tooth. (Torres HO, Ehrlich A: Modern Dental Assisting, 4th Ed. Philadelphia, WB Saunders, 1990, p 97.)

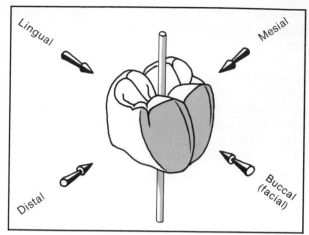

▼ **Figure 4-16**

Axial surfaces of a posterior tooth. (Torres HO, Ehrlich A: Modern Dental Assisting, 4th Ed. Philadelphia, WB Saunders, 1990, p 97.)

Occlusal Surfaces (Fig. 4-17)

The occlusal surface is not an axial surface. It is the horizontal chewing surface of the posterior teeth and is located perpendicular to the axial surfaces. (*Note*: Anterior teeth have *incisal edges,* but these edges are not classified as surfaces.)

Line and Point Angles (Fig. 4-18)

An **angle** is the junction of two or more surfaces of a tooth. A **line angle** is that angle formed by the junction of *two* surfaces of a tooth crown along an imaginary line. Its name is derived by combining the names of the two surfaces (for example, mesiobuccal).

A **point angle** is that angle formed by the junction of *three* surfaces at one point. These angles are described by combining the names of the surfaces forming them (for example, mesiolinguo-occlusal angle).

The anterior teeth have four surfaces, all of which are axial. The posterior teeth have five surfaces—the four axial surfaces plus the occlusal (horizontal) surface.

The axial surfaces are defined as follows:

▼ **Buccal surface.** The axial surface of a posterior tooth positioned immediately adjacent to the cheek (also referred to as the facial surface).

▼ **Labial surface.** The axial surface of an anterior tooth positioned immediately adjacent to the lip (also referred to as the facial surface).

▼ **Facial surfaces.** This term refers, collectively, to both labial and buccal surfaces. Thus, these three terms all refer to that surface of a tooth which is immediately adjacent to the cheeks and lips.

▼ **Lingual surface.** The axial surface of a tooth that faces toward the tongue.

▼ **Distal surface.** The axial surface of a tooth facing away from the midline toward the posterior, following the curve of the dental arch.

▼ **Mesial surface.** The axial surface of a tooth facing toward the midline, following the curve of the dental arch.

Proximal Surfaces

Proximal surfaces are those axial tooth surfaces that are adjacent to each other in the same arch. Mesial and distal surfaces of adjacent teeth in the same arch are proximal surfaces.

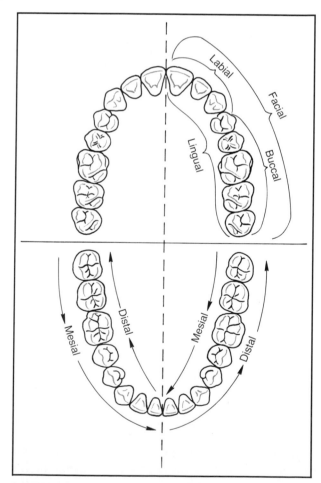

▼ **Figure 4-17**

Axial surfaces of the teeth as they relate to an occlusal view of the dental arches. (Torres HO, Ehrlich A: Modern Dental Assisting, 4th Ed. Philadelphia, WB Saunders, 1990, p 97.)

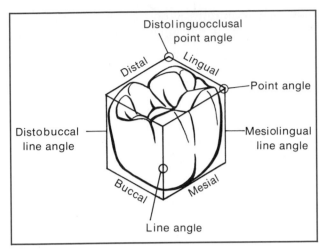

▼ **Figure 4 – 18**

Line and point angles. (Torres HO, Ehrlich A: Modern Dental Assisting, 4th Ed. Philadelphia, WB Saunders, 1990, p 98.)

When combining these words, drop the last two letters of the first word and substitute the letter *o*.

Contours (Figs. 4 – 19 and 4 – 20)

Every segment of a tooth presents curved surfaces except when the tooth is fractured or worn. Although the contour of the different types of teeth may vary, the general principle that the crown of the tooth narrows toward the cervical line holds for all four axial surfaces.

The pronounced curvatures found on the labial or buccal and lingual surfaces of the tooth provide natural sluiceways for the passage of food. This action protects the gingiva from the impact of foods during mastication.

Normal curvature provides the gingiva with adequate stimulation yet protects it from being damaged by food. With inadequate contour, the gingiva may be damaged. With overcontour, the gingiva lacks adequate stimulation.

Contacts

Each tooth crown in the dental arches should be in contact at some point with its adjacent tooth (or teeth) for proper contact relationship.

This proper relationship between adjacent teeth does three things:

1. It serves to keep food from being trapped between the teeth.
2. It helps to stabilize the dental arches by the combined anchorage of all the teeth in either arch in positive contact with each other.
3. It protects the interproximal gingival tissue from trauma during mastication.

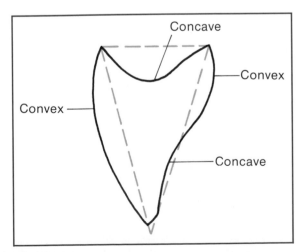

▼ **Figure 4 – 19**

The surfaces of a single tooth are both convex (outward) and concave (inward) curves. (Torres HO, Ehrlich A: Modern Dental Assisting, 4th Ed. Philadelphia, WB Saunders, 1990, p 99.)

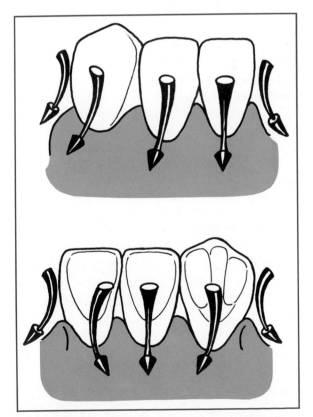

▼ **Figure 4 – 20**

Pronounced curvatures are found on the facial and lingual surfaces of the tooth. (Torres HO, Ehrlich A: Modern Dental Assisting, 4th Ed. Philadelphia, WB Saunders, 1990, p 99.)

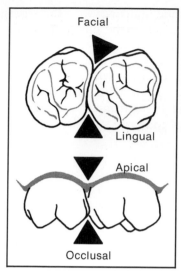

▼ **Figure 4-21**

Embrasures may diverge facially, lingually, occlusally, or apically. (Torres HO, Ehrlich A: Modern Dental Assisting, 4th Ed. Philadelphia, WB Saunders, 1990, p 100.)

The **contact area** is that convex region of the mesial or distal surfaces of a tooth that touches the adjacent tooth in the same arch.

The **contact point** is the exact spot where the teeth actually touch each other. The terms *contact* or *contact area* are frequently used interchangeably to refer to the contact point.

Embrasures

Normally, the teeth within the same arch are arranged in a spatial relationship to each other so that their proximal surfaces contact each other at their greatest convexity (outward curvature). This results in an embrasure, which is a V-shaped space in a gingival direction between the proximal surfaces of two adjoining teeth in contact.

The embrasure may diverge in the following directions: (1) facially, (2) lingually, (3) occlu-

sally, or (4) apically, although normally the interdental papilla of the gingiva fills this embrasure (Fig. 4-21).

Antagonists

The teeth in each arch are arranged in close mesial and distal contact with adjacent teeth to present an unbroken series of occlusal surfaces.

In this arrangement, each tooth in the dental arch has two antagonists in the opposing arch: its class counterpart and the tooth next to it (Fig. 4-22).

The only exceptions to this are the mandibular central incisors and the maxillary third molars, which have only one antagonist.

Because each tooth has two antagonists, the loss of one still leaves one remaining antagonist. This helps to keep the tooth in occlusal contact with the opposing arch and in its own arch relationship at the same time by preventing elongation and displacement through the lack of antagonism.

Overjet and Overbite

The normal overlapping of the maxillary teeth over the mandibular teeth is particularly evident in the anterior region, where the larger maxillary anterior teeth create a wider curvature of the arch.

The horizontal overlap of the maxillary teeth is called **overjet,** and the vertical overlap is known as **overbite** (Fig. 4-23).

Occlusal Form

The cusps and fossae (normal indentations of the occlusal surfaces) produce a mortar-and-pestle action for the effective grinding of food (Fig. 4-24).

The marginal ridge is the highest formation of

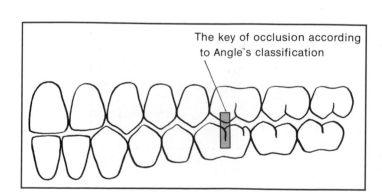

▼ **Figure 4-22**

The antagonistic relationship of the teeth in the dental arches. In normal occlusion, the mesiobuccal cusp of the maxillary permanent first molar occludes in the buccal groove of the mandibular permanent first molar. (Torres HO, Ehrlich A: Modern Dental Assisting, 4th Ed. Philadelphia, WB Saunders, 1990, p 92.)

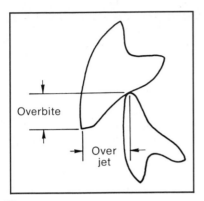

▼ **Figure 4–23**

Overjet is the horizontal overlap of the maxillary teeth. Overbite is the vertical overlap of the maxillary teeth. (Torres HO, Ehrlich A: Modern Dental Assisting, 4th Ed. Philadelphia, WB Saunders, 1990, p 93.)

enamel on the crown of a tooth as the four axial surfaces and the occlusal surface come together.

ANATOMIC LANDMARKS OF THE TEETH

Figure 4–30, which appears at the end of this chapter, is an illustrated glossary of the terms used in describing other anatomic landmarks of the teeth.

OCCLUSION

Occlusion is the contact between the maxillary and mandibular teeth in all mandibular positions and movements.

Centric occlusion occurs when the jaws are closed in a position that produces maximal stable contact between the occluding surfaces of the maxillary and mandibular teeth.

Normal occlusion is the usual or accepted relationship of the teeth in the same jaw and of those teeth in the opposing jaw when the teeth are approximated in centric occlusion .

Malocclusion refers to abnormal or malpositioned relationships of the maxillary teeth to the mandibular teeth when they are in centric occlusion.

Many systems have been developed to classify occlusion; however, the categories established by Dr. Edward H. Angle in early studies of orthodontics are most widely used.

In the Angle system, the first permanent molars were selected for identifying the normal relationship of the mandible to the maxilla.

ANGLE'S CLASSIFICATION OF OCCLUSION AND MALOCCLUSION

Class I (Neutroclusion) (Fig. 4–25)

When the jaws are at rest and the teeth are approximated in centric occlusion, the mandibular arch and the body of the mandible are in normal mesiodistal relationship to the maxillary arch if the following apply:

1. The mesiobuccal (mesiofacial) cusp of the maxillary permanent first molar occludes in the buccal groove of the mandibular first molar.
2. The mesiolingual cusp of the maxillary permanent first molar occludes with the occlusal fossa of the mandibular permanent first molar.

Class I may include the anteriors or individual teeth malaligned in their position in the arch;

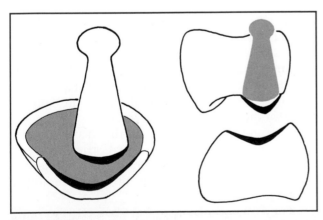

▼ **Figure 4–24**

The occlusal contacts of the cusps and fossae are arranged to produce a mortar-and-pestle action for the effective grinding of food. (Torres HO, Ehrlich A: Modern Dental Assisting, 4th Ed. Philadelphia, WB Saunders, 1990, p 101.)

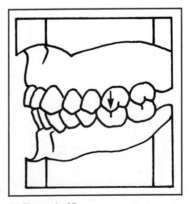

▼ **Figure 4–25**

Class I, or neutroclusion.

however, it is the relationship of the permanent first molars that determines the classification.

Class II (Distoclusion)

The mandibular dental arch and the body of the mandible are in a **distal** relationship to the maxillary arch by half the width of the permanent first molar or by the mesiobuccal width of a premolar. This frequently gives the appearance that the maxillary anterior teeth protrude over the mandibular anteriors.

The mesiobuccal cusp of the maxillary first molar occludes in the interdental space between the mandibular second premolar and the mesial cusp of the mandibular first molar.

Class II, Division 1 (Fig. 4–26)

The lips are usually flat and parted, with the lower lip tucked behind the upper incisors. The upper lip appears short and drawn up over the protruding anterior teeth of the maxillary arch.

The maxillary incisors are in labioversion. (**Labioversion** is the inclination of the teeth to extend facially beyond the normal overlap of the incisal edge of the maxillary incisors over the mandibular incisors.)

Division 1, Subdivision. The distal relationship of the mandibular dental arch, and in some cases the body of the mandible, is not in alignment; it is unilateral or to one side of the opposing teeth of the maxilla. The opposite side of the mandibular

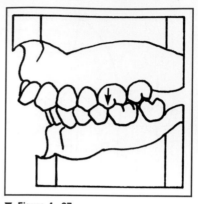

▼ Figure 4–27

Class II, or distoclusion, Division 2.

arch may be in normal relationship with the opposing maxillary teeth.

Class II, Division 2 (Fig. 4–27)

This division includes Class II malocclusions in which the maxillary incisors are not in labioversion. The maxillary central incisors are near normal anteroposteriorly, and they may be slightly in linguoversion. The maxillary lateral incisors may be tipped labially and mesially.

Linguoversion refers to the position of the maxillary incisors as being in back of the opposing mandibular incisors. Normally, the maxillary incisors slightly overlap the mandibular incisors.

Division 2, Subdivision. This is a Class II, division 2 occlusion in which the malocclusion is on one side only (unilateral malocclusion).

Class III (Mesioclusion) (Fig. 4–28)

The mandibular arch and the body of the mandible are in bilateral, **mesial** relationship to the maxillary teeth. This frequently gives the appearance that the mandible protrudes.

The mesiobuccal cusp of the maxillary first molar occludes in the interdental space between the distal cusp of the mandibular first permanent molar and the mesial cusp of the mandibular second permanent molar.

For a malocclusion to be Class III, the body of the mandible must be large or positioned mesially to the maxilla. This results in an abnormal degree of mesial relationship of the mandible to the maxilla.

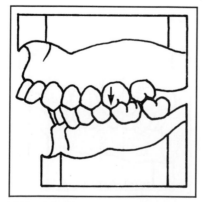

▼ Figure 4–26

Class II, or distoclusion, Division 1.

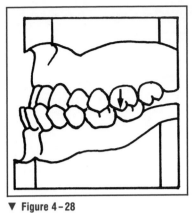

▼ Figure 4-28

Class III, or mesioclusion.

THE UNIVERSAL NUMBERING SYSTEM

In 1968, in an effort to standardize numbering systems, the American Dental Association officially adopted the use of the Universal Numbering System (Tables 4-1 and 4-2).

In this system, the permanent teeth are numbered 1 to 32, starting with the upper right third molar, working around to the upper left third molar, then dropping to the lower left third molar and working around to the lower right third molar.

The primary teeth are lettered, using capital letters *A* through *T* and following the same methodology as for the permanent teeth, starting with the upper right second primary molar and ending with the lower right second primary molar.

On the diagram of a dental chart, the right side of the mouth appears on the left side of the diagram (Fig. 4-29).

Thus, tooth number 1 is in the upper right corner of the diagram, and tooth number 16 is in the upper left corner. Tooth number 17 is in the lower left corner of the diagram, and tooth number 32 is in the lower right corner.

Table 4-1. UNIVERSAL NUMBERING SYSTEM FOR PERMANENT TEETH

	Maxillary Right Quadrant								Maxillary Left Quadrant							
1	2	3	4	5	6	7	8	9	10	11	12	13	14	15	16
Third Molar	Second Molar	First Molar	Second Premolar	First Premolar	Cuspid	Lateral	Central	Central	Lateral	Cuspid	First Premolar	Second Premolar	First Molar	Second Molar	Third Molar
Third Molar	Second Molar	First Molar	Second Premolar	First Premolar	Cuspid	Lateral	Central	Central	Lateral	Cuspid	First Premolar	Second Premolar	First Molar	Second Molar	Third Molar
32	31	30	29	28	27	26	25	24	23	22	21	20	19	18	17
	Mandibular Right Quadrant								Mandibular Left Quadrant							

(Torres HO, Ehrlich A: Modern Dental Assisting, 4th Ed. Philadelphia, WB Saunders, 1990, p 94.)

**Table 4–2. UNIVERSAL NUMBERING SYSTEM
FOR PRIMARY TEETH**

Maxillary Right Quadrant					Maxillary Left Quadrant				
A	B	C	D	E	F	G	H	I	J

Incisors

| Second Primary Molar | First Primary Molar | Cuspid | Lateral | Central | Central | Lateral | Cuspid | First Primary Molar | Second Primary Molar |

| T | S | R | Q | P | O | N | M | L | K |

Incisors

| Second Primary Molar | First Primary Molar | Cuspid | Lateral | Central | Central | Lateral | Cuspid | First Primary Molar | Second Primary Molar |

Mandibular Right Quadrant   **Mandibular Left Quadrant**

(Torres HO, Ehrlich A: Modern Dental Assisting, 4th Ed. Philadelphia, WB Saunders, 1990, p 95.)

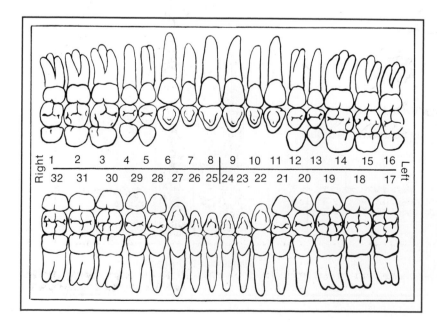

| Right | 1 | 2 | 3 | 4 | 5 | 6 | 7 | 8 | 9 | 10 | 11 | 12 | 13 | 14 | 15 | 16 | Left |
| | 32 | 31 | 30 | 29 | 28 | 27 | 26 | 25 | 24 | 23 | 22 | 21 | 20 | 19 | 18 | 17 | |

▼ Figure 4–29

The permanent teeth as they are represented on the diagrammatic portion of a dental chart. (Courtesy of Colwell Systems, Inc, Champaign, IL.) (Torres HO, Ehrlich A: Modern Dental Assisting, 4th Ed. Philadelphia, WB Saunders, 1990, p 78.)

Cingulum—a bulge or prominence of enamel found on the cervical third of the lingual surface of an anterior tooth.

Cingulum

Cusp—(a) a pronounced elevation on the occlusal surface of a tooth terminating in a conical or rounded surface; (b) any crown elevation which begins calcification as an independent center. A cusp is considered to have an apex and four ridges.

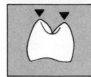
Cusp

Cusp of Carabelli—the "fifth" cusp located on the lingual surface of many maxillary first molars.

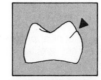
Cusp of Carabelli

Fissure—a fault occurring along a developmental groove caused by incomplete or imperfect joining of the lobes. When two fissures cross they form a *pit.*

Fissure

Fossa—a rounded or angular depression of varying size on the surface of a tooth.

Lingual Fossa—a broad, shallow depression on the lingual surface of an incisor or cuspid.

Lingual fossa

Central Fossa, maxillary molars—a relatively broad, deep angular valley in the central portion of the occlusal surface of a maxillary molar.

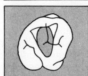
Central fossa– Maxillary molars

Central Fossa, mandibular molars—a relatively broad, deep angular valley in the central portion of the occlusal surface of a mandibular molar.

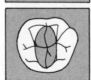
Central fossa– Mandibular molars

Triangular Fossa—a comparatively shallow pyramid-shaped depression on the occlusal surfaces of the posterior teeth, located just within the confines of the mesial and/or distal marginal ridges.

Triangular fossa

Groove—a small linear depression on the surface of a tooth.

Developmental Groove—a groove formed by the union of two lobes during development of the crown.

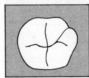
Developmental groove

Supplemental Groove—an indistinct linear depression, irregular in extent and direction, which does not demarcate major divisional portions of a tooth. These often give the occlusal surface a wrinkled appearance.

Supplemental groove

▼ **Figure 4–30**

Illustrated glossary of terms describing anatomic landmarks on individual teeth. (Torres HO, Ehrlich A: Modern Dental Assisting, 4th Ed. Philadelphia, WB Saunders, 1990, pp 118–119.)
Illustration continued on following page

Incisal Edge—formed by the junction of the linguoincisal surfaces of an anterior tooth. This edge does not exist until occlusal wear has created a surface linguoincisally. This surface forms an angle with the labial surface.

Incisal edge

Lobe—a developmental segment of the tooth. As lobes develop they coalesce to form a single unit.

Lobe

Mamelon—a rounded or conical prominence on the incisal ridge of a newly erupted incisor. They are usually three in number, and soon disappear as the result of wear.

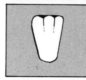

Mamelon

Ridge—a linear elevation on the surface of a tooth. It is named according to its location or form.

Cusp Ridge—an elevation which extends in a mesial and distal direction from the cusp tip. Cusp ridges form the buccal and lingual margins of the occlusal surfaces of the posterior teeth.

Cusp ridge

Incisal Ridge—the incisal portion of a newly erupted anterior tooth.

Incisal ridge

Marginal Ridges—elevated crests or rounded folds of enamel which form the mesial and distal margins of the occlusal surfaces of the posterior teeth and the lingual surfaces of the anterior teeth. Marginal ridges on the anterior teeth are less prominent and are linear extensions from the cingulum, forming the lateral borders of the lingual surface.

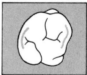

Marginal ridge

Oblique Ridges—elevated prominences on the occlusal surfaces of a maxillary molar extending obliquely from the tips of the mesiolingual cusp to the distobuccal cusp.

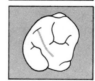

Oblique ridge

Triangular Ridges—prominent elevations, triangular in cross section, which extend from the tip of a cusp toward the central portion of the occlusal surface of a tooth. They are named for the cusp to which they belong. Also described as those ridges which descend from the tip of the cusps and widen toward the central area of the occlusal surface.

Triangular ridge

Transverse Ridges—made up of the triangular ridges of a buccal and lingual cusp which join to form a more or less continuous elevation extending transversely across the occlusal surface of a posterior tooth.

Transverse ridge

Sulcus—an elongated valley in the surface of a tooth formed by the inclines of adjacent cusps or ridges which meet at an angle.

Sulcus

▼ **Figure 4–30** *Continued*

▼ **EXERCISES**

1. The main portion of the tooth structure consists of _____.

   a. cementum
   b. dentin
   c. enamel
   d. pulp

2. The premolars are considered to be _____ teeth.

   a. anterior
   b. posterior

3. The primary dentition contains _____ teeth.

   a. 16
   b. 20
   c. 24
   d. 32

4. Enamel is composed of _____.

   a. prisms
   b. rods
   c. tubules
   d. a or b

5. The _____ arch is fixed and does not move.

   a. mandibular
   b. maxillary

6. The _____ holds the tooth suspended in its socket.

   a. alveolar ridge
   b. cementoenamel junction
   c. periodontal ligament
   d. lamina dura

7. In a _____ malocclusion, the body of the mandible is large or positioned mesially to the maxilla.

   a. Class I
   b. Class II, Division 1
   c. Class II, Division 2
   d. Class III

8. The anatomic crown of a tooth is _____.

   a. fully visible in the mouth
   b. covered with enamel
   c. a and b

9. The contact between the maxillary and mandibular teeth in all mandibular positions and movements is called _____.

    a. embrasure
    b. occlusion
    c. overbite
    d. overjet

10. The permanent dentition contains _____ premolars per quadrant.

    a. one
    b. two
    c. zero

11. _____ is the hardest calcified substance in the body.

    a. Bone
    b. Cementum
    c. Dentin
    d. Enamel

12. The _____ are designed for cutting food without the application of heavy forces.

    a. cuspids
    b. incisors
    c. molars
    d. premolars

13. _____ is living tissue and is capable of repair.

    a. Dentin
    b. Enamel

14. The mesial surface of a tooth is a/an _____ surface.

    a. axial
    b. horizontal
    c. proximal
    d. a and c

15. The permanent first molars erupt at approximately age _____ years.

    a. 4–5
    b. 6–7
    c. 7–8
    d. 9–10

16. A _____ is a rounded or conical prominence on the incisal ridge of a newly erupted incisor.

    a. cingulum
    b. fossa
    c. mamelon
    d. sulcus

17. _____ is the vertical overlap of the maxillary teeth over the mandibular teeth.

    a. Overbite
    b. Overjet

18. A/An _____ is the V-shaped space in a gingival direction between the proximal surfaces of two adjoining teeth in contact.

    a. cingulum
    b. contact point
    c. embrasure
    d. proximal point

19. The tapered end of each root tip is known as the _____.

    a. apex
    b. bifurcation
    c. cementoenamel junction
    d. cervix

20. The _____ surface of a posterior tooth faces toward the tongue.

    a. buccal
    b. facial
    c. labial
    d. lingual

21. _____ is the normal process by which teeth move into occlusion.

    a. Eruption
    b. Exfoliation
    c. Resorption
    d. b and c

22. The distal surface of a tooth faces _____.

    a. away from the midline
    b. away from the tongue
    c. toward the cingulum
    d. toward the midline

23. In the _____ numbering system, the primary teeth are lettered using capital letters *A* and *T*.

    a. International
    b. Palmer
    c. Symbolic
    d. Universal

24. The _____ contains blood vessels, connective tissue, and an extensive nerve supply.

    a. cementum
    b. dentin
    c. enamel
    d. pulp

25. The _____ is/are located in the root of the tooth.

    a. coronal pulp
    b. radicular pulp
    c. pulp horns
    d. b and c

▼ **Criterion Sheet 4-1**

Student's Name _____

Procedure: *IDENTIFY THE TYPES OF TEETH*

Performance Objective:

Given a typodont containing the permanent dentition, the student will identify the types of teeth and state whether each is an anterior or posterior tooth.

		SE	IE
SE = Student evaluation **C** = Criterion met			
IE = Instructor evaluation **X** = Criterion not met			
Instrumentation: Typodont of the permanent dentition			
1. Identified the central and lateral incisors.			
2. Identified the cuspids.			
3. Identified the premolars.			
4. Identified the molars.			
5. Identified the anterior and posterior teeth.			
Comments:			

5 Preventive Dentistry and Nutrition

▼ LEARNING OBJECTIVES

The student will be able to:

1. State the primary goal of preventive dentistry.

2. Describe the use of fluorides in water, fluoride supplements, topical applications, dentifrices, and mouth rinses.

3. Describe dental plaque and state its role in causing dental disease.

4. Describe instructing a patient in the use of disclosing tablets, the Bass technique of toothbrushing, and the use of dental floss.

5. Identify each of the following: interdental cleanser, Perio-Aid, Stimu-u-Dent, oral irrigation devices, and therapeutic oral rinses.

6. Discuss the role of nutrition in preventive dentistry, including giving examples of cariogenic and noncariogenic foods.

7. Discuss the dietary limitations for orthodontic patients, patients with injured anterior teeth, and patients with new dentures.

8. Demonstrate personal oral hygiene.

9. Demonstrate dietary planning for a patient on a soft diet.

OVERVIEW OF PREVENTIVE DENTISTRY

The primary goal of preventive dentistry is to stop the destruction of teeth due to dental caries and the loss of their support through periodontal disease.

However, it is impossible to convince a patient of the value of preventive dentistry if the members of the office team obviously do not believe in and practice it. Therefore, it is essential that each person in the office follow a good dental health program that includes:

▼ Having all required dental work completed.

▼ Carefully following a program of personal oral hygiene.

▼ Routinely practicing good nutrition and recommended general health care procedures.

FLUORIDES

Fluoridated Water

Approximately 1 part per million (ppm) of fluoride in drinking water has been proved a safe and effective means of lowering the incidence of dental caries.

Maximum benefit from such a program may be expected when teeth receive fluoride during the period of formation and eruption. However, the continued use of fluoridated water throughout life is also recommended.

Prescribed Fluoride Supplements

The daily administration of individual dietary supplements of sodium fluoride or acidulated phosphate fluoride may be desirable for young children living where community fluoride programs are not available.

In order to provide maximum benefit to both primary and permanent teeth, the child should receive fluoride supplements on a daily basis from infancy until approximately 13 years of age.

Prescribing dietary supplements of fluoride may be the method of choice for the very young child, whereas topical fluoride application or fluoride mouth rinses are preferable for the older child whose permanent teeth have already erupted.

Children under age 14 who are highly susceptible to caries may benefit from receiving both measures.

Safety of Fluorides

The levels of fluoride in controlled water fluoridation are so low that there is no danger of ingesting an acutely toxic quantity of fluoride from fluoridated water.

However, concentrated fluoride preparations, especially those kept in the home, are of concern. The fatal oral dose has been estimated at from 5 to 10 g of sodium fluoride. Lesser amounts may cause accidental poisoning, and even death, in small children.

As a precautionary measure, it is desirable that no large quantities of sodium fluoride be stored in the home. Therefore, it is recommended that no more than 264 mg of sodium fluoride (120 mg fluoride) be dispensed at one time.

This quantity is sufficient for at least a 4-month period. Each package dispensed should also bear a statement: *Caution — Store out of reach of children.*

Dental Fluorosis

Dental fluorosis, which is also known as *mottled enamel,* may occur in communities that have naturally fluoridated water that contains more than twice the optimum level of fluoride.

Dental fluorosis is characterized by chalky white spots on the teeth; however, not all white spots on the enamel are signs of dental fluorosis.

Topical Application of Fluorides

The topical application of **acidulated phosphate-fluoride** gels has also been demonstrated to have a considerable caries-inhibiting effect in children. (For application procedures, see Chapter 26, "Pediatric Dentistry.")

Fluoride-Containing Toothpastes

Studies have shown that toothpastes (dentifrices) containing **sodium monofluorophosphate** are effective in significantly reducing the decayed, missing, filled surfaces (DMFS) rate, and fluoride-containing dentifrices have been accepted by the Council on Dental Therapeutics of the American Dental Association.

Fluoride Mouth Rinses

Studies evaluating the effectiveness of mouth rinses containing dilute solutions of **sodium fluoride** have shown the usefulness of these agents for children living in nonfluoridated areas.

DENTAL PLAQUE CONTROL

Dental plaque is a sticky, soft, tooth-colored deposit that forms on the teeth near the gingiva and in sheltered areas. It consists chiefly of bacteria and bacterial products; however, it also contains components from oral fluids and food debris.

Evidence indicates that bacteria colonized in dental plaque are a primary factor in dental caries and that the toxic agents produced by these bacteria are directly related to the tissue destruction associated with periodontal disease. Research also indicates that caries and periodontal disease rarely occur in the absence of plaque.

Once plaque has been thoroughly removed, it takes about 24 hours for it to form again. Therefore, the primary goal of plaque control in preventive dentistry is the thorough removal of all plaque at least once daily.

Personal Oral Hygiene (POH)

There are many aspects of plaque control and many means and methods of plaque removal. Because all of the activities that are part of plaque removal can be controlled by the individual, and must be his responsibility, they are grouped together under the title *personal oral hygiene* (POH).

There is no one right method of plaque removal, and personal oral hygiene must remain *personal*. Of the many techniques available, the ones selected must be those that are right for the individual patient.

Disclosing Agents

The thorough removal of dental plaque by home care procedures can be taught more easily if the plaque can actually be visualized (Fig. 5–1).

A number of agents and techniques have been developed for this purpose. A **red disclosing agent** is probably the one most frequently employed in the home. It has the esthetic advantages of being similar in color to the oral soft tissues and of not staining hard tissue significantly.

This disclosing agent is available both as a solution to be painted on the teeth and as artificially sweetened, candy-like wafers. All ingredients are nontoxic and harmless if swallowed.

The patient should be warned that these disclosing agents color the tongue and gingiva as well as the plaque. However, this stain is soon rinsed away by the saliva.

Directions for Use of Disclosing Tablets

1. Crush one tablet between the teeth. This activates the salivary glands and provides enough liquid to swish around in the mouth for at least 30 seconds.
2. Spit the excess liquid into a bowl of running water.
3. Rinse the mouth once or twice with plain water.

The red-colored areas remaining on the teeth indicate plaque, which must be removed. Any pale, film-like area on the teeth is the acquired pellicle.

When the patient is learning proper oral hygiene, disclosing tablets are used daily during the first week or longer. Then they are used on a once-a-week basis and, finally, only as needed to check the effectiveness of the hygiene program.

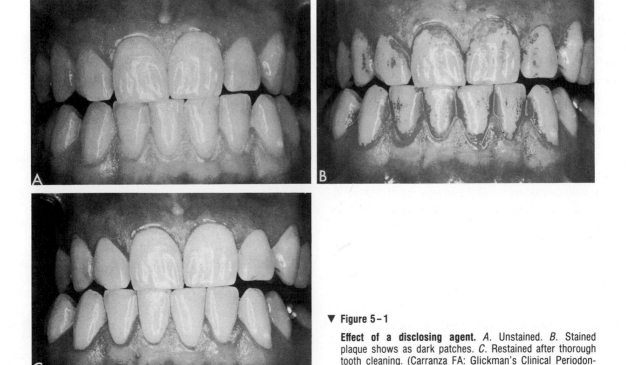

▼ **Figure 5–1**

Effect of a disclosing agent. *A.* Unstained. *B.* Stained plaque shows as dark patches. *C.* Restained after thorough tooth cleaning. (Carranza FA: Glickman's Clinical Periodontology, 7th Ed. Philadelphia, WB Saunders, 1990, p 707.)

Toothbrushes

The primary functional properties of a toothbrush are flexibility, softness, and diameter of the bristles as well as strength, rigidity, and lightness of the handle.

The type of toothbrush recommended depends largely on the method of toothbrushing that is employed, the position of the teeth, and the manipulative skills of the individual. A toothbrush should:

1. Conform to individual requirements in size, shape, and texture.
2. Be easily and efficiently manipulated with safety.
3. Be readily cleaned and aerated.
4. Be impervious to moisture.
5. Be durable.
6. Be inexpensive and therefore easily replaced when worn.

A **powered toothbrush** may be useful for the partially handicapped individuals who cannot readily clean their teeth with a manual brush.

Powered toothbrushes are also helpful for the totally handicapped individuals, who must have their teeth brushed by an attendant, and for young children when adults do the brushing and flossing.

Toothpastes

Toothpastes, which are also known as *dentifrices*, are aids for cleaning and polishing tooth surfaces. Those containing fluorides provide added protection to the tooth. If a dentifrice is to be an effective adjunct to oral hygiene, it must come in intimate contact with the teeth.

This is best achieved by placing the paste *between* the bristles of the toothbrush rather than on top of the bristles, from which large portions of the dentifrice are often displaced before reaching the tooth surfaces.

TOOTHBRUSHING TECHNIQUE

There are many methods of toothbrushing, and each has merits in special situations. However, the Bass method, which is described here, is the one most commonly taught in dental offices.

This method is also known as the *sulcus cleansing method*. (The **sulcus** is the space between the free gingiva and the tooth.)

The Bass Method

Procedure

BRUSHING MAXILLARY TEETH: FACIAL AND FACIOPROXIMAL SURFACES

1. Place the head of a soft-to-medium brush <u>parallel</u> with the occlusal plane with the "tip" of the brush distal to the last molar.

2. Place the bristles at the gingival margin and establish an apical angle of 45 degrees to the long axis of the teeth.

3. Exert gentle vibratory pressure on the long axis of the bristles, and force the bristle ends into the facial gingival sulci as well as into the interproximal embrasures (Fig. 5-2).
   Note: This should produce perceptible blanching of the gingiva. (**Blanching** means to become paler in color.)

4. Activate the brush with a short back-and-forth motion without dislodging the tips of the bristles. Complete 20 such strokes in the same position.
   Note: This cleans the teeth facially within the apical third of their clinical crowns as well as within their adjacent gingival sulci and along their proximal surfaces as far as the bristles reach.

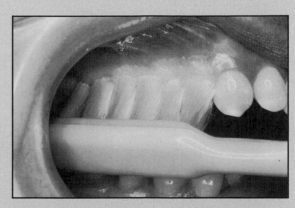

Figure 5-2 Bass method. Correct application of brush should produce perceptible blanching of the gingiva. (Carranza FA: Glickman's Clinical Periodontology, 7th Ed. Philadelphia, WB Saunders, 1990, p 689.)

5   Lift the brush, move it anteriorly, position it so that its "heel" is still distal to the canine eminence, and repeat the process described in steps 1 through 4. (This cleans the premolars and distal half of the cuspid.)

6   Lift the brush and move it so that its tip is mesial to the canine prominence, and repeat the process just described. (This cleans the mesial half of the cuspid and the incisors.)

7   Continue on the opposite side of the arch, section by section, covering three teeth at a time, until the facial and facioproximal surfaces of the entire maxillary dentition are brushed (Fig. 5–3).

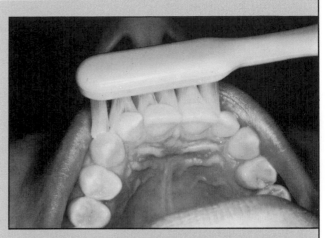

Figure 5–3 Bass method. Clinical aspect of brush position on maxillary incisors. (Carranza FA: Glickman's Clinical Periodontology, 7th Ed. Philadelphia, WB Saunders, 1990, p 461.)

Procedure

BRUSHING MAXILLARY TEETH: PALATAL AND PALATOPROXIMAL SURFACES

1   Engage the brush at a 45-degree apical angle in the molar and premolar areas, covering three teeth at a time. Clean each segment with 20 short back-and-forth strokes (Fig. 5–4).

2   To reach the palatal surface of the anterior teeth, insert the brush vertically.

    Press the "heel" of the brush into the gingival sulci and interproximally at a 45-degree angle to the long axis of the teeth, using the anterior portion of the hard palate as a guide plane. Activate the brush with 20 short up-and-down strokes.

3   If the shape of the arch permits, the brush may be inserted horizontally between the cuspids with the bristles angulated into the gingival sulci of the anterior teeth.

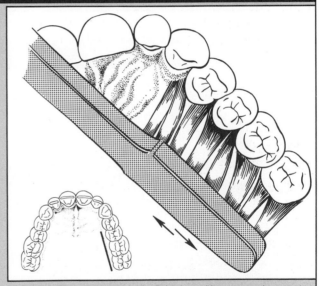

Figure 5–4 Bass method. Palatal position on molars and premolars. (Carranza FA: Glickman's Clinical Periodontology, 7th Ed. Philadelphia, WB Saunders, 1990, p 694.)

Procedure

BRUSHING MANDIBULAR TEETH: FACIAL, FACIOPROXIMAL, LINGUAL, AND LINGUOPROXIMAL SURFACES

1   The mandibular teeth are cleaned in the same way as the maxillary teeth, section by section, 20 strokes in each position.

2   In the anterior lingual region, insert the brush vertically using the lingual surface of the mandible as a guide plane, and with the bristles angulated into the gingival sulci.

3   If space permits, insert the brush horizontally between the cuspids.

Procedure

BRUSHING OCCLUSAL SURFACES

1. Press the bristles firmly on the occlusal surfaces with the ends as deeply as possible into the pits and fissures.

2. Activate the brush with 20 short back-and-forth strokes, advancing section by section until all posterior teeth in all four quadrants are cleaned.

FLOSSING

Dental floss is an effective way to remove plaque from proximal surfaces between the teeth. There are several ways to use dental floss effectively.

The following are guidelines that may be modified according to the patient's preference.

INTERDENTAL CLEANSERS

Special cleaning devices are recommended for proximal cleaning of teeth with large or open interdental spaces, such as those found in periodontally treated dentition. These devices should be easy to handle and should adapt more precisely than dental floss to irregular tooth surfaces.

Interproximal brushes are available in a variety of shapes. For best cleaning efficiency, the diameter of the brush should be slightly larger than the gingival embrasure so that the bristles exert pressure on the tooth surfaces.

These small brushes are inserted interproximally and activated with short back-and-forth strokes in a linguofacial direction.

A **Stim-U-Dent** consists of a soft wooden tip that is triangular in cross section. It is held between the middle finger, index finger, and thumb (Fig. 5–6).

The Stim-U-Dent is then gently introduced in the interdental spaces in such a way that the base

Procedure

FLOSSING TEETH

1. Cut a piece of floss at least 18 inches long. Wrap the excess floss around the middle or index fingers of both hands, leaving a 2- to 3-inch working space exposed.

2. Stretch the floss tightly between the fingers and use the thumb and index finger to guide the floss into place.

3. Gently pass the floss through the contact area with a firm, sideways sawing motion. Do not forcibly snap the floss gingivally past the contact area because this will injure the interdental gingiva.

4. Wrap the floss around the proximal surface of one tooth, at the base of the gingival sulcus. Move the floss firmly along the tooth up to the contact area and gently down into the sulcus again. Repeat this up-and-down stroke five or six times (Fig. 5–5).

5. Carefully move the floss across the interdental gingiva, and repeat the procedure on the proximal surface of the adjacent tooth. Take care not to injure the delicate gingival tissues.

6. When the working portion of the floss becomes soiled or begins to shred, move a fresh area into the working position.

7. Continue throughout the entire dentition, including the distal surface of the last tooth in each quadrant.

8. A "bridge threader" may be used to floss under a fixed bridge.

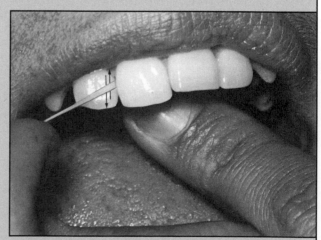

Figure 5–5 Dental flossing. The floss is wrapped around each proximal surface and is activated with repeated up-and-down strokes. (Carranza FA: Glickman's Clinical Periodontology, 7th Ed. Philadelphia, WB Saunders, 1990, p 701.)

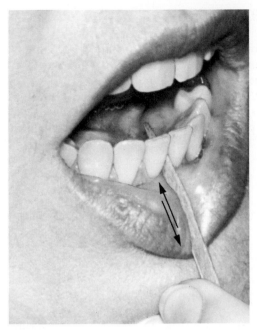

▼ **Figure 5-6**

Wooden tip (Stim-U-Dent). Interproximal cleaning and massage with the moistened wooden tip. (Carranza FA: Glickman's Clinical Periodontology, 7th Ed. Philadelphia, WB Saunders, 1990, p 702.)

surface of the triangle rests on the interproximal gingiva.

The sides of the triangle are in contact with the proximal tooth surfaces. The tip is then repeatedly forced gently in and out of the embrasure.

The **Perio-Aid** consists of a toothpick with a round, tapered end that is inserted in a handle for convenient application. This device is particularly efficient for cleaning along the gingival margin and within gingival sulci or periodontal pockets. Deposits are removed by using either the side or the end of the tip.

Oral Irrigation Devices

Oral irrigators work by directing a high-pressure steady or pulsating stream of water through a nozzle to the tooth surfaces. Oral irrigators clean nonadherent bacteria and debris from the oral cavity more effectively than toothbrushes and mouth rinses. However, water irrigation removes only a negligible amount of stainable plaque from tooth surfaces.

Therapeutic Oral Rinses

The dentist may prescribe an oral rinse containing **chlorhexidine gluconate 0.12 percent** for cer-

tain patients to help control supragingival plaque and reduce gingivitis.

The rinse is generally used twice daily after brushing, and its active ingredient reduces the concentration of some bacteria in the saliva.

This rinse may affect the taste of certain foods, and for this reason it is recommended that the rinse be used after meals. The rinse may also stain the teeth and oral surfaces. Patients using these rinses should be seen regularly for a professional prophylaxis.

THE ROLE OF NUTRITION IN PREVENTIVE DENTISTRY

Foods containing nutrients such as soluble sugars and other refined carbohydrates are readily used by the plaque bacteria. This is one reason why nutrition plays such an important role in preventive dentistry.

Cariogenic Foods

Certain bacteria in dental plaque use the nutrients in sugary foods to produce acids each time these foods are ingested.

This acid attacks the tooth enamel for about 20 minutes, and each occurrence is known as an **acid attack.** Frequent acid attacks may eventually cause the enamel to break down and decay.

Foods that contain the nutrients used by these bacteria in the plaque are said to be **cariogenic.** Foods that are most likely to cause decay are considered to be **highly cariogenic.** Those that do not promote tooth decay are described as being **noncariogenic.**

Guidelines for Cariogenic Foods

1. Only carbohydrate-containing foods are cariogenic. However, many foods, such as catsup, contain carbohydrates in the form of hidden sugars.
2. Simple carbohydrates (which are sugary refined products such as cookies and candy) are more cariogenic than complex carbohydrates (which are found in fresh foods such as fruits and grains).
3. Sticky sweets are more cariogenic than liquid sweets. This is because liquids pass through the mouth more quickly than sticky foods.
4. Cariogenic foods are less damaging when their consumption is limited to mealtime.
5. The frequency and duration of eating sugary

substances may be more important than the quantity eaten.

Snacks and Snack Foods

Snacking on cariogenic food is damaging to dental health. Also, these cariogenic foods contain only empty calories that do not provide essential nutrients. These foods may add excessive calories in the diet without providing the nutrients needed for good health.

Most noncariogenic foods do not create dental problems and are able to contribute essential nutrients to the diet. Table 5–1 shows the sugar content of popular foods that are best avoided as snacks.

The following are suggestions of foods that make nutritionally sound snacks.

▼ **Recommended Snack Foods**

Milk Group. Milk, plain yogurt, and cheese.

Meat Group. Nuts, eggs, lunch meats, and fish.

Vegetable and Fruit Group. Fresh fruits and vegetables, unsweetened fruit and vegetable juices.

Bread and Cereal Group. Popcorn, pretzels, corn chips, potato chips, and sugar-free cereals.

Nonessential Group. Sugar-free gum, sugarless soft drinks, and sugarless gelatin desserts.

Table 5–1. SUGAR CONTENT OF POPULAR FOODS

Food	Approximate Measure	Tsp. of Sugar
Cola	6 oz.	5
Chocolate milkshake	8 oz.	14
Chocolate ice cream soda	Average size	11
Cinnamon bun with raisins	1 average	8
Jelly doughnut	1 average	7
Iced cupcake	1 medium	9
Peach ice cream	1 cup	15
Orange water ice	1/2 cup	19
Apple pie	1/6 of medium pie	14
Chocolate pudding	1/2 cup	9
Raisins	5/8 cup	17
Candy bar	Average	8
Fudge, plain	1″ square	5
Jelly beans	10	4
Lollipop	1 medium	8

(Torres HO, Ehrlich A: Modern Dental Assisting, 4th Ed. Philadelphia, WB Saunders, 1990, p 250.)

SPECIAL DIETS FOR DENTAL PATIENTS

There are times, such as after an extraction or dental injury, when dental patients may temporarily require a modified diet.

It is important that any diet be designed to meet the needs of the body during healing. Also, the patient should be encouraged to return to a well-balanced "normal" diet as soon as possible.

Soft Diet

For most patients, a "soft diet" is a modification of a normal diet that eliminates foods that are difficult to chew.

Unless the dentist prescribes a specific diet for the patient, the following foods from each of the food groups may be suggested:

Milk Group. Milk in all forms, including soft cheeses such as cottage cheese, are recommended. Also good are ice cream, pudding, custards, milk shakes, and yogurt.

Meat Group. In a soft diet, eggs can be eaten in omelet form, poached, soft-boiled, or scrambled. Fried eggs are not usually recommended.

Fish, poultry, or well-cooked meats that are not tough or fibrous can be included; however, meats should be ground or cooked until extremely tender and then cut into very small pieces.

Vegetable and Fruit Group. Foods from this group are particularly important in ensuring that the daily diet contains adequate amounts of vitamin C. Raw vegetables should be omitted from the soft diet. However, well-cooked vegetables, such as asparagus tips, may be included.

Potatoes or potato substitutes (such as mashed, white, or sweet potatoes; macaroni, noodles, or rice) are acceptable. Fried potatoes, roasted potatoes, potato chips, and potato salad should be avoided. Broths, creamed soups, and vegetable soup made with thoroughly cooked and finely diced vegetables and meat are excellent in a soft diet.

Raw fruits, except ripe bananas or very soft mashed fruit with the skin and seeds removed, should be avoided. Canned or cooked fruits, free of tough membranes and seeds, can be used. Fruit juices, tomato juice, gelatin desserts, and sherbet are all good in a soft diet.

Bread and Cereal Group. Hard rolls, sandwiches, waffles, hot breads, and whole grain cereals should be avoided. Cooked and cold cereals, crackers, and enriched bread (without the crust) softened in milk are acceptable in the soft diet.

Postextraction Diet

The special problems faced by patients after dental surgery are the possibility of reduced appetite, a desire to protect the wound site, and a limited capacity for chewing. Depending on the extent of the surgery, the patient may require a liquid or soft diet for the first few days.

The patient should be encouraged to select foods that fully meet his nutritional needs. He should be warned to avoid spicy foods, alcoholic beverages, and hot liquids that may be irritating.

Injured Anterior Teeth

Following injury or treatment of the anterior teeth, the dentist may temporarily restrict the patient's diet so that these teeth are not further damaged. This would mean that the patient is not to eat anything that requires a biting or tearing action by the affected teeth.

The key word for such a diet would be *bite-size,* in that all foods should be cut into small, bite-size pieces before they are eaten. In this diet, sandwiches, hard rolls, toast, tough meats, and raw fruits and vegetables should be eliminated.

The Orthodontic Patient

Very hard foods should be eliminated from the diet of the orthodontic patient because these foods may bend or break brackets or appliances.

Because the bands and appliances make oral hygiene difficult, the orthodontic patient should also take special care to eliminate sticky and cariogenic foods.

Unless given other specific instructions, the orthodontic patient should avoid the following foods: chewing gum, nuts, all sticky candy, cookies, popcorn, pretzels, hard-crusted bread or rolls, and raw carrots and celery.

Apples may be eaten if they are sliced and peeled. There should be no chewing of ice or of chicken or meat bones.

The Patient with Wired Jaws

A patients with a fractured jaw that necessitates wiring the jaws together must obtain all nutrients through a liquid diet.

Because this diet is so limited and because the jaws are usually wired for many weeks, it is advisable to have the patient's diet planned and managed under the supervision of a professional dietician.

The Periodontal Surgery Patient

Following periodontal surgery, the mouth is sore and a periodontal dressing is kept in place. Because of these factors, it is recommended that the patient follow a soft diet and that spicy foods be avoided for several days until healing begins.

The patient must also be careful not to eat foods, such as popcorn, that might fracture or become lodged under the periodontal dressing (Fig. 5–7).

The Patient with New Dentures

The change from natural to artificial teeth may require a period of adjustment as the patient learns how to bite and chew with his new denture.

Thus, the patient may want a liquid or semi-soft diet during the first few days. Then, as the patient tries solid foods, he should cut these into small pieces before eating. The denture wearer will soon learn to eat almost all foods with his new denture and will be able to return to a normal diet.

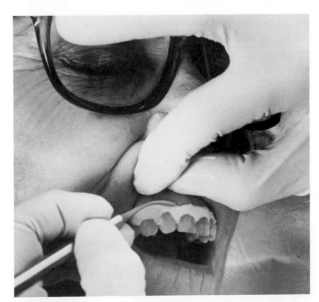

▼ **Figure 5–7**

Following periodontal surgery, the patient must be careful not to eat foods that might become lodged under the periodontal dressing (Torres HO, Ehrlich A: Modern Dental Assisting, 4th Ed. Philadelphia, WB Saunders. 1990, p 816.)

▶ EXERCISES

1. Dental _____ is the sticky, soft, tooth-colored deposit that forms on the teeth.

   a. calculus
   b. caries
   c. cariogenic debris
   d. plaque

2. Toothpaste should be placed _____ the bristles of the toothbrush.

   a. between
   b. on top of

3. With the Bass toothbrushing method, the occlusal surfaces are cleaned with a _____ motion.

   a. rotary
   b. back-and-forth
   c. sweeping
   d. vibrating

4. Foods that are likely to cause decay are considered to be _____ _____ .

   a. cariogenic
   b. noncariogenic

5. A/An _____ works by directing a stream of water through a nozzle to the tooth surfaces.

   a. bridge threader
   b. oral irrigation device
   c. powered toothbrush

6. Dental fluorosis may occur in communities where _____ .

   a. the naturally occurring fluoride level contains more than twice the optimum level of fluoride.
   b. optimal levels of fluoride have been added to the drinking water.

7. A powered toothbrush is recommended for _____ .

   a. people who don't like to brush
   b. the handicapped
   c. young children when adults do the brushing
   d. b and c

8. In the Bass toothbrushing method, the brush is moved with _____ _____ .

   a. a back-and-forth scrubbing motion
   b. a circular motion
   c. an up-and-down scrubbing motion
   d. gentle vibratory pressure

9. A patient with injured anterior teeth should _____.

   a. avoid eating anything that requires a biting or tearing action
   b. follow a soft diet
   c. stay on a liquid diet

10. Therapeutic oral rinses may _____.

    a. affect the taste of certain foods
    b. cause mottled enamel
    c. stain the teeth
    d. a and b

11. Once plaque has been thoroughly removed, it takes about _____ hours for it to form again.

    a. 6
    b. 12
    c. 24
    d. 36

12. Dental floss is moved past the contact point with a _____ motion.

    a. sideways sawing
    b. snapping

13. An oral rinse containing _____ is prescribed to help control supragingival plaque and reduce gingivitis.

    a. chlorhexidine gluconate 0.12 percent
    b. chlorhexidine gluconate 2.0 percent
    c. sodium fluoride
    d. sodium monofluorophosphate

14. As a precautionary measure, it is recommended that no more than _____ mg of sodium fluoride supplements be dispensed at one time.

    a. 100
    b. 223
    c. 264
    d. 296

15. When the patient is learning proper oral hygiene, disclosing tablets should be used _____ during the first week or longer.

    a. twice daily
    b. once daily
    c. on alternate days
    d. once a week

16. Simple carbohydrates, including sugary refined products, are _____ complex carbohydrates.

    a. less cariogenic than
    b. just as cariogenic as
    c. more cariogenic than

17. The recommended concentration of fluoride in drinking water is approximately _____ part(s) per million (ppm).

    a. 1
    b. 10
    c. 15
    d. 100

18. A 6-ounce cola drink contains _____ sugar than an 8-ounce chocolate milkshake.

    a. less
    b. more

19. When using a disclosing agent, the patient should be instructed to _____ _____ .

    a. rub the excess on his lips to disclose any lesions
    b. spit the excess into a bowl of running water
    c. swallow the excess

20. A patient on a soft diet should avoid _____ .

    a. asparagus tips
    b. fruit juice
    c. poached eggs
    d. potato chips

21. A/An _____ consists of a soft wooden tip that is triangular in cross section.

    a. interproximal brush
    b. Perio-Aid
    c. Prophy-Jet
    d. Stimu-U-Dent

22. A patient with his jaws wired together requires a _____ .

    a. diet supervised by a professional dietician
    b. liquid diet
    c. soft diet
    d. a and b

23. A/An _____ consists of a toothpick with a round tapered end that is inserted in a handle for convenient application.

    a. bridge threader
    b. interproximal brush
    c. Perio-Aid

24. Prescribed fluoride supplements may be recommended on a daily basis from birth to approximately _____ years of age.

    a. 5
    b. 8
    c. 13
    d. 18

25. The orthodontic patient should avoid _____.

    a. chewing gum
    b. raw carrots
    c. sticky candy
    d. a, b, and c

▼ **Criterion Sheet 5–1**

Student's Name _____

Procedure: *PERSONAL ORAL HYGIENE*

Performance Objective:

The student will demonstrate competence in maintaining her own oral hygiene.

SE = Student evaluation **IE** = Instructor evaluation	**C** = Criterion met **X** = Criterion not met	**SE**	**IE**
Instrumentation: Disclosing agent, toothbrush, dentifrice, and dental floss			
1. Disclosed plaque with disclosing agent.			
2. Brushed teeth without injury to the gingiva.			
3. Flossed to remove remaining plaque without injury to the gingiva.			
4. Disclosed again to show that all plaque had been removed.			
Comments:			

▼ Criterion Sheet 5-2

Student's Name _____

Procedure: *DIETARY PLANNING FOR A PATIENT ON A SOFT DIET*

Performance Objective:

The student will prepare a written plan for a well-balanced soft diet for 2 days using herself as the patient.

		SE	IE
SE = Student evaluation **IE** = Instructor evaluation	**C** = Criterion met **X** = Criterion not met		
Instrumentation: Plain paper, pen or pencil.			
1. The plan contained only foods acceptable as part of a soft diet.			
2. The plan for each day included food from all four food groups.			
3. The plan did not include excessive empty calories or food high in refined sugar content.			
4. The plan was practical to follow and included varied foods that were appealing to the patient.			
Comments:			

6 Disease Transmission and Pathology

▼ LEARNING OBJECTIVES

The student will be able to:

1. List three types of microorganisms that are of concern in the dental office.

2. State at least two ways in which bacteria are identified, define spores, and name two types of bacteria most commonly found in the mouth.

3. List and describe the three factors that influence the disease-producing capabilities of a pathogen.

4. Describe six forms of disease transmission.

5. State why and how herpes, hepatitis, tetanus, acquired immunodeficiency syndrome (AIDS), and tuberculosis are of concern to dental personnel.

6. Describe the warning signs of periodontal disease.

7. List and describe the five types of periodontitis.

8. Define or describe aphthous stomatitis, acute necrotizing ulcerative gingivitis (ANUG), periapical abscess, periodontal abscess, and periodontal pocket.

OVERVIEW OF DISEASE TRANSMISSION AND PATHOLOGY

The dental assistant must understand the basic causes of diseases and how these diseases are transmitted before she can take the steps necessary to prevent disease transmission. (**Pathology** is the study of disease.)

MICROBIOLOGY

A microorganism is a living organism so small that it can only be seen with a microscope. **Microbiology** is the study of these microorganisms.

Most microorganisms do *not* produce human illness. In fact, they are helpful in many ways. For example, bacteria in the intestinal tract aid in the digestion of food. Yeast ferments wine and makes bread rise.

However, some microorganisms are pathogens. (A **pathogen** is a microorganism that is capable of causing disease.) The pathogens that are of major concern in the dental office are discussed here.

Bacteria

Bacteria are one-celled microorganisms (singular, *bacterium*). Some bacteria are very beneficial; others are pathogens. Bacteria are described or identified in several different ways.

Gram-Positive and Gram-Negative Bacteria

Gram stain is a dye that is used in the study of bacteria. Those bacteria that are stained by the dye are called **gram-positive,** and they appear dark purple under the microscope.

Those bacteria that do not hold the stain are called **gram-negative.** They are almost colorless and nearly invisible under the microscope.

Shapes of Bacteria

Cocci (singular, *coccus*) are spherical or bead-shaped bacteria (Fig. 6–1).

▼ Singly the cocci are known as **monococci.**

▼ The pair-forming cocci are **diplococci.**

▼ The chain-forming cocci are **streptococci.**

▼ Those cocci that form irregular groups or clusters are called **staphylococci.**

▼ Those forming a cuboidal packet of cocci are known as **sarcina;** however, this form is of little medical significance.

Bacilli (singular, *bacillus*) are rod-shaped bacteria. The rod-shaped tubercle bacillus, which causes human tuberculosis, is able to withstand disinfectants that kill many other bacteria.

Spirochetes are bacteria that have flexible cell walls, are capable of movement, and have a wave-like or spiral shape.

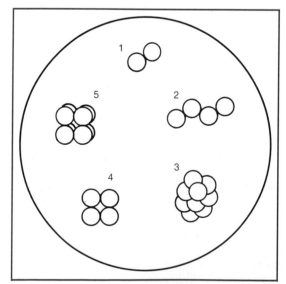

▼ **Figure 6–1**

Diagrammatic representation of the shapes of bacteria. 1, Diplococci; 2, streptococci; 3, staphylococci; 4, gaffkya; 5, sarcina. (Torres HO, Ehrlich A: Modern Dental Assisting, 4th Ed. Philadelphia, WB Saunders, 1990, p 121.)

Lyme disease is caused by a spirochete and is transmitted to humans through the bite of an infected deer tick.

Spores

Some types of bacteria form a protective mucoid coating, called a **capsule** or *slime layer.* This helps the bacteria evade the defense mechanisms of the body. Bacteria with this protection are generally more virulent.

Under unfavorable conditions some bacteria form **endospores,** which are commonly known as *spores.* While in the spore form, the bacteria cannot reproduce or cause disease. However, when conditions are again favorable, the bacteria once more become active and virulent.

Spores represent the most resistant form of life known. Bacteria in the spore stage can survive extremes of heat and dryness and even the presence of disinfectants and radiation.

Aerobes and Anaerobes

Aerobes are a variety of bacteria that must have oxygen in order to grow.

Anaerobes are bacteria that grow in the absence of oxygen and are actually destroyed by oxygen.

Facultative anaerobes are organisms that can grow in either the presence or the absence of oxygen.

Normal Bacterial Populations of the Mouth

Several forms of *Streptococcus,* bacteria that feed on carbohydrates, are the most prominent species in the mouth.

Streptococcus mutans, found in plaque, causes tooth decay (Fig. 6–2).

Lactobacillus is another bacteria that is commonly found in the mouth. It has some strains that are anaerobic and others that are aerobic.

Viruses

A virus invades a host cell, where it replicates (creates copies of itself). The host cell is destroyed as the viruses are released into the body.

Viruses are extremely resistant to efforts to kill them with heat or chemicals. They are also capable of mutation. (**Mutation** means that viruses are able to change their genetic pattern so that they are better suited to current conditions and to resist efforts to kill them.)

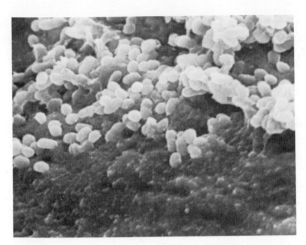

▼ **Figure 6-2**

Streptococcus mutans **in a lesion on an enamel surface** (X 600). (Nester EW, et al: Microbiology, 3rd Ed. Philadelphia, WB Saunders, 1983, p 68.)

Diseases caused by viruses include common colds, influenza, smallpox, measles, chickenpox, herpes, hepatitis, AIDS, rabies, and yellow fever.

Fungi

Fungi are plants, such as mushrooms, yeasts, and molds, that lack chlorophyll (singular, *fungus*).

Candida is a fungus that is part of the normal flora of the skin, mouth, intestinal tract, and vagina. However, it is also capable of causing a variety of infections such as *candidiasis*.

DISEASE-PRODUCING CAPABILITIES

There are three factors that influence the disease-producing capability of a pathogenic organism. These are **host resistance, virulence,** and **concentration.**

Host Resistance

Host resistance is the ability of the body to resist the pathogen. The healthier you are, the better your resistance to disease. Resistance is increased by maintaining good health habits.

When the body is in a lowered state of resistance, it is not strong enough to fight off infection and will succumb to disease more readily.

The state of lowered resistance can result from fatigue, physical or emotional stress, poor nutrition, injury, surgery, impairment of the immune system, or the presence of other diseases.

Immunity

A person who has had a viral disease, such as chickenpox, has acquired immunity. Immunity to some other viral diseases, such as smallpox and hepatitis B, may be acquired through inoculation with an appropriate vaccine.

Immunization is an important part of host resistance. Dental personnel should receive all of the appropriate immunizations and then keep these immunizations up-to-date.

Virulence

Virulence describes the strength or disease-producing capabilities of the pathogen. A virulent pathogen is able to overcome many of the body's defenses—even in a healthy individual.

Concentration

Concentration refers to the number of pathogens that are present. The more pathogens that are present, the better their chances of overwhelming the host and producing disease.

Many of the infection control activities in the dental office are aimed at lowering the risk of infection by reducing the number of pathogens that are present.

DISEASE TRANSMISSION

In a dental practice, there is the danger of disease transmission from:

▼ Patient to the staff.

▼ Staff to the patient.

▼ Patient to patient (through contact with the practice).

As a dental assistant, you have a very important role in preventing disease transmission in the dental office. However, before you can learn how to prevent disease transmission, you must understand how this transmission takes place. (Methods of controlling disease transmission are discussed in Chapter 7, "Infection Control.")

Blood-Borne Pathogens

Blood-borne pathogens are microorganisms that are present in human blood and can cause disease in humans.

These include, but not are not limited to, hepatitis B virus (HBV) and human immunodeficiency virus (HIV), which is the etiologic agent for AIDS.

These diseases are not transmitted by casual contact, such as shaking hands. The intact skin is an excellent protective barrier. It is when this barrier is breached by a cut or scrape that there is danger.

There is risk of transmission of these diseases through a needle-stick injury or a cut caused by a contaminated instrument. There is danger here because your blood may now come into contact with the infected blood.

Droplet Infection

This type of infection is transmitted by the numerous droplets of moisture, containing bacteria or viruses, that are spread as people talk, breathe, sneeze, or cough. When someone sneezes, he sprays contaminated particles out about 8 feet and up about 4 feet.

Of special concern to the dentist and assistant is the mist of bacteria and debris that is produced by the high-speed handpiece with water spray (Fig. 6–3).

Being exposed to this mist is approximately the equivalent of having someone sneeze in your face twice per minute—at a distance of 1 foot.

Indirect Transmission

In the dental office, diseases may be indirectly transmitted by soiled hands and towels, dirty instruments, and even dust.

Also, anything that is touched during patient care is considered **contaminated** and potentially capable of spreading disease through indirect contact. (As used here, *contaminated* means something that may possibly have come into contact with a pathogen.)

This includes instruments, faucet handles, switches, handpieces, drawer handles, medications, dressings, the patient's chart, and even the pen used to make the chart entry.

Self-Infection

In many cases, infective microorganisms are present in the patient's mouth but do not cause infection until they enter the bloodstream. However, an open wound in dental surgery may allow these microorganisms access to the bloodstream, and in this way the patient may actually infect himself.

Operator Infection

Infection from the dentist's or assistant's nose, mouth, or hands may be spread to the patient via droplet infection or by indirect transmission during the operative procedure.

Also, infectious organisms sprayed from the patient's mouth can be transmitted to the dentist or assistant through his or her own nose or mouth or through a break in the skin.

Personal Contact

This mode of transmission, particularly of **sexually transmitted diseases** (STDs), also known as **venereal diseases,** requires direct person-to-person contact.

These diseases include **AIDS, herpes, syphilis,** and **gonorrhea,** and they may produce lesions in the oral cavity.

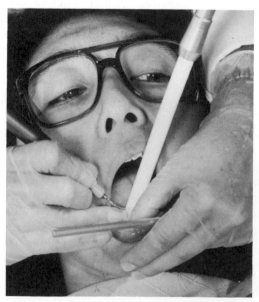

▼ Figure 6–3

Exposure to handpiece and ultrasonic scaler spray is of special concern to the dentist, hygienist, and assistant.

These diseases also can be transmitted through contact with contaminated blood, saliva, or mucous membranes in the mouth.

Carrier Contact

A **carrier** is an individual who harbors in his body the specific organisms of a disease without obvious symptoms and is capable of transmitting this disease to others.

Among carrier-transmitted diseases are **hepatitis, herpes, tuberculosis, typhoid fever,** and **AIDS:**

▼ A carrier may have had the disease and recovered.

▼ A carrier may have been exposed to the disease and may be coming down with it but not yet have obvious symptoms.

▼ A carrier, with natural immunity, may have been exposed to the disease but will never be sick with it.

Having a complete, up-to-date medical history on each patient is helpful in detecting someone who might be a carrier, but this is not 100 percent reliable. Therefore, it is always safer to assume that every patient is a potential carrier.

ORAL PATHOLOGY

Herpes

Herpes Simplex Virus, Type 1 (HSV-1)

Herpes simplex is a viral infection that causes recurrent sores on lips (Fig. 6-4). Because these sores frequently develop when the patient has a cold, or a fever of other origin, the disease has become commonly known as *fever blisters* or *cold sores.*

The herpesvirus, which is highly contagious, usually enters the body early in life. Following an initial childhood infection, the virus of herpes simplex lies dormant, to reappear later in life as the familiar recurring fever blister or cold sore.

A peculiarity of the disease is that in each succeeding attack the sore always develops at the same place. A burning sensation, itching, or feeling of fullness usually is noted about 24 hours before the sore actually appears. The lip becomes swollen and red, and the sore of the herpes is small and covered with a yellow scab.

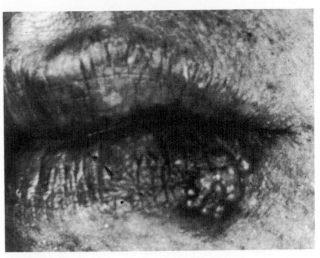

▼ **Figure 6-4**

Cluster of herpetic vesicles ("cold sore"). (Carranza FA: Glickman's Clinical Periodontology, 7th Ed. Philadelphia, WB Saunders, 1990, p 160.)

Fever blisters erupt when the patient's general resistance is lowered. They often occur following illness, trauma, emotional stress, or prolonged exposure to the sun.

Herpes Simplex Virus, Type 2 (HSV-2)

HSV-2, or genital herpes, has become the most common sexually transmitted disease in the United States.

Initial symptoms, which generally appear 2 to 10 days after infection, include tingling, itching, and a burning sensation when urinating. Within a week, clusters of painful blisters develop in the genital area. These sores eventually become crusty and usually heal without scarring.

Once infected, a victim can expect recurrent outbreaks, even though he or she has not been reinfected. The disease can be transmitted only during recurrences.

Herpes Transmission

The major transmission route for the virus is through direct contact with lesions. When lesions are present, the patient may be asked to reschedule his appointment for a time after the lesions have healed. Even when there are no active lesions, there is still the possibility of transmission through saliva.

Because there is no preventive vaccine to protect against herpes, it is essential that precautions be taken to prevent exposure.

Protective eyewear is particularly important because a herpes infection in the eye may cause blindness.

Hepatitis

There are three major viral forms of hepatitis: hepatitis A, hepatitis B, and hepatitis C.

Hepatitis A

Hepatitis A, also known as **infectious hepatitis,** is caused by the hepatitis A virus. The infection most often occurs in young adults and is usually followed by complete recovery. The virus may be spread by contact or through contaminated food or water.

Hepatitis B

Hepatitis B, also known as **serum hepatitis,** is caused by the hepatitis B virus (HBV). The infection may be severe and result in prolonged illness, destruction of liver cells, cirrhosis, or death.

Anyone who has ever had the disease, and some who have been exposed but were not actively ill, may be carriers of the hepatitis B virus.

The virus is transmitted through contact with contaminated blood or body fluids. In the dental office, this could be through direct patient contact. However, the virus may also be spread by contact with instruments or anything contaminated with blood or bloody saliva.

Special Concerns About Hepatitis B. The hepatitis B virus is considered an occupational risk for dental professionals and other health care workers. There is the risk that dental personnel may get HBV from an infected patient.

There is also the risk that infected, or carrier state, dental personnel may infect susceptible patients.

It is to your advantage to be immunized against the hepatitis B virus. Under the Occupational Safety and Health Administration (OSHA) guidelines, the dentist must make immunization available to "exposed" personnel who are directly involved in patient care. (See Chapter 8, "Hazards Management in the Dental Office.")

There are several hepatitis vaccines available. Each is given as a series of three intramuscular injections. (These must be given into the muscular tissue, not into the fatty tissue of the buttock.) Ask your physician or employer which type of vaccine would be best for you.

Prior to immunization, personnel may be tested to determine if they already have been infected with the hepatitis B virus.

An **anti-HBsAG–positive result** indicates that the person is already immune. Anyone who tests as being already immune does not need the vaccine. (HBsAG stands for hepatitis B surface antigen. Anti-HBsAG indicates the presence of an antibody for this antigen.)

An **HBsAG-positive result** indicates that the person is potentially a carrier. Dental personnel who test positive for HBsAG are potential carriers. Because such individuals present a threat to patient health, they must be removed from involvement in patient care.

Hepatitis C

Hepatitis C, formerly known as **non-A/non-B hepatitis,** is caused by the hepatitis C virus (HCV). This is a chronic liver disease that may last for years without causing symptoms.

It is similar to hepatitis B in the mode of transmission. At this time there is no vaccine against the hepatitis C virus.

Tetanus (Lockjaw)

Tetanus, which is also called *lockjaw,* is an extremely dangerous disease that is caused by a spore-forming organism found in soil, dust, or animal or human feces. This microbe is usually introduced into the body through a wound or break in the skin (as in a puncture wound from a soiled instrument).

Any puncture wound should be carefully cleaned and treated promptly. (This is discussed in Chapter 9, "Emergencies in the Dental Office.") Tetanus can be prevented by the administration of a vaccine; however, immunity must be kept current through booster doses. (It is important that dental personnel keep all of the immunizations current.)

AIDS

AIDS is characterized by an irreversible suppression of the immune system and is caused by human immunodeficiency virus.

AIDS is transmitted through blood and contaminated body fluids. Presently there is no vaccine to prevent AIDS or treatment to cure it. However, newer drugs are able to prolong the patient's life expectancy.

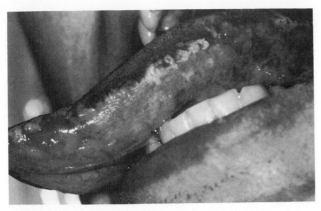

▼ **Figure 6-5**

Hairy leukoplakia is an important early manifestation of acquired immunodeficiency syndrome (AIDS). (Ibsen OAC, Phelan JA: Oral Pathology for the Dental Hygienist. Philadelphia, WB Saunders, 1991, p 212.)

Because the patient's immune system is damaged, opportunistic diseases are of particular concern. (An **opportunistic disease** is one that normally would be controlled by the immune system but that cannot be controlled because the system is not functioning properly.)

The major dental implications of AIDS include HIV-related periodontitis, oral manifestations of Kaposi's sarcoma, candidiasis, hairy leukoplakia, recurring herpes simplex virus, and other opportunistic infections (Fig. 6–5).

Tuberculosis

Until recently, the incidence of tuberculosis was decreasing; however, within the past several years, there has been in increase in the incidence of the disease.

Some individuals who have been exposed to tuberculosis become carriers without ever having actually had the disease.

If the patient is a carrier, or is actively infected, the tubercle bacilli is likely to be present in the mouth and can be spread during dental treatment.

Tuberculosis is caused by *Mycobacterium tuberculosis*. This spore-forming bacterium is so resistant to all efforts to kill it that it is used as the benchmark for rating disinfectants.

The Environmental Protection Agency (EPA)–approved hospital-grade disinfectants used in the dental office *do* kill the tuberculosis bacterium. However, this can happen only when these disinfectants are used properly according to the manufacturer's directions.

There is currently no form of protective immunization against tuberculosis.

Acute Necrotizing Ulcerative Gingivitis (ANUG)

ANUG, also known as *Vincent's infection* and *trench mouth*, is a painful, progressive bacterial infection.

This disease is characterized by **malaise** (a generalized feeling of illness), severe bad breath, and the appearance of grayish or yellowish gray ulcers, which may be found in only a few areas or throughout the mouth.

The affected tissues are so painful that it becomes difficult for the patient to brush his teeth or to chew food.

The onset of this infection is sudden, and in severe cases there may be a rise in temperature, an increased pulse rate, pallor of the skin, insomnia, and mental depression.

Instruction in oral hygiene is not only an important preventive measure but also an essential phase of treatment. The infectious organisms can only successfully invade and grow in tissue whose resistance has been lowered. Therefore, proper diet, rest, and exercise, which lead to the well-being of the individual, can be important preventive measures.

Aphthous Stomatitis

Aphthous stomatitis, which is commonly called *aphthous ulcers* or *canker sores*, is an inflammation with painful sores that may appear anywhere in the oral cavity (Fig. 6–6).

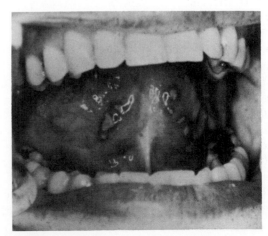

▼ **Figure 6-6**

Aphthous stomatitis. (Courtesy of National Institute of Dental Research, Bethesda, MD.)

They first appear as blisters; however, these rupture after 1 or 2 days to form depressed, spherical ulcers. These ulcers consist of a saucer-like, red or grayish red central portion and an elevated rim-like outer edge.

The aphthous sores tend to heal spontaneously in 10 to 14 days.

Periodontal Disease

Periodontal disease is a generalized term used to describe the many disorders that may affect the tissues surrounding and supporting the teeth. The warning signs of periodontal disease are:

1. Gingival tissues that bleed during tooth brushing.
2. Soft, swollen, or tender gums.
3. Pus between the teeth and gums.
4. Loose teeth.
5. Receding gums.
6. Change in the fit of partial dentures.
7. Shifting or elongated teeth.
8. Persistent bad breath.

Gingivitis

This is an inflammation of the gingival tissues characterized by the typical signs and symptoms of inflammation: swelling, redness, pain, increased heat, and sometimes a disturbance of function.

Usually, the earliest sign of this disorder is a color change of the free gingiva as it turns darker, more red, or blue-red (Fig. 6–7).

This inflammatory process is a result primarily

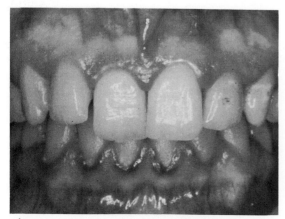

▼ **Figure 6–7**

Chronic gingivitis. The marginal interdental gingivae are smooth, swollen, and discolored. (Carranza FA: Glickman's Clinical Periodontology, 7th Ed. Philadelphia, WB Saunders, 1990, p 110.)

of accumulated plaque or calculus, or both. It is also caused by irritants and injurious agents such as toothbrush bristles, toothpicks, and overhanging margins of restorations.

With effective treatment at this early stage, the gingival tissues return to normal.

Periodontitis

Also commonly known as *pyorrhea*, periodontitis is an inflammatory and destructive disease involving the soft tissue and bony support of the teeth. It is the sequela of untreated or improperly treated gingivitis.

Clinically, periodontitis appears as a severe gingivitis; however, it is differentiated by the degree of severity and by gingival recession, the presence of periodontal pockets, and the loss of supporting bone.

Local irritation caused by poor oral hygiene is the primary cause of periodontal disease, although poorly constructed dental restorations with lack of proper contour, contacts, and margins are equally irritating.

Occlusal trauma, endocrine disturbances, allergy, and some deficiencies may also be contributing factors.

Classification of Periodontitis

The following are the American Academy of Periodontology's definitions of periodontal case types used for diagnostic identification:

1. **Type I Periodontitis.** Also known as **gingivitis,** Type I is inflammation of the gingiva characterized clinically by changes in color, gingival form, position, and surface appearance, and the presence of bleeding and/or *exudate* (fluid, cells, or cellular debris caused by inflammation).
2. **Type II Periodontitis.** Also known as **slight periodontitis,** Type II is a progression of gingival inflammation into deeper periodontal structures and alveolar bone crest, with slight bone loss.
3. **Type III Periodontitis.** Also known as **moderate periodontitis,** Type III is a more advanced stage of Type II, with increased destruction of the periodontal structure with noticeable loss of bone support possibly accompanied by an increase in tooth mobility.
4. **Type IV Periodontitis.** Also known as **advanced periodontitis,** Type IV is further progression of periodontitis with major loss of

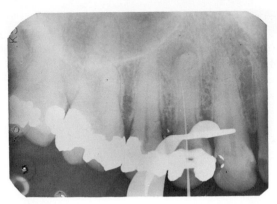

▼ **Figure 6-8**

Radiograph showing bone loss resulting from a periapical abscess. (Note the endodontic file in place and the rubber dam clamp surrounding the tooth.) (Torres HO, Ehrlich A: Modern Dental Assisting, 4th Ed. Philadelphia, WB Saunders, 1990, p 130.)

alveolar bone support usually accompanied by increased tooth mobility. Furcation involvement in multirooted teeth is likely.

5. **Type V Periodontitis.** Also known as **refractory progressive periodontitis,** Type V includes several unclassified types of periodontitis characterized either by rapid bone and attachment loss or by slow but continuous bone and attachment loss.

There is resistance to normal therapy and the condition is usually associated with gingival inflammation and continued pocket formation.

Periodontal Pocket

A periodontal pocket is a pathologically deepened gingival sulcus. It is one of the important clinical features of periodontal disease.

Progressive pocket formation leads to destruction of the supporting periodontal tissues and loosening and exfoliation (loss) of the teeth.

Periodontal pockets may be detected along the mesial, lingual, distal, and/or facial surfaces of the tooth.

Pockets of different depths and types may also occur on different surfaces of the same tooth and on approximating surfaces of the same interdental space.

Abscesses

A **periapical abscess** forms in the bone at the root tip as the result of the infected and dying pulp (Fig. 6-8).

A periapical abscess may cause a severe toothache and requires prompt treatment. (An **abscess** is a localized collection of pus.)

A **periodontal abscess** forms in the gingival tissue (Fig. 6-9). Unless the infection from the periodontal abscess spreads, it does *not* involve the pulpal tissues.

A periodontal abscess may cause toothache, mobility, and eventual loss of the teeth.

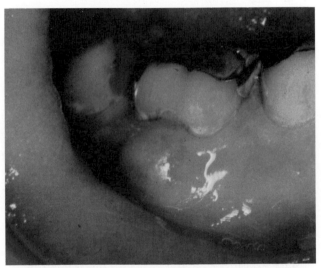

▼ **Figure 6-9**

Chronic periodontal abscess in the wall of a deep pocket. (Carranza FA: Glickman's Clinical Periodontology, 7th Ed. Philadelphia, WB Saunders, 1990, p 232.)

▼ EXERCISES

1. A/An _____ infection in the eye may cause blindness.

   a. aphthous stomatitis
   b. hepatitis B
   c. herpes
   d. tuberculosis

2. *Candida* is a _____.

   a. bacterium
   b. fungus
   c. virus

3. Many infection control activities are aimed at lowering the risk of infection by reducing the _____ of pathogens that are present.

   a. concentration
   b. incubation
   c. virulence
   d. b and c

4. Hepatitis B vaccinations must be given into _____ tissue.

   a. fatty
   b. muscular

5. A _____ pocket is a pathologically deepened gingival sulcus.

   a. gingival
   b. periapical
   c. periodontal
   d. a or c

6. The strength of the disease-producing capabilities of a pathogen is referred to as _____.

   a. concentration
   b. mutation
   c. virulence

7. The EPA-approved hospital-grade disinfectants used in the dental office _____ kill the tuberculosis bacterium.

   a. do
   b. do not

8. _____ is transmitted by carrier contact.

   a. Hepatitis
   b. Herpes
   c. Tuberculosis
   d. a, b, and c

9. Usually the earliest sign of _____ is a color change of the free gingiva as it turns darker, more red, or blue-red.

   a. aphthous stomatitis
   b. gingivitis
   c. HIV periodontitis
   d. periodontitis

10. Hepatitis _____ is a chronic liver disease that may last for years without causing symptoms. At the present time, there is no vaccine against it.

    a. A
    b. B
    c. C
    d. none of the above

11. _____ is a major dental implication of AIDS.

    a. Candidiasis
    b. Hairy leukoplakia
    c. HIV gingivitis
    d. a, b, and c

12. The major transmission route(s) for the herpesvirus is/are through _____ .

    a. a shared drinking glass
    b. direct contact with lesions
    c. transfusions
    d. a, b, and c

13. _____ is of special concern from the spray from the dental handpiece.

    a. Droplet infection
    b. Indirect transmission
    c. Operator infection
    d. Self-infection

14. A thin grayish-white pseudomembrane is typical of _____ .

    a. acute necrotizing ulcerative gingivitis
    b. leukoplakia
    c. measles
    d. trismus

15. _____ transmission requires direct person-to-person contact.

    a. Chickenpox
    b. Hepatitis
    c. Herpes
    d. Tuberculosis

16. _____ are bacteria that require oxygen in order to grow.

    a. Aerobes
    b. Anaerobes
    c. Bacilli
    d. Diplocci

17. Currently, it _____ possible to be immunized against tuberculosis.

    a. is
    b. is not

18. Type _____ periodontitis is further progression of periodontitis with major loss of alveolar bone support usually accompanied by
increased tooth mobility.

    a. II
    b. III
    c. IV
    d. V

19. _____ is commonly referred to as a "cold sore" or
"fever blister."

    a. Aphthous ulcer
    b. Cellulitis
    c. Herpes simplex, Type 1
    d. Herpes simplex, Type 2

20. An anti-HBsAG–positive result indicates that the person _____
_____ .

    a. is already immune
    b. is not immune
    c. is potentially a carrier

21. The patient who has had hepatitis _____ .

    a. is always considered to be a potential carrier
    b. is not considered to be a carrier after 5 years
    c. requires prophylactic antibiotics prior to dental treatment
    d. b and c

22. _____ are chain-forming cocci.

    a. Diplococci
    b. Sarcina
    c. Staphylocci
    d. Streptococci

23. _____ is/are caused by viruses.

    a. AIDS
    b. Common colds
    c. Hepatitis
    d. a, b, and c

24. A/An _____ disease is one that normally would be
controlled by the immune system but that cannot be controlled because the
system is not functioning properly.

    a. opportunistic
    b. pathogenic
    c. systemic
    d. virulent

25. A _____ abscess forms in the bone at the root tip.

    a. periapical
    b. periodontal

7 Infection Control

▼ LEARNING OBJECTIVES

The student will be able to:

1. Define and differentiate between sepsis and asepsis, sterilization and disinfection, disinfectants and antiseptics.

2. Describe the Universal Precautions that must be taken during the treatment of each patient.

3. Describe the use of protective barriers in the operatory.

4. Name and describe the two kinds of sterilization most frequently used in the dental office.

5. Discuss the properties and uses of these disinfectants: glutaraldehyde, chlorine dioxide, iodophors, synthetic phenol compounds, and sodium hypochlorite.

6. Describe the two major sections of the sterilization area and the flow of instruments as they are cleaned and sterilized.

7. Identify the infection control procedures for dental radiography, impressions, and laboratory cases.

8. Demonstrate the use of protective attire for dental personnel, including latex gloves, masks, and protective eyewear.

9. Demonstrate the preparation (cleaning and wrapping) of instruments for sterilization by autoclaving and dry heat.

OVERVIEW OF INFECTION CONTROL

The infection control steps, which are known as **universal precautions**, taken by each member of the dental team are essential in preventing the spread of disease from the patient to the staff or from the staff to the patient.

The necessary precautions must be followed faithfully because it is far easier to prevent a disease than it is to cure it. Worse yet, for some diseases there is not currently a cure available.

IMPORTANT RELATED TERMINOLOGY

Sepsis and Asepsis

The term **sepsis** means the presence of disease-producing microorganisms. **Asepsis** means the condition of being free from pathogenic microorganisms. It also means the steps taken to prevent contact with pathogens.

Because of the sensitive tissues involved, asepsis cannot be achieved within the oral cavity;

however, steps can be taken to reduce the number of pathogens present there and to limit their spread.

Sterilization and Disinfection

Sterilization is the process by which *all* forms of life are completely destroyed in a circumscribed area. This includes all forms of microbial life such as bacteria, fungi, viruses, and bacterial spores.

Sterile is an absolute term—there is no such thing as "partially sterile" or "almost" sterile. All instruments used in intraoral treatment must be sterilized.

Disinfection is the killing of pathogenic agents by chemical or physical means. It does not include the destruction of spores and resistant viruses. The purpose of disinfection is to reduce the microbial population when sterilization is not possible.

Disinfectants and Antiseptics

Disinfectants are applied to inanimate objects such as countertops or equipment. **Antiseptics** are agents that prevent the growth or action of microorganisms and are applied to living tissue.

The terms disinfectants and antiseptics are *not* used interchangeably.

UNIVERSAL PRECAUTIONS

Universal precautions, also known as *infection control procedures*, are the basic steps taken to prevent the transmission of diseases through contact with the dental office.

These steps, which are recommended by the Centers for Disease Control (CDC) and the American Dental Association (ADA), must be taken when treating *all* patients. It is not possible to overemphasize the importance of these precautions. They include:

1. **Protective wear.** All treatment personnel must wear examination gloves, protective masks, and protective eyewear during treatment procedures (Fig. 7–1). For some procedures surgical gowns, aprons, or laboratory coats may also be required.
2. **Sterilization.** All instruments and items used in or near the mouth must be sterilized if possible. Those that cannot be sterilized must be thoroughly disinfected.

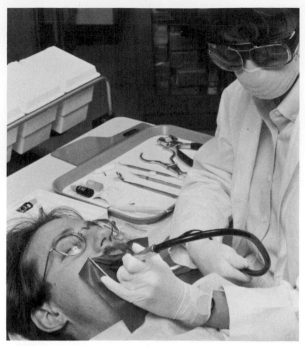

▼ Figure 7–1

Protective barriers are an effective means of preventing disease transmission. (Torres HO, Ehrlich A: Modern Dental Assisting, 4th Ed. Philadelphia, WB Saunders, 1990, p 150.)

3. **Disinfection.** All operatory surfaces that may have been touched or splashed during treatment procedures must be thoroughly cleaned and disinfected with an intermediate or higher level Environmental Protection Agency (EPA)–registered, hospital-grade disinfectant.
4. **Appropriate handling of hazardous waste.** Potentially contaminated waste must be disposed of appropriately. (This is discussed in Chapter 8, "Hazards Management in the Dental Office.")

▼ **Guidelines for Performing Universal Precautions**

1. They must be followed for all patients *as if* the patient were the carrier of a potentially threatening disease.
2. All steps must be completed with 100 percent accuracy each time. Shortcuts or failure to take any of these precautions carefully is dangerous and is not acceptable.
3. Always carry out these steps as if *you* were going to be the next patient to use the operatory or to be treated with these instruments.

PROTECTIVE ATTIRE FOR DENTAL PERSONNEL

Uniforms

According to OSHA regulations that went into effect in March 1992, uniforms that include gowns, laboratory coats, and clinic jackets *may not* be worn out of the office.

The employee may *not* take the contaminated laundry home to be washed. It must be washed at the office or by an outside laundry service. Protective gloves and other appropriate personal protective equipment must be worn when handling contaminated laundry.

Surgical Gowns

The use of surgical gowns, aprons, or laboratory coats is required when splashes to skin or clothing with body fluids are likely to occur (for example, during oral surgery).

Gowns should be made of a fluid-resistant material and protect all areas of exposed skin.

Disposable gowns are discarded after a single use. Cloth gowns are laundered after a single use.

No matter what type of gown is worn, it is used *only* for the treatment of a single patient. It is changed or discarded at the end of that patient visit.

Gloves

Latex Gloves

Latex (rubber) gloves, also known as **exam gloves,** are worn as protection against contact with the patient's body fluids.

These gloves must be worn by the dentist, assistant, or hygienist during all patient treatment in which there is the possibility of contact with the patient's blood, saliva, or mucous membranes.

All gloves are worn only for the treatment of *one* patient. Examination gloves are not washed or disinfected for reuse. During patient care, if a glove is torn or punctured, it is discarded immediately.

The interior of gloves is warm, moist, and dark. It is an ideal breeding ground for bacteria that may already be present or any that gain access through an accident such as a needle stick.

Therefore, the hands must be washed thoroughly with a disinfectant soap prior to gloving and again after removing the gloves. *Chlorhexidine gluconate* is an example of one type of antiseptic soap.

Sterile Latex Gloves

Exam gloves are not sterile and serve strictly as a protective barrier for the wearer. Sterile latex gloves should be worn for invasive procedures such as oral surgery or periodontal treatment.

Sterile gloves are never washed or disinfected for reuse.

Overgloves

Lightweight plastic gloves, also known as *food handler's gloves*, may be worn over latex gloves during procedures that require handling equipment away from the dental chair, for example, taking a radiograph for an endodontic patient during treatment.

These plastic overgloves are not a replacement for wearing or changing latex gloves.

Overgloves are donned prior to performing the secondary procedure and are removed before resuming the patient treatment that was in process. These gloves are discarded after a single use.

Utility Gloves

Utility or heavy-duty household type gloves must also be worn when handling soiled instruments and while cleaning the operatory. Utility gloves may be decontaminated and reused.

▼ Guidelines for Using Gloves

1. Wash hands thoroughly with an **antiseptic soap** before gloving and after removing gloves.

2. If you leave the chair for any reason, wash gloved hands before returning. This time a stronger soap, such as an iodine surgical scrub, may be used, since it does not come in contact with the skin.

3. Wear gloves for one patient only and then discard them. Do not wash and reuse gloves.

4. If gloves are damaged during treatment, remove them immediately, wash hands thoroughly, and reglove before continuing at chairside. (Gloves are effective *only* if they are intact.)

5. When the gloves are removed, wash hands carefully with antiseptic lotion soap to remove the bacterial buildup that may have occurred.

6. Dry the hands thoroughly and discard paper towel.
   Optional: Apply a lotion to maintain healthy skin.

7. Inform the dentist immediately if there is an open sore or wound on your hand.
   Note: You may be asked to refrain from all direct patient care and from handling instruments and equipment until the condition is resolved.

Procedure

HANDWASHING PRIOR TO GLOVING

1. Remove all jewelry. This includes a watch and all rings. Jewelry can harbor microbes, and a rough ring may tear the glove.

2. Use a liquid soap (bar soap transmits germs). This soap should be dispensed with a foot-activated device so that it is not necessary to touch the dispenser.

3. Scrub vigorously with a liquid soap and water to remove surface debris and then rinse.

4. Keep nails short and clean. Be sure to get soap solution under the nails. At the beginning of the day (and more often if necessary), use an orangewood stick and a nail brush to clean soiled areas of the skin and to clean under the fingernails.

5. Use a paper towel to dry hands and then the arms. Discard after use.

6. Use a foot control to regulate the flow of water. If faucets are used, take care not to touch the faucet with your hands. After drying hands, use the towel to turn off the faucets and discard the towel.

Protective Masks and Eyewear

Masks

A mask is worn over the nose and mouth to protect the wearer from possible infection spread by the aerosol handpiece spray. However, once the mask becomes wet, it ceases to be effective.

When placing and removing the mask, touch it only by the edges and elastic or ties. The front of the mask is contaminated.

A clean mask is worn for each patient visit. The mask is discarded after use.

Protective Eyewear for Dental Personnel

There is the danger of damage to the eye from debris, such as a flying amalgam scrap, or from the possibility of a pathogen, such as the herpesvirus, getting into the eye and causing irreparable damage.

Protective eyewear must be goggles or glasses with solid, not perforated, side shields.

Protective Eyewear for Patients

There is also danger to the patient's eyes from handpiece splatter. For this reason, the patient should be provided with protective glasses or be instructed to keep his eyes closed.

Face Shields

A chin-length plastic face shield that protects the entire face from splatter is an acceptable alternative to the use of glasses and masks.

PROTECTIVE BARRIERS

To prevent contamination, any surfaces that are likely to be touched during the dental procedure should be covered with a protective barrier.

This cover should be waterproof and large enough to cover completely the surface being protected.

▼ The light handles may be covered with clear plastic, foil, or a plastic-backed towel. This covering is discarded after use. An alternative is to use removable handle covers that are disinfected and reused.

▼ Clear plastic wrap, or a disposable cover, should be placed over the entire head of the x-ray machine. (Foil is not used for this purpose.)

▼ Countertops, the patient tray, and other work surfaces may be covered with a plastic-backed paper or other barrier.

▼ Sterile gauze sponges may be used to touch containers that must be opened. The sponge is discarded after a single use (Fig. 7–2).

Note: If a container is touched without this protective barrier, the container must be disinfected at the end of the visit.

Placing and Removing Protective Barriers

At the end of the patient visit, used barriers are discarded before removing the latex gloves worn during treatment.

Clean protective barriers are placed after the operatory has been cleaned and disinfected and the utility gloves have been removed.

The details of operatory cleanup and preparation are discussed in Chapter 10, "The Dental Operatory."

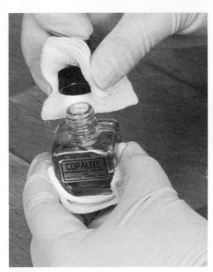

▼ Figure 7-2

Gauze squares may be used to protect against contamination when handling a container or instrument that has not been sterilized. (Torres HO, Ehrlich A: Modern Dental Assisting, 4th Ed. Philadelphia, WB Saunders, 1990, p 336.)

STERILIZATION

The accepted forms of sterilization involve the use of heat above the temperature of boiling water. The three forms of sterilization most commonly used in the dental office are (1) autoclaving, (2) chemical vapor sterilization, and (3) dry heat sterilization.

Ethylene oxide gas sterilization is an accepted form of sterilization; however, because of the time involved (8 to 10 hours per load or overnight) and the toxicity of the fumes, it is not commonly used in dental offices.

Although **boiling water** involves the use of heat, it is *not* an accepted form of sterilization.

AUTOCLAVING

Autoclaving is sterilization by superheated steam under pressure and is the preferred method of sterilization for use in the dental office.

Superheated steam is lighter than air, and as air is eliminated from the autoclave, the steam penetrates the materials in the autoclave in a top-to-bottom flow.

The advantages are that the results are consistently good and that instruments may be wrapped prior to sterilization. The disadvantage is that the steam will rust, dull, or corrode certain metals, especially carbon steel.

The amount of pressure used during autoclaving is usually expressed in terms of *psi* (pounds

per square inch). Most dental autoclaves work at 15 psi at 121°C (250°F).

Flash sterilization involves the use of an autoclave at 30 psi and 132°C (270°F) for 3 minutes for unwrapped loads and 8 minutes for wrapped loads. However, not all autoclaves are

---

Procedure

OPERATING THE AUTOCLAVE

1. Arrange everything within the autoclave to facilitate the top-to-bottom flow of the superheated steam. (Trapped air in the autoclave can prevent proper sterilization.)

   Place large packs, which would block the flow of steam, at the bottom of the autoclave.

   Tilt glass or metal canisters on an angle so that steam may flow in and displace the air.

2. Never overload the autoclave.

   Separate articles and packs from each other by a reasonable space.

   Use suitable wrapping materials to permit a free flow of steam through and around all packs.

3. Take into account the size of the load when calculating the time necessary for sterilization. Timing begins only after full pressure and temperature have been achieved within the chamber of the autoclave.

   Unwrapped loads may be sterilized in 15 minutes.

   Wrapped loads take a *minimum* of 20 minutes.

   A larger load requires more time.

4. Many autoclaves are equipped with automatic controls that start the timing process when the proper temperature and pressure have been achieved.

   If the autoclave does not do this, be sure to allow adequate time for these conditions to be reached *before* starting to time the sterilization cycle.

5. At the end of the sterilization cycle, when the pressure has returned to zero, very carefully open the door of the autoclave to release all remaining vapor.

6. Instruments are dry and ready to remove after 3 to 4 minutes.

designed to reach this pressure and temperature within a short span of time.

The steps in preparing instruments for autoclaving are discussed later in this chapter.

Before operating the autoclave, read the instruction manual carefully. Also, check that all gauges and fluid levels are appropriately set.

Chemical Vapor Sterilization

Chemical vapor sterilization uses a chemical steam instead of water. The advantage is that it does not rust, dull, or corrode metal instruments. The disadvantage is that adequate ventilation is essential because the chemicals used have a strong odor. Also, chemical vapor is not recommended for large loads or tightly wrapped instruments. Chemical vapor sterilization requires 20 to 40 psi at 132°C (270°F) for 20 minutes.

Paper, muslin, and steam-permeable plastic may be used to wrap instruments, but care must be taken not to create packs that are too large to be sterilized throughout.

If instruments are not dry before they are placed in the chemical vapor sterilizer, this increases the amount of water present and the instruments may rust.

Dry Heat Sterilization

Dry heat sterilization is an alternative method for sterilizing instruments that will rust in an autoclave. The advantage is that it does not rust instruments. The disadvantages are that it is time-consuming and is vulnerable to operator error in calculating the correct time.

The steps involved in preparing instruments for dry heat sterilization are discussed later in this chapter.

Sterilization Recommendations

▼ **Stainless steel instruments.** May be autoclaved without damage.

▼ **Non-stainless metal instruments.** Will rust and corrode if autoclaved without adequate protection. These instruments may be dipped in a **corrosion inhibitor solution** (1 percent sodium nitrate) prior to wrapping for autoclaving. An alternative is sterilization by dry heat.

▼ **Autoclavable handpieces.** Handpiece care is discussed in Chapter 12, "Rotary Dental Instruments."

▼ **Autoclavable prophy angles.** Should be sterilized following the manufacturer's directions. Disposable prophy angles are available. These are discarded after a single use.

▼ **Rubber prophy cups and brushes.** Should be discarded after use.

▼ **Stainless steel and tungsten-carbide burs.** May be autoclaved safely.

▼ **Carbon steel burs.** May corrode and should be dipped in a corrosion inhibitor solution prior to autoclaving.

▼ **Metal and heat-resistant plastic evacuators.** May be autoclaved.

▼ **Non–heat-resistant evacuator.** Must be discarded or disinfected using a high-level disinfectant.

▼ **Plastic saliva ejectors.** Are discarded after use.

Procedure

OPERATING THE DRY HEAT STERILIZER

1. When loading the dry heat chamber, permit adequate circulation of air around the articles.

2. Do not add instruments during the sterilization cycle. (Cool instruments lower the temperature of the oven significantly.)

3. Extend the sterilization time for tightly wrapped packs.

4. Start timing *only* after the desired temperature has been reached throughout the load.

5. The following time and temperature combinations are used:
   160°C (320°F) — 120 minutes
   170°C (340°F) — 60 minutes

6. After sterilization, when instruments have cooled, they may safely be removed from the dry heat sterilizer.

▼ **Metal impression trays.** May be sterilized.

▼ **Plastic and custom acrylic impression trays.** Are discarded after use.

▼ **Heat-resistant fluoride gel trays.** May be sterilized.

▼ **Non–heat-resistant fluoride gel trays.** Are discarded after use.

▼ **Glass slabs and dishes, rubber items, and stones.** Can be autoclaved, but must be dry prior to sterilization.

Verifying Sterilization

Process Indicators

Heat-sensitive tapes may be used to seal instrument packages. These tapes change color when they have been exposed to heat. This indicates heat change only and does not ensure that the pack has been exposed to proper sterilization conditions.

Process indicators may also be placed within the pack; however, these still indicate only that the proper temperature was achieved at some time. They do not indicate that it was maintained for the appropriate length of time.

Biological Indicators

Biological indicators, also known as *sporicidal tests*, use spores that are harmless (but highly resistant) as a means of verifying that sterilization has taken place. For most practices, weekly verification is considered adequate.

Biological indicators for monitoring steam autoclave or chemical vapor sterilization contain spores of *Bacillus stearothemophilus*. Indicators for dry heat or ethylene oxide sterilization contain spores of *Bacillus subtilis*.

Each type of biological indicator should be used only to monitor the sterilization method for which it is designed. One common form of biological indicator test consists of *three* strips of special paper impregnated with the appropriate spores.

Two of the strips are placed inside instrument packs in the test load, and the sterilizer is operated under normal conditions. The *third* strip is retained as a control.

After the load has been sterilized, all three strips are cultured. This is usually done by an outside laboratory. (It may be done in the dental office if the appropriate equipment is available.)

The laboratory sends a report that documents cultures at 24, 48, and 72 hours.

▼ A **negative report** indicates that sterilization did occur.

▼ A **positive report** indicates that sterilization did *not* occur. Corrective procedures must be taken immediately.

These reports are kept on file as part of the documentation of the practice infection control program.

DISINFECTION

Based on its effectiveness, a disinfectant is rated by the EPA, described as being **high (hospital-grade), intermediate,** or **low** level.

Anything that goes into the mouth but cannot be sterilized should be disinfected using a high-level disinfectant.

When a disinfecting solution is labeled *tuberculocidal, bactericidal, virucidal,* and *fungicidal* and carries the EPA and ADA acceptance label, it is acceptable for use in dentistry as a high-level disinfectant.

The term **cold sterilization** is sometimes used to describe these disinfecting solutions. This is an erroneous term because these are chemical *disinfectants*. They have an important role; however, they are not a substitute for heat sterilization.

Glutaraldehyde

Glutaraldehyde is a high-level disinfectant used for instruments that cannot be sterilized with heat. This chemical is capable of sterilization *if* there is long enough exposure (from 6 to 10 hours, depending on the product).

However, this method is not a recommended form of sterilization for any instruments that can withstand heat of sterilization.

Glutaraldehydes are available as **neutral, alkaline,** or **acidic solutions.** Each type of glutaraldehyde solution has different properties, and the manufacturer's instructions for mixing and use should be followed exactly.

Those products in the neutral and alkaline range must be activated before use by adding an appropriate buffer. These activated solutions remain active for 14 to 30 days, depending on the preparation.

The term **active life** describes how long a reusable solution remains effective after it has been put into use. The active life of the solution can be altered by incorrect mixing, by dilution from water left on instruments, or by heavy debris and contamination from instruments placed in the solution.

A special color monitor **dipstick** may be used to test the strength of the solution. A solution that is not of the appropriate strength must be replaced immediately.

Glutaraldehydes produce fumes that are very toxic to tissues. Therefore, these chemicals must be used with caution, as follows:

1. Place and remove instruments either while wearing gloves or using sterile transfer forceps. Do *not* put your hand in the solution.
2. Rinse instruments to remove all residue before use in the patient's mouth.
3. Do not use glutaraldehydes routinely as surface disinfectants.

Chlorine Dioxide

Chlorine dioxide is a surface disinfectant that is reported to be effective on operatory surfaces in from 1 to 3 minutes when used in conjunction with a thorough cleaning procedure.

No rinsing or special handling is required; however, chlorine dioxide can be corrosive to metal. Before using it, carefully read and follow the manufacturer's instructions.

Iodophors

Iodophors are available as surgical scrubs (antiseptics) and hard-surface disinfectants. These substances are *not* used interchangeably.

Iodophors are minimally irritating to tissue and do not stain the skin. When used properly, they are effective for surface disinfection in 3 to 30 minutes.

The solutions have a built-in color indicator that changes the amber color to light yellow or clear when the iodophor molecules are exhausted. A fresh solution should be prepared when the amber color disappears.

Because iodophors are inactivated by hard water, they must be mixed using soft or distilled water. Iodophors may corrode or discolor certain metals and may temporarily stain starched clothing.

Synthetic Phenol Compounds

The synthetic phenol compounds approved by the ADA have a broad-spectrum disinfecting action.

When diluted in a 1:32 ratio, they are used for surface disinfection (provided that the surface has been thoroughly cleaned first). Diluted at 1:128, they may be used as a holding solution for instruments.

Sodium Hypochlorite

Sodium hypochlorite, which is common household bleach, can disinfect surfaces in from 3 to 30 minutes. Concentrates ranging from a 1:10 dilution to a 1:100 dilution are considered effective; however, effectiveness depends on the amount of debris present.

Sodium hypochlorite has a strong odor that many find to be objectionable. It is also corrosive to some metals, is caustic to skin and eye, and may eventually cause plastic chair covers to crack.

Sodium hypochlorite solution is not stable and must be mixed fresh each day. To make a 1:10 dilution, mix 1½ cups of bleach with 1 gallon of water. To make a 1:100 dilution, mix ¼ cup of bleach with 1 gallon of water.

INSTRUMENT CLEANING AND STERILIZATION

The Sterilization Area

In the sterilization area instruments are cleaned, sterilized, and prepared for reuse. Most practices organize instruments on "pre-set trays." The preparation of these trays is discussed in Chapter 11, "Dental Hand Instruments."

The sterilization area is divided into the **contaminated** and **clean** sections.

Contaminated Section

The contaminated section usually consists of counter space, storage cabinets for soiled trays, a waste disposal container, the ultrasonic cleaner, and a sink.

Contaminated means that the instruments or supplies have potentially been exposed to a substance that will make them "unclean" or a possible source of infection.

Soiled instruments are returned to the contaminated section of the central sterilization area. Here they may be placed in special cabinets until they can be cleaned and/or instruments may be placed in a holding solution (Fig. 7–3).

Soiled trays or instruments are *never* placed

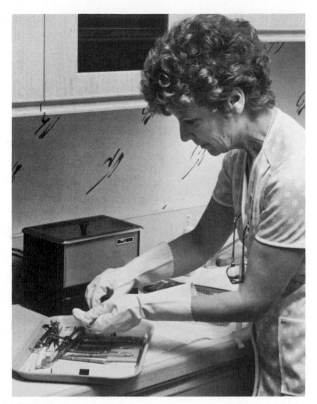

▼ **Figure 7–3**

Soiled instruments are brought into the "contaminated section" of the sterilization area. (Torres HO, Ehrlich A: Modern Dental Assisting, 4th Ed. Philadelphia, WB Saunders, 1990, p 158.)

in the clean area, and soiled and clean instruments are *never* stored in the same cabinet.

Clean Section

The sterilizer is located between the contaminated and clean sections. The clean section is used only for supplies and instruments that have not been contaminated.

This section has counter space, which is used for assembling sterile pre-set trays, and storage space for sterilized instruments and trays.

Limited bulk supplies of materials are stored in this section so that they are readily accessible for placement on pre-set trays or for restocking supplies in the operatories.

Special Precautions in Handling Soiled Instruments

There is a real danger of an accidental needle stick or cut while working with soiled instruments. Always wear heavy utility gloves and handle soiled instruments as little as possible.

Holding Solution (Fig. 7–4)

Holding solutions are used to:

▼ Prevent debris from drying on the instrument.

▼ Minimize the handling of soiled instruments.

▼ Prevent air-borne transmission of dried micro-organisms.

▼ Begin microbial kill on the soiled instruments.

Synthetic phenols, iodophors, and glutaraldehyde are recommended for use as holding solutions. Holding solutions are used in two different ways. In some practices, when you finish using an instrument at chairside, it is immediately placed into a holding solution.

At the end of the procedure, either the entire container of holding solution or the basket liner containing the instruments is removed and taken to the sterilization center.

An alternative is to use the holding solution in the sterilization area. If soiled instruments cannot

▼ **Figure 7–4**

Soiled instruments may be placed in a holding solution. (Torres HO, Ehrlich A: Modern Dental Assisting, 4th Ed. Philadelphia, WB Saunders, 1990, p 158.)

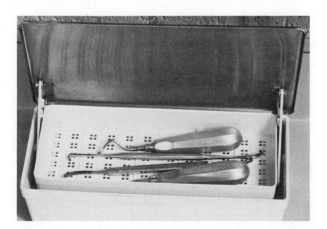

be processed immediately, they are placed in the holding solution as soon as the soiled tray is brought from the operatory.

The instruments are kept in the holding solution until they are processed for sterilization. The use of the holding solution does not replace any of the cleaning or sterilization steps.

Ultrasonic Cleaning

Because of the danger of injury, hand scrubbing of instruments is not recommended. Ultrasonic cleaning effectively removes debris from instruments. This minimizes the amount of handling required to prepare instruments for sterilization. (An ultrasonic cleaner can be seen in the background in Fig. 7–3.)

The ultrasonic cleaner removes the debris from the soiled instruments through the use of the mechanical action of the bursting bubbles, combined with the chemical action of the specialized solutions used in the ultrasonic cleaner.

There are specialized solutions for specific difficult tasks such as removing cements or stains. These are used in small glass beakers that are held in place in the main tank of solution.

Procedure

OPERATING THE ULTRASONIC CLEANER

1 Place the soiled instruments in the ultrasonic cleaner basket.

2 Rinse thoroughly under running water.

3 Drain the basket.

4 Place the basket in the ultrasonic cleaner so that the instruments are completely submerged in this solution.

5 Cover the container (to prevent splatter) and run the cleaner for 5 minutes.

6 After cleaning, remove the basket of instruments and rinse it thoroughly under cool running water to remove all of the ultrasonic solution (Fig. 7–5).

7 If there is any visible debris, scrub the instruments with a brush under running water.
   Alternative: The instruments may also be processed through the ultrasonic cleaner again.
   Note: Always handle soiled instruments with care to avoid a cut, puncture wound, or other injury.

8 At the end of the day, discard the ultrasonic cleaning solution.

9 Wipe the inside of the pan and lid with a cleaning and disinfecting agent. Dilute sodium hypochlorite may be used; however, the manufacturer's instructions must be checked first.

10 Place fresh solution in the ultrasonic cleaner in preparation for use the following day.

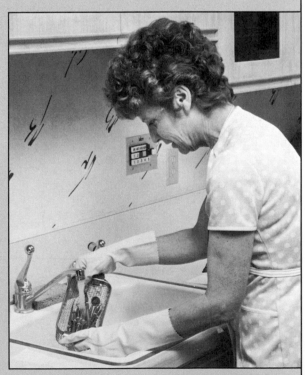

Figure 7–5 Instruments are rinsed thoroughly while still in the ultrasonic basket. (Torres HO, Ehrlich A: Modern Dental Assisting, 4th Ed. Philadelphia, WB Saunders, 1990, p 160.)

Procedure

DRYING THE INSTRUMENTS

1. Instruments must be thoroughly cleaned, rinsed, and dried prior to sterilization.

2. Rinse the instruments thoroughly and place them on a clean paper towel.

3. Use a second paper towel to roll or pat them dry.

4. Discard both towels after this is completed. The instruments are now ready to wrap for sterilization (Fig. 7-6).

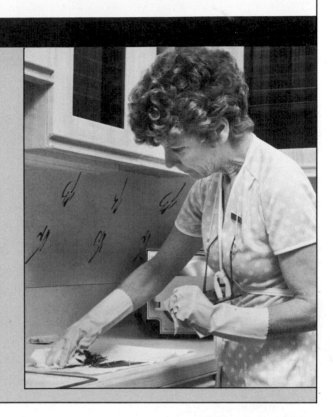

Figure 7-6 Instruments are carefully patted dry prior to wrapping for sterilization. (Torres HO, Ehrlich A: Modern Dental Assisting, 4th Ed. Philadelphia, WB Saunders, 1990, p 160.)

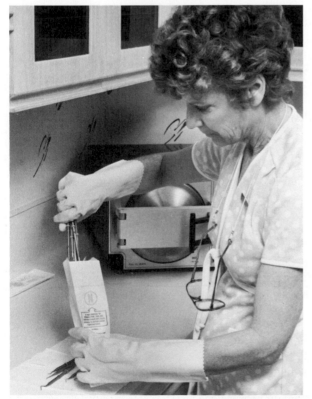

▼ **Figure 7-7**

Instruments are bagged for autoclaving. (Torres HO, Ehrlich A: Modern Dental Assisting, 4th Ed. Philadelphia, WB Saunders, 1990, p 161.)

Wrapping Instruments for Autoclaving

The material used to bag or wrap instruments for autoclaving must be porous enough to permit the steam to penetrate to the instruments (Fig. 7-7).

Cloth such as muslin, paper, or a special nylon film can be used for this purpose. The bag or wrap is sealed with tape because pins, staples, or paper clips make holes in the wrap that allow microorganisms to pass through.

Wrapping Instruments for Dry Heat Sterilization

Aluminum foil, metal, and glass containers may be used in the dry heat oven (Fig. 7-8). The instruments should not be wrapped too tightly because they can puncture the wrapping. Paper and cloth should be used with caution, as they may char.

Handling Sterilized Instruments

Wrapped Instruments

All of the instruments for a given procedure may be bagged or wrapped together. They are stored in this wrapping and opened just prior to use. In the operatory, the bag itself may be used as the sterile field.

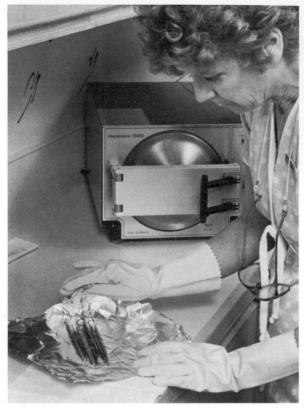

▼ **Figure 7–8**

Instruments are wrapped in aluminum foil for dry heat sterilization. (Torres HO, Ehrlich A: Modern Dental Assisting, 4th Ed. Philadelphia, WB Saunders, 1990, p 161.)

Unwrapped Instruments

Maintaining the sterility of unwrapped instruments is difficult (if not impossible). For this reason, instruments should be wrapped prior to sterilization and kept wrapped until used.

If wrapping is not possible, sterile transfer forceps should be used to remove the instruments from the sterilizer and to move them into and out of storage.

These forceps should be stored in a dry, sterilized container. Both the forceps and the container should be sterilized daily.

SPECIAL CONSIDERATIONS
Handpiece Sterilization

The care and sterilization of handpieces are discussed in Chapter 12, "Rotary Dental Instruments."

Radiography Precautions

Exposing Radiographs

The head of the x-ray machine should be protected with a clear plastic barrier. Switches that are touched during the process must also be protected

(see Figs. 16–1 and 16–2). This can be accomplished by taping a barrier over the switches or using a fresh gauze sponge each time the switch is touched.

The positioning indicating device (PID) is sterilized (if possible) or treated with a high-level disinfectant.

Latex gloves must be worn while exposing the dental x-ray films (see Fig. 16–3). Exposed x-ray films are immediately placed into a plastic cup for safe storage and transfer for processing.

Processing Radiographs

Exposed films have been contaminated with the patient's saliva, and gloves must be worn while processing or handling them. If a "daylight" automatic processor is used (where the hands are placed into the machine through ports), gloves are worn while processing the films.

If films are unwrapped in a darkened area prior to placing them in the processor, the work area is covered with a paper towel and gloves are worn while unwrapping the films.

The unwrapped films are dropped onto this towel, and the contaminated wrappings are immediately discarded. When finished, the gloves are removed and the processing is completed.

The automatic processor should routinely be cleaned and disinfected according to the manufacturer's directions. Surrounding countertops must also be disinfected after use.

Disinfecting Impressions

Follow the manufacturer's recommendation for the disinfection of each type of impression material.

Basic Procedures

At the chair, the impression is rinsed thoroughly, sprayed with a disinfecting solution, and placed in a sealed plastic bag. This isolates the impression and maintains the appropriate humidity. (A damp paper towel may be included to increase the humidity.)

Some dentists prefer to have the impression sprayed with a disinfectant (such as an iodophor) at chairside (Fig. 7–9). The impression is then bagged and sent into the laboratory.

In the laboratory, the impression is removed from the bag and the bag is discarded. If the impression has not already been disinfected, it is disinfected at this time.

Alginate Impressions

Alginate impressions should be disinfected by spraying rather than by immersion because soaking may distort the impression.

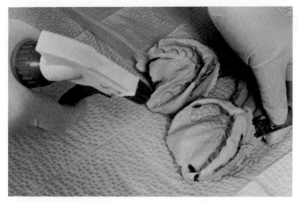

▼ Figure 7–9

Alginate impressions are sprayed with disinfectant. (Torres HO, Ehrlich A: Modern Dental Assisting, 4th Ed. Philadelphia, WB Saunders, 1990, p 164.)

A sodium hypochlorite solution (1:10 dilution) or an iodophor solution (1:213 dilution) may be used for this purpose.

After spraying with the disinfectant, the impression should be left in a sealed plastic bag for the recommended disinfection time.

Polysulfide and Silicone Impressions

Polysulfide and silicone impressions can be disinfected by immersion with any accepted disinfectant product. The length of the immersion time is determined by the manufacturer's recommendations.

Polyether Impressions

Polyether impressions may be adversely affected with disinfection by immersion. These impressions should be sprayed with a disinfectant.

An alternative is immersion in a disinfectant, such as a chlorine compound, that has a short disinfection time (2 to 3 minutes).

Sending Cases to the Laboratory

Blood and saliva should be thoroughly and carefully cleaned from laboratory supplies, materials, and impressions that have been used in the mouth. This includes anything tried in the mouth for fit, occlusion, or aesthetic check (for example, bite rims, counter point balancers, cast framework, and final wax-ups).

These materials must be disinfected before being handled, adjusted, or sent to a dental laboratory. A removable prosthodontic or orthodontic appliance may be disinfected by soaking it for 10 to 30 minutes in a sodium hypochlorite solution.

To determine the best method of disinfection, the instructions provided by the manufacturer of the material being used should be followed.

Cases Returned from the Laboratory

When a case is received from the laboratory, it is unwrapped and all packing materials are discarded. The case is then disinfected and rinsed thoroughly before it is placed in the patient's mouth.

Removable Prosthodontic and Orthodontic Appliances

When an appliance is removed from the patient's mouth, it should be placed directly into a disposable plastic cup and covered with a nontoxic disinfectant.

Laboratory Disinfection

Always wear gloves when working on laboratory cases. If grinding or polishing equipment is used, masks and safety glasses are also necessary.

When polishing, use a clean rag wheel and fresh pumice or other polishing materials for each case. Extreme caution is necessary when working in gloves because they could get caught in equipment such as a grinding wheel or rotary bur.

Working surfaces should be covered with a barrier, such as a large sheet of paper. This is discarded after use on one case.

Laboratory work surfaces should be cleaned regularly with the same system that is used to clean operatory surfaces.

Use separate sets of instruments, attachments, and materials for new prostheses and for those cases that have already been in the mouth. If the bur or instrument may be reused, it should be sterilized before it is used again.

It is recommended that pumice be mixed with dilute sodium hypochlorite (5 parts of sodium hypochlorite to 100 parts distilled water). If the pumice is used on a case that has been in the mouth, it should be discarded after use.

Rag wheels may be washed and then sterilized in an autoclave. As an alternative, a disposable buffing wheel may be used instead of the rag wheel.

The Staff Lounge

In the past, the laboratory, sterilization area, or even a vacant operatory doubled as a staff lounge. However, eating, drinking, smoking, and personal grooming are now *prohibited* in work areas where there is a reasonable likelihood of occupational exposure.

▼ EXERCISES

1. A holding solution is used to ___d___ .

   a. minimize the handling of soiled instruments
   b. prevent debris from drying on the instrument
   c. prevent air-borne transmission of dried microorganisms
   d. a, b, and c

2. When loading the autoclave, large packs are placed at the ___a___
   ___ .

   a. bottom
   b. top

3. ___Antiseptics___ are agents that prevent the growth or action of microorganisms and are applied to living tissue.

   a. Antiseptics
   b. Disinfectants

4. ___Na hypochlorite___ is commonly known as household bleach.

   a. Chlorine dioxide
   b. Quaternary ammonium
   c. Sodium hypochlorite
   d. Synthetic phenol

5. At a temperature of 160°C, dry heat sterilization requires ___b___
   ___ minutes.

   a. 60
   b. 120
   c. 150
   d. 180

6. Latex exam gloves ___d___ .

   a. are sterile
   b. are not sterile
   c. serve only to protect the wearer
   d. b and c

7. Glutaraldehydes ___are not___ routinely used as surface disinfectants.

   a. are
   b. are not

8. When a case is returned from the laboratory, the packing material should be ___a___ .

   a. discarded to avoid cross-contamination
   b. disinfected
   c. saved to return the case to the laboratory
   d. sterilized

9. A color monitor dipstick may be used to test the strength of
_____ solutions.

   a. glutaraldehyde
   b. iodophor
   c. sodium hypochlorite
   d. ultrasonic cleaner

10. For _____, timing does not begin until the controls
show the pressure at 15 psi and the temperature at 121°C.

    a. autoclaving
    b. chemical vapor sterilization
    c. ethylene oxide gas sterilization
    d. flash sterilization

11. After use, rubber prophy cups and brushes are _____.

    a. autoclaved
    b. discarded
    c. disinfected
    d. dry heat sterilized

12. If instruments are not dry before they are placed in the chemical vapor
sterilizer, they may _____.

    a. corrode
    b. fail to be sterilized
    c. rust
    d. a and c

13. When wrapping instruments for dry heat sterilization, they may be wrapped
in _____.

    a. cloth
    b. foil
    c. paper
    d. a, b, or c

14. When wrapping instruments for autoclaving, the pack may be sealed with
_____.

    a. pins
    b. staples
    c. tape
    d. a, b, or c

15. _____ is the condition of being free from pathogenic
microorganisms.

    a. Asepsis
    b. Disinfected
    c. Sepsis
    d. Sterile

16. _____Latex_____ gloves are worn when exposing radiographs.

   a. Latex
   b. No
   c. Surgical
   d. Utility

17. The tape on the instrument pack that turns color in the autoclave indicates that the contents were _____.

   a. disinfected
   b. exposed to heat   *Process Indicators 69*
   c. sterilized
   d. a and b

18. Alginate impressions should be disinfected by _____d_____.

   a. autoclaving
   b. dry heat
   c. soaking
   d. spraying with disinfectant

19. If the object is covered with the solution, glutaraldehyde is capable of _____ in from 6 to 10 hours.

   a. disinfection
   b. sterilization

20. (d)_____ are the basic steps taken to prevent the transmission of diseases through contact with the dental office.

   a. Infection control procedures
   b. OSHA guidelines
   c. Universal precautions
   d. a and c

21. _____b_____ is the process by which all forms of life are completely destroyed in a circumscribed area.

   a. Chemical disinfection
   b. Sterilization
   c. Ultrasonic cleaning

22. _____(a)_____ may be used as a protective cover on the x-ray machine.

   a. Clear plastic wrap
   b. Foil

23. Plastic saliva ejectors are _____(a)_____ after use.

   a. discarded
   b. disinfected
   c. sterlized by autoclaving
   d. sterilized with dry heat

24. Gloves _____(a)_____ required when processing radiographs.

    a. are
    b. are not

25. Nonstainless metal instruments __(a)_____.

    a. may be sterilized safely with dry heat
    b. should be disinfected, not sterilized
    c. will rust and corrode if autoclaved without adequate protection
    d. a and c

▼ **Criterion Sheet 7–1**

Student's Name _____

Procedure: *USING PROTECTIVE BARRIERS*		

Performance Objective:

The student will demonstrate the use of latex gloves, a mask, and protective eyewear, and explain the rationale for the use of each.

SE = Student evaluation **C** = Criterion met	**SE**	**IE**
IE = Instructor evaluation **X** = Criterion not met		
Instrumentation: Antiseptic soap, latex gloves, mask, protective eyewear (for the assistant and patient)		
1. Explained to the patient the need for using protective eyewear during clinical procedures.		
2. Demonstrated handwashing and donning of gloves.		
3. Demonstrated placement of mask and protective eyewear.		
4. Demonstrated removal of gloves and washing of hands.		
Comments:		

▼ Criterion Sheet 7–2

Student's Name _____

Procedure: *PREPARING INSTUMENTS FOR STERILIZATION*

Performance Objective:

The student will demonstrate cleaning instruments in preparation for sterilization.

The student will demonstrate wrapping instruments for autoclaving.

The student will demonstrate wrapping instruments for dry heat sterilization.

	SE	IE
SE = Student evaluation **C** = Criterion met **IE** = Instructor evaluation **X** = Criterion not met		
Instrumentation: Instruments, utility gloves, wrapping materials		
1. Washed hands and donned utility gloves.		
2. Brought soiled instruments into the sterilization area.		
3. Cleaned instruments in ultrasonic cleaner.		
4. Rinsed and dried instruments.		
5. Prepared and wrapped instruments for autoclaving.		
6. Prepared and wrapped instruments for dry heat sterilization.		
Comments:		

8 Hazards Management in the Dental Office

▼ LEARNING OBJECTIVES

The student will be able to:

1. Name and describe the three Occupational Safety and Health Adminstration (OSHA) and Environmental Protection Agency (EPA) programs of primary concern to the dental office.

2. Describe the tasks that may be assigned to employees classified as being at risk for occupational exposure to blood or other potentially infectious materials.

3. Describe the responsibility of the dentist/employer in providing hepatitis B virus (HBV) vaccination for these employees.

4. List and describe the major parts of a program to comply with the OSHA Hazards Communication Regulation.

5. State the purpose and use of Material Safety Data Sheets (MSDS) and labeling requirements.

6. Describe the appropriate handling of acid etch solutions and gels, asbestos, flammable liquids, organic chemicals, gypsum products, formaldehyde, nitrous oxide and oxygen gases, mercury, cast alloys, photographic chemicals, pickling solutions, and visible light-cured materials.

7. Describe the appropriate method of discarding these medical wastes in the dental office: sharps, extracted teeth, items contaminated with blood and saliva.

OVERVIEW OF HAZARDS MANAGEMENT IN THE DENTAL OFFICE

The regulations of major concern in the dental office are:

1. The OSHA infection control program.
2. The OSHA hazard communications regulations.
3. The EPA (and state) medical waste tracking regulations.

The **Occupational Health and Safety Administration** (OSHA) of the U.S. Department of Labor establishes and enforces regulations related to employee safety in the workplace.

The **Environmental Protection Agency** (EPA) deals with issues of concern to the environment and public safety.

In some states there are also state regulations that control these areas. In these situations, the dentist is obligated to comply with the regulation that is most stringent. The dental assistant must also be aware of the employee's role in the implementation of these regulations.

INFECTION CONTROL

In the area of infection control, OSHA requires that the dentist:

1. Perform exposure determination.
2. Develop an infection control plan.
3. Institute a training and education program.
4. Maintain certain records.

Exposure Determination

The OSHA guidelines state that tasks in the dental office should be evaluated according to the degree of occupational exposure risk involved.

These determinations should be based on written job descriptions, and each employee must be notified of the risks associated with his or her position.

Low-Risk Tasks

Employees, such as the receptionist and administrative assistant, who perform only clerical (non-clinical) duties are *not* considered to be at increased risk for occupational exposure.

These duties include answering the telephone, bookkeeping, filing, scheduling, billing, and typing.

At-Risk Tasks

At risk occupational tasks include all procedures or other job-related duties that involve the potential for mucous membrane or skin contact with blood, body fluids, or tissues or a potential for spills or splashes of them.

These tasks include:

▼ Patient treatment procedures.

▼ Radiographic procedures.

▼ Cleaning, disinfection, and sterilization of instruments.

▼ Laboratory procedures that require handling of items contaminated with blood and other potentially infectious materials.

All tasks performed by the dentist, dental hygienist, chairside dental assistant, coordinating as-

sistant, and laboratory technician fall in this category.

The use of all appropriate protective measures is required of these employees.

Hepatitis B Vaccination. Under the OSHA regulations, within 10 working days of initial assignment to a position involving exposure, the dentist/employer is required to offer, at no cost, hepatitis B virus (HBV) vaccinations.

OSHA also requires that the employee be trained regarding hepatitis B and vaccination *prior* to being offered vaccination.

It is necessary to maintain a vaccination record for the employee. If the employee refuses the offer of vaccination, this too must be recorded.

Infection Control Plan

According to the OSHA guidelines, the dentist must establish a written "infection control plan," which incorporates *standard operating procedures* (SOPs) regarding infection control for the tasks in each of these risk categories.

These SOPs should include both the protective equipment and the mandatory work practices necessary to prevent the transmission of disease (Fig. 8–1).

The dentist, or person designated by the dentist, is responsible for monitoring staff compliance with these SOPs. However, *you*, the dental assist-

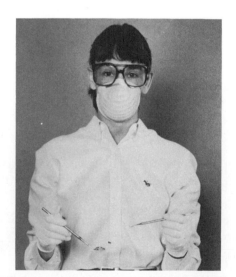

▼ Figure 8–1

Protective garb is an important part of the infection control program.

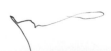

ant, also have a responsibility to follow these guidelines carefully at all times.

Staff Training

Under the OSHA guidelines, the dentist is required to provide an in-office staff training program that includes information regarding modes of disease transmission and methods of infection control. (These topics are discussed in Chapters 6 and 7.)

This training must be provided for new employees and on a periodic basis for all staff members.

Maintaining Records

The dentist is required to maintain records of infection control programs and training sessions.

Exposure Incidents

According to OSHA, an exposure incident means *a specific eye, mouth, other mucous membrane, nonintact skin, or parenteral contact with blood or other potentially infectious materials that results from the performance of an employee's duties.* (**Parenteral** means by injection. This includes any needle-stick injury or cut with a contaminated instrument.) Treatment of such injuries is discussed in Chapter 9, "Emergencies in the Dental Office."

Any such injury should be reported to the dentist immediately. The dentist must maintain records of the incident, name of the source patient, medical treatment provided, and all follow-up procedures.

Follow-up procedures include notifying the source patient and requesting that the patient be tested for human immunodeficiency virus (HIV) and HBV. If the patient refuses or tests positive, the employee should then be examined, tested, and followed up for 6 months.

The employee must be fully informed about the available follow-up procedures. Any employee refusing these follow-up procedures must sign a written "informed refusal" form.

Employee Medical Records

The dentist must establish and maintain an accurate record for each employee covered by the OSHA standard. These records must be maintained for at least the duration of employment plus 30 years.

This is a confidential record, which should include:

▼ The name and social security number of the employee.

▼ A copy of the employee's HBV vaccination records and medical records relative to the employee's ability to receive vaccination.

▼ The circumstances of any exposure incident, including date, location, nature of the incident (such as needle stick), and name of the source patient.

▼ A copy of all results of physical examinations, medical testing, and follow-up procedures as they relate to the employee's ability to receive vaccination or to postexposure evaluation following an exposure incident.

FIRE-SAFETY POLICY

OSHA regulations state that the employer must maintain a written fire-safety policy. This includes the maintenance of fire extinguishers and training employees how to use them.

However, the employer may be exempt from training if the written fire-safety policy requires immediate and total evacuation of employees.

OSHA HAZARDS COMMUNICATION REGULATION

The OSHA Hazards Communication Regulation, often called the *Employee Right To Know Law*, covers the rights of employees to know the potential dangers associated with hazardous chemicals in the workplace.

The goal of this regulation is to ensure that all employees understand the dangers of, and correct procedures for, handling chemicals to which such employees may be exposed during their employment.

Under this regulation, the dentist is required to develop, implement, and maintain a hazards communication program that includes:

1. Training employees in safe handling of hazardous chemicals.
2. Product labeling.
3. Material safety data sheets (MSDS).
4. A written "Hazards Communication Program."

Not all products used in the dental office are covered by this regulation. For example, drugs administered directly to a patient and chemicals that may be purchased by consumers (such as household bleach) are not included.

Although the dentist is responsible for providing the training, *you* are responsible for learning how to handle these materials in a safe manner—and for routinely following these safety precautions. Remember, this is *not* the place to take shortcuts!

Employee Training

The dentist must provide training (1) for all new employees, (2) whenever a new hazardous material is introduced into the workplace, and (3) whenever procedures for safe handling and emergencies are modified.

This training may be provided in a staff meeting, through continuing education and/or audiovisual materials.

The dentist is also required to maintain records of all training sessions and to keep these records on file for at least 5 years. Employees may be asked to sign this record to verify that training was completed as recorded.

Product Labeling

Dental products that are considered hazardous must come from the manufacturer with a label identifying the chemical(s) and containing an appropriate hazard warning. *Pay attention to these warnings.*

If a hazardous substance is transferred to secondary containers, these must be labeled with either a photocopy of the original label or a new handwritten label including all of the manufacturer's information as stated on the original label (for example, if the substance is purchased in a bulk container and is then put into smaller containers for office use).

The exception to this requirement are those products that are identified as being for "immediate use" by the employee who transfers the product.

However, if the product is transferred for later use, or for use by another employee, the new container must be properly labeled with the hazardous substance information.

This means that disinfection materials that are mixed for use and/or are transferred to smaller spray bottles must be clearly labeled.

X-ray tanks must also be labeled with the information contained on the manufacturer's containers of fixer and developer.

Material Safety Data Sheets

The manufacturer must make available material safety data sheets (MSDS) for products that contain a hazardous chemical.

The dentist is required to maintain, for employee use, an up-to-date file of these sheets.

Take time to study these sheets because they contain valuable data concerning precautions and the safe handling of each product.

Each MSDS sheet must contain the following information:

▼ Identification—chemical and common names.

▼ Hazardous ingredient(s).

▼ Physical and chemical characteristics.

▼ Fire and explosion hazard data.

▼ Health hazard data.

▼ Reactivity data.

▼ Spill and disposal procedures.

▼ Protection information.

▼ Handling and storage precautions, including waste disposal.

▼ Emergency and first-aid procedures.

▼ Date of preparation of the MSDS.

▼ Name and address of the manufacturer or supplier.

Written Hazards Communication Program

The written hazards communication program should include the following elements:

▼ A copy of the current OSHA Hazards Communication Regulation posted in the office where employees can see it.

▼ A list of the hazardous chemicals known to be present in the workplace.

▼ MSDS for these substances.

▼ Instructions for appropriate labeling on all containers.

▼ Documentation of a hazards communication training program for the office.

PRECAUTIONS FOR HANDLING HAZARDOUS MATERIALS

Basic Steps for Hazard Reduction

▼ Keep a minimum of hazardous chemicals in the office.

▼ Read the labels and use only as directed.

▼ Store chemicals only in their original, properly labeled containers.

▼ Store according to the manufacturer's directions.

▼ Keep containers tightly covered.

▼ Avoid mixing chemicals unless consequences are known.

▼ Wear protective eyewear and masks. Masks for this purpose should be those approved by the National Institute for Occupational Safety and Health (NIOSH).

▼ Wash hands immediately after removing gloves. (Some chemicals may penetrate gloves.)

▼ Avoid skin contact with chemicals. Immediately wash skin that has come in contact with chemicals.

▼ To minimize chemical vapor in the air, work with good ventilation.

▼ Do not eat or smoke in areas where chemicals are used.

▼ Keep chemicals away from open flames and heat sources.

▼ Have a fire extinguisher available.

▼ Know and use proper cleanup procedures.

▼ Have neutralizing agents available for strong acids and alkaline solutions.

▼ Dispose of all hazardous chemicals in accordance with MSDS instructions and applicable local, state, and federal regulations.

Specific Precautions

Acid Etch Solutions and Gels

Examples include solutions and gels for acid etch techniques associated with placement of composites, sealants, and orthodontic brackets. (These solutions usually contain phosphoric acid.)

Hazards include acid burns with possible sloughing of tissue, and eye damage.

Do:

▼ Handle acid-soaked material with forceps or gloves.

▼ Clean spills with a commercial acid spill cleanup kit.

▼ Avoid skin or soft tissue contact.

▼ In case of eye or skin contact, rinse with a large amount of running water.

Asbestos

Examples include lining material for casting rings and crucibles, and some soldering investments.

Hazards include respiratory diseases and lung disorders.

Do:

▼ Wear gloves, protective eyewear, and NIOSH-approved mask when handling any asbestos-containing material.

▼ Use asbestos substitute.

Flammable Liquids

Examples include solvents such as acetone and alcohol.

Hazards include fire or explosion.

Do:

▼ Store flammable liquids in tightly covered containers.

▼ Provide adequate ventilation.

▼ Have fire extinguishers available at locations where flammable liquids are used.

▼ Avoid sparks or flames in areas where flammable liquids are used.

Organic Chemicals

Examples include alcohols, ketones, esters, solvents, and monomers such as methylmethacrylate and dimethacrylates.

Hazards include fire, allergic manifestations such as contact dermatitis, possible mutagenesis, irritation to mucous membranes, respiratory problems, nausea, liver and kidney damage, central nervous system depression, headache, drowsiness, and loss of consciousness.

Do:

▼ Avoid skin contact.

▼ Avoid excessive inhalation of vapors.

▼ Work in well-ventilated areas.

▼ Use forceps or gloves when handling contaminated gauze or brushes.

▼ Keep containers tightly closed when not in use.

▼ Store containers on flat, sturdy surfaces.

▼ Clean outside surfaces of containers after use to prevent residual material from contacting the next user.

▼ Use a commercially available, flammable solvent cleanup kit in case of spills.

Gypsum Products

Examples include dental plaster and stone.

Hazards include irritation and impairment of the respiratory system, silicosis, and irritation of the eyes.

Do:

▼ Use plaster and other gypsum products in areas equipped with an exhaust system.

▼ Use protective eyewear and NIOSH-approved mask while handling powders or trimming models.

▼ Minimize exposure to powder during handling.

Formaldehyde

An *example* is a component of solutions used in chemical vapor sterilizers.

Hazards include formaldehyde's property as a human carcinogen (routes of entry are through inhalation, ingestion, and skin contact).

Do:

▼ Use only in well-ventilated areas.

▼ Wear household gloves when handling solutions (such as pouring solutions into the sterilizer).

▼ Follow the manufacturer's directions carefully.

▼ If skin contact occurs, immediately wash with soap and water.

Nitrous Oxide and Oxygen Gases

Examples are nitrous oxide and oxygen.

Hazards include fire and explosion of pressurized gas containers. Also, chronic exposure to nitrous oxide may cause spontaneous abortion and other physical problems.

Do:

▼ Secure gas cylinders to prevent tipping.

▼ Avoid having sparks or flames near flammable gases.

▼ Periodically test the entire system for leaks. This includes tanks, lines, nitrous oxide machine, hoses, and masks.

▼ In the operatory, use a scavenging system to remove excess gases not used by the patient.

▼ When placing the nasal hood on the patient, take care to fit it carefully so that there is no leakage.

▼ Maintain adequate ventilation in the dental office.

Mercury

Examples include use in preparing amalgam for restorations.

Hazards include nausea, loss of appetite, diarrhea, fine tremors, depression, fatigue, increased irritability, headache, insomnia, allergic manifestations, such as contact dermatitis, pneumonitis, and nephritis; dark pigmentation of marginal gingiva, and loosening of teeth.

Do:

▼ Work in well-ventilated spaces.

▼ Avoid direct skin contact with mercury.

▼ Store mercury in unbreakable, tightly sealed containers away from any source of heat.

▼ Salvage scrap amalgam; store under photographic fixer solution in a closed container.

▼ Clean up spilled mercury using appropriate procedures and equipment; do not use a household vacuum cleaner.

▼ Place contaminated disposable materials in polyethylene bags and seal.

Special Mercury Considerations

▼ Mercury may be absorbed directly through skin contact or from the inhalation of mercury vapors. The safe mercury vapor level is 0.05 mg in the breathing zone for 8 hours per day, 40 hours per week. Any office that exceeds this limit is considered to be contaminated.

  Urinalysis may be performed to measure the mercury level in the body. The normal level is about 0.015 mg of mercury per liter of urine. The maximum allowable level according to OSHA is 0.15 mg of mercury per liter.

▼ In preparing amalgam, always use preloaded capsules.

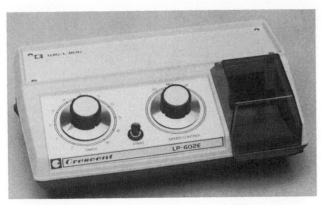

▼ **Figure 8–2**

The protective cover on the amalgamator must be closed during use. This cover, seen to the right of the picture, prevents mercury particles and vapor from escaping during the trituration of amalgam. (Courtesy of Crescent Dental Manufacturing Co, Lyons, IL.)

▼ The amalgamator and capsule should be completely enclosed during trituration (Fig. 8–2). (**Trituration** is the process of mixing mercury and amalgam alloy.)

▼ Reassemble amalgam capsules immediately after dispensing the amalgam mass. The used amalgam capsule is highly contaminated and is a significant source of mercury vapor if left open.

▼ When working with mercury, perform all operations over areas that have impervious and suitably lipped surfaces so as to confine and facilitate recovery of spilled mercury or amalgam.

▼ Clean up any spilled mercury immediately. Droplets may be picked up with narrow-bore tubing connected (via a wash bottle trap) to the low-volume aspirator of the dental unit. Strips of adhesive tape may be used to clean up small spills.

Cast Alloys

Examples include dust and fumes that arise from the melting, grinding, and milling of alloys used to produce cast dental restorations such as full crowns and partial dentures.

Hazards include allergic reactions, and irritation of the eyes and respiratory system.
Do:

▼ Wear gloves, eye protection, and NIOSH-approved mask when casting, polishing, or grinding metallic alloys.

▼ Provide adequate local exhaust ventilation for all operations in casting areas.

▼ Use power suction methods rather than air hoses to remove dust from clothing and to clean machinery.

▼ Dispose of wastes, storage materials, or contaminated clothing in sealed bags.

Photographic Chemicals

Examples include chemicals used to process radiographs.

Hazards include contact dermatitis, and irritation of eyes, nose, throat, and respiratory system from vapors and fine particles of chemicals.
Do:

▼ Use protective eyewear.

▼ Minimize exposure to dry powder during mixing of solution.

▼ Avoid skin contact with photographic processing chemicals and solutions by wearing heavy-duty rubber gloves.

▼ Work in well-ventilated areas.

▼ Clean up spilled chemicals immediately.

▼ If contact occurs, wash off chemicals with large amounts of water and a pH-balanced soap.

▼ Regularly launder clothing that comes in contact with photographic solutions.

▼ Store photographic solutions and chemicals in tightly covered containers in a cool, dark place.

Pickling Solutions

Examples include acids used for pickling a cast restoration.

Hazards include burning of the skin, irritation of the skin and mucous membranes, damage to eyes, and irritation to the respiratory system.
Do:

▼ Wear safety goggles for eye protection.

▼ Use forceps with rubber covers on the tips to hold the object being pickled.

▼ Avoid skin contact by wearing heavy-duty rubber gloves.

▼ Use pickling solutions in well-ventilated areas.

▼ Minimize the formation of air-borne droplets.

▼ Avoid splattering of solution and putting hot objects into the solution.

▼ Store pickling solutions in covered glass containers.

▼ Keep soda lime or a commercial acid spill cleanup kit available in case of spills.

▼ In case of eye or skin contact, rinse with a large amount of running water. Seek medical attention as necessary.

Visible Light-Cured Materials

Examples include visible light-cured restorative materials.

A *hazard* is that repeated exposure to the curing light used with these materials can cause damage to the retina.

Do:

▼ Wear special protective goggles *or* use a special protective shield while using this light (Fig. 8–3).

Additional Precautions for Handling Dental Materials

Changes in the composition of materials may occur for many reasons; however, medical preparations are only of value if they retain their therapeutic activity and identity.

The careful use and handling of medicaments in the dental office is important to ensure that maximum therapeutic activity and reliability are achieved.

The best methods of packaging and storage of any medicinal substance have most likely been

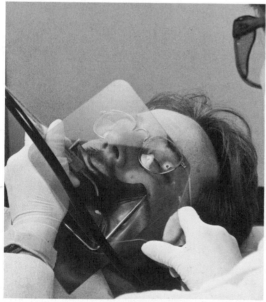

▼ **Figure 8–3**

A protective shield is used with the curing light. As an alternative, the assistant may wear special tinted protective eyewear. (Torres HO, Ehrlich A: Modern Dental Assisting, 4th Ed. Philadelphia, WB Saunders, 1990, p 205.)

determined by the manufacturer. By using their containers and suggestions, therapeutic activity can best be preserved.

Some of the factors present in a dental office that can lead to deterioration of medicaments are discussed subsequently.

Exposure to Air

The effect of direct oxidation from the air may be seen in volatile oils, such as eugenol, resulting in a change of color, viscosity, and odor.

Exposure to Moisture

Moisture can also change the chemical action and composition of drugs such as sodium perborate and aspirin. The drugs should not be used if they show signs of deterioration or chemical change.

Temperature Changes

Heat causes an increase in the rate of reaction and thus increases the rate of deterioration. It also increases the loss of volatile substances such as phenol, eugenol, and eucalyptol or of solvents such as chloroform and alcohol.

Some antibiotics and other pharmaceuticals require refrigerated storage. Follow the manufacturer's instructions carefully.

Freezing affects substances such as local anesthetic solution and radiography processing solution. When shipped in cold weather, these materials should be properly protected to prevent freezing.

Exposure to Light

Light is the prime factor in the deterioration of sodium hypochlorite (household bleach), epinephrine, and hydrogen peroxide. Change in color is one of the most common signs of deterioration.

A basic "safe" policy for the storage of dental medications and materials is to keep them in a dry, cool, dark place where they are not exposed to direct sunlight.

Caution should always be taken to note the expiration date that may be listed on medications. Also, fresh supplies should always be stocked behind the current inventory so that the oldest product is used first.

MEDICAL WASTE MANAGEMENT

In areas where waste disposal is *not* presently regulated by other laws, it is still necessary to comply with the OSHA regulations that cover waste disposal within the dental office. Once the waste leaves the office, it is regulated by the federal Environmental Protection Agency (EPA) and by state and local law.

When covered by more than one regulation, the dentist must comply with the strictest law. It is the responsibility of the dentist to be aware of and comply with those laws that apply to the practice.

Identifying Medical Waste

In the dental office, the following items are considered to be medical waste:

▼ Sharps (injection needles, suture needles, scalpel blades, and dental burs).

▼ Body tissues and extracted teeth.

▼ Blood and blood-soaked items such as bloody cotton rolls and gauze squares.

Under most regulations, the manner of disposal is determined by the amount (weight) of infectious materials to be disposed of. The "average" dentist produces about 1 pound of needles and 1 pound of blood-soaked articles in a 20-day work month.

This places the "average" dental practice in the category of being a small producer of infectious waste, and disposal is regulated accordingly.

The law requires that the dentist maintain records as to the final disposal of this medical waste. This includes documentation as to how, when, and where it was disposed of.

Procedure
SHARPS DISPOSAL

1. Sharps must be discarded into a commercial, puncture-resistant, rigid-sided container.
   These containers must be positioned as close as possible to the point of use.

2. Discard sharps into the container in the operatory, before the soiled instruments are returned to the sterilization area.

3. When the container is full, but not overfilled, it is sealed and discarded in the manner required by law.
   This may be through an approved health care disposal agent or, where permitted, mailed to the manufacturer of the container.

Procedure
MEDICAL WASTE DISPOSAL

1. Handle medical waste only while gloved. Also, organize cleanup to minimize handling of medical waste.

2. As discarded immediately after use, or during cleanup, separate medical waste from noninfectious waste.

3. Discard medical waste into a leak-resistant package that is impervious to moisture.
   The bag or container must be strong enough to prevent tearing or breaking under normal handling conditions.
   Do not overfill the container.
   The container must be clearly labeled *Medical Waste* or display the universal biohazard symbol (Fig. 8–4).

4. Seal the bag or container to prevent leakage during shipping.

5. Prior to shipping, store the containers in a safe place to maintain their integrity and to control odor.

Biohazard

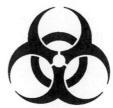

Figure 8–4 The international biohazard label must appear on all containers of hazardous waste.

Procedure
NONINFECTIOUS WASTE DISPOSAL

1. Handle waste products only while gloved.

2. Place noninfectious waste into a container with a plastic liner.
   Noninfectious items are those that are *not* soaked with blood and/or saliva (for example, papers for mixing pads, plastic patient drape.

3. Discard noninfectious waste as regular "trash."

◤ EXERCISES

1. Local anesthetic solution is affected by _____ .

   a. air
   b. freezing
   c. light
   d. b and c

2. OSHA establishes and enforces regulations related to _____
   _____ .

   a. employee safety in the workplace
   b. environmental concerns
   c. patient safety and well-being
   d. a, b, and c

3. Chronic exposure to nitrous oxide may cause _____ .

   a. fine tremors
   b. loosening of teeth
   c. spontaneous abortion
   d. a and c

4. The used amalgam capsule is _____ .

   a. discarded as medical waste
   b. reassembled immediately after dispensing the amalgam mass
   c. reassembled just before returning the tray to the sterilization center
   d. a and c

5. Acetone and alcohol _____ .

   a. are flammable liquids
   b. require adequate ventilation
   c. should be stored in tightly covered containers
   d. a, b, and c

6. When a hazardous substance is transferred to a secondary container, it
   _____ .

   a. does not need to be labeled if it is for immediate use by the employee
      who transfers the product
   b. must always be labeled with a photocopy of the original label
   c. must be properly labeled if transferred for future use
   d. a and c

7. In case of skin contact with the acid etch solutions and gels, the area should
   be _____ .

   a. covered with baking soda
   b. rinsed with a large amount of running water
   c. treated with a commercial acid spill kit
   d. b or c

8. Extracted teeth are discarded as _____ .

   a. medical waste
   b. noninfectious waste
   c. sharps

9. When working with visible light-cured materials, it is necessary to _____.

    a. look away from the light
    b. use a special protective shield
    c. wear special protective goggles
    d. b or c

10. Oxidation resulting from exposure to ___Air___ will cause deterioration in volatile oils such as eugenol.

    a. air
    b. heat
    c. light
    d. moisture

11. Once waste leaves the office it is regulated by _____.

    a. EPA
    b. OSHA
    c. state or local law
    d. a or c

12. Scrap amalgam should be stored under _____ in a closed container.

    a. photographic developer solution
    b. photographic fixer solution
    c. sodium hypochlorite
    d. a, b, or c

13. The _____ deals with issues of concern to the environment and public safety.

    a. ADA
    b. CDC
    c. EPA
    d. OSHA

14. According to OSHA guidelines, the receptionist in a dental office is classified as having a/an ___(b)___ occupational position.

    a. at risk
    b. low risk

15. A needle-stick injury ___d___.

    a. is considered to be an exposure incident
    b. is not reported if the employee is vaccinated
    c. must be reported to the dentist immediately
    d. a and c

16. When there are state federal regulations covering a practice activity, the dentist must comply with _____.

    a. the federal regulations
    b. the state regulations
    c. whichever regulations are most stringent

17. A chairside assistant who is at risk for exposure to hepatitis B _____.

    a. may work during the 2- to 6-month period it takes to complete the necessary vaccine injections

    b. must be offered hepatitis B vaccination free of charge

    c. must maintain a vaccination record

    d. a, b, and c

18. When mixing gypsum powder or trimming models, a/an _____ _____ should be worn.

    a. OSHA-approved mask

    b. NIOSH-approved mask

    c. protective eyewear

    d. b and c

19. Sharps are discarded _____.

    a. in the operatory

    b. when the soiled instruments are returned to the sterilization area

20. Material safety data sheets are provided by the _____.

    a. ADA

    b. EPA

    c. manufacturer

    d. MSDS

21. According to OSHA guidelines, staff members who regularly take radiographs and sterilize instruments are considered to be occupationally _____.

    a. at risk

    b. low risk

22. Sharps are discarded in a _____.

    a. puncture-resistant, rigid-sided container

    b. sealed plastic bag

    c. sterile container

    d. a and c

23. Discarded dental burs are classified as _____.

    a. medical waste

    b. noninfectious waste

    c. sharps

24. The safe mercury vapor level is _____ mg in the breathing zone for 8 hours per day, 40 hours per week.

    a. 0.05

    b. 0.50

    c. 1.00

    d. none of the above

25. The dentist is required to provide hazardous material training _____.

    a. for new employees

    b. whenever a new hazardous material is introduced into the workplace

    c. whenever procedures for safe handling and emergencies are modified

    d. a, b, and c

9 Emergencies in the Dental Office

▼ LEARNING OBJECTIVES

The student will be able to:

1. Describe the types of emergencies that might be encountered in a dental office.

2. Describe the basic staff qualifications for managing medical emergencies.

3. Describe types of supplies that might be found in a minimal emergency kit.

4. Differentiate between administering oxygen and the use of positive-pressure ventilation.

5. State the six basic emergency steps to be taken until help arrives.

6. Describe the emergency treatment for anaphylactic shock, angina pectoris, diabetic acidosis, insulin shock, and an epileptic seizure.

7. List the five classifications of fractured teeth and describe the treatment for evulsed teeth.

8. Demonstrate the treatment for syncope, hyperventilation, and postural hypotension when the patient feels faint.

9. Demonstrate and describe the steps to be taken in treating a needle-stick injury.

OVERVIEW OF EMERGENCIES IN THE DENTAL OFFICE

The types of emergencies that may be encountered in the dental office include a full variety of medical emergencies, plus dental emergencies such as fractured teeth.

A medical emergency could arise for a patient. It is also possible that a member of the dental staff might be in need of emergency aid. In either situation, the dentist and staff must be capable of providing prompt and appropriate care.

EMERGENCY PREPAREDNESS

Emergency preparedness is the key to providing emergency care smoothly, efficiently, and calmly even in a highly stressful situation. Without this, there is the danger of frightening the patient and compounding the seriousness of the situation.

The following preparedness steps must be practiced on a routine basis before there is an emergency situation.

Emergency Information

Emergency information must be posted next to each telephone in the office. This includes local emergency numbers (usually 911) for emergency medical services (EMS) and police and fire departments. In addition, it is important to post the names and telephone numbers of at least two nearby physicians.

Basic Staff Qualifications

All dental personnel are expected to obtain and maintain a current certificate in **cardiopulmonary resuscitation (CPR), basic first aid**.

Staff members must also be proficient in the **Heimlich maneuver** to aid a choking victim.

Establishing an Emergency Routine

The dentist must establish a clearly documented emergency routine. The documentation should include a description of the location and use of the emergency kits and supplies.

It should also contain a description of the role of each staff member in an emergency.

Practicing the Emergency Routine

The emergency routine must be practiced regularly (at least twice a year), so that everyone is certain of his or her role in any type of emergency.

These practice sessions should include cross-training so that staff members can assist each other as needed.

Vital Signs Chap 14

Taking and recording vital signs is an important part of emergency preparedness. This is discussed in Chapter 14, "The Dental Examination."

Patient Observation

Ongoing observation of the patient's condition (for all patients) is an important part of emergency preparedness.

While the dentist is concentrating on the dental treatment, the assistant must be alert to changes in the patient's condition and look for any sudden change in physical appearance such as indications of pain, distress, sweating, pallor, loss of consciousness, or difficulty in breathing.

EMERGENCY MEDICAL SUPPLIES

Emergency medical supplies are organized as a portable tray or kit. These kits are stored where they are readily available from any area of the office. There may be one kit in central supply, or there may be an emergency kit in each operatory.

The dentist decides which drugs are included in the emergency kit (Fig. 9–1). Staff members should learn the use of each drug and know how to prepare it for administration. (Most injectable emergency drugs are supplied in prefilled syringes.)

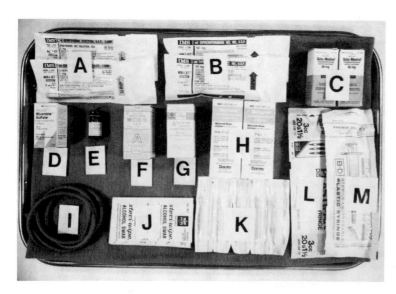

▼ **Figure 9–1**

Sample emergency drug and equipment tray for use in the dental office. *A,* Epinephrine; *B,* diphenhydramine; *C,* methylprednisolone; *D,* mephentermine; *E,* nitroglycerin; *F,* morphine; *G,* atropine; *H,* metaproterenol; *I,* tourniquet; *J,* alcohol sponges; *K,* needles; *L,* 3-ml syringe; *M,* 5-ml syringe. (From McCarthy FM: Medical Emergencies in Dentistry. Philadelphia, WB Saunders, 1982, p 280.)

The drugs in the emergency kit have an expiration date. These dates must be reviewed and the drugs updated on a regular basis. Also, if any supplies have been used, they must be replaced promptly. A member of the office staff may be assigned the responsibility of keeping these drugs up-to-date and in adequate supply.

Minimal Emergency Kit

The following are the minimum emergency drugs and devices for a dental office as recommended by McCarthy:*

1. Oxygen source.
2. Positive-pressure ventilation capability.
3. Aromatic ammonia ampules (for use in syncope).
4. Preloaded syringes of epinephrine (for use in severe allergic reactions).
5. Nitroglycerin tablets (for use in case of angina pectoris).
6. Tourniquets (if needed for intravenous injections).
7. Sugar packets or tablets (for treatment of hypoglycemia).
8. Padded tongue blade (for use in epileptic seizures).

Oxygen

One hundred percent oxygen (O_2) is an excellent agent for the resuscitation of a patient who is unconscious but still breathing.

After a few minutes on 100 percent oxygen, a patient should regain consciousness and begin to feel relaxed, less apprehensive, and able to react normally to his surroundings.

If the dentist administers nitrous oxide–oxygen relative analgesia, these units provide a ready source of oxygen for emergency use (Fig. 9–2).

Sterile masks in adult and child sizes should be stored in each operatory so that a clean mask for the emergency patient can be placed quickly on the oxygen unit.

If these units are not available, portable units with *two* tanks of oxygen may be stored conveniently near the dental operatories. The unit can be rolled into a particular dental operatory in a medical emergency.

* Adapted from McCarthy F: Essentials of Safe Dentistry for the Medically Compromised Patient. Philadelphia, WB Saunders, 1989.

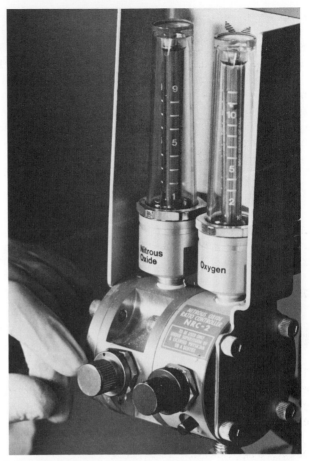

▼ **Figure 9–2**

The nitrous oxide–oxygen unit is a source of oxygen for emergency use. (Torres HO, Ehrlich A: Modern Dental Assisting, 4th Ed. Philadelphia, WB Saunders, 1990, p 282.)

Note: The oxygen cylinder (tank) is green. An "E" size tank provides approximately 78 liters of oxygen per minute for half an hour. A reserve tank of oxygen should also be available for the treatment of emergency situations (Fig. 9–3).

Positive-Pressure Ventilation

Positive-pressure ventilation is used to force air into the lungs of the patient who is not breathing. This may be accomplished with an Ambu bag, such as the one shown in Figure 9–4.

The Ambu bag without an oxygen connection is used to force atmospheric air into the lungs. An Ambu bag connected to an oxygen source is used to force oxygen enriched air into the lungs.

To use the Ambu bag, place the mask firmly over the patient's mouth, chin, and nose to make a tight seal. Stabilize the mask with the thumb and forefinger of the hand. With the other hand, squeeze the self-inflating bag at a rate of once

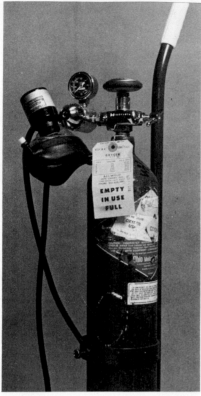

▼ Figure 9-3

Emergency oxygen supply. Shown here is a green E-cylinder of oxygen. (From McCarthy FM: Medical Emergencies in Dentistry. Philadelphia, WB Saunders, 1982, p 282.)

every 5 seconds for an adult and once every 3 seconds for a child.

If nitrous oxide–oxygen units are available, the oxygen and reservoir bag from these units may be used for positive-pressure ventilation with 100 percent oxygen. However, oxygen should be administered in this manner only by someone with specialized training (Fig. 9-4).

BASIC EMERGENCY STEPS

Whenever there is a medical emergency in the practice, no matter how seemingly minor, the dentist must be notified immediately. Once on the scene, the dentist takes control of the situation and gives directions for the patient's care.

Unless the nature of the emergency is clearly defined, the following are the appropriate first-response steps to take until the dentist or other help arrives:

1. Place the patient in a supine position.
2. Determine that the patient has an open airway.
3. Determine the presence or absence of spontaneous breathing.
4. Administer oxygen.

5. Monitor vital signs.
6. Be prepared to assist in further emergency treatment.

MEDICAL EMERGENCIES

Syncope

Syncope, also known as *fainting*, is a temporary loss of consciousness due to a temporary insufficient blood supply to the brain.

This is the most common medical emergency encountered in the dental office. Although it may seem like a minor problem, the symptoms of syncope may also indicate a larger emergency. In addition to prompt response, it is important to be prepared in case additional treatment is required.

Symptoms

The patient becomes pale, perspires and feels distressed, weak, dizzy, and nauseated.

Procedure

RESPONDING TO A SYNCOPE EMERGENCY

1. Lower the patient in the dental chair to a supine position with the feet elevated higher than the head. (This causes the blood to flow away from the stomach and toward the brain.)

2. Fracture an ampule of spirits of ammonia in a gauze square and waft this gently under the patient's nostrils. (The strong odor causes the patient to inhale quickly and thus receive additional oxygen.)
   Note: Do not hold the spirits of ammonia directly under the nostrils, because the ammonia vapors may irritate the membranes of the nasal passages.

3. Administer oxygen if necessary.

4. Record vital signs.
   Note: The patient usually regains consciousness within 1 or 2 minutes.

Hyperventilation

In the dental office, a patient who is nervous about his treatment may hyperventilate. (**Hyperventilation** is an increase in the rate or depth of

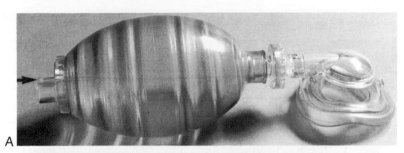

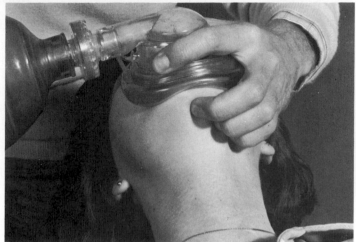

▼ **Figure 9-4**

Devices for positive-pressure ventilation. *A.* Bag-valve-mask device. The self-inflating bag enables the rescuer to deliver atmospheric air to the victim. Oxygen-enriched air may be administered by attaching the oxygen tube to the opening at the back of the bag device. (*See arrow to left of photo.*) *B.* Proper use of the bag-valve-mask device requires the rescuer to maintain head tilt and an air-tight seal of the mask with only one hand. (From McCarthy FM: Medical Emergencies in Dentistry. Philadelphia, WB Saunders, 1982, p 283.)

breathing that results in a deficit of carbon dioxide in the blood.)

Symptoms

The patient may appear nervous or anxious; although the patient may not be aware of it, he increasingly breathes deeper and faster.

The patient may complain of a feeling of suffocation, tightness in the chest, and dizziness.

Procedure

RESPONDING TO A PATIENT WHO IS HYPERVENTILATING

1. Place the patient in a comfortable upright position.

2. Do *not* administer oxygen to this patient.

3. The dentist then instructs the patient to inhale and hold the breath for several seconds before exhaling. (This increases the carbon dioxide level.)
Alternative: Give the patient a paper bag and instruct him to breathe in and out of the bag. The bag is not forced over the patient's face, and a plastic bag is never used for this purpose.

Postural Hypotension

Postural, or *orthostatic*, hypotension may occur when the patient has been in a supine position in the dental chair for a long time (for example, after 2 or more hours of a long appointment).

Symptoms

An abrupt change in position, such as suddenly being moved into an upright position, may cause lightheadedness and fainting.

To avoid such adverse reactions, all patients should always be positioned upright very slowly.

Procedure

RESPONDING TO THE PATIENT WHO FEELS FAINT

1. Immediately reposition the patient in the supine position.

2. After a few minutes, slowly return the patient to an upright position.

3. If the patient still feels dizzy and faint, immediately lower him to the supine position once again.

4. Administer oxygen if necessary.

Procedure

RESPONDING TO THE PATIENT WHO HAS LOST CONSCIOUSNESS

1. Position patient in supine position.
2. If patient does not revive after assuming the supine position, tilt his head back (chin up) and check his breathing.
3. If breathing is not normal, do a triple airway check:
   Clear the oral cavity.
   Clear the airway.
   Check for breathing.
4. Administer oxygen.
5. Check blood pressure. The patient's physician should be advised if the patient has had difficulty regaining normal vital signs.

Allergic Reactions

The patient may suffer an allergic reaction to local anesthetic solution or the medications used in dental treatment.

A severe allergic reaction, known as **anaphylactic shock**, is a life-threatening crisis that requires *immediate* response.

Procedure

RESPONDING TO THE PATIENT WHO IS HAVING AN ALLERGIC REACTION

1. Place the patient in a supine position and administer oxygen.
2. The dentist administers epinephrine by injection. (Prepared syringes should be included in the emergency kit.)
   Epinephrine, a vasopressor with an antihistamine action, is the drug used most frequently in the treatment of anaphylactic shock. (Epinephrine is discussed in Chapter 18, "Pharmacology and Pain Control.")
3. Be prepared to perform CPR or other emergency treatment for an obstructed airway.

Symptoms

The patient may exhibit any number of symptoms including the signs of shock, large itching hives, and localized swelling in the airway and larynx, which may result in respiratory distress.

Heart Disease

Symptoms

Angina pectoris is characterized by episodes of spasmodic, choking, or suffocating chest pain.

Nitroglycerin, which is a vasodilator, may be used to relieve an angina attack. This is administered by placing a tablet under the tongue. Here it is rapidly absorbed into the blood, and the effects should be evident within 90 seconds.

A **myocardial infarction**, commonly known as a *heart attack*, is also characterized by severe compressing, squeezing, chest pain, which is *not* relieved by nitroglycerin.

Both conditions are serious, and both require immediate treatment by qualified medical personnel.

Procedure

RESPONDING TO THE PATIENT EXPERIENCING CARDIAC SYMPTOMS

1. Keep the patient as calm, quiet, and comfortable as possible. (The patient will probably be most comfortable in a seated position.)
2. The dentist may administer oxygen.
3. The dentist may administer nitroglycerin.
4. Be prepared for complications including cardiac arrest.

Diabetes Mellitus

In the diabetic patient, medical complications may occur if the prescribed routine for diabetes is not followed.

Symptoms

Diabetic acidosis and insulin shock are two of the most serious complications.

Diabetic acidosis, also known as *hyperglycemic coma*, occurs because of an abnormally increased level of sugar in the blood. This may occur because the patient has eaten too much sugar-containing food, has not taken enough insulin, or has an infection.

Diabetic acidosis can lead to convulsions, coma, and death. The clinical signs of diabetic acidosis include:

▼ Acetone breath (smelling like fruit).

▼ Warm, dry skin and dry mouth.

▼ Rapid and weak pulse.

▼ Air hunger, rapid deep breathing.

▼ Unresponsiveness to questioning.

▼ Unconsciousness.

Insulin shock, also known as *hypoglycemia*, is a condition in which a high level of insulin causes a decrease in blood sugar (glucose). This decreases the glucose supply to the brain, and unconsciousness may follow. The patient's symptoms include:

▼ Clammy skin.

▼ Sweating.

▼ Vertigo (dizziness).

▼ Confusion.

Procedure

RESPONDING TO THE PATIENT WITH A DIABETIC EMERGENCY

1. If the patient is conscious, ask when he ate last and whether he has taken his insulin.

2. In **diabetic acidosis,** the patient has probably eaten but has not taken his insulin.

   This patient needs insulin and other medical care immediately.

3. When **insulin shock** is present, the patient has probably taken his insulin but has not eaten an adequate meal.

   The patient should be offered sugar, candy, orange juice, ginger ale, or other sugar-containing foods, and a physician should be called immediately.

4. If the patient is unconscious and you are not sure whether he is suffering from diabetic coma or insulin shock, place a sugar cube under his tongue.

   If the condition is insulin shock, there will be less chance of brain cell damage.

Epilepsy

Symptoms

Epileptic seizures can be classified into two general types: petit mal and grand mal.

Petit mal seizures are mild and are brief in duration, sometimes lasting only a few seconds. A patient having a petit mal seizure may seem merely to be staring into space.

Grand mal seizures are severe, usually with loss of consciousness followed by violent contractions of the muscles caused by abnormal stimulation to the brain cells controlling the muscular system. These seizures may last several minutes.

Overfatigue and anxiety increase the possibility of a seizure. To avoid this, the epileptic patient should be scheduled for treatment early in the day.

Procedure

RESPONDING TO THE PATIENT WHO IS HAVING A SEIZURE

1. Protect the patient from self-injury. The patient may be moved out of the dental chair and onto the floor.

2. If time, place a heavily padded tongue depressor or folded towel between the patient's teeth so that he does not bite his tongue. (Never put the fingers in the patient's mouth; during the seizure the patient's jaw closes with great force.)

3. Attempt to maintain a free airway for the patient, but do *not* put your fingers in the patient's mouth.

4. As he regains consciousness, turn the patient on one side so that any secretions are not aspirated into the lungs.

5. Do not give the patient anything to eat or drink until he is fully alert.

6. Allow the patient to rest. Keep him warm and do not ask questions.

CARE OF A NEEDLE-STICK INJURY

Any needle-stick injury, puncture, and/or cut caused by a soiled needle or instrument is potentially infectious and very serious.

All needle sticks and puncture wounds should receive the following immediate first-aid treatment.

Procedure

FIRST AID FOR A NEEDLE-STICK INJURY

1. Squeeze the wound to cause it to bleed.

2. Clean the wound under running tap water.

3. Disinfect the wound with a recommended skin disinfectant.

4. Report the injury to the dentist or supervisor immediately so that additional care and follow-up may be provided.

5. Complete appropriate exposure incident reports. (These are discussed in Chapter 8.)

DENTAL EMERGENCIES

Hemorrhage

During dental treatment, particularly oral surgery, the tissues of the oral cavity may be injured causing hemorrhage (excessive bleeding). The control of this bleeding is discussed in Chapter 30, "Oral Surgery."

Injuries to the Teeth and Mouth

Accidents involving injuries to the mouth (when the patient is brought to the dental office) may involve teeth that are evulsed, extruded, or fractured (Fig. 9–5).

Evulsed, also known as *avulsed*, means torn away or knocked out by force. **Extruded** means forced forward or outward. **Fractured** means broken.

Such injuries may be accompanied by lacerations (cuts) of the lips, gingiva, or cheeks and damage to the alveolar bone.

These patients are in pain and should be seen as soon as possible even if this means having to reschedule a waiting patient. (Even in the event of an emergency, if the patient is a child, it is necessary to receive consent from the parent or guardian.)

Examination of Injured Teeth

Histories

If this is a new patient, a medical history and other background information must be gathered. If this is a returning patient, this information should be updated (see Chapter 14, "The Dental Examination.")

The dentist also needs information concerning the accident, including how long ago it occurred. (Time is essential in treating an injured tooth.)

Radiographs

As ordered by the dentist, radiographs of the injured tooth or teeth are exposed and processed immediately on the patient's arrival.

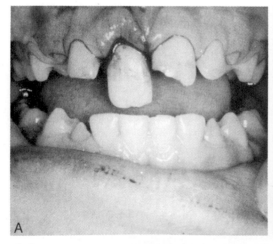 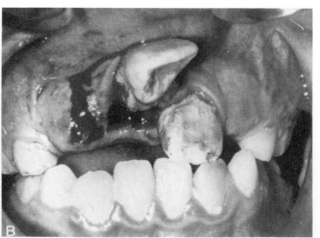

▼ Figure 9–5

Injured teeth. *A.* An extruded tooth in which the tooth is partially dislocated from its socket. *B.* A tooth that is displaced laterally from its socket. (From Pinkham JR: Pediatric Dentistry: Infancy Through Adolescence. Philadelphia, WB Saunders, 1988, p 173.)

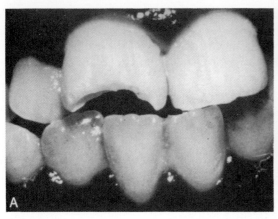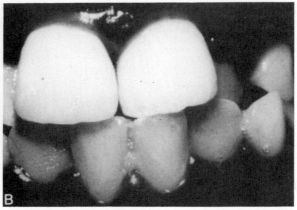

▼ Figure 9-6

A simple fracture and repair. *A.* A fractured permanent anterior tooth. *B.* The same tooth repaired using an acid-etch composite restoration. (From Pinkham JR: Pediatric Dentistry: Infancy Through Adolescence. Philadelphia, WB Saunders, 1988, p 411.)

Clinical Examination

The injured tooth or teeth are examined using percussion (tapping) and thermal and pulp testing (vitalometer). These tests are discussed in Chapter 29, "Endodontics."

Evulsed Teeth

The person who calls the office regarding an emergency involving an evulsed tooth is advised to do the following:

1. Attempt to find the tooth.
2. Wrap the tooth in a clean cloth moistened with water. Some dentists recommend a mild saline (salt) solution or milk as an alternative.
3. Bring the patient to the office *immediately.*
4. When the patient arrives, he is escorted immediately into an operatory and the dentist is informed of his arrival.
5. The dentist checks the evulsed tooth to see if it can be reimplanted (put back) into the original socket and stabilized with a splint. (The lapse of time from evulsion of a tooth to reimplantation into its socket should be no more than 30 minutes.)
6. If the tooth can be saved, it is repositioned in the arch and splinted and/or cemented into place.

Classification of Fractured Teeth

▼ **Class 1**. Simple fracture of the enamel of the crown (Fig. 9-6).

▼ **Class 2**. Extensive fracture of the enamel and dentin, including injury to the pulp.

▼ **Class 3**. Extensive fracture of the crown, exposing the pulp of the tooth.

▼ **Class 4**. Traumatized tooth, nonvital.

▼ **Class 5**. Tooth lost owing to trauma (injury).

Treatment of Fractured Teeth

The treatment or lack of treatment of a fracture is dictated by the extent of the injury.

Class 1. A Class 1 fracture may be smoothed with a sandpaper disc and left alone. Another option is to restore the tooth with a composite restoration.

In either case, the patient is advised to treat the tooth carefully for several days and is instructed to report to the office immediately if the fractured tooth becomes sensitive.

Class 2. A larger Class 2 fracture may be treated with a palliative (soothing) substance and a temporary crown. Later when it is obvious that the pulp is not permanently damaged, the tooth may be restored with a full permanent crown.

Class 3. Class 3 fractures, with more extensive pulpal involvement may be treated by placing calcium hydroxide and zinc oxide–eugenol (ZOE) cement or intermediary restorative material (IRM) over the tooth within a celluloid or stainless steel crown form.

The vitality of the pulp is checked in 6 to 8 weeks. If the pulp has recovered, the fractured tooth may be restored.

If the pulp has not recovered, endodontic treatment will be necessary. This is discussed in Chapter 29, "Endodontics."

▼ EXERCISES

1. _____(a)_____ is characterized by episodes of spasmodic, choking, or suffocating chest pain.

   a. Angina pectoris
   b. Diabetic acidosis
   c. Hypoglycemia
   d. Myocardial infarction

2. During treatment, the assistant should watch the patient for indications of ____(d)____.

   a. difficulty breathing
   b. loss of consciousness
   c. pain
   d. a, b, or c

3. A needle-stick injury should be ____(c)____.

   a. bandaged immediately
   b. ignored
   c. squeezed to make the wound bleed

4. A Class _____ fracture involves fracture of the crown and injury to the pulp.

   a. 1
   b. 2
   c. 3
   d. 4

5. The oxygen cylinder tank is ____green____.

   a. blue
   b. green

6. _____(d)_____ is commonly called fainting.

   a. Anoxia
   b. Cerebrovascular accident
   c. Hyperventilation
   d. Syncope

7. The time lapse for reimplanting an evulsed tooth is no more than _____ minutes.

   a. 15
   b. 30
   c. 45
   d. 60

8. An _____(d)_____ tooth has been completely torn out of the mouth.

   a. avulsed
   b. evulsed
   c. extruded
   d. a or b

9. If the diabetic patient's breath smells like fruit, he is probably suffering from
   (b) diabetic acidosis

   a. anaphylaxis
   b. diabetic acidosis
   c. insulin shock
   d. petit mal seizure

10. The epileptic patient should be scheduled for dental treatment _____ .

    a. early in the day
    b. immediately after eating
    c. later in the day
    d. time of day is not important

11. Positive-pressure ventilation is used with the patient who _____ _____ .

    a. complains of chest pain
    b. has fainted
    c. is not breathing
    d. a and b

12. A patient who is nervous about his treatment may _____*(a)*_____ .

    a. hyperventilate
    b. hypoventilate

13. _____*(c)*_____ is frequently used to treat anaphylaxis.

    a. Atropine
    b. Dextrose
    c. Epinephrine
    d. Nitroglycerin

14. All dental staff members are expected to know _____*(d)*_____ .

    a. basic first aid
    b. cardiopulmonary resuscitation
    c. the Heimlich maneuver
    d. a, b, and c

15. When a patient regains consciousness after a seizure, _____*(a)*_____ .

    a. give him nothing to eat or drink until he is fully alert
    b. give him sugar water drink
    c. insist that he walk around to improve his circulation
    d. a and c

16. Emergency information to be posted by the telephone includes phone numbers for _____*(d)*_____ .

    a. local emergency medical response
    b. police and fire
    c. two nearby physicians
    d. a, b, and c

17. A patient may be predisposed to postural hypotension as a result of _____ _d_ .

    a. long appointments
    b. sudden upright position
    c. supine position for long periods
    d. a, b, and c

18. _____ _c_ _____ is administered as treatment for angina pectoris.

    a. Glucose
    b. Morphine
    c. Nitroglycerin
    d. Sublingual sugar

19. A Class 2 fracture is treated with _____.

    a. a soothing substance
    b. a temporary crown
    c. endodontic treatment
    d. a and b

20. A padded tongue blade is used for the patient who is experiencing _____ _b_ _____ .

    a. angina
    b. a seizure
    c. insulin shock
    d. syncope

21. A puncture wound _____ _d_ _____ .

    a. is potentially very serious
    b. must be reported to the dentist or supervisor
    c. should be squeezed to make it bleed
    d. a, b, and c

22. The Ambu bag is squeezed at the rate of once every _5_ _____ seconds for an adult.

    a. 3
    b. 4
    c. 5
    d. 10

23. Emergency kit supplies should be renewed and updated _____ _(c)_ .

    a. after each use
    b. on a regular basis
    c. a and b

24. Sugar may be administered to increase the level of glucose in the blood of the ___insulin shock___ patient.

    a. diabetic acidosis coma.
    b. epileptic
    c. insulin shock   hypoglycemia
    d. hypotensive

25. If the patient becomes pale, perspires, and feels dizzy, he is probably suffering from ___*Syncope*___ .

    a. anaphylaxis
    b. hyperventilation
    c. syncope
    d. b or c

▼ Criterion Sheet 9–1

Student's Name _____

Procedure: *PROVIDING EMERGENCY CARE FOR A PATIENT WITH SYNCOPE*

Performance Objective:

The student will demonstrate emergency care for a patient in a state of syncope in the dental chair.

Another student will play the patient. The patient is breathing and has no visible signs of injury or distress.

SE = Student evaluation **IE** = Instructor evaluation	**C** = Criterion met **X** = Criterion not met	**SE**	**IE**
Instrumentation: First-aid kit, spirits of ammonia ampule, and gauze sponges			
1. Asked patient, "Are you all right?" The patient did not respond.			
2. Called for help.			
3. Placed patient in supine position with his head slightly lower than his feet.			
4. Crushed ammonia ampule and wafted near patient's nostrils.			
5. Reassured patient as he regained consciousness.			
Comments:			

▼ **Criterion Sheet 9–2**

Student's Name _____

Procedure: *PROVIDING EMERGENCY CARE FOR A PATIENT WITH HYPERVENTILATION*

Performance Objective:

The student will demonstrate emergency care for a patient who is hyperventilating. Another student will play the patient. The patient is breathing rapidly and feels faint.

	SE	IE
SE = Student evaluation **IE** = Instructor evaluation **C** = Criterion met **X** = Criterion not met		
Instrumentation: First-aid kit and paper bag		
1. Reassured patient.		
2. Called for help.		
3. Placed patient in upright position.		
4. Asked patient to inhale and hold the breath for several seconds. Patient was unable to cooperate.		
5. Instructed patient to breathe in and out of paper bag until the symptoms were gone.		
Comments:		

10 The Dental Operatory

▼ LEARNING OBJECTIVES

The student will be able to:

1. Identify the major pieces of equipment found in the dental operatory.
2. Describe the use and care for each of these pieces of equipment.
3. Describe the morning and evening routines for operatory care.
4. Describe the correct seated position of the operator and assistant at chairside.
5. Demonstrate seating the patient, placing the patient in the supine position, and restoring the patient to an upright position.
6. Demonstrate operatory care between patients to ensure infection control.

OVERVIEW OF THE DENTAL OPERATORY

Dental operatories, also referred to as *treatment rooms*, are the dynamic areas of the dental office. It is here that all dental procedures are performed.

Most dental offices include two or more identically equipped operatories. The layout of these operatories and placement of the equipment, accessories, and supplies in them are important in maximizing efficiency and maintaining a smooth patient flow throughout the day.

DENTAL OPERATORY EQUIPMENT

Each operatory contains the same essential equipment: mobile and/or fixed cabinets with sinks, a lounge-type dental chair, two operating stools, a dental unit (or units), an operating light, an x-ray unit, and a view box (Figs. 10–1 and 10–2).

Having the equipment in the same location in each operatory makes it easier for the dental team to go back and forth from one operatory to another during patient care.

Dental Chair

The contour of the lounge-type dental chair is designed to support the patient's body comfortably at the head, shoulders, buttocks, and knees and to accommodate a wide range of body sizes (Fig. 10–3).

The arms of the chair support the patient's arms and elbows without strain. For greater ease in seating the patient, one arm of the chair should be raised out of the way and repositioned after the patient is seated.

Most chairs have an adjustable and removable doughnut-shaped headrest. To provide greater flexibility of positioning, the patient is asked to move his head within the headrest.

Controls placed at the base or side of the chair make it possible to raise and lower the overall height of the chair. The dental chair may be swiveled from side to side on its base by adjusting levers on the base.

The **back rest control, foot rest control**, and **automatic positioning and return control**

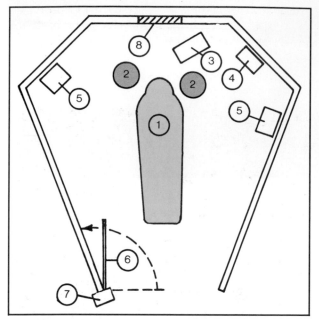

▼ **Figure 10-1**

Dental operatory diagram showing the basic equipment. *1,* Dental chair/patient; *2,* stools—dentist, to right of patient, assistant to left; *3,* mobile unit cart; *4,* x-ray unit (wall mount); *5,* sinks; *6,* lead barrier; *7,* control panel of x-ray unit (outside of operatory); *8,* view box (recessed wall mount). (Torres HO, Ehrlich A: Modern Dental Assisting, 4th Ed. Philadelphia, WB Saunders, 1990, p 325.)

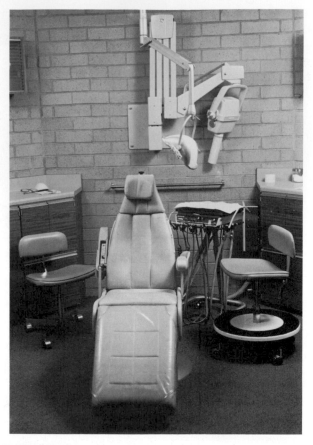

▼ **Figure 10-2**

Fully equipped dental operatory with a mobile unit prepared to receive the dental patient. (Torres HO, Ehrlich A: Modern Dental Assisting, 4th Ed. Philadelphia, WB Saunders, 1990, p 340.)

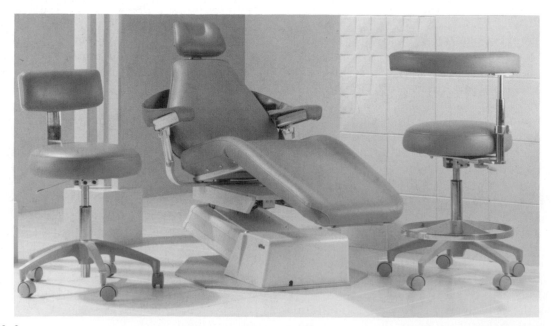

▼ **Figure 10-3**

Lounge type dental chair. Shown here with an operator's stool (to the left of the photo) and an assistant's stool (to the right of the photo). (Courtesy of A-dec, Newberg, OR.)

are located on the side of the head of the chair or on the chair back (Fig. 10–4).

These controls make it possible to place the patient in a range of positions from sitting upright to a reclining position. The position of the patient is determined by the procedure to be performed.

Proper seating includes adjusting the back and leg support, the headrest, and the overall height of the chair to ensure that the patient's head is positioned in the headrest over the operator's lap.

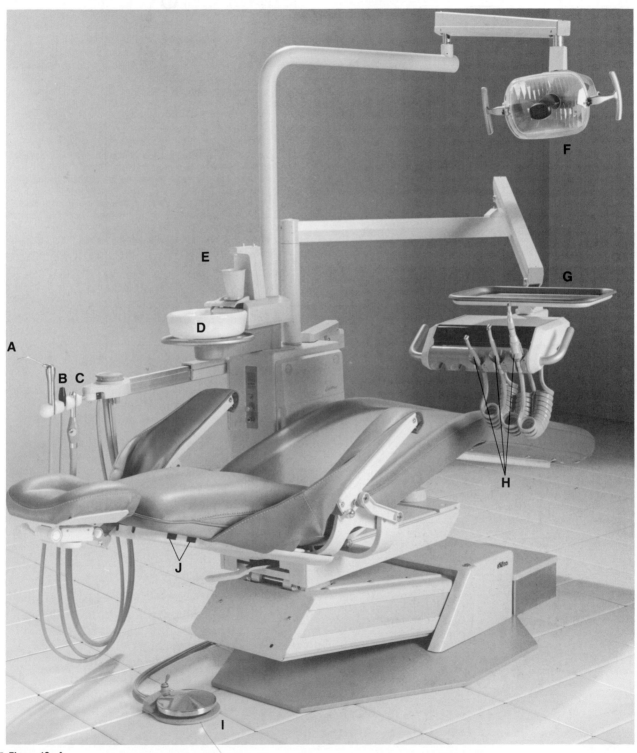

▼ **Figure 10–4**

Dental chair with chair-mounted equipment. *A*, Air-water syringe; *B*, saliva ejector housing; *C*, HVE receptacle; *D*, cuspidor; *E*, cup filler; *F*, operating light; *G*, bracket tray; *H*, handpieces; *I*, rheostat; *J*, chair adjustment switches. (Courtesy of A-dec, Newberg, OR.)

to operate handpieces

Supine Position

Most dental treatment is provided with the patient in a supine (reclining) position. (**Supine** means positioned lying on the back with the face up.)

For this position, the head of the chair is tilted back and the foot is raised so that the patient is comfortably reclined with the nose and knees at approximately the same level (Fig. 10–5).

Figure 10–5 shows the patient in the supine position. Figure 10–6 shows the positioning of the operator and assistant in relation to the seated patient.

In the **subsupine position,** the patient's head is positioned lower than the legs. Some patients find this position uncomfortable, and it is used only when necessary for selected procedures.

Care of the Dental Chair

The air syringe should be used to blow away the small bits of debris, such as chips of dental cements and other materials, that may cling to the inner surfaces of the dental chair.

Attention to this detail is important because a patient notices such things on entry into the operatory. If the patient sees dirt here, he may assume the entire office is unclean.

The upholstery and the enamel or metal surfaces of the dental chair and stools should be cared for regularly following the manufacturer's recommendations.

Operator's Stool

As shown on the left in Figures 10–2 and 10–3, the operator's stool should include the following features:

1. A broad base with castors to provide stability and mobility.

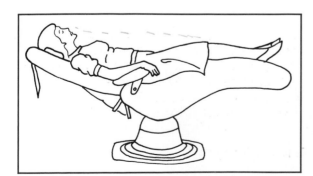

▼ **Figure 10–5**

Patient reclining in a supine position. (Torres HO, Ehrlich A: Modern Dental Assisting, 4th Ed. Philadelphia, WB Saunders, 1990, p 338.)

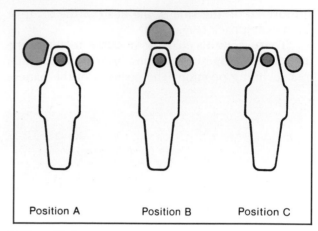

Position A   Position B   Position C

▼ **Figure 10–6**

Diagrams illustrating positioning of dental team and patient. The operator's stool is shown in gray, the assistant's position is shown in pink, and the red circle represents the position of the patient's head.

Position A. Operator's stool is straight-on to the chair. The operator is perpendicular to the dental chair with the feet placed vertically under the head of the chair.

Position B. Operator's stool is directly behind the patient's head. The operator is parallel with the dental chair with the feet pointed toward the foot of the chair under the patient's head.

Position C. Operator's stool is parallel to the chair. The operator's legs are parallel with the side of the dental chair with the feet pointed to the back wall of operatory. (Torres HO, Ehrlich A: Modern Dental Assisting, 4th Ed. Philadelphia, WB Saunders, 1990, p 351.)

2. A padded seat to provide adequate support of the buttocks and thighs without cutting off circulation to the legs.
3. A back support that is adjustable vertically and horizontally to support the lumbar area of the operator's back. (The lumbar region is the inward curved portion of the back.)
4. Adjustable chair back height, to approximately 16 inches from seat to floor.
5. An adjustable seat, from a minimum of 14 inches to a maximum of 21 inches from the floor.

Seated Position of the Operator

1. The operator is seated in a relaxed, unstrained position with elbows close to the sides, shoulders parallel to the floor, and the field of operation at elbow height.
2. When seated, the operator's knees are slightly above hip level, the feet are flat on the floor, and the back is straight.
3. The patient's head in the headrest of the dental chair is positioned over the operator's lap. The patient's body is positioned slightly toward the operator's side of the dental chair.
4. This enables the operator to maintain a focal distance of at least 14 inches while holding the

head relatively erect and with the eyes focused downward.

In some instances, the operator's head may be lowered to no more than a 15-degree angle.

Assistant's Stool

As shown on the right in Figure 10–2, the assistant's stool should include the following features:

1. An adjustable seat and back to provide total support of the back and buttocks.
2. A broad, flat rim near the base of the stool to support the feet. This support permits circulation of blood to the feet and legs when in a seated position.
3. As shown in Figure 10–3, the assistant's stool may include an arched extension from the back of the stool to the front. This extension provides support at the level of the assistant's abdomen when leaning forward toward the operating field.

Seated Position of the Assistant

1. The assistant is seated in a relaxed position 4 to 5 inches higher than the operator (Fig. 10–7).
2. When the patient is reclining in the dental chair, the assistant's hips are level with the patient's shoulders. As the assistant faces the patient, the thighs are parallel with the patient's upper body.
3. The assistant is seated well back onto the seat of the stool with the stool back adjusted properly to provide support to the back. The feet are placed firmly on the flat circular platform at the base of the stool.
4. The assistant is able to see the field of operation with slight positioning of the head only, without bending the back.
5. The assistant is able to reach the dental unit and instrument tray easily and may also reach objects placed nearby on a countertop by pivoting slightly to the right or left.
6. The assistant is out of the operator's line of vision while performing oral evacuation and other assisting duties.

Operatory Cabinets

The operatory design includes mobile cabinets, fixed wall-mounted cabinets, or a combination of both.

These cabinets provide working surfaces and storage space for frequently used small equip-

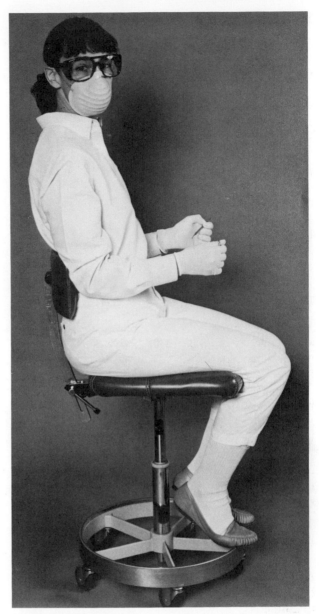

▼ **Figure 10–7**

Assistant demonstrating proper seated position. (Torres HO, Ehrlich A: Modern Dental Assisting, 4th Ed. Philadelphia, WB Saunders, 1990, p 339.)

ment, such as the amalgamator, plus a limited quantity of dental materials and other supplies.

The fixed or mobile cabinet on the assistant's side may include a movable section, with a sliding top and drawers, which serves as an adjunct to the delivery system (Fig. 10–8).

Supplies in the Cabinets

A limited "emergency" set of sterile instruments may also be stored here to be used for replacement of an instrument accidentally dropped during treatment.

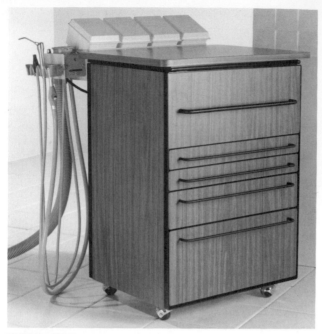

▼ **Figure 10–8**

Mobile cabinet with instrumentation mounted at the left. (Courtesy of A-dec, Newberg, OR.)

However, the major supplies of instruments and materials are stored in the central supply and sterilization area, where they are placed on sterile pre-set trays.

The following items are *examples* of materials and extra sterile instruments found in the various compartments of the mobile cabinet.

▼ **Recessed area under the movable top of the mobile cabinet or top drawer**: Dental cements, composites, calcium hydroxide, zinc oxide–eugenol, isopropyl alcohol, petroleum jelly, preloaded amalgam capsules.

▼ **Compartment area at rear of cabinet**: Sterile cotton rolls, 2 × 2 inch gauze squares, cotton pellets, dental floss, topical and local anesthetic supplies, hemostatic solutions, and retraction cord.

▼ **First drawer**: Sterile mouth mirrors (2), explorers (2), cotton (college) pliers (2), periodontal probes, disposable syringes (sterile), plastic instruments, amalgam carriers, condensers, and carvers. (In some mobile cabinets, a large first drawer is used to recess the amalgamator.)

▼ **Second drawer**: Rubber dam material, punch, rubber dam forceps, dam frame, ligatures, crown and bridge scissors, carbide burs, diamond, and polishing stones.

▼ **Third drawer**: Accessories for stabilizing dental film in the patient's oral cavity during film

exposure, stock "temporary" crowns, crown remover, and shade guides.

▼ **Fourth drawer**: Bulk impression material, mixing pads, mixing bowls, spatulas, water measuring devices, sterile or disposable impression trays, peripheral and utility waxes, wax spatula, laboratory knife, a portable Bunsen burner or alcohol torch, and folder of matches.

Maintaining Infection Control

Should it be necessary to remove anything from a drawer during treatment, precautions must be taken to maintain infection control. Otherwise, the gloved hand and anything touched by it is contaminated.

Prior to opening a drawer while gloved, a light plastic overglove must be put on. The glove is removed and discarded immediately after use.

An alternative is to use a sterile gauze square to grasp the drawer handle. The gauze square is discarded after a single use.

Care of Dental Cabinets

Cabinet tops must be kept clean and free of miscellaneous equipment and supplies. The cabinet surfaces and handles are thoroughly cleaned and disinfected after each patient visit.

This equipment is also polished periodically following the manufacturer's instructions.

Dental Units

Some dental practices use a single dental unit with accessories available to both the operator and the assistant.

A **fixed unit** (which cannot be moved) is placed to the left and slightly forward of the dental chair. Figure 10–4 shows a dental chair with all essential equipment attached directly to it.

A **mobile unit**, such as the one shown in Figure 10–9, may be moved as needed. The type of unit shown here is frequently used for "rear delivery" (behind the patient's head) of equipment and supplies.

When a single unit is used, the assistant may work on a mobile cart that is positioned near the knees to provide easy access and a working surface.

Other practices use separate mobile units for the operator and assistant.

Operator's Unit

The separate operator's unit is equipped with both a high-speed and a low-speed handpiece, an air-

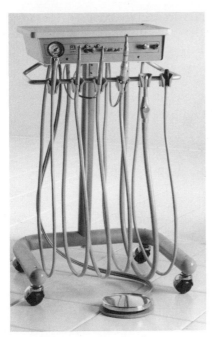

▼ **Figure 10-9**

"Duo cart" for rear delivery is used by both dentist and assistant. Instrumentation includes air-water syringe, three handpieces, high-volume evacuator, a saliva ejector, and all necessary controls. (Courtesy of A-dec, Newberg, OR.)

water syringe, and a vacuum attachment (for oral evacuation) (see Fig. 10-4). (Handpieces are discussed in Chapter 12, "Rotary Dental Instruments.")

The operator's unit is positioned so that the operator may use all equipment with minimal reaching motions.

Assistant's Unit

The separate assistant's unit contains an air-water syringe and oral evacuation attachments (for high-volume evacuation and a saliva ejector). This unit may also contain a cuspidor and a cup filler (see Fig. 10-4).

The assistant's unit, mobile cabinet, or portable cart with instrument tray and materials is moved into position on the assistant's side of the dental chair.

The cabinet top, or the assistant's cart, is positioned with the instrument tray over the knees of the assistant.

Care of Dental Units

The laminated wood and metal portions of the units should be maintained according to the manufacturer's recommendations.

Routine care between patient visits includes cleaning and disinfection of surfaces. A plastic protective barrier may also be placed over the unit and/or the hose attachments.

Operatory Sinks

It is essential that both the operator and the assistant wash their hands before gloving and again after the gloves are removed. To ensure easy access, the operatory is equipped with two sinks, one on the operator's side and one on the assistant's side.

Each sink is equipped with disposable towels, a nonallergenic liquid-soap solution, and hypoallergenic dusting powder.

If the operatory sinks are not equipped with foot or electronic water controls, the faucet handle is grasped with a paper towel. The towel is discarded after a single use.

Care of Operatory Sinks

The sinks and surrounding area must be kept free of splatter and clean in appearance. The chrome trim should be kept shining and spotless after each patient visit.

ASSOCIATED EQUIPMENT

Cup Filler

It is a courtesy to the patient to provide a cup of water, to rinse his mouth prior to and at the end of the treatment.

A fresh cup is put out for each patient. This is filled with mouthwash or water as needed. During operatory cleanup, the cup is emptied and discarded.

Air-Water Syringe

The air-water syringe may be used in three ways. It can deliver (1) a stream of water, (2) a stream of air, or (3) a combined spray of air and water.

The temperature of the air and water is variable. The assistant should learn to keep the temperature at an even, warm level that is neither too hot nor too cold.

Important: The air-water spray should not be used in the oral cavity when a soft tissue wound, such as the socket from an extraction, is present.

Use of the spray at this time may disturb the initial clot formation. It may also force infected material into the tissues or bloodstream.

Care of the Air-Water Syringe

Air-H₂O Syringe tip

At the end of the patient visit, the air-water syringe should be run for 30 seconds to flush it out. Then, if possible, the tip should be removed and sterilized and a clean tip used for each patient.

If the tip cannot be sterilized, it should be wiped thoroughly clean and then placed on the bracket table or tray.

Here it is sprayed with disinfectant to keep it thoroughly wet for at least 2 minutes. Then it is wiped clean with gauze sponges or paper towels.

Operating Light

The operating light may be suspended from the ceiling or attached to the chair. This light is very bright and is adjusted to avoid shining it in the patient's eyes.

Care of the Operating Light

The operating light handle is protected from contamination with a removable barrier, and this is the only part of the light that is touched while gloved.

During operatory cleanup, this contaminated barrier is removed and a fresh one is placed.

When cool, the lens of the light is wiped free of smudges, using a mild detergent and a soft cloth. This is done only when the light is cool—touching the warm lens with a damp cloth could cause it to break.

Central Air Compressor

A large central air compressor is used to provide compressed air for the three-way syringe and for the air-driven handpieces.

Because of the noise level and for safety reasons, the compressor system is placed outside the operatory. However, it must be accessible for maintenance by the office staff on a regular basis.

One of the major maintenance needs is to check for the condensation of moisture in the compressor tank and in the tubing leading into the operatories and laboratory.

Moisture in the compressed air line causes the formation of sediment and algae, which ruin the precision parts of the air-driven handpieces. It may also cause the debris to be ejected into the patient's mouth.

Condensation builds up as the temperature of the air changes throughout the day. It is removed by "bleeding" the jet opening near the main compressor connection (or the end of the tubing) onto a sterile gauze square. No instrument is connected to the air line during this procedure.

Regular maintenance of the entire compressor is important, and the manufacturer's recommendations should be followed. One staff member should be responsible for seeing that maintenance of the compressor is accomplished on a routine basis.

Oral Evacuation Systems

The *use* of the saliva ejector and oral evacuation systems is discussed in Chapter 13, "Oral Evacuation and Instrument Transfer." Following are procedures for the *care* of these systems.

Saliva Ejector

A sterile disposable saliva ejector is used for a single patient. It is discarded at the end of that patient's visit.

The housing of the saliva ejector is cleaned and disinfected during the operatory cleanup routine.

The small screen near the top of the saliva ejector tubing should be removed daily and rinsed thoroughly to clear it of any debris.

To clean the tubing, the saliva ejector is turned on. Clean, warm water is run through the tubing. Periodically, a disinfecting and deodorizing solution may be added to this rinse water to prevent an accumulation of odorous material. A sodium hypochlorite (bleach) solution may be used to sanitize the tubing.

High Volume Evacuator

The high volume evacuator (HVE) tip, which is placed in the patient's mouth, is removable and may be reused after it has been sterilized. A fresh, sterile tip is provided for each patient.

The receptacle for the HVE (not the tip) is cleaned and disinfected during the operatory cleanup routine. The hoses to the central vacuum compressor are cleaned with warm water after each use. They too should be regularly rinsed with a cleaning solution, such as sodium hypochlorite (bleach), to prevent odors from forming.

Cuspidor

The dental unit usually includes a cuspidor, which is automatically flushed with running water. Although it has this rinse feature, the cuspidor must be cleaned and disinfected during the operatory cleanup routine.

An alternative is a small portable cuspidor, which may be handed to the patient while he is in a reclining position.

A portable cuspidor resembles a funnel with tubing that is attached to the oral evacuation system. This too must be cleaned and disinfected during the operatory cleanup routine.

Central Vacuum Compressor

The central vacuum compressor is used for the oral evacuation system, and it too requires regular care. The vacuum tank, or debris container, requires daily attention following the manufacturer's instructions.

Nitrous Oxide – Oxygen System

The use of nitrous oxide – oxygen is discussed in Chapter 18, "Pharmacology and Pain Control." Only the care of the system is discussed here.

If the office has a wall-installed nitrous oxide and oxygen delivery system, the main storage of the nitrous oxide and oxygen tanks is locked away from the main area of the dental office.

This is done for safety purposes, and the security of this storage system is most important. Also, the operation and content of the individual supply tanks must be checked frequently throughout the day.

Dental X-Ray Unit

Dental radiography is discussed in Chapters 15 and 16, "Fundamentals of Dental Radiography" and "Dental Radiography: Paralleling Techniques." Only care of the equipment is discussed here.

Prior to the patient visit, the x-ray unit is covered with a protective plastic barrier. This may be plastic wrap covering only the position-indicating device (PID) or a large plastic bag covering the entire x-ray head (see Fig. 16–1 and 16–2). A metallic wrap barrier is *not* placed on the x-ray unit.

If the x-ray unit was used during the patient visit, the contaminated barrier is removed and discarded as part of the operatory cleanup. A fresh barrier is then placed for the next patient.

This equipment also requires periodic polishing and care according to the manufacturer's instructions. Prior to this cleaning, the unit is disconnected from the electrical socket.

View Box for Radiographs

A view box used to read and diagnose radiographs is placed in the cabinetry or wall of the operatory. It consists of a bright white light source with frosted glass cover.

The glass surface of the view box must be kept free of smudges and dust by wiping it with a soft cloth. If touched during treatment, it must be disinfected with other surfaces during operatory cleanup.

THE BETWEEN-PATIENTS ROUTINE

Operatory cleaning and disinfection are always accomplished while wearing heavy-duty utility gloves.

Any operatory surfaces that may have been touched or contaminated during the patient visit must be cleaned and disinfected between every patient visit.

If in doubt as to whether a surface was contaminated, *clean and disinfect it.* The surfaces to be routinely cleaned and disinfected include:

▼ Light handles.

▼ Chair switches.

▼ Tubing on handpieces, syringe, and oral evacuation system.

▼ Air-water syringe.

▼ Handpieces.

▼ Ultrasonic scaler.

▼ Bracket table or tray.

▼ X-ray head (if used).

▼ Operatory cabinet or cart surfaces.

▼ Work tubs or drawer pulls.

▼ View box.

▼ Anything touched during patient care.

Patient Chart

The dentist reviews the patient's chart and radiographs prior to beginning treatment. However, in order to avoid contamination of the patient chart, it should not be touched once treatment begins.

1. At the end of the visit and while still gloved, enter today's treatment on a piece of paper.
2. After the latex gloves have been removed, use a

different pen to copy this treatment information onto the patient's chart.

3. Discard the contaminated note paper and disinfect the pen or pencil that was used to make that note.

4. The patient's mounted radiographs are removed from the view box after the assistant's gloves have been removed and the hands have been scrubbed.

5. The patient's chart and radiographs are then returned to the business office.

Operatory Care

Procedure

PREPARING THE OPERATORY

While Still Gloved for the Patient Visit

1. Discard all disposables (follow guidelines outlined in Chapter 7 for handling hazardous waste).

2. Remove the barriers used during the last patient visit.

3. Place soiled instruments on the tray to be returned to the "contaminated section" of the sterilization area. (The care of soiled instruments is discussed in Chapter 11, "Dental Hand Instruments.")

4. Remove the latex gloves and thoroughly scrub and dry your hands. If necessary, complete entries on patient chart.

While Wearing Utility Gloves

1. Put on utility gloves before beginning to clean the operatory.

2. **Surface cleaning:** Thoroughly clean the surfaces to remove all debris by spraying the surface with a cleaner and scrubbing vigorously (Fig. 10–10). A special sponge or brush or paper towels may be used for this purpose. If gauze sponges are used, they should be either the 3- or 4-inch size. (The 2-inch size is too small to do this effectively.) Gauze sponges are discarded; brushes are discarded or sterilized.

3. **Surface disinfection:** Next spray or sponge the surface again with the disinfecting solution (Fig. 10–11). This time, leave it moist and keep it moist for the manufacturer's recommended exposure time. This is usually 2 to 10 minutes.

    Caution: When working with a disinfectant carefully read the manufacturer's directions for dilution and use. Pay special

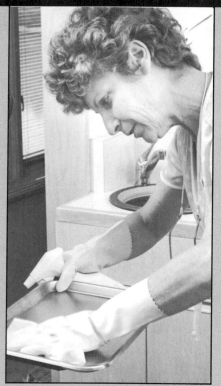

Figure 10–10 Contaminated surfaces are sprayed with a cleaner and scrubbed vigorously. (Torres HO, Ehrlich A: Modern Dental Assisting, 4th Ed. Philadelphia, WB Saunders, 1990, p 156.)

attention to any precautions such as warnings about surfaces that it may stain or corrode. Also take care not to mix materials that might cause a chemical reaction or toxic fumes.

4. *Optional:* Finally, vigorously wipe and clean the disinfected surfaces with a fresh paper towel or large gauze sponges. This step removes any residual disinfectant and remaining pathogens. This step is optional because some dentists prefer to leave the residual disinfectant in place.

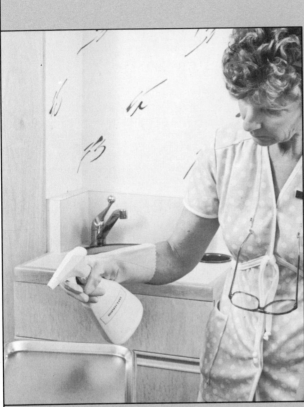

Figure 10–11 Surfaces are sprayed with a disinfectant and left moist. (Torres HO, Ehrlich A: Modern Dental Assisting, 4th Ed. Philadelphia, WB Saunders, 1990, p 157.)

After Removing Utility Gloves

1. Remove utility gloves and wash hands.
2. Place clean barriers in the operatory (Fig. 10–12).
3. If the radiographs for the previous patient have not been removed, take them down at this time and return them to the business office.

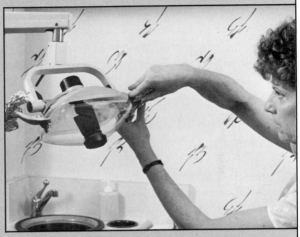

Figure 10–12 Fresh protective barriers are placed after utility gloves have been removed. (Torres HO, Ehrlich A: Modern Dental Assisting, 4th Ed. Philadelphia, WB Saunders, 1990, p 157.)

Prepared Operatory

▼ The between-patient routine has been completed so that the operatory is clean and ready for the next patient (see Fig. 10–2).

▼ The appropriate pre-set tray and other supplies are in place; however, the pre-set tray is not opened until the operator is ready to begin treatment for the patient.

▼ The patient's chart, radiographs and laboratory case are in place in the operatory (Fig. 10–13).

▼ The dental chair is in its lowest position, with the back upright and the arm raised on the side of admitting the patient.

▼ Equipment is placed away from the path of entry of the patient and dental team.

THE PATIENT VISIT

Admission of the Patient

1. Greet the patient in the reception area by name, and ask that he follow you to the operatory.

2. Bring the patient's coat and other personal items into the operatory; place them within the patient's view but out of the way of treatment.
3. In an effort to make the patient feel more comfortable and relaxed, you may attempt to make pleasant conversation (Fig. 10–14). However, if the patient obviously does not want to talk, this should not be forced.
4. Answer any questions about impending treatment honestly and within the scope of your knowledge. If in doubt, defer the question to the dentist.

Seating the Patient

1. Seat the patient and adjust the controls *before* donning gloves for an examination or operative procedure.
2. Ask the patient to sit on the edge of the dental chair and swing his legs into position. The patient should be positioned so that buttocks and shoulder blades are flush against the back of the chair.
3. Lower the chair arm.
4. Depending on the intended treatment, the patient is draped with a disposable towel and possibly with a plastic drape (Fig. 10–15 *A, B*).

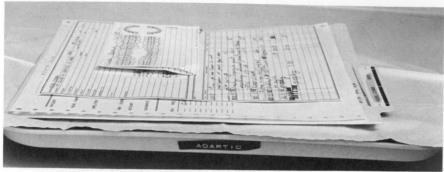

▼ **Figure 10–13**

Covered pre-set tray and the patient's chart ready to be carried into the operatory. (Torres HO, Ehrlich A: Modern Dental Assisting, 4th Ed. Philadelphia, WB Saunders, 1990, p 343.)

5. After the patient is advised of chair movement, slowly adjust the chair into the proper position for the operator to proceed with the dental treatment.

Adjusting the Operating Light

1. When the patient is seated, and before donning gloves, turn on the operating light and position it with the light showing on the patient's chest or lap—approximately 36 inches below the patient's mouth.
2. After preparing the patient, wash your hands thoroughly. Don clean latex gloves before assisting in patient care.
3. Slowly adjust the light upward to illuminate the

oral cavity. Take care to touch only the protective barrier on the light handle.
4. When properly positioned, the light illuminates the area to be treated without projecting shadows of the operator's or assistant's hands onto the oral cavity.

Dismissal of the Patient

1. When treatment has been completed, the dentist or assistant gives the patient postoperative instructions, if any.
2. Slowly return the chair to the upright position and at the same time return the chair to its lowest position.

    Caution: It is important that the chair be raised slowly (and that the patient be encouraged to get up slowly). Otherwise, the sudden change in position may cause the patient to feel faint.
3. Check the patient's face and clothing, making certain that there are no debris or smudges.
4. Remove the towel and drape and raise the chair arm (Fig. 10–16).
5. While the patient is still seated, return any personal belongings.
6. Courteously assist the patient from the chair, if necessary, and escort him to the business office.

DAILY MAINTENANCE ROUTINE FOR THE CHAIRSIDE ASSISTANT

Morning Routine (Opening of Office)

1. Arrive 30 minutes prior to the opening of the office for the day. Change into a fresh uniform at the office. Because of the possible danger of spreading contamination, the uniform is *not* worn outside the office.
2. Check thermostat for proper "climate control" throughout the office.

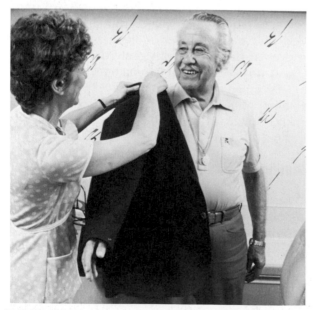

▼ **Figure 10–14**

The assistant greets the patient and helps to make him comfortable. (Torres HO, Ehrlich A: Modern Dental Assisting, 4th Ed. Philadelphia, WB Saunders, 1990, p 346.)

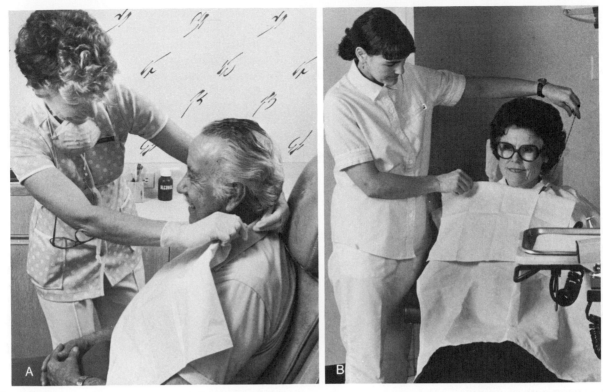

▼ **Figure 10-15**

Draping the patient. *A.* For most treatment, the patient is draped with a disposable, plastic-backed patient towel. *B.* For procedures such as impressions or ultrasonic scaling, the patient is covered first with a large plastic drape and then with the patient towel. (Torres HO, Ehrlich A: Modern Dental Assisting, 4th Ed. Philadelphia, WB Saunders, 1990, p 347.)

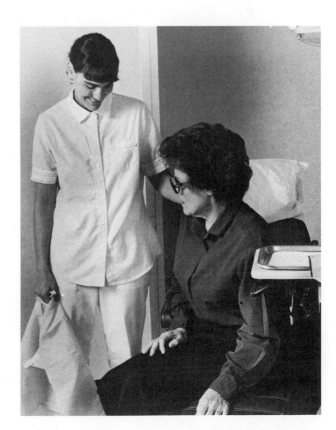

▼ **Figure 10-16**

The back of the chair is raised slowly, the towel and drape are removed, and the patient is dismissed. (Torres HO, Ehrlich A: Modern Dental Assisting, 4th Ed. Philadelphia, WB Saunders, 1990, p 347.)

3. Turn on the central air compressor and the central vacuum units. Check for condensation of moisture in compressor and vacuum units and lines and "bleed" these lines if necessary.
4. Turn on the master switch of the dental and x-ray units.
5. Dust operatories and equipment.
6. Check operating light for function and position.
7. Check the operatory to be certain that basic materials and instrument trays are ready for seating the first patient.
8. Check that the position of the dental unit and chair, operating stools, and operating light are correct for entry of the patient.
9. Recheck the appointment schedule of patients for the day to be certain that the pre-set trays, patients' records, radiographs, and laboratory cases are available as needed for the planned treatment.

Evening Routine (Closing of Office)

1. After dismissal of the last patient, follow the between-patient routine. Take special care to be certain that all areas and equipment in the operatories are thoroughly cleaned.
2. Return soiled instruments to the sterilization area, where they are cleaned and sterilized.
3. Wear heavy-duty gloves as you empty waste receptacles and place fresh plastic liners.
4. Restock consumable "supplies," including paper towels and soap, with a supply adequate for the next day.
5. Rinse the tubing of the central vacuum compressor with clear water, disinfecting solution, or both. Also check the compressor for accumulation of waste and turn off the master switch.
6. Turn off x-ray units and dental units.
7. Clean the sterilization area. This includes changing solutions, disinfecting work surfaces, and discarding waste.
8. Check the appointment schedule for the next day to see that necessary laboratory work has been completed for delivery to the patient. Also, make sure that all necessary patient records are ready, including radiographs.
9. Leave the operatories ready for use in the morning.
10. Change out of uniform and check for fresh uniform for the next day. Check for clean and polished shoes to ensure their neatness.
11. Readjust the "climate control" in the office and turn off all lights except night light.
12. Secure office (lock all windows and doors).

▼ EXERCISES

1. At the end of the patient visit, soiled barriers are removed _____ _____.

   a. before donning utility gloves
   b. before the patient is dismissed
   c. while still gloved from the patient visit
   d. while wearing utility gloves

2. Any operatory surfaces that may have been touched during the patient visit must be cleaned and disinfected _____.

   a. at least twice a day
   b. at the end of the day
   c. before the next patient

3. When properly seated, the assistant is _____.

   a. at eye level with the operator
   b. four to five inches higher than the operator
   c. seated with his or her feet flat on the floor
   d. b and c

4. The lens of the operating light is wiped free of smudges _____ _____.

   a. immediately after use
   b. only when the light is cool

5. During treatment, a drawer may be opened _____.

   a. if the gloved hand is rinsed before returning to the chair
   b. using a gauze square to grasp the drawer handle and discarding it after use
   c. while wearing a light plastic overglove, which is discarded after use
   d. b or c

6. When cleaning the operatory, the assistant wears _____.

   a. latex gloves
   b. overgloves
   c. the gloves from the prior procedure
   d. utility gloves

7. The _____ unit contains high-speed and low-speed handpieces.

   a. assistant's
   b. operator's

8. A _____ c _____ barrier is placed on the x-ray unit.

   a. metallic wrap
   b. permanent
   c. plastic

9. The HVE tip is _____.

    a. discarded after use
    b. disinfected during operatory cleanup
    c. sterilized for reuse
    d. b or c

10. In a _____ position, the patient's head is lower than his legs.

    a. subsupine
    b. supine

11. Use of the air-water spray when there is an open wound in the oral cavity may _____.

    a. cause extensive bleeding
    b. force infected material into the bloodstream
    c. force infected material into the tissue
    d. b and c

12. Sodium hypochlorite is used to clean the tubing for the _____ _____.

    a. compressor
    b. high-volume evacuator
    c. saliva ejector
    d. b and c

13. The air-water syringe may be used to deliver _____.

    a. air
    b. air-water spray
    c. water
    d. a, b, and c

14. The _____ unit is equipped with handpieces, an air-water syringe and a vacuum attachment.

    a. assistant's
    b. operator's

15. When the patient is seated, the operating light is positioned _____.

    a. 36 inches below the patient's mouth
    b. at the patient's forehead
    c. near the patient's chin
    d. to illuminate the oral cavity

16. At the end of the day, the assistant should wear _____ while emptying waste receptacles and placing fresh liners

    a. overgloves
    b. utility gloves
    c. no gloves are necessary for this acitivity

17. The controls of the chair are adjusted _____ donning treatment gloves.

    a. after
    b. before

18. The central air compressor is used to provide air for the _____ _____ .

    a. air-driven handpieces
    b. air-water syringe
    c. oral evacuation system
    d. a and b

19. The entry on the patient's chart is made _____ .

    a. after gloves have been removed
    b. while still gloved from the procedure
    c. while wearing utility gloves

20. Clean barriers are placed _____ .

    a. after removing utility gloves
    b. after the next patient is seated
    c. while still wearing utility gloves

▼ Criterion Sheet 10–1

Student's Name _____

Procedure: *IDENTIFYING OPERATORY EQUIPMENT*

Performance Objective:

The student will identify and state the use of each of the pieces of operatory equipment listed below.

SE = Student evaluation IE = Instructor evaluation	C = Criterion met X = Criterion not met	SE	IE
Instrumentation: A fully equipped operatory or a clear photograph.			
1. Identified the dental chair.			
2. Identified the operator's stool.			
3. Identified the assistant's stool.			
4. Identified the operating light and x-ray view box.			
5. Identified the cup filler and cuspidor.			
6. Identified the HVE and saliva ejector holders.			
7. Identified the dental units (fixed or mobile).			
Comments:			

▼ Criterion Sheet 10–2

Student's Name _____

Procedure: *SEATING AND POSITIONING THE PATIENT*

Performance Objective:

The student will demonstrate seating and draping the patient.

The student will demonstrate placing the patient in a supine position and returning the patient to an upright position.

Another student will play the patient.

	SE	IE
SE = Student evaluation **C** = Criterion met **IE** = Instructor evaluation **X** = Criterion not met		
Instrumentation: Lounge-type dental chair, patient drape, patient towel, and towel clip.		
1. **Before the patient entered:** _____ Lowered the chair. _____ Placed the back in an upright position. _____ Raised the chair arm on the entrance side. _____ Cleared patient's path of all hoses, switches, and equipment.		
2. **Admitted patient:** _____ Seated patient. _____ Draped patient. _____ Provided patient with safety glasses. _____ Informed patient that chair was to be reclined. _____ Gradually lowered chair back until patient was in supine position. _____ Maintained patient comfort.		
Comments:		

▼ Criterion Sheet 10–3

Student's Name _____

Procedure: *BETWEEN-PATIENT OPERATORY CARE*

Performance Objective:

The student will demonstrate removing soiled instruments, surface cleaning and disinfection, and placing clean barriers.

		SE	IE
SE = Student evaluation **IE** = Instructor evaluation	**C** = Criterion met **X** = Criterion not met		
Instrumentation: Latex gloves and soiled instruments (from patient visit), utility gloves, cleaning solution, paper towels, disinfectant solution, materials for clean barriers.			
1. **While still gloved from the patient visit:** _____ Discarded all disposables and waste. _____ Removed barriers used during the visit. _____ Placed soiled instruments on tray. _____ Returned tray to "soiled section" of the sterilization area. _____ Removed latex gloves and scrubbed and dried hands.			
2. **While wearing utility gloves:** _____ Cleaned all potentially contaminated surfaces. _____ Disinfected these surfaces.			
3. **After removing utility gloves:** _____ Removed gloves and washed and dried hands. _____ Placed clean barriers. _____ Positioned equipment ready for patient visit.			
Comments:			

11 Dental Hand Instruments

▼ LEARNING OBJECTIVES

The student will be able to:

1. Identify and describe the three major parts of most hand instruments.
2. Identify and state the function of the three instruments found in the basic setup used for all dental procedures.
3. Identify and state the function of at least 10 dental hand instruments.
4. Demonstrate the preparation of a sterile pre-set tray for a restorative procedure.

OVERVIEW OF DENTAL HAND INSTRUMENTS

The term **hand instrument** refers to one that is used under hand direction and application, as opposed to a rotary instrument, which is motor-driven or air-driven. (Rotary instruments are discussed in Chapter 12, "Rotary Dental Instruments.")

Each type of hand instrument comes in several designs and sizes. It is important that you learn to identify these instruments quickly and accurately.

You must also be aware of the position-of-use for each instrument so that you can pass it to the dentist in the correct position. (This is discussed in Chapter 13, "Oral Evacuation and Instrument Transfer.")

HAND INSTRUMENT DESIGN

The basic components of most dental hand instruments are the handle (or shaft), the shank, the blade or nib, and the tip or working end of the instrument. The overall length of these instruments is approximately 6 inches (Fig. 11–1).

Parts of Hand Instruments

Handle (Shaft)

The handle, or shaft, of the instrument is designed and shaped so that the operator may grip it securely while gloved.

Shank

The shank is the tapered portion of the instrument connecting the handle and the blade. The shank is angled to provide access to the tooth to be operated. It may be:

▼ **Straight** (no angle).

▼ **Monangled** (one angle).

▼ **Binangled** (two angles).

▼ **Triple-angled** (three angles).

Blade Or Nib

The blade, or nib, begins at the end of the last angle of the shaft and continues to become the working portion of the instrument.

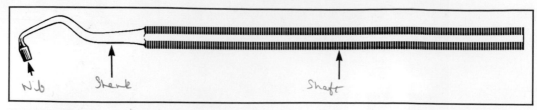

Nib *Shank* *Shaft*

▼ Figure 11–1

Basic parts of a dental hand instrument. Shown here is a back-action amalgam condenser. (Courtesy of Hu-Friedy, Chicago, IL.)

A **blade** is beveled (angled and sharpened) to form a cutting edge. The sharpness and the angle of the instrument are a vital part of its design.

A **nib** forms a smaller, blunt working surface. The nib may be smooth or serrated. (**Serrated** means rough, marked with notches like the teeth of a saw.)

Although there is a distinct difference, the terms blade and nib, or tip, are often used interchangeably.

Double-Ended Instruments

A **double-ended instrument** has a shank and nib or blade on both ends of the handle. This is done to increase the efficiency of use and to reduce the number of instruments required during a procedure.

Many instruments are designed as "pairs" with a left and right version, which permits the operator to reach all areas of the tooth. These "pairs" are usually provided as a single double-ended instrument.

BASIC SETUP

The basic setup for almost every dental procedure includes one or two mouth mirrors, an explorer, and cotton pliers (are also known as *college pliers*).

Mouth Mirrors

Small, plain, or magnifying mirrors (½ to 1 inch in diameter) are used to reflect the operating field, to retract the tissue and tongue, and to protect the tissue from injury during operation.

Mouth mirrors may be designed with the mirror either on the front or on the reverse side for front and back viewing (Fig. 11–2A).

Explorers

Explorers are used to examine tooth surfaces to detect minute breaks in the pits and fissures and to detect defective margins of restorations.

These instruments are made of fine, flexible

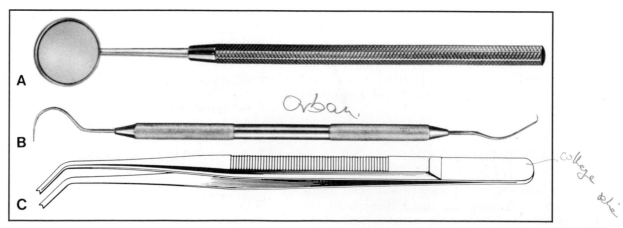

Orban. *College plie*

▼ Figure 11–2

The basic setup. *A.* Mouth mirror. *B.* Explorer (double-ended), *C.* College pliers. (Courtesy of Hu-Friedy, Chicago, IL.)

steel with very sharp points. They are available in straight or curved forms and come as single-ended or double-ended instruments (Fig. 11–2*B*).

Cotton Pliers

Cotton pliers, also known as *college pliers*, are designed with plain or serrated points. These enable the operator to perform many functions, such as picking up, holding, and placing medicaments, cotton pellets, and cotton rolls (Fig. 11–2*C*).

INSTRUMENTATION FOR RESTORATIVE PROCEDURES

Restorative dentistry, which is also called *operative dentistry*, involves the preparation and placement of dental cements, amalgam, composite, and cast restorations.

The hand instruments described in this section are those used most frequently in procedures. The use of these instruments is further explained in the appropriate chapters.

Excavators

Excavators have sharpened edges and are used for the removal of carious dentin. Some excavators may also be used in carving amalgam before it hardens.

A spoon excavator is similar in shape to a household spoon, with the difference that the entire margin of the spoon is tapered and sharpened (Fig. 11–3*B*, *C*).

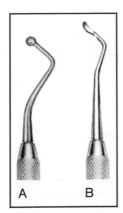

▼ **Figure 11–3**

Excavators. *A.* Spoon excavator. *B.* Oval spoon excavator. (Courtesy of Hu-Friedy, Chicago, IL.)

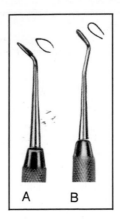

▼ **Figure 11–4**

Cleoid-discoid. *A.* Cleoid. *B.* Discoid. (Courtesy of Hu-Friedy, Chicago, IL.)

Cleoid-Discoid

These instruments also have sharpened edges that are designed to dig out the carious dentin of a decayed tooth and to remove excess material during the carving of an amalgam restoration.

A **cleoid** has a nib in the form of a claw, which is sharpened to a point. A **discoid** is a disc-shaped excavator with sharpened edges (Fig. 11–4). The cleoid and discoid may be placed on the same handle to form a double-ended cleoid-discoid instrument.

Chisels

Chisels are used to remove undermined enamel or dentin from a carious tooth. Chisels, which are similar to a carpenter's wood chisel with a very small, sharp blade, are used only in a *push* motion (Fig. 11–5*A*).

Hatchets

Hatchets are used primarily to prepare retentive areas, sharpen internal line angles, and remove hard caries.

A dental hatchet is similar to a wood hatchet in that the angle of its cutting edge is at a right angle to the axis of the blade (Fig. 11–5*B*). The hatchet is used in a cleaving action.

Hoes

Hoes are used for removing hard caries and forming the line angles on anterior teeth.

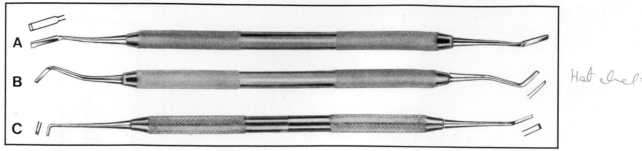

Hatchel

▼ **Figure 11-5**

Hand cutting instruments. *A.* Binangle chisel. *B.* Hatchet. *C.* Hoe. (Courtesy of Hu-Friedy, Chicago, IL.)

A dental hoe, which is similar to a garden hoe with the blade placed at right angles to the long axis of the instrument handle, must be used only with a *pull* motion (Fig. 11–5*C*).

Angle Formers

An angle former, which has a blade that is sharpened on three sides, is used for defining line angles, obtaining retentive form in dentin, and placing bevels on enamel margins (Fig. 11–6*A*).

Margin Trimmers

A margin trimmer, also known as a *gingival margin trimmer* (GMT), is used primarily to properly bevel the gingival enamel margins of cavity preparation for amalgam restorations, inlays, or onlays (Fig. 11–6*B*).

The margin trimmer is similar to the enamel hatchet except that the cutting edge is at an angle to the blade. Also, the blade is curved slightly to provide accessibility to the mesial *or* distal area of the tooth.

Amalgam Carriers

An amalgam carrier is an instrument with a hollow tip and a spring mechanism that is used to pick up, carry, and place the freshly mixed amalgam (Fig. 11–7).

Amalgam Condensers

An amalgam condenser, also known as a *plugger*, is used to pack and condense the freshly mixed amalgam into the cavity preparation before the material hardens (Fig. 11–8).

▼ The surface of the condenser nib may be either serrated or plain.

▼ To enable the operator to reach all tooth surfaces, the shank of the condenser is available in different angulations.

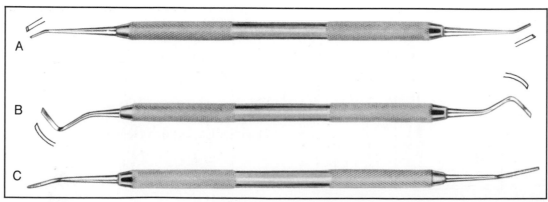

▼ **Figure 11-6**

Hand cutting instruments. *A.* Angle former. *B.* Margin trimmer. *C.* Wedelstaedt amalgam file. (Courtesy of Hu-Friedy, Chicago, IL.)

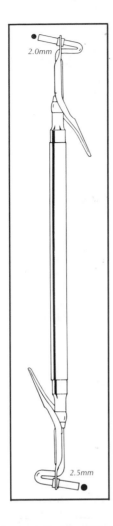

▼ **Figure 11–7**

Double-ended amalgam carrier. The "2.0 mm" end is the "regular end." The "2.5 mm" end is the "large end." (Courtesy of Hu-Friedy, Chicago, IL.)

▼ The operator uses several different condensers in different nib sizes and shapes while "packing" the amalgam into a single restoration.

Carvers

Carvers are used to shape the amalgam before it hardens in the final set. In this process, the operator carves the occlusal surface of the restoration so

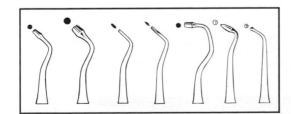

▼ **Figure 11–8**

An assortment of amalgam condensers. (Courtesy of Hu-Friedy, Chicago, IL.)

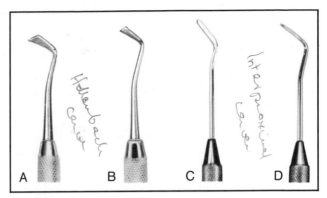

▼ **Figure 11–9**

Assorted amalgam carvers. *A* and *B.* Hollenback carvers. *C* and *D.* Interproximal carvers. (Courtesy of Hu-Friedy, Chicago, IL.)

that it resembles the occlusal surface of the natural tooth (Fig. 11–9).

Knives and Files

Knives and files are used to trim away excess filling material or to smooth off overhanging margins of metal restorations (see Fig. 11–6*C*, Fig. 11–10).

Plastic Instruments

These instruments, which are usually made of metal, are called "plastic instruments" because they are used to shape and mold restorative materials while they are still plastic (soft) (Fig. 11–11).

Burnishers

A burnisher, which has a nib with a smooth beveled edge, is used to burnish the margin of the restoration and the enamel.

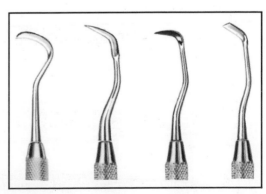

▼ **Figure 11–10**

Assorted knives. These are used for trimming away excess restorative material. (Courtesy of Hu-Friedy, Chicago, IL.)

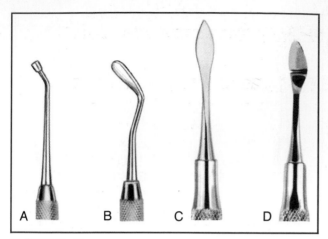

▼ **Figure 11-11**

Plastic instruments. *A* and *B*. Woodson plastic instrument (both ends). *C* and *D*. Cosmetic contour instrument (both ends) used with composite restorative materials. (Courtesy of Hu-Friedy, Chicago, IL.)

Burnishing is the process of smoothing a metal surface by rubbing. This is usually done before the material hardens and while it is still workable.

Commonly used burnisher designs are in the form of a ball, football, or egg. Each design comes in several sizes (Fig. 11-12).

The **beaver tail burnisher** is used to smooth the interproximal surface of a restoration. It is also used in the application of the rubber dam.

Spatulas

Spatulas of various sizes and shapes, with flexible or stiff blades, are used to mix materials such as cements and impression materials (Fig. 11-13).

Spatulas are made of steel, stellite steel, agate, plastic, and wood. In the laboratory, a wooden-handled spatula is used to mix plaster or dental stone.

PRE-SET TRAYS

Pre-set trays are color-coded trays containing all of the sterile instruments and supplies needed for a given procedure.

For example, there are special trays for amalgam restorations, composite restorations, crown and bridge preparation, oral surgery, and endodontic treatment.

Since each operator has specific instrument preferences, the operator's choice determines which instruments are to be included in a tray.

The covered pre-set tray is brought into the operatory during preparation for the patient's visit and is unwrapped just prior to beginning the procedure (Fig. 11-14).

A practice should have several of each kind of tray setup so that there are enough instruments available for use while the others are being sterilized.

Color-Coded Instruments

Two color-coded bands may be used on the instruments to speed sorting and placement of sterilized instruments on the tray.

▼ The first band, placed on the handle of the instrument, indicates the procedure (for example, blue for amalgam instruments).

▼ The second band indicates the position of the instrument in the setup.

Instrument Placement on the Tray

The sterile instruments are organized on the tray from left to right in the **sequence of use**. This placement facilitates handing the instruments to the operator in their proper sequence.

In preparing the tray, the first instrument to be used for the procedure is positioned as the first

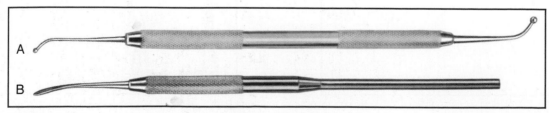

▼ **Figure 11-12**

Burnishers. *A*. Ball burnisher. *B*. Beaver tail burnisher. (Courtesy of Hu-Friedy, Chicago, IL.)

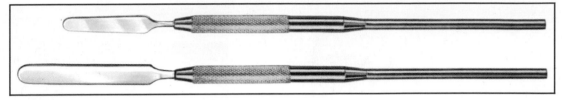

▼ **Figure 11-13**

Cement spatulas. (Courtesy of Hu-Friedy, Chicago, IL.)

instrument on the left side of the tray. The remaining instruments are arranged from left to right in the order of use.

Tray Preparation

The trays are prepared and stored covered in the *clean* section of the central sterilization area until carried into the operatory as needed.

Wrapped Instruments

All of the instruments for a given procedure may be bagged or wrapped together for sterilization. After sterilization, the instruments are stored in this wrapping. This is the best way to maintain instrument sterility, for once the package has been opened, sterility is no longer assured.

In the operatory, the bag itself may be used as the sterile field. The gloved assistant arranges the

instruments on the inside of the used wrapping just prior to the beginning of the procedure. Many practices use this system for surgical instruments.

Sterile disposables, such as gauze sponges, cotton rolls, and pellets, may be added to the pack prior to sterilization, or they may be added to the tray just prior to use.

Another option is the sterilization of instruments in a covered metal tray, such as the one shown in Figure 11-15. After sterilization, the box is kept covered and is opened just prior to use.

Unwrapped Instruments

After the instruments and trays have been cleaned and sterilized, the tray is reassembled for reuse. This takes place only in the "clean" portion of the sterilization area.

Unwrapped sterile instruments are handled only with sterile transfer forceps (Fig. 11-16). These should be used to remove the instruments

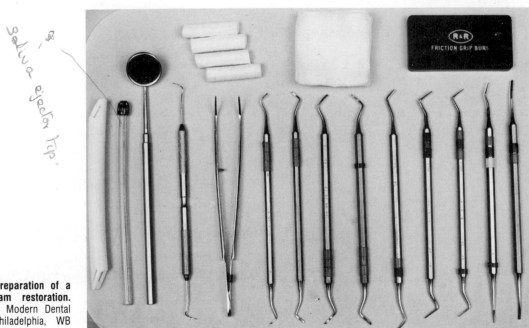

▼ **Figure 11-14**

Pre-set tray for the preparation of a tooth for an amalgam restoration. (Torres HO, Ehrlich A: Modern Dental Assisting, 4th Ed. Philadelphia, WB Saunders, 1990, p 366.)

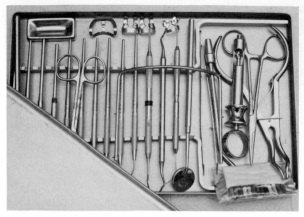

▼ **Figure 11-15**

A pre-set metal endodontic tray with cover. (Torres HO, Ehrlich A: Modern Dental Assisting, 4th Ed. Philadelphia, WB Saunders, 1990, p 161.)

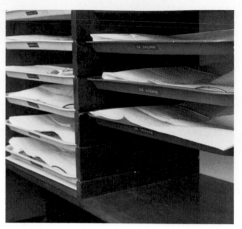

▼ **Figure 11-17**

Covered pre-set trays are stored in a cabinet until ready to be used. (Courtesy of the University of the Pacific School of Dentistry, San Francisco, CA.)

from the sterilizer (or storage) and to arrange them on the pre-set tray.

The transfer forceps should be stored in a dry, sterilized container. Both the forceps and the container should be sterilized daily.

After the instruments have been placed, disposable supplies, such as cotton rolls and gauze squares, are added. The completed tray is covered with a sterile towel or cover and placed in a special cabinet in the *clean* section until it is taken into the operatory for use (Fig. 11-17).

Reminder: Soiled Trays

The tray of soiled instruments is returned from the operatory only to the *contaminated* section of the sterilization area (Fig. 11-18).

These soiled trays may be temporarily stored in a special cabinet until the instruments are cleaned and sterilized and the trays reassembled.

Soiled trays are *not* placed in the *clean* section or stored in the same cabinet with clean trays containing sterile instruments.

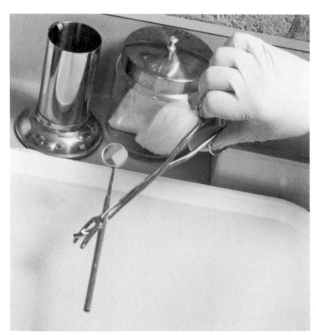

▼ **Figure 11-16**

Unwrapped sterile instruments are handled only with sterile transfer forceps. The sterile holder for these forceps is shown in the upper left portion of the photograph.

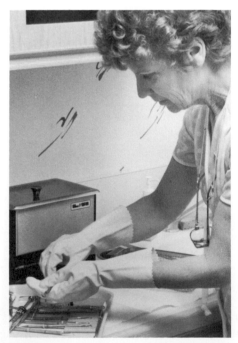

▼ **Figure 11-18**

Soiled instruments are returned only to the contaminated section of the sterilization area.

▼ EXERCISES

1. A/An _____ has a nib in the form of a claw, which is sharpened to a point.

   a. angle former
   b. explorer
   c. cleoid
   d. discoid

2. A plastic instrument is so named because it is made of plastic.

   a. true
   b. false

3. A _____ is used to mix impression materials.

   a. burnisher
   b. plastic instrument
   c. spatula

4. A/An _____ is used in the application of rubber dam.

   a. angle former
   b. beaver tail burnisher
   c. discoid
   d. interproximal knife

5. The nib of a condenser may be _____.

   a. serrated
   b. smooth
   c. sharpened
   d. a or b

6. Commonly used burnisher shapes include _____.

   a. ball
   b. football
   c. egg
   d. a, b, and c

7. When color coding instruments, the first band indicates the _____.

   a. procedure
   b. position of the instrument in the setup

8. Transfer forceps are stored in a _____.

   a. dry container
   b. holding solution
   c. sterile container
   d. a and c

9. A _____ has a cutting edge that is at a right angle to the axis of the blade.

   a. carver
   b. chisel
   c. hatchet
   d. hoe

10. Unwrapped sterile instruments are placed on the instrument tray using _____.

    a. a clean hand
    b. a gloved hand
    c. sterile transfer forceps

11. An amalgam condenser is also known as a _____.

    a. burnisher
    b. carver
    c. plugger
    d. a or c

12. Soiled trays are returned to the _____ section of the sterilization area.

    a. clean
    b. contaminated

13. A Woodson is a/an _____.

    a. amalgam condenser
    b. amalgam carver
    c. burnisher
    d. plastic instrument

14. The edges of an excavator are _____.

    a. rounded
    b. sharpened

15. The _____ mm end of an amalgam carrier is known as the "regular" end.

    a. 2.0
    b. 2.5

16. Sterile disposable items may be added to the pack or tray prior to _____.

    a. sterilization
    b. use
    c. a or b

17. The shank of a hand instrument is the _____.

    a. blade end
    b. nib end
    c. portion connecting the handle and blade
    d. portion grasped by the operator's hand

18. A/An _____ is an instrument made of flexible steel with a very sharp point used to examine tooth surfaces.

   a. carver
   b. cleoid
   c. explorer
   d. spatula

19. A _____ is beveled and sharpened to form a cutting edge.

   a. blade
   b. nib

20. An amalgam _____ is used to place the freshly mixed amalgam in the cavity preparation.

   a. carrier
   b. carver
   c. condenser

▼ Criterion Sheet 11-1

Student's Name _____

Procedure:	*IDENTIFYING THE BASIC SETUP INSTRUMENTS, SPATULAS, AND PLASTIC INSTRUMENTS*

Performance Objective:

The student will identify and state the use of the basic setup instruments, spatulas, and plastic instruments.

SE = Student evaluation **IE** = Instructor evaluation	**C** = Criterion met **X** = Criterion not met	**SE**	**IE**
Instrumentation: Basic setup instrumentation, spatulas, and plastic instruments			
1. Identified the three instruments for the basic setup. Stated the use of each.			
2. Identified the spatulas. Stated the use of the spatulas.			
3. Identified the plastic instruments. Stated the use of the plastic instruments.			
Comments:			

▼ Criterion Sheet 11–2

Student's Name _____

Procedure: *IDENTIFYING DENTAL HAND INSTRUMENTS*

Performance Objective:

The student will identify and state the use of five dental hand instruments. Instruments to be selected by the instructor.

	SE	IE
SE = Student evaluation **C** = Criterion met **IE** = Instructor evaluation **X** = Criterion not met		
Instrumentation: A group of five dental hand instruments.		
1. Instrument name: Instrument use:		
2. Instrument name: Instrument use:		
3. Instrument name: Instrument use:		
4. Instrument name: Instrument use:		
5. Instrument name: Instrument use:		
Comments:		

▼ Criterion Sheet 11-3

Student's Name _____

Procedure: *PREPARING PRE-SET TRAYS*

Performance Objective:

Provided with an instrument list and the appropriate assorted instruments, the student will prepare a sterile pre-set instrument tray.

		SE	IE
SE = Student evaluation **IE** = Instructor evaluation	**C** = Criterion met **X** = Criterion not met		
Instrumentation: Tray, tray cover, instrument list, "sterile" instruments, disposable supplies.			
1. Disinfected tray and placed clean cover.			
2. Placed instruments on tray ready for use.			
3. Added disposable supplies to tray.			
4. Prepared tray for storage.			
5. Maintained sterility throughout tray preparation.			
Comments:			

12 Rotary Dental Instruments

▼ LEARNING OBJECTIVES

The student will be able to:

1. Describe the major uses of rotary instruments in dentistry.
2. Differentiate between high-speed and low-speed handpieces.
3. Identify and state at least one use of each of the following: straight handpiece (SHP), right-angle handpiece (RAHP), and contra-angle handpiece (CAHP).
4. State the three major pieces of information needed in order to identify a bur.
5. Demonstrate identifying dental burs, stones, points, and discs.
6. Demonstrate preparation for use, bur changing, and caring for a high-speed handpiece.
7. Demonstrate cleaning, sterilizing, and caring for a contra-angle handpiece and a right-angle handpiece.

OVERVIEW OF ROTARY DENTAL INSTRUMENTS

The term **rotary dental instruments** describes dental handpieces that are used to hold and turn the cutting instruments, which are commonly referred to as *burs*.

Together, the dental handpiece and bur are like the industrial power drill and bit used to prepare holes and grooves in wood and metal. Perhaps this is why many patients refer to the dental handpiece and bur as the "drill."

Rotary instruments have many uses in dentistry, including:

▼ During the steps in cavity preparation (these are described in Chapter 21, "Amalgam Restorations").

▼ Reducing and reshaping the teeth in preparation for the placement of crowns and other cast restorations.

▼ Removing old amalgam or cast restorations that must be replaced.

▼ Polishing the teeth.

▼ Polishing recently placed restorations.

DENTAL BURS

A dental bur consists of three parts. These are the shank, neck, and head (Fig. 12–1*A*).

▼ The **shank** is the part of the bur that fits into the handpiece. The length of the shank depends on the specific function of the bur. For example, the shanks on laboratory and surgical burs are longer than those on the burs used for restorative dentistry.

▼ The **neck** is the narrow portion of the bur that connects the shank and the head.

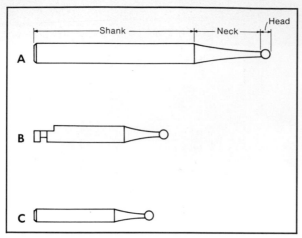

▼ **Figure 12–1**

Basic design of burs. *A.* Straight shank of a bur used in a straight handpiece. *B.* Latch-type bur for use in a contra-angle handpiece. *C.* Friction grip bur for use in a contra-angle handpiece. (Torres HO, Ehrlich A: Modern Dental Assisting, 4th Ed. Philadelphia, WB Saunders, 1990, p 313.)

▼ The **head** of the bur is the cutting portion. These are manufactured in many sizes, shapes, and materials.

Bur Identification

Each bur is designed for a specific purpose. The following information is necessary so that the correct bur is selected for each use:

1. The shank type (friction grip or latch-type).
2. The type of bur (carbide steel, plain steel, or diamond).
3. The bur head shape and size number.

Shank Types

The shape of the shank is designed to fit into a specific handpiece.

▼ **Straight handpiece burs** have a straight shank. In catalog descriptions, these are abbreviated as SH (straight handpiece) or HP (handpiece) (see Fig. 12–1*A*).

▼ **Latch type burs** with a notched shank. In catalog descriptions, these are abbreviated as LA (latch-type angle) or RA (right-angle latch-type) (see Fig. 12–1*B*).

▼ **Friction grip burs** have a smooth shank. In catalog descriptions, these are described as FG (friction grip); FGS, FGSS, or FG-SS (friction grip short shank); and FG-SU (friction grip surgical shank) (see Fig. 12–1*C*).

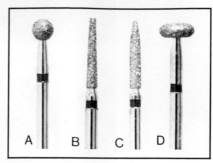

▼ **Figure 12–2**

Sample shapes of diamond burs. *A.* Round. *B.* Flat end taper. *C.* Flame. *D.* Wheel contour. Notice the identifying band on the shank. (Courtesy of Midwest Dental Products Corp, Des Plaines, IL.)

Bur Types

Carbide steel burs, which are often referred to simply as *carbides*, operate efficiently at high speeds and retain their sharp edges over repeated usage. For these reasons, carbide burs are favored in operative dentistry.

Plain steel burs may be used in removing carious tooth structure and dentin but are not effective in the removal or reduction of enamel. When used incorrectly, they generate heat, which may damage the tissues of the tooth and cause discomfort to the patient. Much laboratory work is accomplished using steel burs.

Diamond stones are burs in which the cutting portion is covered with bits of industrial diamonds. These burs are used in the high-speed handpiece as a fast and effective means of cutting the hard tissue of a tooth.

The head shapes of diamond stones are similar in design to those of carbide burs. However, diamond burs have their own number designation for the head size and shape. Also, as shown in Figure 12–2, some diamond burs are identified by a colored band on the shank.

Sizes and Shapes of Bur Heads

Each bur shape comes in several different sizes, which are represented by a series of numbers. The lower the number in a series, the smaller the bur head size.

Amalgam Preparation

As the name implies, these burs are used primarily in the preparation of amalgam restorations. The commonly used sizes of amalgam restoration burs are numbers 245 and 246 (Fig. 12–3).

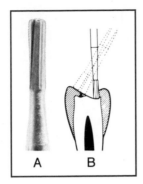

▼ **Figure 12–3**

Amalgam preparation bur. *A.* Shape of the bur. *B.* The bur in use. (Courtesy of Midwest Dental Products Corp, Des Plaines, IL.)

Round

During cavity preparation, round burs may be used to remove carious tooth structure. Round burs are also used to open the pulp chamber of a tooth in preparation for endodontic treatment.

The commonly used sizes of round burs range from numbers ¼ to 10 (Fig. 12–4*A*).

Inverted Cone

This bur is shaped like a cone with the top cut off. The commonly used sizes for inverted cone burs range from numbers 33½ to 37L (L indicates long) (Fig. 12–4*B*).

Fissure Burs

The term **fissure** means groove, and these burs are characterized by grooves. The sides of the **straight fissure bur** are parallel. The sides of a **taper fissure bur** converge toward the tip end of the bur.

Both plain and taper fissure burs may be either plain-cut or cross-cut (Figs. 12–4*C,D* and 12–5).

Cross-cut fissure burs, which are also known as *dentate burs*, have cuts along the blade surfaces like the teeth of a saw. These cross-cuts give the bur additional cutting ability (Figs. 12–4*E,F* and 12–5).

Plain fissure burs do not have cross-cuts.

▼ The commonly used sizes for **plain straight fissure burs** range from numbers 56 to 58L.

▼ The commonly used sizes for **cross-cut straight fissure burs** range from numbers 556 to 588L.

▼ The commonly used sizes for **plain taper fissure burs** range from numbers 169 to 171L.

▼ The commonly used sizes for **cross-cut taper fissure burs** range from numbers 699 to 701L.

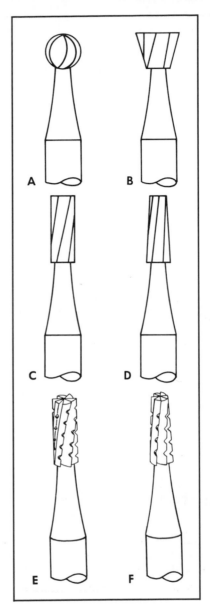

▼ **Figure 12–4**

Basic shapes of burs. *A.* Round. *B.* Inverted cone. *C.* Straight fissure—plain. *D.* Taper fissure—plain. *E.* Straight fissure—crosscut. *F.* Taper fissure—crosscut. (Torres HO, Ehrlich A: Modern Dental Assisting, 4th Ed. Philadelphia, WB Saunders, 1990, p 317.)

The **end-cutting bur** is similar in design to the straight fissure bur, with the exception of the cutting portion, which is placed on the *end* of the bur only. The commonly used sizes of end-cutting burs are numbers 957 and 958.

Trimming and Finishing Burs

Trimming and finishing burs, also referred to as *T and F burs*, are designed for trimming, shaping, and finishing all restorative materials; however, this term is most commonly applied to the burs used for trimming and finishing composite resto-

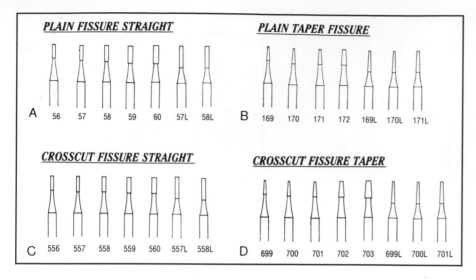

▼ **Figure 12-5**

Size range for fissure burs. (Courtesy of Miltex Instrument Co, Lake Success, NY.)

rations. (Composite restorations are discussed in Chapter 22, "Cosmetic Dentistry.")

These burs are available in a variety of shapes and sizes, which have their own range of identification numbers (Fig. 12-6).

Frequently these burs are described by the number of blades on the head. The more blades there are, the finer the finish. Thus, a 30-bladed bur, also known as a *fine finishing bur*, produces a smoother finish than does a 12-bladed bur.

OTHER ROTARY INSTRUMENTS

Points and Stones

Points and stones, which are usually identified by their color, are used for polishing and finishing restorations. They are available in a variety of materials, sizes, and shapes.

White stones and points are used for finishing composite and porcelain restorations.

Brown and **green** stones and points are used for finishing and polishing porcelain, composites, and gold and amalgam restorations (Fig. 12-7).

Gray stones and points are used for polishing nonprecious metals.

Pink stones and points are used in the laboratory for finishing metal restorations.

Discs and Mandrels

A **mandrel**, which is shaped like the shank of a bur, serves as a mounting device for discs and wheels.

The smooth-shank mandrel fits into a straight

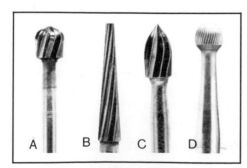

▼ **Figure 12-6**

Assorted trimming and finishing burs. *A.* T & F 12-bladed round. *B.* T & F 12-bladed cone. *C.* T & F 12-bladed flame. *D.* F.F. 30-bladed ball. (Courtesy of Midwest Dental Products Corp, Des Plaines, IL.)

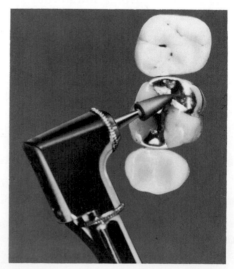

▼ **Figure 12-7**

Mounted stone, in latch-type, low-speed handpiece, used for polishing an amalgam restoration. (Courtesy of Shofu Dental Corp, Menlo Park, CA.)

handpiece. The notched-type mandrel fits into a contra-angled handpiece.

Some discs and wheels snap onto the head of the mandrel. Others are held in place with a screw set in the head of the mandrel.

Disposable discs are made of abrasive materials such as sand, garnet, Carborundum, or cuttlefish embedded on a metal or paper backing, with a hole in the center to be held by a mandrel.

These discs may be used in finishing cavity preparations and on restorations that need to be polished or reduced in contour (Fig. 12–8).

The discs are flat and round with the material placed on the inside (safe outside) or the outside (safe inside) or on both sides of the disc.

Discs are routinely identified by their diameter, the material impregnated on the surface, the type and size of grit, and the design fitting a certain type of mandrel.

Carborundum Discs or Stones

Carborundum, a type of abrasive made of silicon carbide, is bonded into the shape of a disc or a stone, mounted on a mandrel.

The Carborundum disc or stone is used mostly in the laboratory to separate metallic restorations or bridgework and castings.

A **Jo Dandy disc**, also known as a *Damascus disc*, is a sharp carbide disc designed to cut metallic restorations or castings. The disc is thin and very brittle and is discarded at once if damaged.

Rubber Polishing Wheels and Discs

Soft or hard rubber polishing wheels and discs are manufactured by impregnating abrasive material

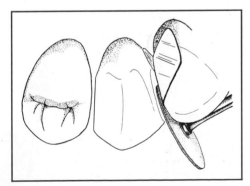

▼ Figure 12–8

Use of a thin disk to clear a proximal contact. (Baum L, Phillips RW, Lund MR: Operative Dentistry, 3rd Ed. Philadelphia, WB Saunders, 1985, p 436.)

into the processed rubber. They are prepared for use with a mandrel, or they may be premounted on a mandrel by the manufacturer. They are available in fine, medium, or coarse grit.

These wheels and discs are ordered according to the type of grit, the size, and an indication for mounting on a mandrel or the unmounted type.

Bur Care

The following are the basic steps for the care of all burs, diamond burs, polishing points, and stones.

1. Burs may be presoaked *briefly* to prevent debris from drying on them. Do not soak carbide burs longer than 20 minutes because the chemicals in the disinfecting solution may dull or weaken the burs.
2. To remove debris prior to sterilization, rinse and brush the burs with a nylon or brass bristle brush. (A stiff metal brush is not used because this would dull cutting edges.)
3. As an alternative, debris can be removed from the bur with a rubber eraser.
4. Burs may be ultrasonically cleaned if inserted in a bur block or holder to prevent damage to the blades from rubbing or vibrating against each other or any hard surface or material.
5. Burs can be sterilized by dry heat, chemiclave, hot oil, or autoclaving.
6. Prior to autoclaving, the burs must be dipped in a corrosion inhibitor and then placed in an autoclavable bur block.

Bur Removal Tool

The bur removal tool that was used during treatment is cleaned and disinfected as part of the operatory cleanup procedure.

DENTAL HANDPIECES

Dental handpieces are described by their speed expressed as the number of revolutions per minute (rpm) and by their shape.

High-Speed Handpieces

High-speed handpieces rotate at a speed ranging from 100,000 to 800,000 rpm. The contra-angle design of the head of the handpiece makes it

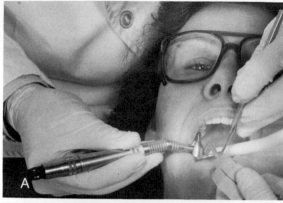

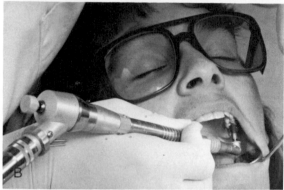

▼ **Figure 12–9**

High-speed and low-speed handpieces have many uses in dentistry. *A.* The high-speed handpiece in use during a cavity preparation. *B.* The low-speed handpiece, with a right-angle adaptor, in use during a prophylaxis procedure.

possible to gain access to all areas of the mouth (Fig. 12–9*A*).

High-speed handpieces, which are air driven, are used when the rapid and efficient cutting of tooth structure is important.

To avoid overheating, the handpiece sprays an air-water coolant on the tooth during the prepara-

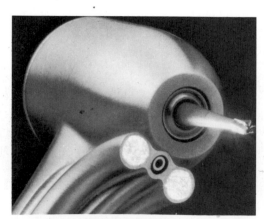

▼ **Figure 12–10**

Fiberoptic light for complete illumination of the operating field. (Courtesy of Midwest Dental Products Corp, Des Plaines, IL.)

tion. This is known as the **washed-field technique** and is described in Chapter 13, "Oral Evacuation and Instrument Transfer."

To ensure better visibility, some high-speed handpieces have a fiberoptic light, which is built into the head. This projects a beam of light from the head of the handpiece directly onto the bur and tooth under preparation (Fig. 12–10).

Low-Speed Handpieces

Low-speed handpieces, which rotate at a speed ranging from 6000 to 10,000 rpm, are used both in the operatory and in the dental laboratory (see Fig. 12–9*B*).

Adapters are used with the low-speed handpiece so that it may function as a straight handpiece (SHP), a contra-angle handpiece (CAHP), or a right-angle handpiece (RAHP).

Straight Handpieces (SHP)

The straight handpiece adapter, which is *not* angled, holds burs in the low-speed handpiece. In the operatory, the dentist may use it with finishing burs, sandpaper discs, and other abrasives to finish or polish the anterior teeth (see Fig. 12–15*A*).

However, the straight handpiece is used primarily in the dental laboratory with burs, abrasive stones, or discs to trim custom trays or to adjust and polish cast restorations and appliances (see Fig. 1–8).

The low-speed laboratory handpiece may be belt driven. This uses a round belt and pulley between the motor and the handpiece (Fig. 12–11).

Contra-Angle Handpieces (CAHP)

The contra-angle handpiece attaches to the low-speed straight handpiece to form an extension

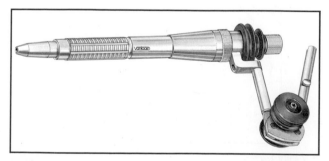

▼ **Figure 12–11**

A straight handpiece with pulley and belt for laboratory use. (Courtesy of Miltex Instrument Co, Lake Success, NY.)

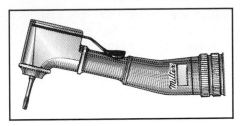

▼ **Figure 12-12**

Latch-type, contra-angle handpiece with bur in place. (Courtesy of Miltex Instrument Co, Lake Success, NY.)

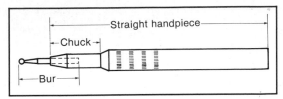

▼ **Figure 12-14**

Diagram of a straight handpiece with the bur mounted in the chuck. (Torres HO, Ehrlich A: Modern Dental Assisting, 4th Ed. Philadelphia, WB Saunders, 1990, p 325.)

with an angle that is greater than 90 degrees at the working tip. This angulation provides better access to the posterior teeth (Fig. 12–12).

The contra-angle handpiece may be used with a round bur during the final stages of a cavity preparation to remove carious dentin. It is also used with abrasive stones or discs to polish restorations and appliances.

Right-Angle Handpieces (RAHP)

The right-angle handpiece attaches to the low-speed straight handpiece to form an extension with a right angle (90 degrees) at the working tip.

The right-angle handpiece is mostly used for cleaning and polishing during the prophylaxis procedures. For this reason, it is often referred to as a *prophy angle.*

In one style, the rubber prophy cup and the bristle brush snap over a ball-like projection on the head of the right-angle handpiece. In another design, they come with a screw attachment that screws into the end of a right-angle handpiece (Fig. 12–13).

Positioning Cutting Instruments Within the Handpiece

In an industrial power drill, a **chuck** is used to hold the cutting instrument in place. In the dental

drill, a chuck is also used to securely position the bur, or other rotary cutting instruments, in the head of the handpiece.

Dental drills use different types of chucks to hold the bur in place. These are referred to as latch-type and friction-grip.

In a **straight** handpiece, the chuck is mechanically tightened to hold the bur in place (Figs. 12–14 and 12–15).

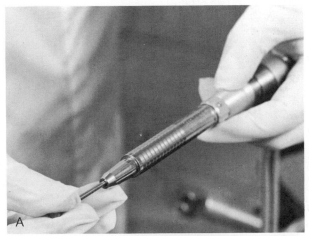

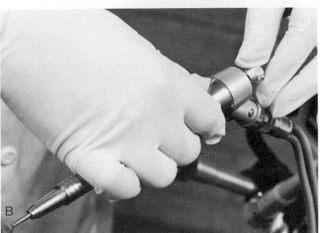

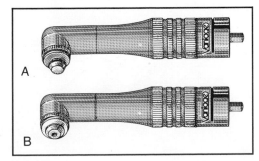

▼ **Figure 12-13**

The right-angle handpieces. *A.* With snap-on tip. *B.* With screw-on tip. (Courtesy of Miltex Instrument Co, Lake Success, NY.)

▼ **Figure 12-15**

Mounted stone used in the straight handpiece. *A.* The assistant places the bur in the handpiece. *B.* The chuck is tightened to hold the bur firmly in place. (Torres HO, Ehrlich A: Modern Dental Assisting, 4th Ed. Philadelphia, WB Saunders, 1990, p 326.)

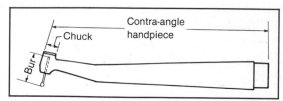

▼ **Figure 12-16**

Diagram of a contra-angle handpiece with bur mounted in the chuck. (Torres HO, Ehrlich A: Modern Dental Assisting, 4th Ed. Philadelphia, WB Saunders, 1990, p 327.)

A **latch-type** handpiece has a latch that fastens around a notch in the shank of the bur to hold it securely in place. Generally, but not always, low-speed contra-angle handpieces use latch-type burs.

A handpiece that holds a **friction-grip bur** has a chuck that holds the shank of the bur securely in place when tightened (Fig. 12-16). Friction-grip burs are used in high-speed and some low-speed handpieces.

Procedure

ATTACHING THE DENTAL HANDPIECE

1. Attach the handpiece to the tubing extension of the dental unit.

2. Tighten the threaded housing and give the handpiece a gentle tug to check that it is properly attached to the tubing (Figs. 12-17 and 12-18).

3. Adjust the pressure gauges if necessary.

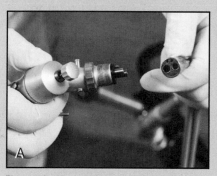
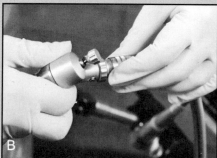
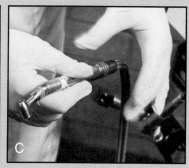

Figure 12-17. Attaching the handpiece. *A.* The assistant prepares to attach the handpiece to the tubing. *B.* The threaded housing is tightened. *C.* The tubing is tugged gently to be certain that the handpiece is attached properly. (Torres HO, Ehrlich A: Modern Dental Assisting, 4th Ed. Philadelphia, WB Saunders, 1990, p 365.)

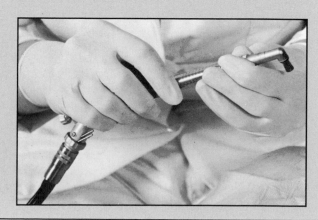

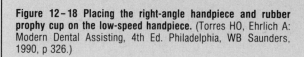

Figure 12-18 Placing the right-angle handpiece and rubber prophy cup on the low-speed handpiece. (Torres HO, Ehrlich A: Modern Dental Assisting, 4th Ed. Philadelphia, WB Saunders, 1990, p 326.)

The handpiece that holds a friction-grip bur comes with a **bur inserting-removal** tool, which is used when placing and removing the bur from the handpiece. (Some high-speed handpieces are equipped with a lever that makes this tool unnecessary.)

HANDPIECE PREPARATION AND BUR CHANGING

The exact steps in the preparation of the handpiece for use depend on the manufacturer's instructions. The procedures shown on pages 188 and 189 are the general steps to be followed in handpiece preparation and use.

HANDPIECE MAINTENANCE

Dental handpieces are expensive precision pieces of equipment. To protect the handpiece, each one must regularly receive the preventive care as recommended by the manufacturer.

The manufacturer's instructions for each handpiece are very specific. Read and follow these directions carefully.

Procedure

USING THE HANDPIECE

1. Extract a sufficient length of air tubing so that the tubing comfortably reaches across the patient's chest and to the operator's hand.

2. Lock the tubing in a nonretractable position.

3. Gently tug to determine that the tubing is firmly locked.

4. Pass the handpiece to the operator with the left hand in the position of use.
   The bur is pointed upward for a maxillary preparation.
   The bur is pointed downward for a mandibular preparation.

HANDPIECE CARE AND STERILIZATION

In addition to routine maintenance, handpieces must be cleaned and sterilized after each use. The following are general guidelines for between-pa-

Procedure

PLACING AND CHANGING THE BUR

1. At the beginning of the procedure, select and place the first bur (as specified by the operator).

2. Tug gently to determine that the bur is firmly in place.

3. When changing a bur, first remove the used bur and then place the new one (Fig. 12–19).

4. Tug gently to determine that the bur is firmly in place.

Figure 12–19 Changing burs. *A.* The assistant uses the bur changer to remove the used bur. *B.* The assistant prepares to place the next bur in the handpiece. (Torres HO, Ehrlich A: Modern Dental Assisting, 4th Ed. Philadelphia, WB Saunders, 1990, p 366.)

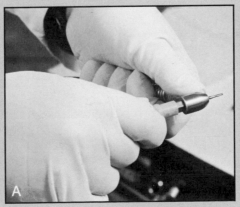
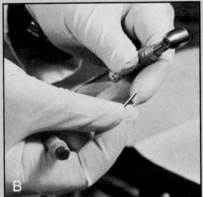

tient care for high-speed and low-speed handpieces and attachments (contra-angle, right-angle, and straight).

Handpieces that cannot be sterilized must be disinfected very carefully. However, handpieces should not be soaked in disinfecting solution because these chemicals can corrode and damage the handpiece.

Procedure

CLEANING THE HANDPIECE

Flush and Remove

1. Wear gloves while handling soiled handpieces (Fig. 12–20).

2. At the end of each patient visit, to flush the water hose run the handpiece over the cuspidor for 30 seconds.

3. Remove the handpiece from the air and water hose. (Some manufacturers recommend leaving the bur in place; others specify that it should be removed.)

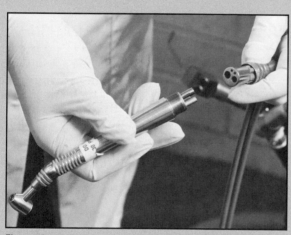

Figure 12–20 Soiled handpieces are handled only while wearing gloves. (Torres HO, Ehrlich A: Modern Dental Assisting, 4th Ed. Philadelphia, WB Saunders, 1990, p 330.)

Scrub and Dry

1. Scrub the exterior surface of the handpiece with a cleaning solution to remove soil and debris. A gauze, sponge, or clean brush may be used for this purpose.

2. Rinse away solution and residue by scrubbing under clean tap water. (Do not immerse the handpiece.)

3. Thoroughly dry the handpiece using gauze, paper towel, or air from the syringe.

Lubricate and Operate

1. Lubricate the handpiece using only the lubricant recommended by the manufacturer.

2. Run the handpiece briefly to remove excess lubricant. (If a bur has been in place, remove it.)

3. Remove the handpiece.

Procedure

STERILIZING THE HANDPIECE

1. Place the handpiece in a sterilization bag.

2. Sterilize the handpiece according to the manufacturer's directions.

   Most manufacturers recommend autoclaving or chemical vapor sterilization.

   Dry heat and "flash sterilization" that exceeds 275°F should *not* be used.

3. Leave the handpiece in the autoclave bag for storage.

4. If recommended by the manufacturer, lubricate the handpiece again after sterilization and prior to use.

5. Clean the fiberoptic light-transmitting surfaces on both ends of the fiberoptic handpiece with isopropyl alcohol before reconnecting the handpiece to the hose (Fig. 12–21).

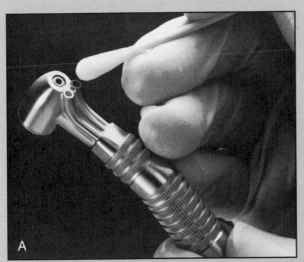
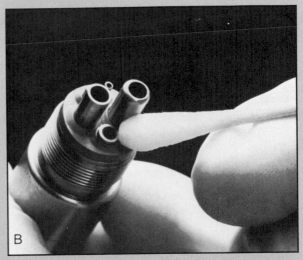

Figure 12–21 Both ends of the fiberoptic light surface are cleaned with a cotton swab wet with isopropyl alcohol. (Courtesy of Midwest Dental Products Corp, Des Plaines, IL.)

Procedure

DISINFECTING THE HANDPIECE

1. Wipe the handpiece thoroughly clean.
2. Place it on the bracket table or tray.
3. Spray it with disinfectant.
4. Keep it thoroughly wet for at least 2 minutes.

5. Wipe thoroughly clean with gauze sponges or paper towels. (Some operators prefer to leave the disinfectant on the handpiece.)

Procedure

CLEANING AND LUBRICATING THE CONTRA-ANGLE HANDPIECE

1. Mount the contra-angle handpiece on the bench motor in the laboratory.
2. Place the working end of the handpiece into a small bottle of **handpiece cleaning solvent**. (Latch type: latch is left open.)
3. Run the handpiece forward and then backward in the cleaner solvent for approximately a minute in each direction. (This will remove the soil and debris lodged in and on the handpiece.)

4. Turn the motor off. Remove the handpiece from the solvent and wipe it dry with a soft, clean cloth.
5. To lubricate the handpiece after sterilization, mount it on the bench motor and run backward and forward in **handpiece lubricating oil**.
6. Remove the handpiece, wipe it dry, and place it in storage for further use.

Procedure

CLEANING AND LUBRICATING THE RIGHT-ANGLE HANDPIECE

1. Mount the right-angle handpiece on the bench motor in the laboratory.

2. Place the working end of the handpiece into a small bottle of **handpiece cleaning solvent.**

3. Run the handpiece backward and forward for 1 minute in each direction.

4. Remove the handpiece from the cleaner and wipe dry with a soft, clean cloth.

5. Remove the handpiece from the bench motor and disassemble the handpiece, using the special wrench furnished by the manufacturer.

6. Following sterilization, take the parts of the disassembled handpiece from the sterilizer and place them on a clean tray.

7. Place heavy lubricant, usually petroleum jelly or a commercial lubricant, on the gears of the handpiece before it is reassembled.

   Note: The heavy lubricant is essential because it prevents the wear of the gears caused by the abrasives used during polishing.

8. Wipe the handpiece dry and place it in storage for further use.

▼ EXERCISES

1. A _high speed_ handpiece rotates at a speed ranging from 100,000 to 800,000 rpm.

   a. high-speed
   b. low-speed

2. Handpieces may be sterilized by _____.

   a. autoclaving
   b. dry heat in excess of 275°F
   c. flash sterilization
   d. a, b, or c

3. _____ are used for polishing and finishing restorations.

   a. Mandrels
   b. Points
   c. Stones
   d. b and c

4. A _a   b_ handpiece is also referred to as a prophy angle.

   a. contra-angle
   b. right-angle
   c. straight

5. When cleaning a handpiece, it _____ be soaked to remove soil.

   a. may
   b. may not

6. Some _b_ burs are identified by a colored band on the shank.

   a. carbide steel
   b. diamond
   c. latch-type
   d. plain steel

7. The fiberoptic of the handpiece is cleaned with _____.

   a. handpiece cleaning solvent
   b. isopropyl alcohol
   c. sodium hypochlorite
   d. a or b

8. Burs _____ routinely discarded after a single use.

   a. are
   b. are not

9. A fine finishing bur has _____ blades on the head.

   a. 5
   b. 12
   c. 30
   d. 60

10. A right-angle handpiece is lubricated with _____.

    a. handpiece lubricating oil
    b. petroleum jelly
    c. a or b

11. The _____ of the bur is that portion that fits into the handpiece.

    a. head
    b. neck
    c. shank

12. In a _____ handpiece the chuck is mechanically tightened to hold the bur in place.

    a. friction-grip
    b. latch-type
    c. straight

13. Petroleum jelly may be used to lubricate the moving parts of the _____ handpiece.

    a. contra-angle
    b. high-speed
    c. right-angle
    d. straight

14. _____ burs are in the size range numbers ¼ to 10.

    a. Amalgam
    b. Round
    c. Straight fissure
    c. Taper fissure

15. Burs may be sterilized by _____.

    a. autoclaving
    b. chemiclave
    c. dry heat
    d. a, b, or c

16. A straight handpiece is used primarily _____.

    a. in the dental laboratory
    b. to clean and polish the teeth
    c. with latch-type burs

17. A _____ is a mounting device used with rotary discs and wheels.

    a. chuck
    b. friction grip
    c. latch
    d. mandrel

18. _____ steel burs are favored for use in operative dentistry.

    a. Carbide
    b. Plain

19. ___White___ stones and points are used for finishing composite and porcelain restorations.

   a. Gray — *Non precious metal*
   b. Green
   c. Pink — *metal restoration in lab*
   (d.) White

20. Burs may be cleaned by _____.

   a. brushing with a nylon or brass bristle brush
   b. placing the burs in a holder and using the ultrasonic cleaner
   c. removing debris with an eraser
   (d.) a, b, or c

▼ Criterion Sheet 12–1

Student's Name _____

Procedure: *IDENTIFYING BURS, STONES, POINTS, AND DISCS*

Performance Objective:

The student will identify 10 burs, stones, points, or discs.

		SE	IE
SE = Student evaluation **IE** = Instructor evaluation	**C** = Criterion met **X** = Criterion not met		
Instrumentation: An assortment of burs, stones, points, and discs selected by the instructor.			
1. Name:			
2. Name:			
3. Name:			
4. Name:			
5. Name:			
6. Name:			
7. Name:			
8. Name:			
9. Name:			
10. Name:			
Comments:			

▼ Criterion Sheet 12-2

Student's Name _____

Procedure: *PREPARATION, USE, AND CARE OF A HIGH-SPEED HANDPIECE*

Performance Objective:

The student will demonstrate attaching the high-speed handpiece to the dental unit, placing and removing a bur, passing the handpiece to the operator, and caring for the handpiece.

Prior to this performance, the student will have seen a demonstration and had an opportunity to ask questions regarding all of these steps for this particular handpiece.

SE = Student evaluation **IE** = Instructor evaluation	**C** = Criterion met **X** = Criterion not met	**SE**	**IE**
Instrumentation: A friction grip bur, bur remover-seating tool, and high-speed handpiece in a dental operatory setting. (Appropriate infection control barriers will be used during all procedures actually performed on a patient.)			
1. Attached the handpiece to the dental unit. Tightened threaded housing.			
2. Determined that the handpiece was securely attached. Adjusted pressure gauges as necessary.			
3. Placed the bur in the handpiece. Determined that the bur was seated securely.			
4. Extracted sufficient length of tubing for the handpiece. Determined that the tubing was firmly locked.			
5. Passed the handpiece to the operator in the position of use.			
6. Handled the soiled handpiece only while wearing gloves. Flushed and removed the handpiece from the dental unit.			
7. Cleaned, lubricated, and prepared the handpiece for sterilization.			
8. Sterilized, prepared, and stored the handpiece.			
Comments:			

▼ Criterion Sheet 12-3

Student's Name _____

Procedure: *CLEANING, STERILIZING, AND LUBRICATING CONTRA-ANGLE AND RIGHT-ANGLE HANDPIECES*

Performance Objective:

The student will demonstrate cleaning, sterilizing, and lubricating contra-angle and right-angle handpieces.

Prior to this performance, the student will have seen a demonstration and had an opportunity to ask questions regarding all of these steps for these handpieces.

		SE	IE
SE = Student evaluation **IE** = Instructor evaluation	**C** = Criterion met **X** = Criterion not met		
Instrumentation: Utility gloves; contra-angle and right-angle handpieces; and cleaning, disinfecting, and lubricating supplies.			
1. Donned utility gloves.			
2. **Contra-angle handpiece:** Removed handpiece from the dental unit. Scrubbed and dried the handpiece. Cleaned and lubricated the handpiece. Prepared and sterilized the handpiece. Lubricated, operated, and stored the handpiece for future use.			
3. **Right-angle handpiece:** Removed handpiece from the dental unit. Scrubbed and dried the handpiece. Cleaned and lubricated the handpiece. Disassembled and autoclaved the handpiece. Lubricated and reassembled the handpiece. Prepared and stored the handpiece for future use.			
Comments:			

13 Oral Evacuation and Instrument Transfer

▼ LEARNING OBJECTIVES

The student will be able to:

1. Describe the four operating zones and the uses of each.
2. State the precautions for use of the high volume evacuator (HVE) tip.
3. Demonstrate assembling, adjusting, and positioning of the HVE tip in each area of the oral cavity.
4. Demonstrate retraction of the cheeks, tongue, and lips.
5. Demonstrate passing instruments in the position of use.
6. Demonstrate the exchange of instruments, handpieces, and materials at chairside.

OVERVIEW OF ORAL EVACUATION AND INSTRUMENT TRANSFER

Proper positioning of the team, the smooth transfer of instruments, and effective oral evacuation and retraction to maintain a clear field of operation are all important elements in providing quality patient treatment.

Washed Field Technique

With the **washed field technique,** a fine air-water mist is sprayed from the tip of the handpiece. This removes debris, dissipates the heat of cutting the preparation, reduces the possibility of injury to the tooth pulp, and minimizes any discomfort that might be caused by this heat.

With the washed field technique, the assistant uses high volume evacuation to remove the water and debris from the patient's oral cavity.

Direct and Indirect Vision

Throughout the procedure, the operator must be able to see the field of operation clearly. To accomplish this, the operator uses either direct or indirect vision.

With **direct vision,** the operator is able actually to see the tooth or tissues being operated.

With **indirect vision,** the operator uses a mouth mirror to reflect a view of the operating field (Fig. 13–1).

Throughout each procedure, the assistant must take care to stay clear of the operator's field of vision.

THE OPERATING ZONES

The use of operating zones, based on the "clock concept," aids the operator and assistant in working smoothly together during instrument transfer and oral evacuation.

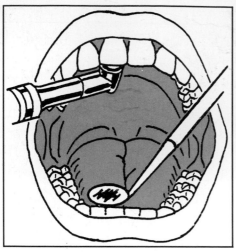

▼ **Figure 13-1**

Using a mouth mirror for indirect vision. (Torres HO, Ehrlich A: Modern Dental Assisting, 4th Ed. Philadelphia, WB Saunders, 1990, p 351.)

In the **clock concept**, an imaginary circle is placed over the dental chair, with the patient's head at the center of the circle. The circle is numbered like a clock, with the top of the circle at 12 o'clock.

Static Zone

The static zone (Fig. 13-2, Area A), between 11 and 2 o'clock, is reserved for large equipment, such as the mobile dental unit and instrument cart. This is referred to as **rear delivery.**

The rare exception to this, known as the *12 o'clock position,* is when the operator needs to be positioned behind the patient's head.

When an object is heavy or a material might be objectionable if held near the patient's face, it may be passed or held in the static zone. In addition, anesthetic injection syringes are sometimes passed to the operator from this zone so that the patient will not be alarmed at the sight of the syringe.

If the assistant is called away from chairside for any length of time and the coordinating assistant is busy elsewhere, the assistant's cart may be placed horizontal to the back of the patient's head, thus providing the operator with access to instruments, materials, and the high volume evacuator (HVE).

Transfer Zone

The transfer zone (Fig. 13-2, Area C) is from 4 to 8 o'clock. It is used for passing and receiving instruments over the chest and at the chin of the patient. This action is also referred to as front delivery.

In **front delivery,** the assistant passes and receives the handpiece, instruments, and materials to and from the operator in the transfer zone near the area of the patient's chin and lower face area.

The handpiece, air-water syringe, and saliva ejector tubings are passed over the patient's upper chest area.

Operator's and Assistant's Zones

The placement of the operator's and assistant's zones depends on whether the operator is left-handed or right-handed.

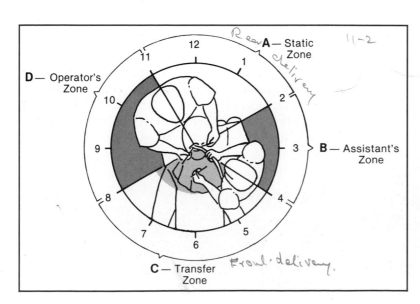

▼ **Figure 13-2**

Clock concept positions of patient, operator, and assistant for four-handed dentistry. The patient's head is center of the clock. *A.* Static zone (11-2 o'clock). *B.* Assistant's zone (2-4 o'clock). *C.* Transfer zone (4-8 o'clock). *D.* Operator's zone (8-11 o'clock). (Torres HO, Ehrlich A: Modern Dental Assisting, 4th Ed. Philadelphia, WB Saunders, 1990, p 350.)

Right-Handed Operator

The right-handed operator is seated to the right of the patient. This places the operator's zone between 8 and 11 o'clock (Fig. 13–3).

When working with a right-handed operator the assistant's zone is between 2 and 4 o'clock (see Fig. 13–2, Area B).

Left-Handed Operator

The left-handed operator is seated to the left of the patient. This places the operator's zone between 1 and 4 o'clock (Fig. 13–4).

When working with a left-handed operator, the assistant's zone is between 8 and 10 o'clock.

THE AIR-WATER SYRINGE

During oral evacuation, the air-water syringe is held in the assistant's left hand. By pressing the buttons in the appropriate combination, the air-water syringe can be used to spray:

▼ Air and water to cool the tooth.

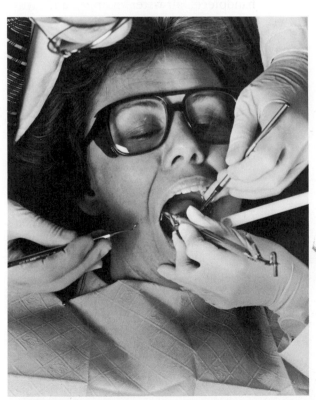

▼ **Figure 13–3**

A right-handed operator is seated to the right of the patient. (Torres HO, Ehrlich A: Modern Dental Assisting, 4th Ed. Philadelphia, WB Saunders, 1990, p 350.)

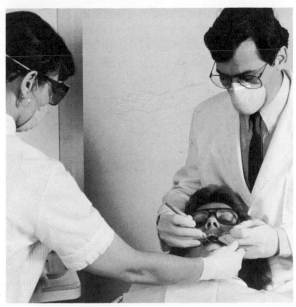

▼ **Figure 13–4**

A left-handed operator is seated to the left of the patient. (Torres HO, Ehrlich A: Modern Dental Assisting, 4th Ed. Philadelphia, WB Saunders, 1990, p 350.)

▼ Water to rinse debris from the site.

▼ Air to dry the teeth or tissues.

HIGH VOLUME ORAL EVACUATION

The primary goal of oral evacuation is to keep water from accumulating in the patient's mouth and/or hindering the operator's vision. However, the HVE tip is also used to keep the tongue and cheek away from the field of operation.

HVE Precautions

The high volume evacuation system works on a vacuum principle (like a vacuum cleaner). If the tip "grabs" (adheres to) the soft tissues of the oral cavity, it can cause serious damage. The following precautions should be heeded when using the HVE tip:

1. Place the HVE tip very carefully and gently to avoid injury to these delicate tissues.
2. If the tip does grab the tissues, lower your arm and slightly rotate the angled opening of the tip until the vacuum (suction) is broken.
3. If this action does not free the tissue, turn the vacuum control off immediately. This breaks the suction and avoids further trauma to the tissue.

4. To avoid triggering the gag reflex (on the soft palate), always place the HVE tip firmly (but gently) on the gingiva, tissues of the hard palate, or tongue. Also, it helps to keep the tip moving.

HVE Tip

The plastic or metal HVE tip is contoured with a slanted opening at each end so it will adapt to the anterior and posterior areas of the maxillary or mandibular arches (Fig. 13–5).

Anterior Placement

The opening of the end for anterior placement is slanted in an obtuse angle (greater than 90 degrees).

When operating on an anterior tooth, the posterior end of the tip is placed into the handle, so that the anterior end extends ready for use.

Posterior Placement

The opening of the opposite end, for posterior placement, is slanted in an oblique angle (less than 90 degrees).

When operating on a posterior tooth, the anterior end of the tip is placed into the handle, so that the posterior end extends ready for use.

Holding the HVE Handle and Hose

In order to position and control the tip as needed, follow these steps:

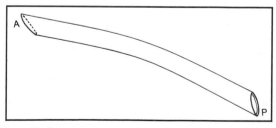

▼ **Figure 13–5**

The HVE tip. A, Anterior opening for placement in the anterior position. P, Posterior opening for placement in the posterior position. (Torres HO, Ehrlich A: Modern Dental Assisting, 4th Ed. Philadelphia, WB Saunders, 1990, p 352.)

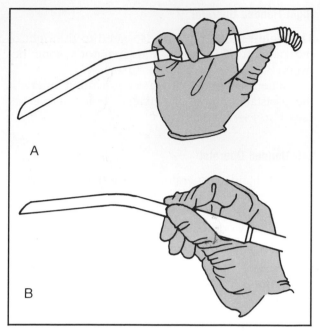

▼ **Figure 13–6**

Techniques for grasping HVE tip. *A.* Reverse palm-thumb grasp. Tubing is tucked under arm close to the body when using this position. *B.* Conventional technique for holding HVE tip, using a modified pen grasp (wand position). (Torres HO, Ehrlich A: Modern Dental Assisting, 4th Ed. Philadelphia, WB Saunders, 1990, p 352.)

1. At the beginning of treatment, place a sterile HVE tip firmly into the HVE handle.
2. Using a modified pen grasp or the reverse palm-thumb grasp, hold the handle in the right fist (Fig. 13–6).
3. Tuck the hose extension under the right arm close to the side of the body.

HVE TIP PLACEMENT

Placement of the HVE tip varies to accommodate the use of the handpiece in the different quadrants of the mouth (Fig. 13–7).

At the beginning of the procedure, the HVE tip is placed so that the slanted opening is used to retract the cheek or tongue.

After the HVE tip has been positioned, the operator will place the mouth mirror, dental instrument, or handpiece.

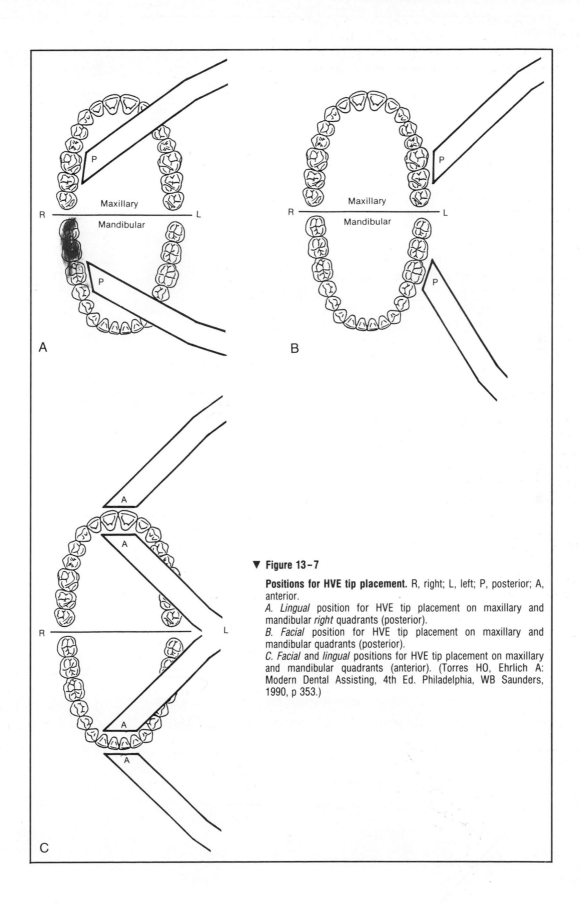

▼ **Figure 13-7**

Positions for HVE tip placement. R, right; L, left; P, posterior; A, anterior.
A. Lingual position for HVE tip placement on maxillary and mandibular *right* quadrants (posterior).
B. Facial position for HVE tip placement on maxillary and mandibular quadrants (posterior).
C. Facial and *lingual* positions for HVE tip placement on maxillary and mandibular quadrants (anterior). (Torres HO, Ehrlich A: Modern Dental Assisting, 4th Ed. Philadelphia, WB Saunders, 1990, p 353.)

Procedure

HVE TIP PLACEMENT, MAXILLARY RIGHT QUADRANT (Fig. 13-8)

1. The operator approaches the maxillary right quadrant from the 11 o'clock position and uses indirect vision to observe the field of operation.

2. Position the HVE tip on the palatal surface near the right maxillary teeth.

3. Hold a mouth mirror in the left hand. This may rest on the tongue and mandibular incisors to remind the patient to keep his mouth open.

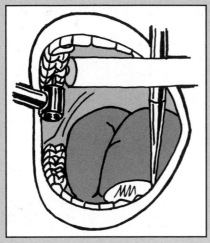 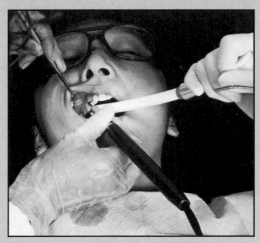

Figure 13-8 HVE tip placed for maxillary right quadrant preparation. (Torres HO, Ehrlich A: Modern Dental Assisting, 4th Ed. Philadelphia, WB Saunders, 1990, p 354.)

Procedure

HVE TIP PLACEMENT, MAXILLARY LEFT QUADRANT (Fig. 13-9)

1. The operator approaches the maxillary left quadrant from the 11 o'clock position and uses indirect vision to observe the field of operation.

2. Turn the slanted opening of the tip so that the extreme part of the tip surface is pointed toward the distal surface of the tooth being operated.

3. Place the HVE tip on the occlusal surface of the tooth posterior to the tooth being operated.
   Alternative: Place the HVE tip toward the facial surface of that tooth.

4. *Optional:* Rest a mouth mirror, or the fingers of the left hand, on the mandibular anteriors or the tongue to prevent the patient from closing his mouth.

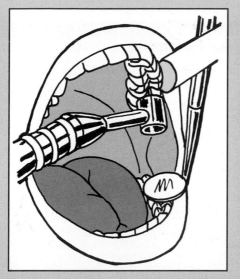

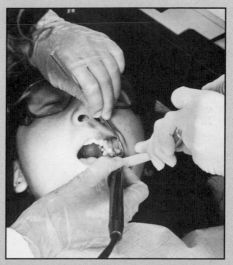

Figure 13-9 HVE tip placed for maxillary left quadrant preparation. (Torres HO, Ehrlich A: Modern Dental Assisting, 4th Ed. Philadelphia, WB Saunders, 1990, p 354.)

Procedure

HVE TIP PLACEMENT, MANDIBULAR RIGHT QUADRANT (Fig. 13-10)

1. The operator approaches the mandibular right quadrant from the 8 to 9 o'clock position and uses either direct or indirect vision to observe the field of operation.

2. Place the HVE tip at the lingual surface of the teeth, slightly posterior to the tooth being operated, when possible.

3. Use the extension of the vacuum tip as an aid in depressing the tongue.

4. If the patient's tongue is extremely active, use a mouth mirror in the left hand. Place the mirror firmly on the tongue or under the right side of the tongue to retract the tongue toward the left side of the mouth.

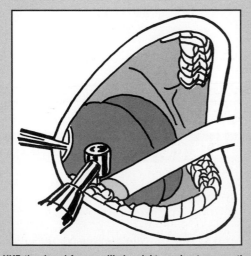

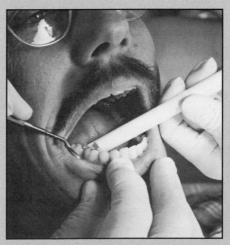

Figure 13-10 HVE tip placed for mandibular right quadrant preparation. (Torres HO, Ehrlich A: Modern Dental Assisting, 4th Ed. Philadelphia, WB Saunders, 1990, p 355.)

Procedure

HVE TIP PLACEMENT, MANDIBULAR LEFT QUADRANT (Fig. 13-11)

1. The operator may approach the mandibular left quadrant from the 11 o'clock position.

   Alternative: The operator may approach from the 9 o'clock position. If so, for easier access, the patient's head can be turned slightly to the right.

2. Place the HVE tip at the extreme left corner of the mouth, retracting the cheek during the process. Place the opening of the vacuum tip along the facial surface of the teeth.

3. *Alternative placement:* Position the HVE tip from across the oral cavity, from right to left, with the vacuum hose across the chest of the patient and the tip placed lingual to the patient's tongue.

4. The operator retracts the tongue with the mouth mirror.

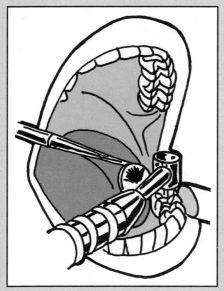
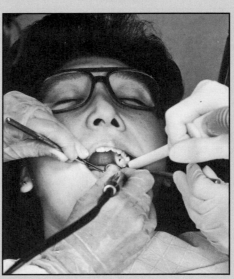

Figure 13-11 HVE tip placed for mandibular left quadrant preparation. (Torres HO, Ehrlich A: Modern Dental Assisting, 4th Ed. Philadelphia, WB Saunders, 1990, p 355.)

Procedure

HVE TIP PLACEMENT, MAXILLARY ANTERIOR TEETH (Fig. 13-12)

Facial Approach Preparation

1. The operator may approach from the 9 o'clock position for a facial surface preparation of the anterior teeth.

2. Place the HVE tip at the anterior palatal surface of the teeth. The slanted opening is against the palatal surfaces near the rugae or near the incisal edge of the teeth being prepared.

3. *Alternative placement:* Place the vacuum tip on the facial surface below the handpiece.

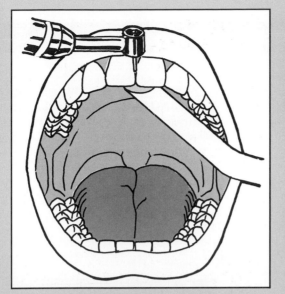
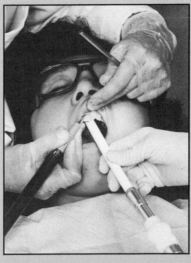

Figure 13-12 HVE tip placed for maxillary anterior facial preparation. The HVE tip is placed to the lingual. (Torres HO, Ehrlich A: Modern Dental Assisting, 4th Ed. Philadelphia, WB Saunders, 1990, p 356.)

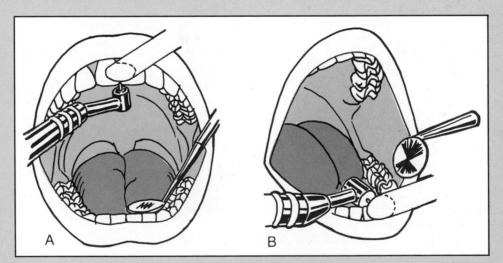

Figure 13-13 HVE tip placed for anterior palatal and lingual preparations. *A.* Tip placed at maxillary facial area. *B.* Tip placed at mandibular facial area. (Torres HO, Ehrlich A: Modern Dental Assisting, 4th Ed. Philadelphia, WB Saunders, 1990, p 356.)

Palatal Approach Preparation

1. The operator approaches from the 11 o'clock position, using the mouth mirror placed for an indirect palatal view of the teeth (Fig. 13-13*A*).

2. After the operator is in position, place the HVE tip on the facial surface of the teeth.

Procedure

HVE TIP PLACEMENT, MANDIBULAR ANTERIOR TEETH

Facial Approach Preparation

[1] The operator may approach from the 9 o'clock position.

[2] Place the HVE tip lingual to the anterior mandibular teeth (Fig. 13–14).

Lingual Approach Preparation

[1] The operator approaches from the 11 or 12 o'clock position (see Fig. 13–13B).

[2] Gently stretch the lower lip away from the teeth to form a trough between the lower lip and the facial-labial surfaces of anterior teeth.

[3] Place the HVE tip in this trough.

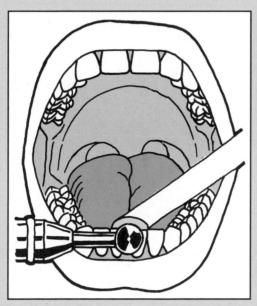 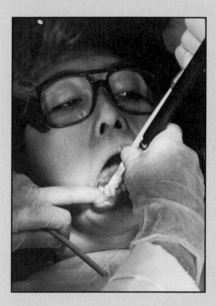

Figure 13–14 HVE tip placed for mandibular anterior facial preparation. The HVE tip is placed to the lingual. (Torres HO, Ehrlich A: Modern Dental Assisting, 4th Ed. Philadelphia, WB Saunders, 1990, p 356.)

THE SALIVA EJECTOR

During certain preparations, the operator may prefer to work in a dry field. At these times, a disposable plastic saliva ejector may be used to keep the saliva level under control, hold the tongue away from the field of operation, and make the patient more comfortable.

The saliva ejector may also be used when the field must be kept dry for placement of a material that will take a long period to set.

Saliva Ejector Placement

1. While gloved, contour the saliva ejector into a **J** shape to fit comfortably over the lip at the angle of the patient's mouth.
2. Extend the tubing for the saliva ejector from the dental unit to a length that will prevent the tubing from retracting or pulling on the patient's lip.
3. Place the saliva ejector in the tubing end.
4. Position the saliva ejector comfortably under

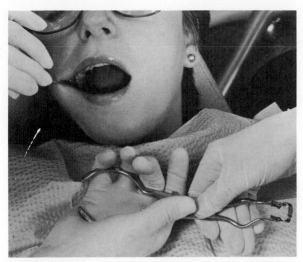

▼ **Figure 13–15**

The operator uses a mirror to retract with the right hand while receiving a palm grasp instrument in the left hand. (Torres HO, Ehrlich A: Modern Dental Assisting, 4th Ed. Philadelphia, WB Saunders, 1990, p 357.)

the patient's tongue on the side *opposite* where the operator is working.

TONGUE AND CHEEK RETRACTION

The operator or assistant may use the index finger to retract the patient's tongue or cheeks. The HVE tip and a mouth mirror are frequently used for

tongue and cheek retraction (Fig. 13–15). (**Retract** means to pull back or hold away from.)

During retraction, the HVE tip or mouth mirror must be held firmly so that it does not slip or cause patient discomfort.

INSTRUMENT GRASPS

Common positions for grasping dental hand instruments are the **pen grasp, inverted pen grasp, palm grasp, palm-thumb grasp**, and **modified palm-thumb grasp**.

Pen Grasp

Figure 13–16*A* shows how the assistant holds a pen grasp instrument as she prepares to pass it to the operator.

Figure 13–16*B* shows how the operator holds a pen grasp instrument in the position of use. Note that the index finger, third finger, and thumb grasp the handle (shaft) of the instrument.

Inverted or Reverse Pen Grasp

In the inverted or reverse pen grasp, the index finger, third finger, and thumb support the instrument in a manner similar to the pen grasp.

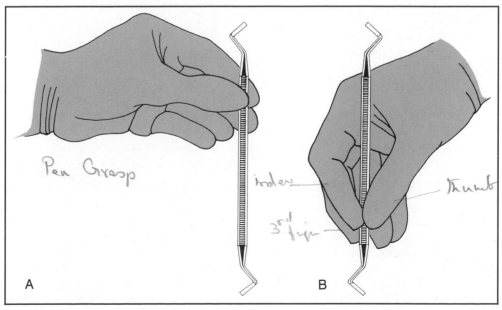

▼ **Figure 13–16**

Pen grasp instruments. *A.* The assistant holds a pen grasp instrument in position to pass it to the operator. *B.* The operator holds a pen grasp instrument in the position of use. (Courtesy of Colwell Systems Inc, Champaign, IL.)

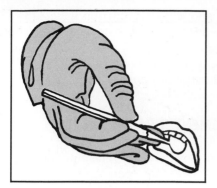

▼ **Figure 13–17**

Inverted or reverse pen grasp. The fulcrum is on the lower teeth. The slight clockwise rotation of the wrist creates a reverse pen grasp. (Torres HO, Ehrlich A: Modern Dental Assisting, 4th Ed. Philadelphia, WB Saunders, 1990, p 359.)

The difference is the slight clockwise rotation of the wrist, which places the hand slightly on the side (Fig. 13–17).

Palm Grasp

The palm grasp may be used to hold the handles of a rubber dam clamp forceps or surgical forceps (Fig. 13–18).

In the palm grasp, the instrument is held in the palm of the hand, with all five fingers surrounding and supporting the instrument.

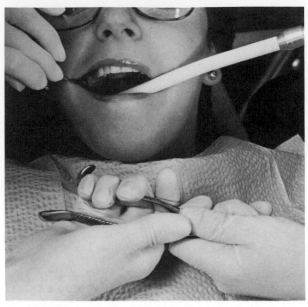

▼ **Figure 13–18**

Palm grasp instrument exchange. (Torres HO, Ehrlich A: Modern Dental Assisting, 4th Ed. Philadelphia, WB Saunders, 1990, p 359.)

Figure 13–19A shows how the assistant grasps the instrument near the junction of the handles (near the beaks) as she passes it to the operator.

Figure 13–19B shows how the operator holds the palm grasp instrument in the position of use.

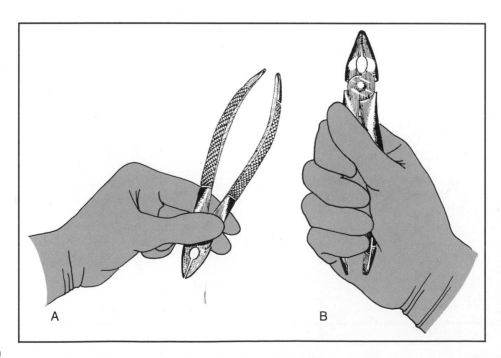

▼ **Figure 13–19**

Palm grasp instruments. A. The assistant holds a palm grasp instrument ready to pass it to the operator. B. The operator holds the instrument in the position of use. (Courtesy of Colwell Systems Inc, Champaign, IL.)

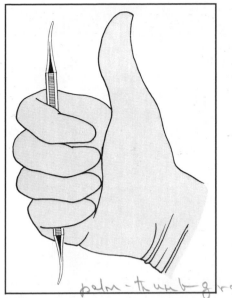

▼ **Figure 13–20**

Instrument as it is held in a palm-thumb grasp by the operator. (Courtesy of Colwell Systems Inc, Champaign, IL.)

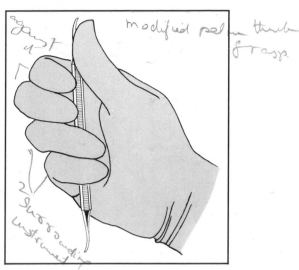

▼ **Figure 13–22**

The instrument as it is held by the operator in a modified palm-thumb grasp. (Courtesy of Colwell Systems Inc, Champaign, IL.)

Palm-Thumb Grasp

In the palm-thumb grasp, the instrument is held firmly by four fingers, with the handle deep in the palm of the hand.

Figure 13–20 shows the palm-thumb grasp applied on an enamel chisel.

The blade of the instrument may be held upward, supported by the thumb, to allow a thrust action in applying the blade to the tooth surface (Fig. 13–21).

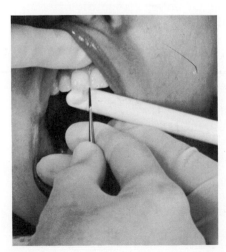

▼ **Figure 13–21**

Palm-thumb grasp instrument in use. (Torres HO, Ehrlich A: Modern Dental Assisting, 4th Ed. Philadelphia, WB Saunders, 1990, p 361.)

Modified Palm-Thumb Grasp

In the modified grasp, two fingers surround the instrument and two are placed against it. This provides more ease of movement than the regular palm-thumb grasp (Fig. 13–22).

INSTRUMENT EXCHANGE

Basic Principles

▼ During a successful instrument transfer, the operator's fingers do not move from the fulcrum, and the operator's eyes do not move from the field of operation. (A **fulcrum** is the support base that the operator establishes and maintains while using an instrument; see Fig. 13–23).

The operator passes the used instrument and receives the new instrument with the hand that is *not* used to establish the fulcrum.

▼ Each instrument is transferred to the operator's hand in the **position of use** so that it is ready to use (Fig. 13–24). (The position of use is determined by how and where the instrument is to be used.)

▼ Instrument and materials are exchanged in the transfer zone near the patient's chin. (This prevents instruments or materials from being dropped on the patient's face.)

▼ The assistant anticipates the operator's needs

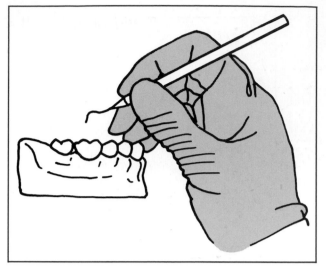

▼ **Figure 13-23**

Establishment of a fulcrum. The operator uses the fourth and little fingers to stabilize the hand on the dental arch near tooth to be prepared. (Torres HO, Ehrlich A: Modern Dental Assisting, 4th Ed. Philadelphia, WB Saunders, 1990, p 361.)

and is ready to pass the next instrument at a signal from the operator.

▼ With a smooth motion, the used instrument is received and the instrument being transferred is placed firmly in the operator's hand.

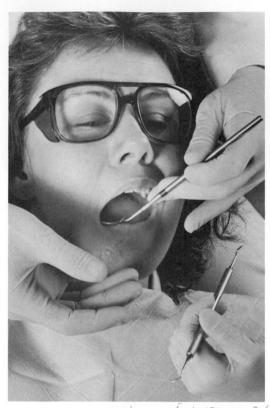

▼ **Figure 13-24**   *Inverted pen grasp*

The assistant passes the instrument to the operator in the position of use. It is shown here with the working end turned upward for use on a maxillary tooth. (Torres HO, Ehrlich A: Modern Dental Assisting, 4th Ed. Philadelphia, WB Saunders, 1990, p 361.)

Procedure

ASSISTING WITH A PROCEDURE

Handpiece Instrument Exchange

1. At the beginning of the procedure, pick up the mouth mirror and explorer. Simultaneously pass the mirror to the operator's left hand and the explorer to the operator's right hand. (**Simultaneous** means to happen at the same time.)

2. Pick up and position the HVE tip with the right hand.

3. Hold the handpiece in the left hand and extend the little finger of that hand to receive the explorer from the operator's right hand. (The operator retains the mouth mirror in the left hand.)

4. Extend the handpiece to the operator in the area of exchange. After passing the handpiece, replace the explorer on the instrument tray and pick up the air-water syringe.

Instrument Exchange

1. With the right hand, continue to hold and use the HVE tip. Put down the air-water syringe.

2. With the left hand, use the index finger and thumb to pick up the next instrument to be used. This instrument is grasped at the end *opposite* the working end (Fig. 13-25).

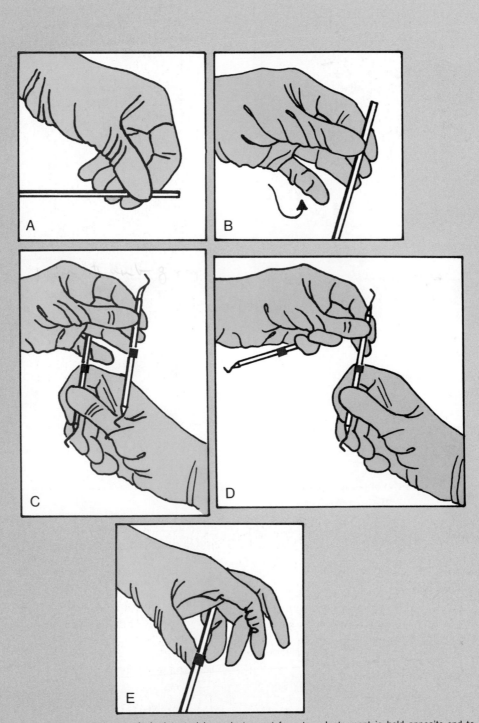

Figure 13-25 Steps in instrument exchange. *A.* Assistant picks up instrument from tray. Instrument is held opposite end to be used. *B.* New instrument is held with thumb, and index and third fingers ready for passing. Little finger is extended to receive used instrument (arrow). *C.* Passing position. Instrument is aligned with used instrument in operator's hand. *D.* Operator receives new instrument with the nib in position of use. Assistant *palms* used instrument after receiving it. *E.* The thumb is used to rotate the used instrument into position for placement on the tray *or* to pass to operator for reuse. (Torres HO, Ehrlich A: Modern Dental Assisting, 4th Ed. Philadelphia, WB Saunders, 1990, p 363.)

Continued

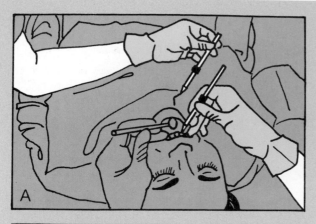

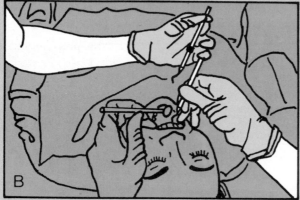

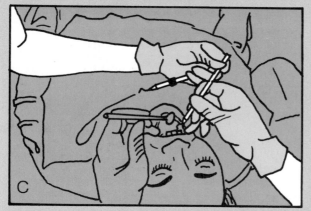

Figure 13-26 Instrument exchange (topical view). *A.* Assistant aligns new instrument with used instrument at chin of patient. Notice *fulcrums* of the operator's right and left hands. *B.* Operator maintains the fulcrum of the right hand. Assistant grasps used instruments with fourth and little fingers of left hand. Operator retains fulcrum of left hand holding the mouth mirror. *C.* Assistant places new instrument in position of use in operator's right hand and palms the used instrument in the left hand. Operator receives instrument while maintaining fulcrum of right hand. Operator's left hand has retained fulcrum with mouth mirror in position. (Torres HO, Ehrlich A: Modern Dental Assisting, 4th Ed. Philadelphia, WB Saunders, 1990, p 364.)

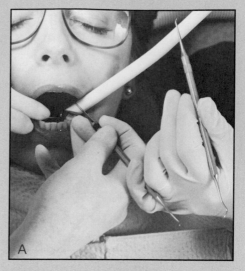

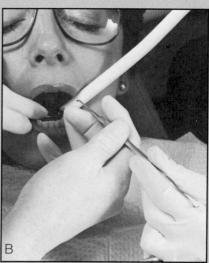

Figure 13-27 Instrument pick up and palming during exchange. *A.* The assistant takes the used instrument with the little finger and swings it toward the palm of the hand. *B.* The assistant passes the new instrument in the position of use. (Notice the end of the used instrument extending between the assistant's fourth and fifth fingers.) (Torres HO, Ehrlich A: Modern Dental Assisting, 4th Ed. Philadelphia, WB Saunders, 1990, p 365.)

3 Move the instrument into position so that it is grasped with the index and third fingers and thumb and is ready to be passed to the operator (Fig. 13-26).

4 Hold the new instrument in the transfer zone parallel to the instrument in use — and out of the operator's way.

Note: The operator signals for an instrument exchange by maintaining the fulcrum and with a pivotal action rotates the hand away from the patient's oral cavity. This positions the used instrument so that the assistant can grasp it with the little finger (Fig. 13-27).

5 Use the little finger to pick up the used instrument. Brace the used instrument securely against the palm of the hand

with the fourth and little fingers. (This is called **palming** the instrument.)

6 Simultaneously extend the new instrument to the operator in the position of use.

7 Return the used instrument to its original position on the tray.

Procedure

MATERIALS EXCHANGE

1 After the material is mixed and ready, transfer the placement instrument to the operator's right hand.

2 Use the right hand to hold the bulk material receptacle close to the transfer area.

3 Use the left hand to hold the air syringe to dry the area for application and placement of the material.
Alternative: Hold a gauze square in the left hand so that the operator may wipe excess material from the applicator instrument.

▼ EXERCISES

1. When working in the ___mandibular rt quad___ quadrant, the operator approaches from the 8 to 9 o'clock position and uses either direct or indirect vision.

   a. mandibular left
   b. mandibular right
   c. maxillary left
   d. maxillary right

2. The _____ grasp is used for surgical forceps.

   a. palm
   b. palm-thumb
   c. pen
   d. reverse pen

3. With ___(b)___ vision, the operator uses a mouth mirror to view the operating field.

   a. direct
   b. indirect

4. At the beginning of the procedure, the assistant transfers the _____ _____ to the operator's left hand.

   a. air-water syringe
   b. explorer
   c. handpiece
   d. mouth mirror

5. Immediately after the assistant receives the used instrument, it is ___(palming)___ with the fourth and little fingers.

   a. braced against the palm of the hand
   b. handed to the coordinating assistant
   c. replaced on the tray
   d. a or b

6. If the assistant is called away from chairside for any length of time, the assistant's cart may be placed in the ___STATIC___ zone.

   a. assistant's
   b. operator's
   c. static
   d. transfer

7. In front delivery, the assistant passes and receives instruments and handpieces in the ___Transfer___ zone.

   a. static
   b. transfer

8. When working with a right-handed operator, the assistant is seated between _____ o'clock.

   a. 1 and 4
   b. 2 and 4
   c. 8 and 10
   d. 8 and 11

9. The assistant receives a used instrument from the operator with the
   _____ .

   a. little finger of the left hand
   b. little finger of the right hand
   c. thumb, index, and third fingers of the left hand
   d. thumb, index, and third fingers of the right hand

10. Dental materials are exchanged in the _____Transfer_____ zone. *Front-Delin 4-8 o'clock*

    a. assistant's
    b. operator's
    c. static
    d. transfer

11. When using oral evacuation in the _____(a)_____ quadrant, the
    HVE tip is placed at the extreme left corner of the mouth, retracting the
    cheek in the process.

    a. mandibular left
    b. mandibular right
    c. maxillary left
    d. maxillary right

12. During instrument exchange, the assistant holds the new instrument in the
    transfer zone ____parallel____ to the instrument in use.

    a. at a right angle
    b. immediately next
    c. parallel
    d. perpendicular

13. When passing a palm grasp instrument, the assistant holds it _____
    _____ .

    a. firmly by the handles
    b. near the junction of the handles
    c. securely in the palm of her right hand
    d. a and c

14. A left-handed operator is seated to the _____ of the
    dental chair.

    a. left
    b. right

15. A/An _____ is an example of an instrument that is used
    in a palm-thumb grasp.

    a. enamel chisel
    b. explorer
    c. extraction forceps
    d. rubber dam forceps

16. To avoid stimulating the gag reflex on the soft palate, the HVE tip should be
    placed gently against the tissue.

    a. true
    b. false

17. _____ may be used for tongue and cheek retraction.

    a. A mouth mirror
    b. The HVE tip
    c. The index finger
    d. a, b, and c

18. Using the clock concept, the _____ zone is located between 11 and 2 o'clock.

    a. assistant's
    b. operator's
    c. static
    d. transfer

19. During oral evacuation, the assistant holds the _____ in the left hand.

    a. air-water syringe
    b. HVE tip
    c. local anesthetic syringe
    d. used instrument

20. When a saliva ejector is used, it is positioned _____ the side where the operator is working.

    a. next to
    b. opposite

21. _____ is the support base that the operator establishes and maintains while using an instrument.

    a. A fulcrum
    b. A stabilizer
    c. Rear delivery
    d. The pen grasp

22. When the assistant picks up the next instrument from the tray, it is grasped _____ .

    a. firmly in the palm of her hand
    b. in the middle of the handle
    c. in the position of use
    d. opposite the end to be used

23. Rubber dam forceps are held in an (a) _____ grasp.

    a. inverted pen grasp
    b. palm
    c. palm-thumb
    d. pen

24. When using the HVE tip for anterior placement, the end with an angle _____ 90 degrees is placed into the handle.

    a. greater than
    b. less than

25. The HVE tip is held with a ———————————— grasp.

    a. fist
    b. modified pen
    c. reverse palm-thumb
    d. b or c

▼ Criterion Sheet 13–1

Student's Name ————————————————————————————

Procedure: *USE OF ORAL EVACUATION AND AIR-WATER SYRINGE*

Performance Objective:

The student will demonstrate placement and use of the HVE tip and air-water syringe for the area under treatment.

The operator is seated at the 9 to 10 o'clock position. The assistant is seated at the 2 to 3 o'clock position. The patient is seated in a supine position.

		SE	IE
SE = Student evaluation **IE** = Instructor evaluation	**C** = Criterion met **X** = Criterion not met		
Instrumentation: Dental unit, sterile HVE tip, mouth mirror, and air-water syringe. (Appropriate infection control barriers will be used during all procedures actually performed on a patient.)			
1. Held air-water syringe in left hand. Held HVE tip in right fist using a reverse palm grasp. Held the vacuum hose close to body.			
2. Positioned the HVE tip for the **mandibular left quadrant.** Demonstrated evacuation of the quandrant.			
3. Positioned the HVE tip for the **mandibular right quadrant.** Demonstrated rinsing and evacuation of the quadrant.			
4. Positioned the HVE tip for the **maxillary left quadrant.** Demonstrated rinsing and evacuation of the quadrant.			
5. Positioned the HVE tip for the **maxillary right quadrant.** Demonstrated rinsing and evacuation of the quadrant.			
6. Positioned the HVE tip for the **mandibular anteriors.** Demonstrated rinsing and evacuation of the area.			
7. Positioned the HVE tip for the **maxillary anteriors.** Demonstrated rinsing and evacuation of the area.			
Comments:			

▼ Criterion Sheet 13–2

Student's Name _____

Procedure: *INSTRUMENT EXCHANGE*

Performance Objective:

The student will demonstrate the exchange of dental instruments with another student acting as the operator.

The operator is seated at the 9 o'clock position. The assistant is seated at the 2 o'clock position. The patient is in a supine position.

	SE	IE
SE = Student evaluation **C** = Criterion met **IE** = Instructor evaluation **X** = Criterion not met		
Instrumentation: Basic setup, spoon excavator, extraction forceps, and root elevator. (Appropriate infection control barriers will be used during all procedures actually performed on a patient.)		
1. Simultaneously picked up mouth mirror in right hand and explorer in left hand.		
2. Simultaneously passed the mirror to the operator's left hand and the explorer to the operator's right hand in position of use.		
3. **Pen grasp.** Picked up the spoon excavator in left hand. Received used instrument with little finger of left hand, palmed it. Passed spoon excavator to the operator in the position of use. Returned used instrument to the instrument tray.		
4. **Palm thumb grasp.** Picked up the root elevator in left hand. Received used instrument, palmed it. Passed the root elevator to the operator in the position of use. Returned used instrument to the instrument tray.		
5. **Palm grasp.** Picked up extraction forceps with left hand. Received used instrument. Passed the forceps to the operator in the position of use. Returned used instrument to the instrument tray.		
Comments:		

14 The Dental Examination

The student will be able to:

1. Describe the basic components of a complete dental examination.
2. Describe the function of treatment plans and the case presentation visit.
3. List and describe Black's classification of cavities.
4. State where the left and right sides of the dental arches appear on anatomic and geometric dental diagrams.
5. Demonstrate taking the patient's vital signs.
6. Demonstrate charting a dental examination using the symbols commonly employed to record dental conditions and treatment.

OVERVIEW OF THE DENTAL EXAMINATION

Complete dental care begins with a thorough examination and careful diagnosis. Based on this information, the dentist can develop a treatment plan and present it to the patient.

The following are the basic components necessary for thorough dental examination:

▼ Personal information.

▼ Medical history.

▼ Dental history.

▼ Vital signs.

▼ Oral examination.

▼ Radiographs and photographs (see Chapter 15, "Fundamentals of Dental Radiography," and Chapter 16, "Dental Radiography: Paralleling Technique").

▼ Study casts (see Chapter 17, "Alginate Impressions and Diagnostic Casts").

Unless otherwise indicated, these parts of the examination are described later in this chapter.

Diagnosis and Treatment of the Emergency Patient

Often the patient's first contact with the practice is an emergency call for the relief of pain. When this happens, the patient should be seen as quickly as possible.

At the beginning of the visit, basic information including a medical history and personal data must be gathered. Radiographs may also be required. Then the dentist will diagnose the patient's condition and provide emergency treatment necessary to relieve the patient's discomfort.

If the emergency patient has a regular dentist, he is then referred back to his original dentist for ongoing care.

If the emergency patient does *not* have a regular dentist and if he requests continued treatment, he is rescheduled so that a complete diagnosis can be made and a case presentation can be prepared.

Treatment Plans and the Case Presentation

The dentist studies the diagnostic aids and data gathered during the examination. Based on this information, he formulates one or more treatment plans and cost estimates for the patient.

▼ An **"optimal" treatment plan** is one in which all necessary dental care is provided, using the very best options, regardless of cost.

▼ A **"holding" treatment plan** is one in which all necessary dental care is provided, but making some changes in the planned treatment to accommodate the patient's special needs and financial situation.

The case presentation visit, which is usually scheduled for 15 to 30 minutes, usually takes place in the dentist's private office or consultation room. The patient's radiographs, study casts, chart, treatment plans, and fee estimates are prepared and placed in the consultation room prior to the appointment.

At this time, the dentist explains the diagnosis and proposed treatment plans and answer the patient's questions. After the patient has accepted one of the treatment plans, the administrative assistant helps the patient make the necessary financial arrangements and schedule appointments for the completion of treatment.

INFECTION CONTROL REMINDER

It is essential that each staff member follow the universal precautions of infection control without deviation during all patient treatment. These procedures are discussed in Chapter 7, "Infection Control."

DATA GATHERING

Personal Information

Personal information includes the patient's full name, address, age, employment, dental insurance, and referral source.

This information is gathered on a patient registration form, such as the one shown in Figure 14–1, and is used to help the administrative assistant in making financial arrangements and in collecting the fees owed to the dentist.

Patient Chart

The patient chart, which is also known as the *clinical record*, is a written record of all examination findings and treatment provided for the patient (Fig. 14–2). Financial information is *not* included in the patient chart.

This is an important legal record. All treatment entries must be complete and clearly written in ink. Although the assistant may make the entry, it should be initialed by the individual performing the procedure.

Medical History

New patients are requested to complete a medical history form prior to initial treatment. Returning patients are asked to update their medical history information. This is usually accomplished before the patient is escorted to the operatory.

This form includes questions concerning the patient's medical history, present physical condition, chronic conditions, allergies, and all medications that the patient is taking (Fig. 14–3).

This information helps the dentist evaluate the patient's physical condition and to be alert to the need for any special treatment. Based on data from the medical history, the dentist may order medical laboratory tests such as blood tests or a biopsy.

The dentist may also wish to consult the patient's physician regarding health problems such as a heart condition or chronic illnesses.

Dental History

The patient's dental history offers important clues concerning previous dental care, how recently the patient has received dental treatment, the frequency of dental visits, and the patient's attitude concerning the importance of dental care.

Vital Signs

Vital signs, which are indicators of a patient's health, may be recorded as part of the examination, prior to routine care, and/or in the event of an emergency.

The assistant may be given the responsibility of obtaining and recording the vital signs when preparing a patient for dental treatment. These vital signs include:

▼ Pulse rate.

▼ Respiration rate.

▼ Temperature.

▼ Blood pressure.

PATIENT REGISTRATION FORM

Responsible Party __James_____ __A._____ __Gridley_____
First Name   Initial   Last Name

Address __670 Northridge Terrace_____

City __Champaign_____   State __IL_____   Zip Code __61820_____

Phone: (Home)__351-4498_____   (Work)__322-0987_____

Employer __Champion Automotive Supply_____

Address __9000 Broad Street, Champaign, IL 61820_____

Name & Address of Nearest Relative (not living with you)_____

_____ Phone _____

Referring Physician __Dr. Grace Hardy_____

Family Member Information

First Name	Last Name	Sex	Relationship* I–S–C–O	Birthday
Pt. #				
(1) James	Gridley	M	I	04/05/55
(2) Ruth	Gridley	F	S	11/30/56
(3) Lisa	Gridley	F	C	06/20/83
(4) Ben	Gridley	M	C	10/01/85

Please list additional members on reverse.   *I = Insured, S = Spouse, C = Child, O = Other Dependent

Dental Insurance Information

Subscriber Name __James A. Gridley_____   S.S.#__890-49-5381_____   Pt.#__1_____

Carrier Name & Address __Equitable_____
__2000 Tower Place, New York, NY 10003_____

Group Name __Champion Auto_____   Group Number __CH-23000_____

Does this plan cover all family members? __X__ Yes ____No

If no specify those __NOT__ Covered.

ASSIGNMENT OF BENEFITS	RELEASE OF INFORMATION
I authorize payment of dental benefits to myself or the named provider for professional services rendered. Signed _James A. Gridley_ Date 1/9/xx (Subscriber)	I authorize the release of any dental information necessary to process this claim. Signed _James A. Gridley_ Date 1/9/xx (Patient, or parent if Minor)

▼ Figure 14-1

A patient registration form. (Courtesy of Colwell Systems, Inc, Champaign, IL.)

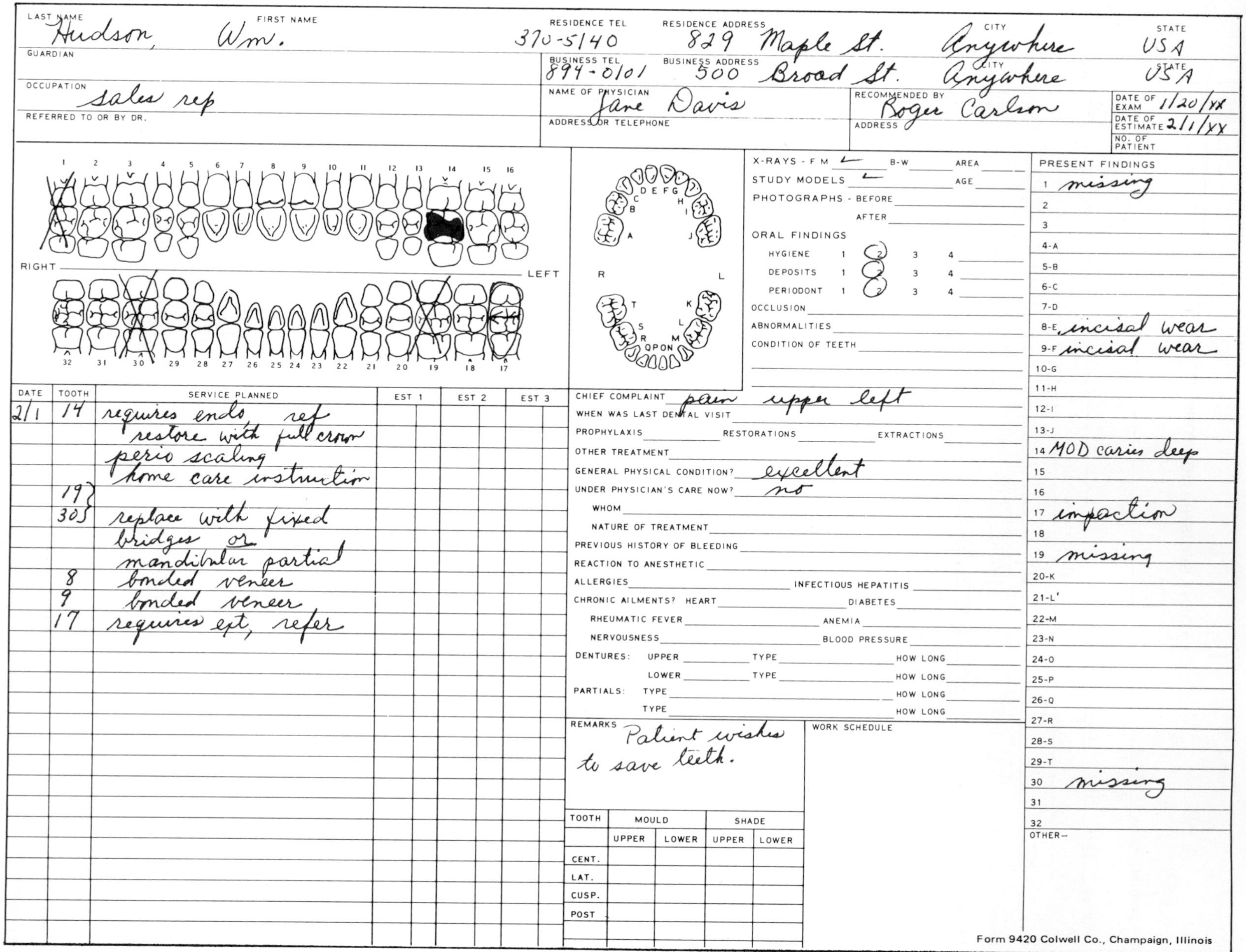

LAST NAME Hudson, FIRST NAME Wm. | RESIDENCE TEL 370-5140 | RESIDENCE ADDRESS 829 Maple St. | CITY Anywhere | STATE USA

GUARDIAN | BUSINESS TEL 894-0101 | BUSINESS ADDRESS 500 Broad St. | CITY Anywhere | STATE USA

OCCUPATION sales rep | NAME OF PHYSICIAN Jane Davis | RECOMMENDED BY Roger Carlson | DATE OF EXAM 1/20/xx

REFERRED TO OR BY DR. | ADDRESS OR TELEPHONE | ADDRESS | DATE OF ESTIMATE 2/1/xx | NO. OF PATIENT

1 2 3 4 5 6 7 8 9 10 11 12 13 14 15 16

RIGHT — LEFT

32 31 30 29 28 27 26 25 24 23 22 21 20 19 18 17

D E F G H I J C B A R L T K S L R M Q P O N

X-RAYS - F M ✓ B-W AREA

STUDY MODELS ✓ AGE

PHOTOGRAPHS - BEFORE

AFTER

ORAL FINDINGS

HYGIENE 1 (2) 3 4

DEPOSITS 1 (2) 3 4

PERIODONT 1 (2) 3 4

OCCLUSION

ABNORMALITIES

CONDITION OF TEETH

DATE	TOOTH	SERVICE PLANNED	EST 1	EST 2	EST 3
2/1	14	requires endo, ref			
		restore with full crown			
		perio scaling			
		home care instruction			
	19 }				
	30 }	replace with fixed			
		bridges or			
		mandibular partial			
	8	bonded veneer			
	9	bonded veneer			
	17	requires ext, refer			

CHIEF COMPLAINT pain upper left

WHEN WAS LAST DENTAL VISIT

PROPHYLAXIS RESTORATIONS EXTRACTIONS

OTHER TREATMENT

GENERAL PHYSICAL CONDITION? excellent

UNDER PHYSICIAN'S CARE NOW? no

WHOM

NATURE OF TREATMENT

PREVIOUS HISTORY OF BLEEDING

REACTION TO ANESTHETIC

ALLERGIES INFECTIOUS HEPATITIS

CHRONIC AILMENTS? HEART DIABETES

RHEUMATIC FEVER ANEMIA

NERVOUSNESS BLOOD PRESSURE

DENTURES: UPPER TYPE HOW LONG

LOWER TYPE HOW LONG

PARTIALS: TYPE HOW LONG

TYPE HOW LONG

REMARKS Patient wishes to save teeth.

WORK SCHEDULE

TOOTH	MOULD UPPER	MOULD LOWER	SHADE UPPER	SHADE LOWER
CENT.				
LAT.				
CUSP.				
POST				

PRESENT FINDINGS

1	missing
2	
3	
4-A	
5-B	
6-C	
7-D	
8-E	incisal wear
9-F	incisal wear
10-G	
11-H	
12-I	
13-J	
14	MOD caries deep
15	
16	
17	impaction
18	
19	missing
20-K	
21-L'	
22-M	
23-N	
24-O	
25-P	
26-Q	
27-R	
28-S	
29-T	
30	missing
31	
32	
OTHER—	

Form 9420 Colwell Co., Champaign, Illinois

▼ **Figure 14-2**

The patient's dental chart. This side of the chart shows the dentist's initial findings and treatment plan. All treatment provided is recorded on the reverse side. (Courtesy of Colwell Systems, Inc, Champaign, IL.)

Date _____

Name _James A. Gridley_   Date of Birth _04/05/55_

Address _670 Northridge Terrace, Champaign Ill_   Telephone _357-4498_

Business Address _____   Business Phone _322-0987_

    Soc. Sec. No. _____

Patient Name

PATIENT MEDICAL HISTORY

Physician _Dr. Grace Hardy_   Office Phone _322-0643_   Home Phone _____

Approximate date of last physical examination _One year_

		Yes	No
1.	Are you under any medical treatment now?	☑	☐
2.	Have you had any major operations? If so what?	☐	☑
3.	Have you ever had a serious accident involving head injuries?	☐	☑
4.	Have you had any adverse response to any drugs including penicillin?	☐	☑
5.	Has a physician ever informed you that you had: A Heart Ailment?	☑	☐
6.	High Blood Pressure?	☑	☐
7.	Respiratory Disease?	☐	☑
8.	Diabetes?	☐	☑
9.	Rheumatic Fever?	☐	☑
10.	Rheumatism or Arthritis?	☐	☑
11.	Tumors or Growths	☐	☑
12.	Any Blood Disease?	☐	☑
13.	Any Liver Disease?	☐	☑
14.	Any Kidney Disease?	☐	☑
15.	Any Stomach or Intestinal Disease?	☐	☑
16.	Any Venereal Disease?	☐	☑
17.	AIDS?	☐	☑
18.	Yellow Jaundice or Hepatitis?	☐	☑
19.	Do you have night sweats accompanied by weight loss or cough?	☐	☑
20.	Are you on a diet at this time?	☑	☐
21.	Are you now taking drugs or medications?	☑	☐
22.	Are you allergic to any known materials resulting in hives, asthma, eczema, etc.?	☐	☑
23.	Are you in general good health at this time?	☑	☐
24.	Have any wounds healed slowly or presented other complications?	☐	☑
25.	Are you pregnant?	☐	☑
26.	Do you have a history of fainting?	☐	☑
27.	Have you ever had any X-RAY TREATMENTS (other than diagnostic)?	☐	☑

PATIENT DENTAL HISTORY

		Yes	No
28.	Do you have pain in or near your ears?	☐	☑
29.	Do you have any unhealed injuries or inflamed areas in or around your mouth?	☐	☑
30.	Have you experienced any growth or sore spots in your mouth?	☐	☑
31.	Does any part of your mouth hurt when clenched?	☐	☑
32.	Have you ever had Novocaine anesthetic?	☑	☐
33.	Any reactions or allergic symptoms to Novocaine?	☐	☑
34.	Any difficult extractions in the past?	☐	☑
35.	Prolonged bleeding following extractions in the past?	☐	☑
36.	Trench Mouth?	☐	☑
37.	Do your gums bleed?	☐	☑
38.	Have you ever had instruction on the correct method of brushing your teeth?	☑	☐
39.	Have you ever had instructions on the care of your gums?	☑	☐
40.	Do you chew on only one side of your mouth? If so why?	☐	☑
41.	Do you at the present time have any dental complaints?	☐	☑
42.	Do you habitually clench your teeth during the night or day?	☐	☑
43.	When was your last full mouth X-RAY taken? _6 months ago_ Where? _____	☐	☑
44.	Any part of your mouth sore to pressures or irritants (cold, sweets, etc.)	☐	☑
	If so locate _____		

Signature _James A. Gridley_

FORM 9879 COLWELL SYSTEMS, INC., CHAMPAIGN, IL 61820

▼ **Figure 14–3**

Medical history form. (Courtesy of Colwell Systems, Inc, Champaign, IL.)

[Handwritten notes at top of page: Pulse = 72 per/out. Child – 80 – 100. Temp. 37°C or 98·6°F child. Resp 16–18 respiration/out. 24–28 resp/wt]

Procedure

TAKING VITAL SIGNS

1. Wash hands before beginning to take the patient's vital signs. Gloves and mask are not required for these procedures.

2. Record the information promptly and clearly on the patient's chart.

3. After completing these tasks, clean all equipment and return it to its proper place.

4. Wash hands again.

Pulse

The pulse is the rhythmic expansion of an artery as the heart beats. The radial artery on the inner surface of the wrist (thumb side) is the most commonly used site for taking the pulse.

Procedure

TAKING A PULSE

1. Place the index and third fingers of the hand lightly on the wrist between the radius (bone on the thumb side) and the tendon as the pulse is taken (Fig. 14–4).

2. Using a watch that indicates seconds, count the pulse for 30 seconds, and double the number of beats. An alternative is to count the pulse for a full minute.

3. Record the pulse rate immediately.
   The normal pulse rate in adults is between 60 and 80 heart beats per minute.
   In children, the rate is between 80 and 100 heart beats per minute.

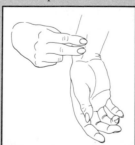

Figure 14–4 Taking the patient's pulse in the wrist. (Torres HO, Ehrlich A: Modern Dental Assisting, 4th Ed. Philadelphia, WB Saunders, 1990, p 449.)

Respiration Rate

To count the respiration rate, observe the rise and fall of the patient's chest as he inhales (breathes in) and exhales (breathes out). One complete respiration includes one inhalation and one exhalation.

Procedure

COUNTING RESPIRATION RATE

1. Count the rate of respiration for ½ minute and multiply by two. An alternative is to count it for 1 full minute.

2. Promptly record the respiration rate.
   The normal respiration rate for a relaxed adult is 16 to 18 breaths per minute.
   The normal respiration rate for a child is 24 to 28 breaths per minute.

3. Unusual breath odors may indicate a respiratory illness or other abnormalities. If unusual odors are observed, note them on the patient's chart.

Temperature

The patient's body temperature may be taken with an electronic thermometer or with a glass thermometer.

To ensure the sterility of either type of thermometer, a disposable plastic cover is placed over the portion that is put under the patient's tongue. This cover is discarded after one use.

The procedure for taking the patient's temperature orally with a glass thermometer is on page 227.

Blood Pressure

The term **blood pressure** refers to the systolic and diastolic values of arterial pressure.

Procedure

TAKING A TEMPERATURE

1 Place a disposable plastic sheath over the bulb end of the thermometer, which will be placed in the patient's mouth (Fig. 14–5).

2 Hold the thermometer by the end near the high gradations (*not* the tip). Shake it gently until the mercury has been forced down into the tip.

3 Place the tip of the thermometer gently under the patient's tongue next to the lingual frenum.

4 Instruct the patient to close his lips on the thermometer and to refrain from talking or from moving it out of the mouth.

5 Leave the thermometer in place for 3 to 5 minutes, then remove the thermometer from the patient's mouth.

6 Read the thermometer immediately before it cools or the reading will not be accurate.

To obtain the best reading, hold the thermometer horizontally by the end near the high gradations, not by the bulb end.

Rotate the thermometer slowly at eye level until the column of mercury is clearly visible (Fig. 14–6).

7 Record the reading immediately as a number. For most patients the normal reading is 98.6°F (37.0°C).

8 Discard the plastic sheath and shake down the thermometer.

Disinfect the thermometer with 70 percent isopropyl alcohol or other acceptable germicidal agent.

Store the thermometer in a sterile container for future use.

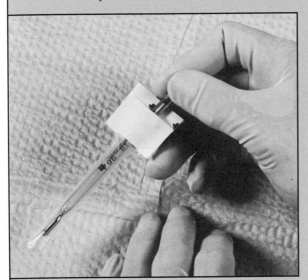

Figure 14–5 A disposable plastic sheath is placed over the glass thermometer prior to use. After use, the sheath is discarded and the thermometer is disinfected. (Torres HO, Ehrlich A: Modern Dental Assisting, 4th Ed. Philadelphia, WB Saunders, 1990, p 455.)

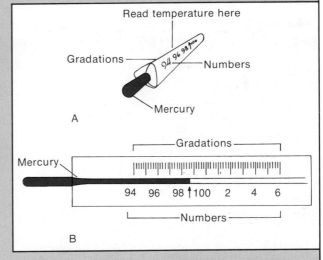

Figure 14–6 Components for reading a glass thermometer. (Torres HO, Ehrlich A: Modern Dental Assisting, 4th Ed. Philadelphia, WB Saunders, 1990, p 455.)

Systolic pressure is the highest pressure exerted on the circulatory system by the contraction of the heart.

Diastolic pressure is the lowest pressure of the circulatory system, which occurs as the heart relaxes.

Systolic and diastolic pressures are measured and recorded in terms of millimeters of mercury (mm Hg) above atmosphere pressure. This is recorded with the systolic value over the diastolic value. For example, 136/80 means systolic pressure of 136 and diastolic pressure of 80.

The normal adult range for blood pressure is 110/60 to 140/90. As age increases, the blood pressure gradually increases: a 6-year-old child may normally have a reading of 90/60, whereas it would not be unusual for a 60-year-old man to have a reading of 140/90.

Sphygmomanometers

Blood pressure is measured using a stethoscope and a sphygmomanometer. The stethoscope is used to listen to the sounds made by the blood as it moves through the artery.

A sphygmomanometer, which is commonly referred to as a *blood pressure cuff*, consists of a gauge attached to an inflatable bladder. The bladder is enclosed in a cloth cuff with a closure (usually nylon tape [Velcro]) to hold it in place.

A **mercury sphygmomanometer** provides readings on a column of mercury.

An **aneroid sphygmomanometer** provides reading on a dial that is directly attached to the cuff. This type of equipment is shown in Figures 14–8 and 14–9.

Korotkoff Sounds

Korotkoff sounds are a series of sounds as the result of the blood rushing back into the brachial artery that has been collapsed by the pressure of the blood pressure cuff.

As the pressure in the cuff is slowly released, the stethoscope picks up a clear, sharp tapping sound that grows louder and then softens to a murmur as the flow of blood expands the artery to its former shape.

▼ **Phase I**: There is the sudden occurrence of a clear, sharp, snapping sound that grows louder.

▼ **Phase II**: The sound is softened and becomes prolonged into a murmur.

▼ **Phase III**: The sound again becomes crisper and increases in intensity.

▼ **Phase IV**: There is distinct abrupt muffling of the sound.

▼ **Phase V**: This is the point at which the artery is fully open and the sound disappears.

Procedure

PLACING OF THE BLOOD PRESSURE CUFF AND STETHOSCOPE

1 Seat the patient in the dental chair in a supine or sitting position.

   Allow the patient to rest quietly for a few minutes before having his blood pressure recorded.

   Explain to the patient what is to be done and why the blood pressure reading is important.

2 Extend the patient's arm (left or right) and support the elbow on the arm of the chair.

   The palm should be facing upward.

   The patient's arm (at the elbow) should be at the same level as the heart. (If the arm is higher than the heart, a false low reading may be obtained.)

   If the patient's sleeve is tight, it should be loosened. (A tight sleeve may partially compress the brachial artery.)

3 Place the blood pressure cuff lightly on the patient's arm with the inflatable "bladder" over the inner area of the upper arm near the brachial artery, approximately 2 cm above the antecubital space.

   The **antecubital space** (fossa) is the small groove on the inner arm (just above

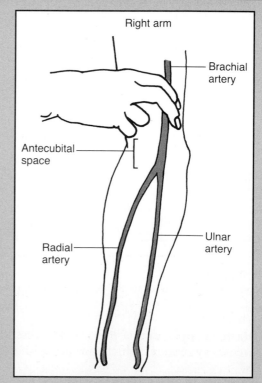

Figure 14–7 Locating the antecubital space with the fingers. (Torres HO, Ehrlich A: Modern Dental Assisting, 4th Ed. Philadelphia, WB Saunders, 1990, p 452.)

the elbow) and at the level of the left ventricle of the heart (Fig. 14–7).

4 Use one hand to stabilize the end of the cuff just above the elbow.

With the other hand, wrap the cuff smoothly around the upper arm over the brachial artery with the gauge facing you.

Use the closure to hold the cuff securely in place. Allow some space between the cuff and the arm to permit inflation as air enters the cuff.

5 Expel all air from the cuff by opening the valve of the bulb on the end of the tubing and pressing the cuff gently.

6 Place the earpieces of the stethoscope in the ears so the earpieces are facing anteriorly. This position of the earpieces is more comfortable and closes out distracting noises while taking the blood pressure.

7 Place the diaphragm of the stethoscope at the medial side of tendon and over the brachial artery just below the lower border of the cuff and on the antecubital space (Figs. 14–8 and 14–9).

8 Hold the diaphragm with the thumb, and place the fingers under the patient's elbow. This ensures that there is no gap between the skin and the diaphragm.

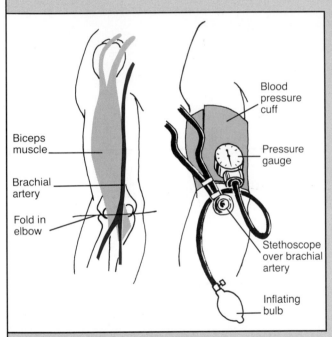

Figure 14–8 Positioning the blood pressure cuff and stethoscope. (Torres HO, Ehrlich A: Modern Dental Assisting, 4th Ed. Philadelphia, WB Saunders, 1990, p 453.)

Labels: Biceps muscle, Brachial artery, Fold in elbow, Blood pressure cuff, Pressure gauge, Stethoscope over brachial artery, Inflating bulb

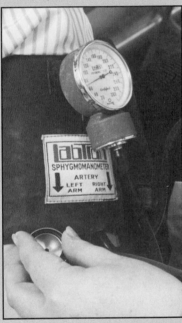

Figure 14–9 The diaphragm of the stethoscope is placed just below the border of the blood pressure cuff. (Torres HO, Ehrlich A: Modern Dental Assisting, 4th Ed. Philadelphia, WB Saunders, 1990, p 454.)

Procedure

OBTAINING THE BLOOD PRESSURE READING

1 Place the palm of the right hand over the rubber inflation bulb. Rotate the valve screw (opening adjustment) using the fingers and thumb to check the closure of the valve vent.

Turning the screw clockwise closes the valve.

Turning the screw counterclockwise opens the valve.

Continued

2 Feel the pulse in the wrist or just below the antecubital space.

3 Check placement of the stethoscope diaphragm and listen for the sound of the pulse.

Pump the bulb to inflate the cuff until the sound of the pulse can no longer be heard.

This will be approximately 20 to 30 mm Hg above the previously measured systolic pressure.

4 Check the reading on the gauge of the blood pressure apparatus.

The reading may be as high as 160 to 170 mm Hg as the last sound of the pressure is heard.

5 Slowly release the valve screw of the rubber bulb.

Permit the pressure to drop in the gauge at 2 mm Hg per second.

Two millimeters represents one notch on the mercury or aneroid gauge.

6 While listening with the stethoscope, pump the bulb to inflate the cuff.

The reading on the gauge should be 10 to 20 points above the reading acquired when testing the apparatus (170 to 180).

7 Listen with the stethoscope as you *slowly* open the bulb and release the pressure on the cuff

The pressure in the gauge will drop approximately 2 mm with each beat of the heart.

8 Note the registration of the first sharp, tapping sound as you lower the air pressure in the cuff.

This is the systolic pressure.

9 Slowly continue to deflate the apparatus by releasing the air in the cuff.

Deflate until the last sound of the heart beat is heard.

This is the diastolic pressure.

10 When the blood pressure reading has been completed, quickly deflate the cuff and gently remove it.

11 Clean the stethoscope earpieces and diaphragm by wiping with a disinfectant. Store all equipment carefully.

Recording the Blood Pressure Reading

The patient's blood pressure must be recorded immediately to avoid forgetting the reading.

A blood pressure (BP) reading is recorded as *right arm patient seated* (RAS) or *left arm patient seated* (LAS). The pressure is expressed as a fraction.

For example, *RAS.BP 120/70* means that the blood pressure was recorded on the right arm of a seated patient. The systolic pressure was 120 mm Hg, and the diastolic pressure was 70 mm Hg.

Repeated Blood Pressure Readings

The blood pressure reading may be taken two or three times to obtain an accurate or average reading. If the patient appears to be apprehensive at the time of the first reading, wait a few minutes to permit him to relax.

The blood pressure cuff can remain on the arm in a loosened position after the first reading is obtained in case another reading is needed or during a prolonged operative or surgical procedure.

THE ORAL EXAMINATION

A thorough examination includes the hard and soft tissues of the neck, face, lips, and oral cavity. The purpose of this examination is to determine deviations from normal and to identify any condition or disease, such as oral cancer, that may be present.

Instrumentation

▼ Basic setup.

▼ Gauze squares, 4 × 4 inch.

▼ Periodontal probe.

▼ Dental floss.

▼ Patient chart.

▼ Pencils—black, blue, red, green.

Procedure

PERFORMING THE ORAL EXAMINATION

1 As the patient enters the operatory, observe his general appearance, height, weight, posture, gait (manner of walking), skin tone, speech, and response to directions.

These are important diagnostic signs that indicate the general health of the patient.

Make a notation on his chart if the patient appears to have difficulties in any of these areas.

2 The assistant seats and drapes the patient.

The operator explains the procedure to the patient and performs the examination.

The assistant records the findings as dictated by the operator.

3 The operator examines the patient's face and neck to detect:

Abnormalities such as distortions, lumps, or swelling.

The texture, color and flexibility, and continuity of tissue of the lips.

Unusual swelling in the lymph nodes of the head, neck, and face (Fig. 14–10).

Difficulty opening or closing the mouth, pain and tenderness, or unusual sounds in the temporomandibular joint (TMJ).

Abnormal oral habits including bruxism, thumb sucking, tongue thrust swallow, and mouth breathing.

4 The operator examines the tissues lining the oral cavity including the labial frena, Stensen's duct, the hard and soft palates, and the uvula.

5 To examine the tongue, the patient is requested to extend his tongue.

The operator holds a sterile 4 × 4 inch gauze square, grasps the tip of the tongue, and gently pulls it forward while examining the top and sides of the tongue (Fig. 14–11).

To enable the operator to examine the undersurface of the tongue and the floor of the mouth, the patient is asked to touch the tip of the tongue to the palate.

6 To check the occlusion, the patient is asked to open and close his mouth normally. If deviations from normal occlusion are detected, a more extensive examination of the occlusion is indicated.

7 The operator examines the gingival tissues to determine the depth of the gingival sulcus and the epithelial attachment. (Periodontal charting is described in Chapter 28, "Periodontics.")

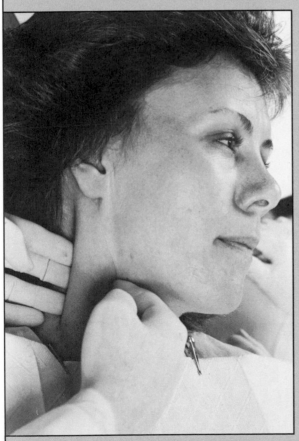

Figure 14–10 The operator examines the right cervical chain of lymph nodes. (Torres HO, Ehrlich A: Modern Dental Assisting, 4th Ed. Philadelphia, WB Saunders, 1990, p 456.)

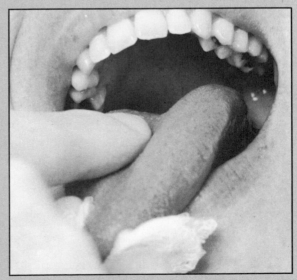

Figure 14–11 Examining sides of the tongue. The operator gently examines the top and sides of the tongue.

BLACK'S CLASSIFICATION OF CAVITIES

The classification and description of cavities was developed by G. V. Black in about 1900. Black's original classification included Classes I through V. Class VI was added later (Fig. 14–12).

These classifications are used by the dentist to describe the types and locations of carious lesions and existing restorations that are found during the examination of the teeth.

Class I—Pit and Fissure Cavities

Class I cavities occur in the pits and fissures (natural indentations) of the teeth in the following sites:

1. Occlusal surfaces of premolars and molars.
2. Occlusal two thirds of the facial surfaces of mandibular molars.

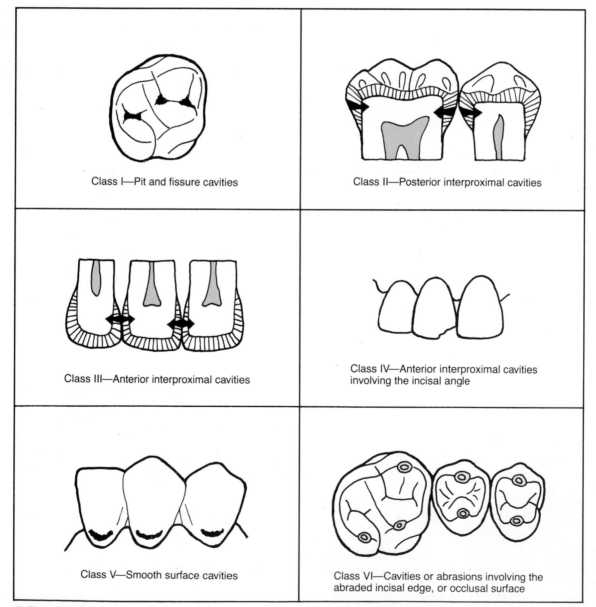

Class I—Pit and fissure cavities

Class II—Posterior interproximal cavities

Class III—Anterior interproximal cavities

Class IV—Anterior interproximal cavities involving the incisal angle

Class V—Smooth surface cavities

Class VI—Cavities or abrasions involving the abraded incisal edge, or occlusal surface

▼ Figure 14–12

Black's classification of cavities.

3. Occlusal one third of the lingual surfaces of the maxillary molars.
4. Lingual surfaces of maxillary incisors most frequently in the pit near the cingulum.

Class II — Posterior Interproximal Cavities

Class II cavities occur in the proximal surfaces of premolars and molars that may undermine the occlusal surface.

Class III — Anterior Interproximal Cavities

Class III cavities occur in the proximal surfaces of incisors and cuspids.

Class IV — Anterior Interproximal Cavities Involving the Incisal Angle

Class IV cavities occur in the proximal surfaces of incisors and cuspids and involve the incisal angle.

Class V — Smooth Surface Cavities

Class V cavities occur in the gingival third of the facial (or lingual) surfaces of any tooth.

Class VI — Cavities or Abrasions Involving the Abraded Incisal Edge or Occlusal Surface

Class VI cavities or abrasions involve the incisal edge of anterior teeth or the occlusal surfaces of posterior teeth. (**Abraded** means worn away.)

EXAMINATION OF THE TEETH

Using an explorer, mouth mirror, dental floss, or periodontal probe (as needed), the operator examines each tooth and the surrounding tissues in detail.

This includes the facial, lingual, mesial, distal, and occlusal or incisal surfaces of each tooth.

The operator notes carious lesions, existing restorations, recurrent caries, excessive wear, fractures, impactions, missing teeth, and other abnormalities.

To give the operator a better view, the assistant may be asked to rinse or to dry the teeth with warm air from the air-water syringe.

When recording the examination of the teeth, the dentist's findings are recorded using the Universal Numbering system (see Chapter 5), a charting diagram, charting symbols, and abbreviations.

▼ The dentist begins the examination with tooth number 1 and works around the dental arches to tooth number 32. (For children these are teeth A to T.)

▼ As the dentist dictates these findings, the assistant records them using the appropriate symbols, color codes, and abbreviations.

▼ To verify accuracy, the assistant may be asked to read back the findings as they have been recorded.

Charting Diagrams

In a charting diagram, the teeth are arranged as if you were looking at them from a position on the patient's tongue.

Thus, the right quadrants are on the left side of the page and the left quadrants are on the right side of the page.

Radiographs are usually mounted in the same order so that the chart and radiographs are parallel in their representation.

Figure 14–13 shows an "anatomic" representation of the permanent and primary teeth in which the diagram resembles the tooth surfaces.

Figure 14–14 is a "geometric" representation of the permanent and primary teeth. Here circles are used to indicate the surfaces of the teeth.

Figure 14–15 shows specialized occlusal view diagrams that may also be used.

Charting Symbols

Charting symbols are used to represent visually various conditions and restorations. These symbols are used on the "tooth diagram" portion of the patient's chart.

There are many informal systems of charting symbols. For example, in some systems an **X** is used to indicate a missing tooth. In other systems, a single slash **/** is used for this purpose.

In some systems, a tooth that is to be extracted is indicated with two parallel lines (as seen in Fig. 14–13). In other charting systems, a tooth to be extracted may be marked with an **X** (as seen in Fig. 14–12).

Each dentist has individual preferences, and it is important to learn to use the dentist's preferred system.

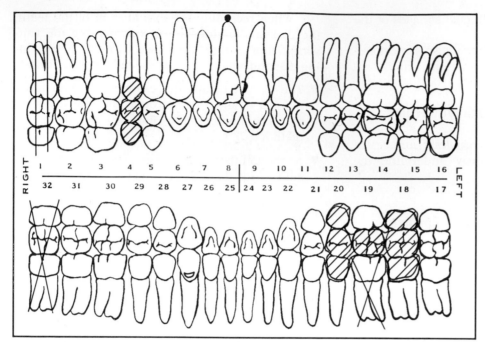

▼ **Figure 14-13**

Tooth diagram portion of a dental chart showing conditions and restorations present. 1—To be extracted. 4—Completed endodontic treatment, restored with a full crown. 8—MI fracture, periapical abscess. 9—M composite restoration. 14—MOD amalgam restoration. 16—Impacted, mesial drift. 19—Missing, replaced with a three-unit bridge with teeth 18 and 20 as abutments. 27—Class V caries. 32—Missing. (Courtesy of Colwell Systems, Inc, Champaign, IL.)

▼ **Figure 14-14**

Geometric diagram used to chart mixed dentition. All of the permanent first molars (3, 14, 19, 30) have erupted. So too have the maxillary central incisors (8 and 9), and the mandibular central and lateral incisors (23, 24, 25, 26). All of the primary centrals and laterals (D, E, F, G, N, O, P, Q) have been lost naturally. Primary tooth A is marked for extraction. (Courtesy of Colwell Systems, Inc, Champaign, IL.)

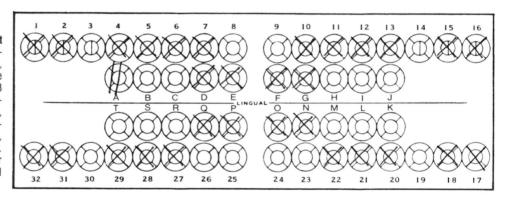

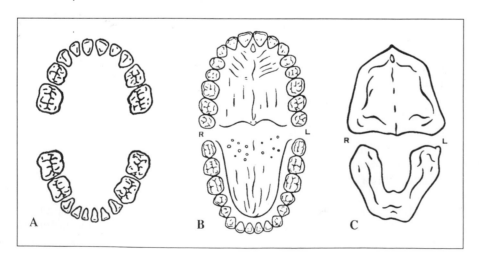

▼ **Figure 14-15**

Special dental diagrams showing occlusal views. *A.* The primary dentition. *B.* The permanent dentition. *C.* Edentulous maxillary and mandibular arches. (Courtesy of Colwell Systems, Inc, Champaign, IL.)

Color Coding

Some operators also use a color coding system to indicate restorations and defects. The following are some of the most commonly used color codes:

▼ Decay is outlined in pencil on the tooth surface involved.

▼ When the tooth is restored, the area is filled in with the appropriate color.

▼ A completed amalgam is colored in with a blue pen or pencil.

▼ Gold restorations are colored in red.

▼ Composite restorations may be *shaded* in green to distinguish the difference in restorative material.

▼ If a present restoration must be replaced, the involved area is *outlined* in the color corresponding to the color of the intended restoration.

Charting Abbreviations

Abbreviations are used to indicate a single surface or a combination of tooth surfaces. (Review the names of the tooth surfaces in Chapter 4.)

▼ Single Surfaces Abbreviations

B	buccal
D	distal
F	facial (to describe both buccal and labial surfaces)
	I — incisal
L	lingual
M	mesial
O	occlusal

Combinations of Surfaces

When "naming" a combination of the tooth surfaces, a new term is formed. This is done by dropping the last letter(s) of the first word of the combination, and changing the word ending to "o." For example, mesial changes to mesio when combined with occlusal: mesio-occlusal.

However, when dictating these findings, the dentist simply gives the letters involved. For example, an MI fracture to describe the mesioincisal fracture of an anterior tooth.

▼ Combination Abbreviations

BO	bucco-occlusal
DI	distoincisal
DO	disto-occlusal
LO	linguo-occlusal
MI	mesioincisal
MO	mesio-occlusal
MOD	mesio-occlusodistal

Treatment Abbreviations

Many abbreviations are used when recording the treatment provided to the patient. Again, each dentist has his or her personal preferences.

When in doubt about the meaning or use of an abbreviation, it is far better to spell out completely what has taken place.

▼ Common Treatment Abbreviations

Amal	amalgam
Br	bridge
C & B	crown and bridge
Com	composite
CR	crown
X	extraction
Fo	foil
G	gold
GI	gold inlay
In	inlay
MandFD or LFD	mandibular (or lower) full denture
MandPD or LPD	mandibular (or lower) partial denture
MFD or UFD	maxillary (or upper) full denture
MPD or UPD	maxillary (or upper) partial denture
M	missing
PFM	porcelain fused to metal
PJC	porcelain jacket crown
PI	porcelain inlay

▼ EXERCISES

1. A/An _____ is a Class II cavity involving the mesial, occlusal, and distal surfaces.

   a. DOM
   b. MOD
   c. ODM
   d. OMD

2. The normal body temperature for the average adult is _____ °F.

   a. 97.6
   b. 98.1
   b. 98.6
   d. 99.6

3. On a charting diagram, the right quadrants are on the _____ side of the diagram.

   a. left
   b. right

4. To determine the pulse in the patient's wrist, palpate the _____ artery.

   a. brachial
   b. facial
   c. radial
   d. ulnar

5. The abbreviation PFM stands for _____.

   a. patient faints momentarily
   b. porcelain filling on mesial
   c. porcelain fused to metal
   d. protrusive forward movement

6. In a/an _____ charting diagram, circles are used to indicate the surfaces of the teeth.

   a. anatomic
   b. geometric
   c. universal

7. The normal respiration rate for a child is _____ breaths per minute.

   a. 16-18
   b. 22-26
   c. 24-28
   d. 28-30

8. To examine the tongue, the operator uses a/an _____ to pull the tongue forward gently.

   a. cotton plier
   b. explorer
   c. sterile gauze square
   d. a and c

9. The normal range of blood pressure for an adult ＿＿＿＿＿＿＿＿＿ from 110/60 to 140/90.

   a. is
   b. is not

10. When using color coding with charting symbols, a gold restoration is recorded in ＿＿＿＿＿＿＿＿＿＿.

    a. black
    b. blue
    c. green
    d. red

11. A DI fracture of a central incisor is described as a Class ＿＿＿＿＿＿＿ cavity.

    a. II
    b. III
    c. IV
    d. VI

12. The abbreviation for a mandibular full denture is ＿＿＿＿＿＿＿＿＿＿＿.

    a. LFD
    b. LPD
    c. ManFD
    d. a or c

13. After use, a glass thermometer is ＿＿＿＿＿＿＿＿＿＿.

    a. autoclaved
    b. discarded
    c. disinfected

14. When charting an examination, decay is outlined in ＿＿＿＿＿＿＿＿ on the tooth diagram.

    a. ink
    b. pencil
    c. green
    d. red

15. When obtaining a blood pressure reading, the stethoscope disc is placed on the ＿＿＿＿＿＿＿＿＿.

    a. brachial artery
    b. brachial vein
    c. carotid artery
    d. carotid vein

16. According to Black's classification, Class ＿＿＿＿＿＿＿＿＿＿ cavities involve the proximal and possibly occlusal surfaces of posterior teeth.

    a. I
    b. II
    c. III
    d. IV

17. The bladder of the blood pressure cuff is placed over the _____ _____ area of the upper arm.

    a. back
    b. inner
    c. side away from the body
    d. side next the body

18. Abraded surfaces, involving the incisal edges and occlusal surfaces of the teeth, are classified as Class _____.

    a. III
    b. IV
    c. VI
    d. VII

19. When examining the teeth of an adult patient, the dentist begins with tooth number _____

    a. 1
    b. 32
    c. A
    d. a or c

20. _____ pressure is the highest pressure exerted on the circulatory system by the contraction of the heart.

    a. Diastolic
    b. Systolic

21. A medical history includes information about the patient's _____ _____.

    a. current medications
    b. medical history
    c. present physical condition
    d. a, b, and c

22. Counting the respiration rate is based on _____.

    a. each time the patient inhales
    b. each time the patient exhales
    c. one inhalation and one exhalation

23. If a present restoration must be replaced, the involved area of the diagram is _____.

    a. filled in with ink
    b. highlighted in red
    c. outlined in the color corresponding to the intended restoration
    d. shaded in black

24. According to Black's classification, a facial (F) cavity on a smooth surface is a Class _____ cavity.

    a. I
    b. III
    c. IV
    d. V

25. The charting abbreviation "F" includes both the buccal and labial surfaces.

    a. true
    b. false

▼ Criterion Sheet 14–1

Student's Name _____

Procedure: *OBTAINING AND RECORDING VITAL SIGNS*		
Performance Objective: The student will demonstrate obtaining and recording a patient's pulse, respiration rate, temperature, and blood pressure. Another student will act as the patient.		

SE = Student evaluation **C** = Criterion met **IE** = Instructor evaluation **X** = Criterion not met	**SE**	**IE**
Instrumentation: Sphygmomanometer, stethoscope, thermometer, patient's chart, pencil, and paper.		
1. Gathered necessary equipment.		
2. Washed hands.		
3. Informed patient of the procedure.		
4. Accurately obtained and recorded pulse.		
5. Accurately obtained and recorded respiration rate.		
6. Accurately obtained and recorded temperature.		
7. Accurately obtained and recorded blood pressure.		
8. Washed hands again.		
9. Properly maintained and stored all equipment.		
Comments:		

Criterion Sheet 14–2

Student's Name _____

Procedure: *RECORDING THE DENTAL EXAMINATION*

Performance Objective:

The student will demonstrate recording the dental examination using the symbols and abbreviations specified by the dentist (or instructor).

	SE	IE
SE = Student evaluation **C** = Criterion met **IE** = Instructor evaluation **X** = Criterion not met		
Instrumentation: Patients chart (with tooth diagram), colored pencils.		
1. Accurately recorded diagnostic information as dictated by the dentist.		
2. Used appropriate symbols.		
3. Used appropriate color coding.		
4. Used appropriate abbreviations.		
5. Accurately read findings back to the dentist.		
Comments:		

15 Fundamentals of Dental Radiography

▼ LEARNING OBJECTIVES

The student will be able to:

1. State the principles of radiation safety as applied to dental radiography.

2. Describe the ALARA (As Low As Reasonably Achievable) principle, plus the responsibilities of the dentist and dental assistant as they relate to dental radiography.

3. Discuss the biological and cumulative effects of x-radiation on human tissues.

4. Define the maximum permissable dose (MPD) of ionizing radiation to occupational workers and explain the necessity of monitoring of dental personnel regarding their exposure to x-radiation.

5. Explain and discuss the hazards of primary, secondary, and scatter radiation.

6. Describe the need for operatory shielding, patient protection and operator protection, as related to exposure to radiation.

7. Name and describe the major components of the dental x-ray unit.

8. Describe these variables that are applied in dental radiographic technique: Milliamperage, kilovoltage, exposure time, and length of the position indicator device (PID).

9. Explain the need for fast speed film and name the sizes and composition of film used for intraoral dental radiographs.

10. List and discuss the properties of exposed and processed dental radiographic film and the criteria related to diagnostic-quality radiographs.

11. Define vertical and horizontal angulation as they are related to producing dental radiographs.

12. List the essential anatomic landmarks as applied to intraoral dental radiography.

OVERVIEW OF FUNDAMENTALS OF DENTAL RADIOGRAPHY

Dental radiographs are aids to the dentist in the diagnosis of conditions of the patient's dentition and supportive structures.

Radiographs produced by the application of principles of radiation safety, along with sound technical skill on the part of the operator, result in diagnostically acceptable radiographs commonly referred to as "dental x-rays."

A **complete radiographic survey** (CRS) provides a minimum of *two* views of each area of each tooth of the dentition.

For the average adult, this usually involves at least 18 radiographs (including 2 bite-wings of the premolars and 2 bite-wings of the molars). However, the dentist must determine the number of radiographs in the series according to the needs of the patient.

Radiographs are taken *only* when indicated and with the patient's permission. If a patient refuses radiographs, he may be asked to sign a release stating that he understands the potential consequences of his refusal.

PRODUCING X-RADIATION

Naturally occurring background radiation and other forms of environmental radiation are evident in our everyday lives.

Additional radiation, beyond that found in nature, is primarily emitted by x-ray machines, radioactive isotopes, and other materials used for diagnostic and therapeutic purposes.

Electromagnetic radiations are made of units of pure energy called **photons,** which have no mass or weight.

X-rays, visible light, and radio waves are all forms of electromagnetic radiation. **Electromagnetic waves** are energy waves that travel at the speed of 186,000 miles per second.

All forms of electromagnetic radiation are grouped according to their wavelengths. Together they are referred to as the **electromagnetic spectrum.** Different wavelengths within this spectrum have different uses.

At one end of the spectrum are the long wavelengths such as radio and television waves. At the opposite end of the spectrum are the short wavelengths such as gamma rays and x-rays.

The differences in wavelengths are important when considering x-radiation sources because:

▼ The *shorter* the wavelength, the *greater* the ability of the radiant energy to penetrate matter: Human tissue in this instance. Dental x-radiation equipment generates useful short waves of energy.

▼ The *longer* the wavelength, the *weaker* the penetrative power of the radiant energy. Therefore, properly functioning dental x-ray equipment is collimated and filtered to prevent emitting radiation of nonuseful long wavelengths.

The **collimator** is a leaded apparatus with a small opening. The opening in the collimator controls the size of the x-ray beam emitted from the head of the machine.

The **filters** are layers of aluminum placed in the head of the x-ray unit near the collimator to filter out nonuseful radiation of long wavelengths.

SPECIFIC RADIATION HAZARDS

Primary Radiation

Primary radiation, also known as the *primary beam,* is the central beam emitted from the x-ray unit tube head. It travels in a straight line and contains the powerful short waves.

These short waves in the primary beam expose the film to produce the diagnostically useful radiograph.

Secondary Radiation

Secondary radiation is given off by all matter exposed to radiation. For example, during the exposure of dental x-ray film, adjacent tissues become irradiated. This irradiation may continue to expose the film and harm the adjacent tissues.

Scatter Radiation

Scatter radiation is radiation that has been deflected from its path during the impact with matter. The scatter radiation is deflected in all directions and is impossible to confine.

As the patient is exposed to radiation, the radiation scatters on impact and travels to all parts of the body as well as throughout the operatory.

During this process, x-ray photons interact with electrons of the atoms of the irradiated tissue. The result is scatter radiation, which has less energy and an increased wavelength and is of no use in dentistry.

Without adequate protective barriers, the operator and persons standing or sitting nearby all may be affected by exposure to scatter radiation.

Leakage Radiation

Scatter radiation may also be caused by the leaking of low-intensity wavelengths from the opening of the collimator in a poorly filtered x-ray beam. This radiation is not diagnostically useful; however, it is dangerous.

The head of the x-ray unit should be checked regularly to detect any leakage of radiation. If there is a problem, the unit must be taken out of service and corrected immediately before additional films are exposed.

Some states have regulations regarding the installation, inspection, and operation of new x-ray equipment. Some states also require periodic inspections of all x-ray equipment. These functions are conducted by the state department of health, usually for a small fee.

TISSUE SENSITIVITY TO RADIATION

All human cells are sensitive to some degree to the effects of radiation. However, the most sensitive cells are those that are more specialized and reproduce more quickly.

As shown in the following chart, the relative sensitivity of cells and tissues to radiation is listed beginning with the most sensitive.

▼ Tissue Sensitivity to Radiation

1. In pregnancy, the cells of the embryo
2. Blood-forming tissue (bone marrow), white and red blood cells
3. Gonadal tissue
4. Thyroid tissue
5. Epithelial tissue of the alimentary canal
6. Gastrointestinal tissue
7. Tissue of the cornea of the eye
8. Mature bone tissue
9. Mature nerve tissue
10. Muscle tissue

Individual Sensitivity

Pregnant Women

Prior to an exposure to x-radiation, all women of child-bearing age should be tactfully questioned as to the possibility of being pregnant.

If the gametes (sex cells) are exposed to ionizing radiation, mutation may occur. (**Mutation** is the development of tissue abnormality—for example, abnormal growth.)

The most sensitive of all human tissues is the fetus, particularly during the first 3 months of pregnancy. If possible, the dentist may prefer to postpone all radiographs during this period.

Children

Children, whose tissues are rapidly growing and developing, are also extremely sensitive to radiation. (Remember, rapidly developing tissues are much more sensitive than are "mature cells," which are not in the process of rapid change.)

To calculate exposure time for children, reduce the adult exposure time by about one third. (Follow the manufacturer's instructions on exposure time for dental film.)

The Elderly

The exposure time for the elderly may also be reduced because of the thinness of bones as a result of osteoporosis. Also, the repair mechanism of the body becomes less effective with advancing age, and therefore less exposure to x-radiation is indicated.

Radiation Therapy

The dentist will exercise particular caution in the case of patients receiving radiation therapy. If the treatment has been extensive, recent, or currently in progress, the dentist may decide to forego dental radiographs.

Cumulative Effects of Ionizing Radiation

The effects of radiation are cumulative. That is, repeated exposure causes a cumulative (increasing) effect. This is identified as the **long-term effect.**

The **latent period** is the time before the results of the cumulative effects of radiation are manifested and become visible to the eye.

An accidental intense exposure is described as an **acute dose,** and it can be fatal. An acute dose is usually followed by a short latent period.

However, the results of the acute dose may be manifested within a matter of hours or days. One of the first clinical symptoms of this is **erythema,** a reddening of the skin similar to sunburn.

The dental staff must never assume that the patient has *not* had recent exposure to radiation. Questions about exposure to radiation must be addressed routinely and tactfully as part of the total medical history for all patients.

Also, it is important that information on exposure to x-radiation be updated and recorded on the patient's treatment record at each subsequent appointment.

RADIATION LIMITS

Maximum Permissible Dose

The term maximum permissible dose (MPD) is used to describe the exposure that occupationally exposed dental personnel (the dentist, assistant, or hygienist) may safely receive.

MPD is considered to be the dose of radiation to the whole body that produces very little chance of bodily or genetic injury. For the general population (nonoccupational), exposure is described as *dose limit*.

In a year, the MPD for a dental occupational worker is 5 rem (radiation equivalent man) or 0.05 Sv (sieverts). Because the effects of radiation are cumulative, an age-based formula is also used.

For the general public, pregnant radiation workers, and those workers under 18 years of age, a maximum permissible dose of 0.5 rem is suggested. This is about one tenth that of a dental occupational worker. For this reason, no person under 18 should be permitted to expose film for radiographs.

Personnel Monitoring

A film monitoring service is used to provide radiation monitoring for all members of the dental office staff functioning in or near the operatories.

The **dosimeter badge** monitoring device is worn at all times when in the dental office. It measures the amount and type of radiation to which each individual is exposed in the working environment.

The dosimeter badge should *not* be worn out of the office, since doing this could lead to overexposure to various factors and result in a false reading.

The periodic report on radiation monitoring should become a permanent record for the office staff. Also, each staff member should receive a copy of the periodic report of his or her own radiation record.

RADIATION SAFETY PRECAUTIONS

Exposure to x-radiation is hazardous and cumulative in its effect on human tissues; therefore, certain principles of radiation safety must prevail.

The ALARA Principle

ALARA stands for *As Low As Reasonably Achievable*. This concept endorses the use of the lowest possible exposure of the patient (and operator) to x-radiation to produce a diagnostically acceptable radiograph.

Adherence to the ALARA principle means that every available method of reducing exposure to x-radiation is used to minimize potential risks for patients and for dental personnel.

Responsibilities of the Dentist

1. The dentist prescribes only those radiographs that are diagnostically necessary.
2. The dentist assumes responsibility for having all radiographic equipment installed and maintained in safe working condition. This includes the x-ray unit, processing equipment, accessories, and "E" speed dental film.
3. The dentist assumes responsibility for having all personnel who expose radiographs adequately trained, properly credentialed, and appropriately supervised.

The dentist and the assistant must be fully informed of current state regulations applying to the dental assistant exposing radiographs.

Some states have formal testing requirements for licensure or registration of dental auxiliaries in radiographic technique and radiation safety.

Responsibilities of the Dental Assistant

1. The dental assistant obtains radiographs only when directed by, and under the general supervision of, the dentist.
2. The dental assistant must be properly trained and have met state licensure or registration requirements before exposing x-ray film on patients.
3. The dental assistant must understand and apply radiation hygiene precautions.
4. The dental assistant must demonstrate competency in radiation exposure techniques that will produce the best possible diagnostic yield with the least possible exposure of the patient and operator to x-radiation.
5. The dental assistant must perform these duties to the best of her ability to protect the patient from unnecessary exposure required in retaking films of poor quality.

Federal Legislation

The *Consumer–Patient Radiation Health and Safety Act* was enacted into law in 1981. This legislation addresses the qualification of dental auxiliaries who operate radiation-emitting equipment and expose dental radiographs.

Under this act, each state is required to inform the federal Secretary of Health and Human Services how it complies with the Act and qualifies dental personnel (assistants and hygienists) to operate dental x-ray equipment within the state.

To qualify, the operator (dental assistant) may be required to be a currently Certified Dental Assistant or to have passed a course in dental radiographic technique and radiation safety.

Each auxiliary is advised to check his or her State Board of Dentistry for regulations regarding operators of dental radiographic equipment.

Operatory Shielding

The dental x-ray unit should be located at the most distant point possible from the heavy traffic in the dental office.

The staff and patients in the adjacent areas are protected from the effects of x-radiation by operatory walls constructed of at least two ⅝ inch thicknesses of gypsum sheet rock or 1/16 inch-thick sheets of lead embedded in the wall. (Lead is used here because of its ability to block the passage of x-radiation.)

The operator stands outside of the operatory behind a lead-lined door or wall. This barrier must be large enough to shield the operator from the top of the head down to and including the feet.

A leaded glass window in this shield protects the operator while permitting observation of the patient during exposure of the film. Leaded glass prevents the passage of x-radiation.

X-Ray Control Panel

The control panel and timer switch must be positioned so that the operator may make all adjustments and exposures while standing behind a protective barrier.

An alternative is to have the timer switch on an extension cord. This enables the operator to press the button while standing behind protective shielding at a safe distance from the source of radiation (minimum of 6 feet).

Patient Protection

Protection for the patient is provided by the proper placement of the lead apron and lead thyrocervical collar (Fig. 15–1).

These protective devices are carefully placed on the patient prior to the first exposure and are left in position until the last film is exposed.

The apron covers the chest and gonadal areas of the patient. The thyrocervical collar is placed

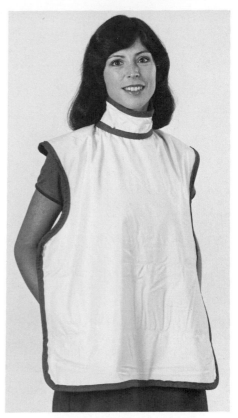

▼ **Figure 15–1**

Lead apron and thyrocervical collar on radiography patient. (Torres HO, Ehrlich A: Modern Dental Assisting, 4th Ed. Philadelphia, WB Saunders, 1990, p 375.)

snug to the patient's throat (up to the chin) to cover the thyroid and parathyroid glands.

When not in use, the lead apron and collar must be placed *unfolded* on a support rod in the operatory. (Folding damages the lead apron and collar, allowing radiation to penetrate through the cracks when in use.)

The patient's fingers are used to hold the film *only* if positioning accessories will not stabilize the film. At no time should the operator, or any member of the staff, hold film in the mouth of the patient.

If the patient is an infant or toddler, a member of the patient's family may be used—but then only in an emergency. The family member and child must be draped with a lead apron.

Operator Protection

The operator must *always* keep away from the primary beam of the x-ray unit and from secondary and scatter radiation. If not behind the protective barrier, the operator must stand at least 6 feet away from the head of the x-ray unit.

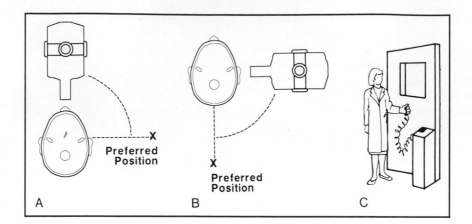

▼ **Figure 15-2**

Preferred positions for operator. *A.* The X in this diagram shows the preferred position for the operator for exposure of an anterior film. The region between the tubehead and the X is also considered safe for the operator when standing behind a protective barrier. *B.* The X indicates the preferred position for the operator behind a protective barrier when a posterior film is exposed. *C.* The operator standing behind a protective lead-walled barrier. (Adapted from Miles DA, Van Dis ML, Jensen CW, Ferretti A: Radiographic Imaging for Dental Auxiliaries. Philadelphia: WB Saunders, 1989, p 3.)

At this distance, the operator should be positioned behind and to the right or left of the head of the patient opposite the opening of the position-indicator device (PID). This places the operator at a 135-degree angle to the x-ray beam (Fig. 15-2).

THE DENTAL X-RAY MACHINE

The dental x-ray machine should be of a late manufacturing date and equipped with a control panel that is mounted outside the operatory. The machine should have an electronic timer and have the potential for 65 to 95 kVp and 10 to 15 mA.

Master Switch

By law, the x-ray machine must have a separate master switch that controls or cuts off electricity to the machine. However, the x-ray machine may safely be left on all day because it does *not* produce x-radiation until the electronic timer is set and fired.

Electronic Timer

As a safety device, the timer operates only while the switch is being pressed and automatically cuts off the electrical current as soon as the switch is released.

This automatic cutoff of electrical current when the switch is released is referred to as the "dead man's switch." The timer automatically resets itself after each exposure.

Controls

The three major variables found on the machine control panel are **milliamperage** (mA), **kilovoltage** (kV), and **exposure time.**

The manner in which these adjustments are made varies from machine to machine. It is important that you become familiar with these controls before trying to operate the machine.

The setting selected for these variables is influenced by several factors, including the film speed and the exposure technique, plus specifics about the individual patient and the area to be radiographed. Check with the dentist before operating the dental x-ray unit as to the milliamperage, kilovoltage, and exposure time preferred.

These settings must be reviewed carefully, and the settings on the x-ray unit must be checked carefully *prior* to exposing a radiograph.

Milliamperage

An **ampere** is the unit of measure for the electrical current. A **milliampere** (mA) is one thousandth of an ampere. The **milliamperage meter** on the machine registers the milliamperage used.

The milliamperage determines the **quantity** (amount) of potential x-radiation by changing the amount of electrons in the central beam.

A higher milliamperage increases the amount of radiation. A lower milliamperage decreases the amount of radiation.

Amperage is controlled by the **milliamperage regulator.** Dental x-ray units usually operate in the range of 7.5, 10, to 15 mA: 10 mA is the setting most commonly used for dental radiographs.

The amount of exposure that the patient actually received is expressed in **milliampere seconds** (mAs).

To calculate the milliampere seconds, the milliamperage used is multiplied by time of exposure (mA × time = mAs). Adding the number of exposures is used to record total exposure data on the patient's clinical record.

Kilovoltage

A volt is a unit of electrical potential. A **kilovolt** (kV) is equal to 1000 volts.

The **kilovoltage peak** (kVp) identifies the maximum potential of the central beam of radiation as the current is activated.

The kilovoltage used determines the **quality** (penetrating power) of the central beam. The higher the kV, the greater the penetrating power, the shorter the exposure time, and the longer the range of the gray scale.

The lower the kV, the less the penetrating power, the longer the exposure, and the shorter the gray scale range. The result is few differences of shades of gray.

The **kilovolt meter** on the control panel of the x-ray unit registers the kilovoltage used. Most dental x-ray machines have a kVp potential of 55 to 120 kVp. The most commonly used settings are between 70 and 90 kV.

The Gray Scale

A longer range of the gray scale is capable of distinguishing between densities of varying types of tissue. The longer gray scale is desirable because it provides a higher diagnostic quality film, which includes more definitive density and contrast in the radiograph.

The longer gray scale includes more steps, or shades, of gray to provide finer distinction between softer tissues, semi-hard tissue, and hard tissues of the teeth and their supporting structures.

Exposure Time

The **electronic timer** of the x-ray machine automatically controls the flow of electricity to generate x-radiation.

Some timers are calibrated in seconds and fractions of seconds. Other units are calibrated with gradations called **impulses.**

An impulse is a fraction of a second, and 30 impulses equal ½ second. Most electronic timer controls register a maximum of 60 impulses.

The exposure time is affected by the radiographic technique, the type of x-ray film, the tissues being radiographed, the age and condition of the patient, and the target film distance (TFD) being used.

Position-Indicator Device

The position-indicator device (PID) is an extension placed on the tube head at the collimator attachment. Its purpose is to guide and limit the amount of radiation.

To minimize the amount of radiation exposure to the patient, the PID is lead-lined or made of a material that is impervious to passing radiation.

The shape of the PID may be cylindrical or rectangular, and its open end is positioned against the patient's face during film exposure. The rectangular PID limits the beam size to that of a number 2 size (periapical) dental film (Fig. 15–3).

The length of the PID provides an extension of 8, 12, or 16 inches from the anode of the x-ray unit to the patient's skin.

The length of the PID selected depends on the radiographic technique being used and on the desired target film distance.

The **target film distance** (TFD), or *skin film distance* (SFD), is the distance from the source of the x-radiation to the object being radiographed.

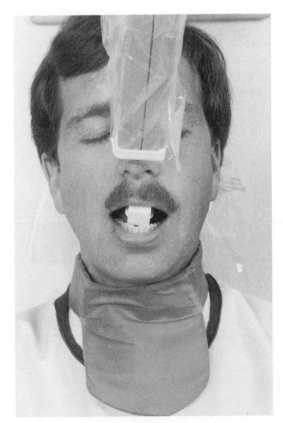

▼ Figure 15–3

A rectangular PID guides and limits the amount of radiation.

Accessories

Accessories are designed to assist in the placement and stabilization of the dental film. The XCP instruments for the paralleling technique, which are shown in Figures 15–3 and 15–4, are designed and patented by the Rinn Corporation, Elgin, IL. The small angular holders are designed by the Stabe Manufacturing, Rinn Corporation, Elgin, IL.

Film placement and PID alignment with accessories may vary. When using any accessory, carefully follow the manufacturer's directions for use, placement, and sterilization.

DENTAL X-RAY FILM

Film Packet

Individual dental films are packaged in a light-tight packet that is made of either plastic or paper. Inside the packet the film is positioned between an inner lining of two sheets of black paper (Figs. 15–5 and 15–6).

A sheet of lead foil is located at the "back" of the packet, that is, next to the side of the packet with a tab opening. The lead foil protects the film from secondary radiation, which would cause the film to fog. It also protects the tissue surrounding the area being radiographed from unnecessary exposure.

The back of the packet has a tab opening that is used to remove the film for processing. This side is always placed next to the tongue or palate and *away* from the tooth being radiographed.

The front, pebbly, or smooth side of the film packet has a small **embossed dot**, or "raised bump." This side is always placed *toward* the PID.

When placing the film in the oral cavity, the dot should also be positioned toward the occlusal

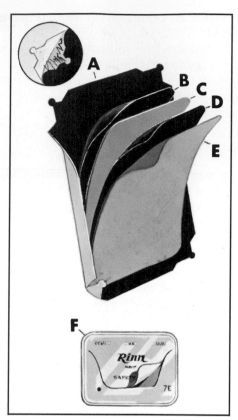

▼ **Figure 15–5**

Dental film packet. *A.* Saliva-proof paper or plastic outer wrapper. *B.* Black paper to protect film from light damage. *C.* Dental film. *D.* Second sheet of black paper. *E.* Foil backing to protect film from excess secondary radiation. *F.* Dot on tab side of envelope to indicate that the opposite side of the film must be placed toward the source of radiation. (Courtesy of Rinn Corporation, Elgin, IL.)

surface, or the incisal edge of the teeth being radiographed. This placement of the dot prevents imposition of an artifact, which could appear to be an abscess, on the apex of a tooth. (An **artifact** is a structure or appearance that is not normally present in the radiograph. Artifacts are produced by artificial means.)

The exceptions for placement of the dot are for:

1. The mandibular right molar area (to avoid superimposition of the dot on the retromolar area).
2. Bite-wing exposures.

In both these cases, the dot is placed toward the apices on the mandibular teeth because the mandibular teeth have fewer roots.

Dual Film Packets

Dual film packets contain *two* pieces of film between the black paper lining. This makes it possible to produce an exact duplicate set of the films without exposing the patient to additional radiation.

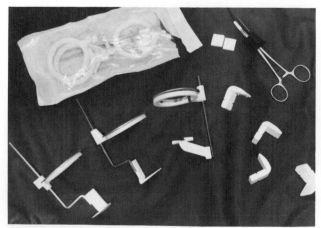

▼ **Figure 15–4**

Sterile accessories for holding dental film.

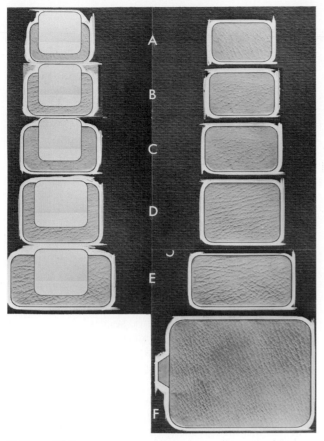

▼ **Figure 15-6**

Types of intraoral dental x-ray film. *A* through *E*. Dental films with bite-wing tabs (left) and without tabs (right). *A* through D. Periapical films. *A*. No. 00 pedodontic ($^{13}/_{16}$″ × 1¼″) *B*. No. 0 pedodontic ($^{7}/_{8}$″ × 1⅜″) *C*. No. 1 narrow ($^{15}/_{16}$″ × 1⁹/₁₆″) *D*. No. 2 standard (1¼″ × 1⅝″) *E*. No. 3 bite-wing (1¹/₁₆″ × 2⅛″) *F*. No. 4 occlusal (2¼″ × 3″). (Courtesy of Rinn Corporation, Elgin, IL.)

Since original radiographs are important records that should not be allowed to leave the office, dual packets should be used when the dentist anticipates needing radiographs for insurance purposes or for referral to a specialist.

Film Speed

The film speed (the film's sensitivity to radiation) determines the amount of x-radiation needed to produce a diagnostic-quality radiograph. The faster the film speed, the smaller the amount of x-radiation needed for exposure.

Film speed is rated according to standards adopted by the American National Standards Institute (ANSI). The standards institute is an independent body that determines the quality and speed of dental film.

The manufacturer dates and labels the film box with the film speed and recommended settings for exposure when using the film.

The recommended speed for dental radio-

graphs is the "E" speed film. This speed further reduces the exposure of the patient to ionizing radiation.

Intraoral Film Sizes

Intraoral films are used to produce **periapical, bite-wing,** and **occlusal** radiographs. The film size selected for each of these exposures depends upon the area being radiographed and the size of the patient's oral cavity.

A **periapical** radiograph is a vertical or horizontal view of the teeth. The radiograph records the crown, roots, and supporting structures. Periapical film (size numbers 0, 1, and 2) is commonly used for this purpose.

A **bite-wing** radiograph records the crowns and interproximal regions of maxillary and mandibular teeth on the same film. Film size numbers 1, 2, and 3 may be used for this purpose; however, number 3 film, which is most frequently used for bite-wing radiographs, is longer than number 2 film.

An **occlusal** radiograph shows an entire arch on one film. Film size number 4 is commonly used for this purpose. (*Note:* Occlusal films are usually supplied in a dual pack containing two films.)

Film Storage

All dental films should be stored so that they are protected from light, heat, moisture, chemicals, aromatic substances, and scatter radiation.

Film kept in the operatory or near the x-ray unit should be stored in a lead box, preferably off the floor to prevent the absorption of moisture.

The operator should never leave either exposed or unexposed films in the path of the central beam or scatter radiation because this additional "exposure" can fog the film and render it useless as a radiograph.

X-ray films have a limited shelf life and should not be used beyond the expiration date printed on the box.

If long-term storage of x-ray film is necessary, the unopened packages may be stored in the refrigerator. Prior to use, the films are allowed to warm gradually to room temperature.

INTRAORAL TECHNIQUE BASICS

In the **paralleling technique,** which is discussed further in Chapter 16, "Dental Radiography: Paralleling Technique," the film packet and x-ray beam are at right angles (90 degrees) to one another, with the film packet placed parallel to the long axis of the tooth.

There are three major factors that must be taken into consideration with this technique. These are **PID length and exposure time, vertical angulation,** and **horizontal angulation.**

PID Length and Exposure Time

The paralleling technique uses a PID of 12 to 16 inches in length. If changing from a shorter to a longer PID, the exposure time must be increased.

According to the **inverse square law,** the intensity of the radiation is inversely proportional to the square of the distance. (**Inverse** means opposite or reverse effect.)

When the distance is doubled, the intensity of radiation is only one fourth the intensity at the original distance. Therefore, the exposure time must be adjusted accordingly.

For example, to expose a film with a 16-inch PID requires more exposure time than would the same film used with an 8-inch PID. When making exposure time recommendations, some film manufacturers may express the distance as **focus-film distance** (FFD) or as **target-film distance** (TFD).

Position Indicator Distance PID

Vertical Angulation

Adjustments of both the vertical and the horizontal angulation of the x-ray tube head are necessary so that the PID is positioned correctly.

Vertical angulation (VA) refers to up and down (raising and lowering) movements. Vertical angulation determines how accurately the length of the object being radiographed is reproduced in the radiograph.

Changes in vertical angulation are similar to those changes in shadows caused as the sun moves throughout the day.

At noon, when the sun is directly overhead, the shadow is foreshortened (shorter). **Foreshortened images,** those that appear shorter than the actual object, are caused by *too much* vertical angulation.

At 4 P.M., as the sun moves toward the horizon, the shadow is elongated (lengthened). **Elongated images,** those that appear longer than the actual object, are caused by *too little* vertical angulation.

Vertical angulation is determined by the degree of angulation *above* and *below* the neutral "0" (zero) degree on a 360-degree circle. With the patient sitting upright, a line parallel with the floor, such as the occlusal plane, is at zero.

An increase in vertical angulation from the zero position is indicated by a plus sign (+). To produce this, the head of the unit is raised and the opening of the PID is pointed *downward* rather than parallel with the floor.

A decrease in vertical angulation from the zero position is indicated by a minus sign (−). To produce this, the head of the unit is lowered and the PID opening is pointed *upward* rather than parallel with the floor.

Horizontal Angulation

Horizontal angulation (HA) refers to back and forth movements on a plane that is parallel with the floor. Proper horizontal angulation projects the proximal surfaces of the adjacent teeth on the film without overlapping the surfaces.

For example, on the radiograph the mesiodistal contacts of the first and second molars are *touching* at the natural contact point and not overlapping each other. The exception is crowded dentition, in which the teeth actually *are* overlapped in the dental arch.

When adjusting horizontal angulation, the head of the unit moves *only* on a 360-degree axis (circle) around the head of the patient. The plane parallel with the floor still holds at zero (Fig. 15–7).

The horizontal angulation should be placed to direct the central beam accurately on the long axis of a tooth or **through the contacts** of two adjacent teeth determined by the dentist for diagnosis.

If the horizontal angulation is too distal (pointed too sharply from the back), the resultant image shows the distal tooth overlapping the one mesial to it. For example, the first maxillary molar appears to be superimposed over the second premolar.

If the horizontal angulation is too mesial

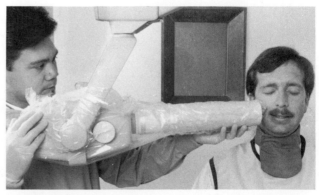

▼ Figure 15–7

Checking the horizontal angulation of the PID and placement of the film for a bite-wing radiograph.

360°

(pointed too sharply from the front), the reverse occurs, and the premolars overlap the mesial of the first maxillary molar.

ANATOMIC LANDMARKS

Knowledge of anatomic landmarks is important for correct angulation and radiographic technique. These landmarks are shown in Figure 15–8.

A **canthus** is either corner, or angle, of the eye where the upper and lower eyelids meet. The **inner canthus** is the angle where eyelids meet adjacent to the nose. The **outer canthus** is the junction of the eyelids at the outer corner of the eye, closest to the temple.

The **ala** is the winged flare of the nostril as it meets the cheek. The **tragus** is the small prominence of tissue located anteriorly at the middle of the opening of the ear. The **ala–tragus line** is an

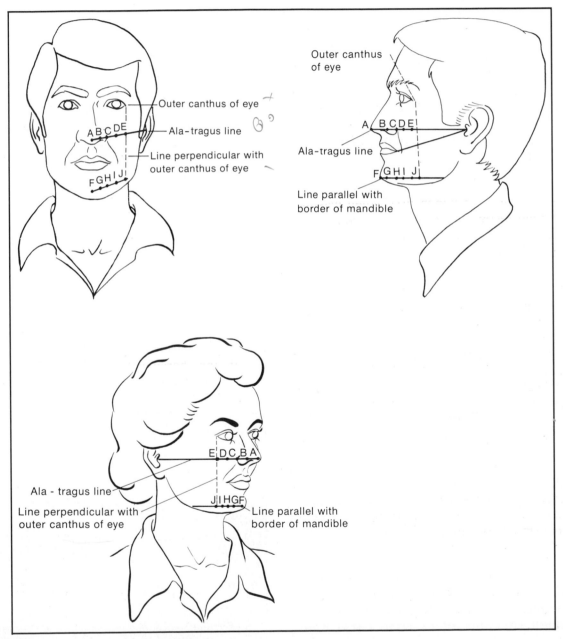

▼ **Figure 15–8**

Landmarks of the face for radiographic projection. *A.* Placement of the PID for projection of the maxillary centrals and laterals. *B.* Placement of the PID for projection of the maxillary laterals. *C.* Placement of the PID for projection of the maxillary cuspids. *D.* Placement of the PID for projection of the maxillary premolars. *E.* Placement of the PID for projection of the maxillary molars. *F.* Placement of the PID for projection of the mandibular centrals and laterals. *G.* Placement of the PID for projection of the mandibular laterals. *H.* Placement of the PID for projection of the mandibular cuspids. *I.* Placement of the PID for projection of the mandibular premolars. *J.* Placement of the PID for projection of the mandibular molars. (Torres HO, Ehrlich A: Modern Dental Assisting, 4th Ed. Philadelphia, WB Saunders, 1990, p 390.)

imaginary line drawn from the ala of the nostril to the middle of the opening of the ear.

The **border of the mandible** is a margin of compact bone on the lower margin of the mandible. This area appears opaque on, or near, the apex of the mandibular teeth.

THE PROPERTIES OF DEVELOPED RADIOGRAPHS

Once a dental x-ray film has been exposed and processed, it is called a radiograph. The inherent properties of dental radiographs include **density, contrast, detail,** and **definition.**

Density

A radiograph appears similar to a photo negative — all areas of white, gray, and black that form shades of gray.

Density is the degree of blackness of the processed radiograph. It is apparent by the amount of light transmitted through a radiograph when placed near an illuminated source, such as an x-ray view box.

Note: When describing a radiograph, the term density *(blackness)* is not the same when describing density *(nonpermeability)* of tissues.

Contrast

Contrast is the difference in density (darkness and lightness) of various areas of the radiograph. The different densities of tissue structure are recorded as varying degrees of blackness (shades of gray) on the radiograph. Something is said to be **opaque** when it has the ability to block the passage of light.

Radiopaque tissues are those dense structures that do *not* permit the passage of x-radiation through them onto the film.

The more radiopaque a structure, the lighter it appears on the radiograph. For example, enamel appears clearer (whiter) compared with the less dense pulpal chamber. A metallic restoration, particularly a gold crown, appears totally white.

Radiolucent is the term used to describe *less* dense tissues and materials that do permit the x-radiation to pass through onto the dental film.

The more radiolucent a structure, the darker the image appears on the radiograph. For example, a composite restoration is less dense than

dentin or enamel and appears as darker shades of gray.

Detail and Definition

Detail and definition relate to the ability of the film to reproduce sharp outlines of the objects radiographed. This is often referred to as the quality of the film. Movement of the patient or the tube head may blur the sharpness or detail of the objects, thus ruining the radiograph.

Criteria for Diagnostic-Quality Radiographs

It is important that each film exposed be of the highest possible diagnostic quality. This is technically referred to as the highest yield in diagnostic quality. The criteria for diagnostic-quality radiographs are listed in the following chart.

▼ Criteria for Diagnostic-Quality Radiographs

The radiograph should include:

1. Adequate contrast and definition to define clearly the detail and structure of the teeth and surrounding area being radiographed.

2. An accurate reproduction of the long axis of the tooth or teeth. The overall measurement on the radiograph must be the same as that of the natural tooth.

3. At least ¼ inch of alveolar bone beyond the apex of the tooth. A periapical radiograph should also include a margin of ⅛ to ¼ inch between the crown of the tooth and the edge of the radiograph.

4. On the posterior radiographs, the occlusal plane presented as straight or slightly curved upward toward the distal area.

5. The adjacent teeth and their contacts shown without overlapping.

6. A clear image of the periodontal space including the alveolus, tissue adjacent to the tooth, and the trabeculae of the bone.

7. An accurate representation of anatomic landmarks within the area of the teeth being radiographed.

8. Accurate location of pathologic conditions when situated in proximity to the teeth being radiographed.

9. Accurate location of an impacted tooth and its position relative to other structures in the dental arch.

▼ EXERCISES

1. The use of the lead apron protects the patient's _____ from exposure to ionizing radiation.

   a. gonadal tissues
   b. pituitary tissue
   c. tonsilar tissue
   d. thyroid and parathyroid glands

2. A lateral view of the crowns and two thirds of the cervical area of the roots of the teeth are presented in a/an _____.

   a. bite-wing
   b. extraoral
   c. occlusal
   d. periapical

3. The ALARA principle refers to the _____ radiation exposure of the film during radiographic technique.

   a. highest possible
   b. intermittent
   c. lowest possible
   d. moderate

4. The _____ are the cells most sensitive to the effects of radiation.

   a. cells of the embryo
   b. dentin of the tooth
   c. mature nerve tissue
   d. retina of the eye

5. The effects of exposure to radiation are _____ to human tissues.

   a. cumulative
   b. nonirritating
   c. sedative
   d. soothing

6. In radiation, _____ is the term used for measuring exposure of occupational workers.

   a. LPD
   b. MPD
   c. rad

7. The _____ period is the time between exposure to x-radiation and visible changes in the tissues.

   a. dormant
   b. initial
   c. erythmatic
   d. latent

8. Monitoring of occupational workers to radiation is made possible through the _____.

   a. dosimeter badge
   b. exposure plus age
   c. exposure period
   d. MPD

9. The ability of the x-ray beam to penetrate hard and soft tissues is made possible by using the _____ wavelength.

   a. greater
   b. higher
   c. longer
   d. shorter

10. _____ radiation is that given off by matter after it is exposed to radiation.

    a. Gamma
    b. Primary
    c. Scatter
    d. Secondary

11. To prepare the x-ray operatory with maximum shielding from x-radiation, the walls are lined with two _____5/8"_____ inch thicknesses of sheet rock.

    a. ⅛
    b. ¼
    c. ½
    d. ⅝

12. Protective devices used in dental radiography during exposure of film include a _____.

    a. lead apron
    b. lead thyrocervical collar
    c. plastic PID
    d. a and b

13. _____Vertical_____ angulation determines how accurately the length of the object being radiographed is reproduced in the radiograph.

    a. Distal
    b. Horizontal
    c. Lateral
    d. Vertical

14. At a minimum, the operator of the x-ray unit must stand 6 feet behind and to the left or right away from the _____ of the x-ray machine.

    a. control panel
    b. electrical switch
    c. head
    d. PID

15. The acceptable standard material used in construction of the PID is
_____.

    a. hard rubber
    b. lead
    c. plastic

16. The milliamperage meter of the x-ray unit control panel measures the
_____.

    a. amount of radiation
    b. penetration of the x-ray beam
    c. speed of the electrons
    d. time of exposure

17. The measurement of the patient's exposure to x-radiation is represented by
the _____.

    a. kilovoltage
    b. kVp
    c. mAs
    d. milliamperage

18. The kilovoltage meter of the control panel measures the _____
_____ of the central beam.

    a. amount of electrons
    b. exposure time
    c. penetrating power

19. The embossed "dot" on the film packet is always placed in the oral cavity
_____ the PID.

    a. away from
    b. toward

20. The long axis view of the tooth is produced by a _____
radiograph.

    a. bite-wing
    b. extraoral
    c. occlusal
    d. periapical

21. The component of the x-ray machine that limits the size of the x-ray beam is
the _____.

    a. collimator
    b. exposure switch
    c. kilovolt meter
    d. milliamperage meter

22. Layers of aluminum placed in the head of the x-ray unit to reduce the
nonuseful radiation to the patient is the _____.

    a. collimator
    b. extension arm
    c. filter
    d. PID

23. The sheet of lead foil placed in the film packet is to limit the amount of secondary radiation to the surrounding tissues.

    a. true
    b. false

24. At least _____ of an inch of tissue around the apices of the tooth should be evident in a periapical radiograph.

    a. ⅟₃₂
    b. ⅟₁₆
    c. ⅛
    d. ¼

25. _____ radiation is the harmful, nonuseful radiation that can be stopped by protective barriers for the patient and the operator.

    a. Leakage
    b. Primary
    c. Secondary

16 Dental Radiography: Paralleling Technique

▼ LEARNING OBJECTIVES

The student will be able to:

1. Describe the use of the paralleling technique in dental radiography.

2. State the role of quality assurance in dental radiography.

3. Describe the characteristics and uses of periapical, bite-wing, occlusal, and panoramic dental radiographs.

4. Describe the maxillary and mandibular anatomic landmarks that are evident in radiographs of these areas.

5. Identify the causes of the following errors in exposing and processing dental radiographs: foreshortened image, elongated image, overlapping of the image, cone cutting, bending of film, lightness of radiograph, darkness of radiograph, fogging of film, blurred image, saliva stain, double exposure, herringbone effect, superimposed objects, spots or streaks, static electricity, and scratches on the film.

6. Demonstrate seating and preparing a patient for dental radiography, including observing the universal precaution infection control steps.

7. Demonstrate, on a dental radiography manikin, exposure of a complete series of dental radiographs using the paralleling technique.

8. Demonstrate producing occlusal radiographs of the maxillary and mandibular dental arches on a dental radiographic manikin.

OVERVIEW OF DENTAL RADIOGRAPHY: PARALLELING TECHNIQUE

The paralleling technique for producing radiographs uses the rule of **paralleling of objects**. That is:

1. The film must be aligned parallel with the buccal plane of the teeth being radiographed. (The **buccal plane** [facial plane] is the alignment of the teeth as they face toward the cheek and lips.)

2. The paralleling technique generally uses a long, 12- to 16-inch, position-indicator device (PID).

3. The film is positioned so that the tooth or teeth to be radiographed are centered on the film.

4. When radiographing a single tooth, the film packet is placed parallel with the long axis of that tooth. The central beam is projected at a right angle to the film packet.

5. The opening of the PID is aligned so that it covers the teeth and film to be exposed.

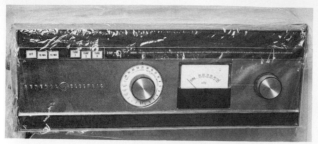

▼ Figure 16-1

X-ray unit control panel draped with plastic for infection control protection.

Universal Precautions

When exposing and processing radiographs, it is essential that all of the necessary universal precautions be carefully followed (Figs. 16-1 through 16-3). The precautions as applied to radiography are discussed in Chapter 7, "Infection Control."

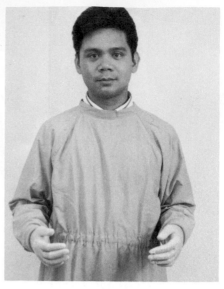

▼ Figure 16-3

Operator wearing infection control protective garb prior to exposing radiographs.

Quality Assurance in Dental Radiography

A quality assurance policy is established and followed to ensure that maximum diagnostic-quality radiographs are produced with a minimum of x-radiation exposure.

1. The dentist prescribes only those exposures that are required for diagnostic purposes.
2. All operators are properly trained and credentialed in the safe and efficient operation of the dental x-ray unit and processing equipment.
3. The radiographic equipment is maintained in an accurate and a safe operating condition.
4. Adequate holding accessories are available to eliminate the need for the patient or others to stabilize the film in the oral cavity.
5. Only fast speed "E" radiographic film is used for periapical and bite-wing exposures.
6. A policy is in place as to the number of allowable retakes of film on an individual patient. If an exposure is particularly difficult, someone with additional expertise needs to assist the operator.
7. Processing equipment and solutions are fresh and maintained at the proper temperature.
8. Processed radiographs are mounted properly and correctly dated and identified.

Quality Assurance Film

A quality assurance film is exposed and processed daily to verify that all parts of the dental radiography system are working properly.

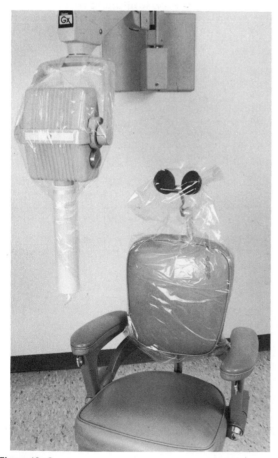

▼ Figure 16-2

X-ray unit head and dental chair draped for infection control protection.

The first step is to expose using a **step wedge**. (A step wedge is an object composed of several graduated pieces of aluminum placed so that each successive piece is shorter, thus producing the step effect.)

The dental film is laid, tab side down, on a flat surface in the operatory. The step wedge is laid over the x-ray film, and the PID is brought down near the step wedge. The exposure time is similar to that of a bite-wing radiograph.

Following exposure, the film is processed. The processed radiograph should show an object with varying shades of gray from the differing thickness of the step wedge (Fig. 16–4).

If the film is of good quality, it is taped to the view box in the operatory as the daily quality control film. If there is a variation of quality, adjustments are made as necessary.

▼ Check the temperature of the processing solutions.

▼ Check the quality of the processing solutions.

▼ If necessary, change the solutions. If solutions are changed, another quality assurance film is exposed and processed.

▼ Check the processing procedure to determine that there were no variations.

▼ Check the quality of the x-ray film to determine whether it passed its expiration date.

▼ Check the controls on the dental x-ray unit to determine that all controls and procedures are correct. If the machine is not working properly, it must be shut down and repaired immediately.

PREPARING THE PATIENT FOR FILM EXPOSURE

Prior to seating the patient, review "Checklist for Exposing Film."

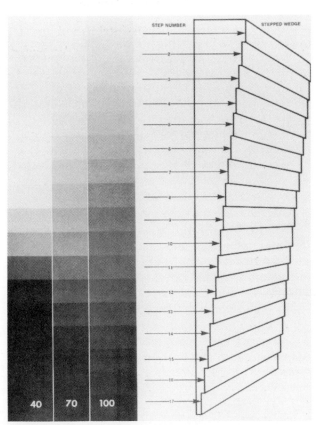

▼ **Figure 16–4**

Radiographs exposed using a step wedge. (The step wedge is shown on the right.) Those radiographs taken at 40 kV are predominately black and white and have a short scale of contrast. Those taken at 100 show many shades of gray and a long scale of contrast. (Miles DA, et al: Radiographic Imaging for Dental Auxiliaries. Philadelphia, WB Saunders, 1989, p 91.)

▼ **Checklist for Exposing Film**

1. Assemble all necessary equipment and films prior to seating the patient.

2. Seat and position the patient. Place lead apron and thyrocervical collar.

3. Scrub hands, dry thoroughly, and don latex gloves.

4. Ask patient to remove any removable dental appliance or other object, such as glasses or jewelry, that might interfere with exposing the radiograph.

5. Check machine controls: master switch on; mA, kV, and electronic timer. Set electronic timer for selected exposure time.

6. Select film to be exposed, and position patient's head for placement of this individual film.

7. Position the PID near the patient's face, close to the area of exposure. Approximating the PID position prior to placing the film helps to reduce patient discomfort.

8. Place film; make final adjustment of PID.

9. Expose the film, remove it from the patient's mouth, and wipe it free of saliva.

10. Repeat these steps until all prescribed films have been exposed.

11. Identify exposed films, and store them safely until processed.

12. If no other treatment is indicated at this visit, return the patient's belongings and reschedule as necessary.

Procedure

PREPARING THE PATIENT FOR FILM EXPOSURE

Instrumentation

1 Patient's chart.

2 Basic setup.

3 Latex gloves.

4 Sterile film holding accessories.

5 Required number and sizes of x-ray films (packaged to maintain sterility until used).

6 Cup with patient identification information (to store exposed films).

7 Facial tissues.

8 High volume evacuator (HVE) tip.

Prior to Seating the Patient

1 Turn on the x-ray unit (if it is not already on), and check the basic settings (mA, kV, and exposure time).

2 Assemble instrumentation, including the necessary dental x-ray films, bite blocks, and other sterile auxiliary aids. To avoid overexposure or fogging, place the unexposed films in a labeled receptacle outside the operatory near the controls.

3 Label a paper or plastic cup with the patient's name, the date, and the number of exposed films.

This container, placed outside the operatory, is used for temporary storage of each exposed film.

4 Lower the dental chair, with the arm raised, and move all wires and hoses out of the patient's way.

5 Check that the patient's chart is available and ready to record the number of films, total kVp, and total dental x-ray exposure (mAs).

If the patient is a referral, the prescription for radiographs from the referring dentist should be filed with the patient's records.

Seating the Patient

1 Position the patient upright in the dental chair with the head resting firmly on the headrest of the dental chair. The midline of the body should be perpendicular to the floor (Fig. 16–5).

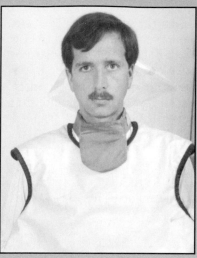

Figure 16–5 Patient seated upright and draped with lead apron and thyrocervical collar.

2 For **maxillary radiographs,** the patient's head is positioned so that the occlusal plane of the maxillary teeth is parallel to the floor.

For **mandibular radiographs,** the patient's head is positioned so that the occlusal plane of the mandibular teeth is parallel to the floor when the patient's mouth is open slightly.

3 Place the lead apron and thyrocervical collar over the patient.

4 Ask the patient to remove his glasses, if he is wearing any, as well as any removable partial or complete dentures (unless the dentures are needed to stabilize the film).

Female patients are asked to remove lipstick, earrings, and hair ornaments if these will interfere with the projection of x-radiation.

Instructions to the Patient

1 The patient is instructed to close his eyes during each film exposure. (Closing the eyes aids in protecting these sensitive tissues from exposure to x-radiation.)

2 The patient is instructed to hold his breath momentarily and not move during exposure of the film. Any movement causes a blurred image on the radiograph.

Managing the Gag Reflex

If the patient is apprehensive or begins to gag, positive statements and involving him in conversation during the preliminary arrangements may take his mind off the procedures and lessen the tendency to gag. If this fails, a topical anesthetic may be used to control the gagging sensation.

This topical anesthetic is supplied as a flavored liquid.

The patient is instructed to "swish this around" in the mouth before spitting out the excess into the cuspidor.

THE PARALLELING TECHNIQUE

Maxillary Left Quadrant

The lingual roots of the **maxillary teeth** are positioned on an incline, in varying degrees of angulation, toward the midline of the palate.

Therefore, to obtain a true projection of the long axis of the tooth, the size number 1 or 2 film is frequently placed *across* the midline of the maxillary arch—on the *opposite* side of the arch of the teeth to be radiographed.

For maxillary films, the patient's head is positioned so that the occlusal plane of the maxillary teeth is parallel with the floor.

Central and Lateral

Periapical film (size number 1) is placed *vertically* and parallel to the long axis of the left central and lateral (Fig. 16–6). The raised film dot is placed at the incisal edge.

For plus (+) vertical angulation, the PID is positioned parallel with the extension of the holding device and perpendicular to the long axis of the teeth and film. Using the rectangular PID, the device is positioned vertically to cover the film.

Horizontal angulation is accomplished by centering on the central and lateral, with the open end of the PID placed on the ala–tragus line directly over the central lateral contact.

The central and lateral are centered on the radiograph. The distal of the right central and the mesial of the left cuspid will also appear on the radiograph.

If the anterior area of the maxillary arch is wide enough to accommodate film placement, a

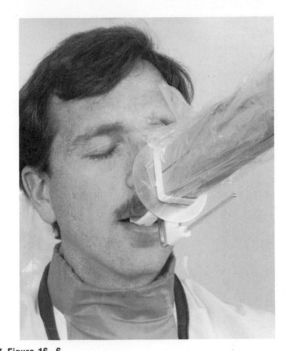

▼ **Figure 16–6**

Placement of the PID and XCP instrument for maxillary left central-lateral radiograph. Note rectangular PID.

projection of both maxillary anteriors may be obtained.

Cuspid

Periapical film (size number 2) is placed *vertically* and parallel to the long axis of the cuspid. The raised dot is at the incisal edge. The cuspid must be centered on the film, with the tip of the crown approximately 1 mm above the incisal margin of the film (Fig. 16–7).

The plus (+) vertical angulation of the PID is determined by placing the central beam perpendicular to the film and long axis of the cuspid.

The PID is brought into position for the horizontal angulation with the center of the rectangular opening placed vertically near the ala of the nose.

The cuspid is centered on the radiograph, and the mesial of the first premolar and the distal of the lateral are also visible.

Premolars

Periapical (size number 2) film is placed *horizontally* and aligned with the occlusal surface of the premolars. From 1.5 to 2 mm of film margin will

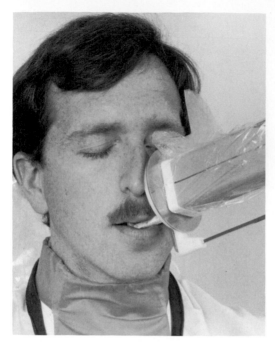

▼ **Figure 16-7**

Placement of the PID and XCP instrument for maxillary left cuspid radiograph.

show at the occlusal edge of the radiograph. The raised dot is placed at the occlusal surface (Fig. 16–8).

For vertical angulation, the PID is brought in toward the premolar area and aligned parallel with the angle of the film holder. The central beam is centered slightly under the zygoma. (The **zygoma** is the bony process forming the outer margin of the cheek.) The rectangular opening of the PID is placed horizontally to cover the film in this exposure.

If the vertical angulation of the PID and central beam is too high, the zygoma is superimposed on the apices of the premolars, resulting in an indistinct image of the teeth.

The horizontal angulation is focused on a line perpendicular to the center of the pupil of the left eye down on the ala–tragus line. The film is centered within the opening of the PID.

The first and second premolars are centered on the radiograph, with the contacts open. The distal of the cuspid and the mesial of the first molar are also visible.

Molars

Periapical film (size number 2) is placed *horizontally* so that the first and second molars are centered on the film. The raised dot is at the occlusal surface.

The vertical angulation of the PID is in line with the ala–tragus line as it crosses a line perpendicular with the outer canthus of the eye (Fig. 16–9).

The horizontal angulation of the central beam should be situated under the zygomatic arch. The opening of the PID encompasses the film.

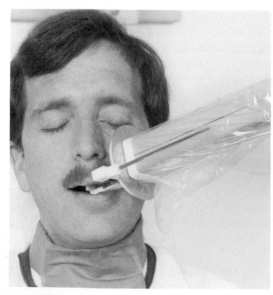

▼ **Figure 16-8**

Placement of the PID and XCP instrument for maxillary left premolar radiograph.

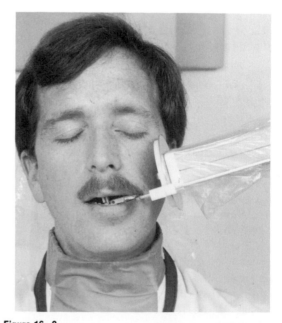

▼ **Figure 16-9**

Placement of the PID and XCP instrument for maxillary left molar radiograph.

The first and second molars are in the center of the radiograph, with the distal of the second premolar visible on the anterior border and the third molar visible on the distal portion of the radiograph.

Third Molar and Tuberosity

Periapical film (size number 2) is placed *horizontally* and slightly more distally than the previous exposure. The raised dot is at the occlusal edges.

The vertical angulation is practically the same as for the molar projection. The horizontal angulation is slightly distal (3 to 4 mm) to the outer canthus of the eye on the ala–tragus plane.

This exposure gives a distal oblique angulation, which displays the condition of the tuberosity area posterior to and including the third molar.

This particular projection is excellent for locating impacted third molars. (The second and first molars are distorted on this radiograph because of the extreme distal projection.)

Maxillary Right Quadrant

When placing and exposing film in the maxillary right quadrant, begin with the central and lateral and go on to the third molar area and tuberosity in the same manner as for the left side of the maxillary dentition. The landmarks for film and PID placement remain the same as for the left quadrant.

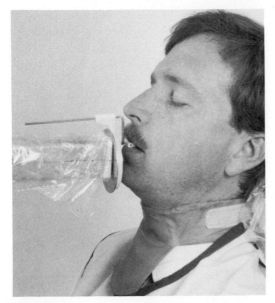

▼ **Figure 16–10**

Placement of the PID and XCP instrument for mandibular left central radiograph.

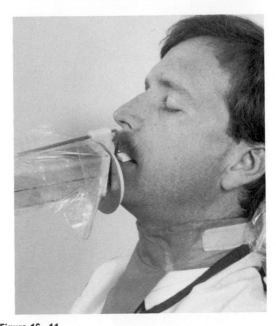

▼ **Figure 16–11**

Placement of the PID and XCP instrument for mandibular left lateral radiograph.

Mandibular Left Quadrant

The patient's head is positioned so that the occlusal plane of the mandibular teeth is parallel with the floor when the patient's mouth is open. This involves moving the headrest slightly backward.

The accurate exposure of the mandibular teeth is accomplished by placing the film packet *close* to the lingual surface of the respective teeth.

The film is placed in the lingual fold, near the mylohyoid ridge or the lingual frenum of the anterior area of the floor of the mouth, depending on the teeth to be radiographed.

Central and Lateral

Periapical film (size number 1 or 2) is placed *vertically,* aligned with the long axis of the teeth. The raised dot is placed at the incisal edges (Figs. 16–10 and 16–11).

Care must be taken to place the film lightly across the lingual frenum in the anterior floor of the mouth. The margin of the film above the incisal edges of the teeth should be approximately 2.5 mm.

The PID is brought to the area of the chin, with the vertical angulation at a minus (−) degree from zero. The opening of the PID circles the area, with the teeth and the film in alignment with the exact center of the PID opening.

The horizontal angulation is placed at the

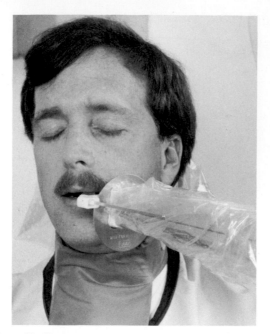

▼ **Figure 16–12**

Placement of the PID and XCP instrument for mandibular left cuspid radiograph.

middle, or slightly to the left of the midline, of the chin.

The left central and lateral are in the center of the radiograph, with the right central incisor and left cuspid visible on the margins of the radiograph.

Cuspid

Periapical film (size number 2) is placed *vertically* so that it is aligned with the long axis of the cuspid. The raised dot is at the incisal edge (Fig. 16–12).

The PID is placed perpendicular to the film and the long axis of the cuspid. A minus vertical angulation is selected, with the position of the PID opening centered on the cuspid and the film.

A horizontal angulation is maintained to ensure covering of the film and cuspid area by the opening of the PID. The cuspid is centered on the film, with the incisal margin appearing 2 mm from the edge of the radiograph.

The left lateral incisor and first premolar are also visible on the radiograph.

Premolars

Periapical film (size number 2) is placed *horizontally* in the arch. Because of access to the area, the film is aligned close to and parallel with the teeth in the mandible for this radiograph (Fig. 16–13).

The margin of the film above the occlusal

surfaces of the teeth should measure approximately 1.5 to 2 mm. The raised dot is placed at the occlusal surfaces. The patient is instructed to bite on a disposable bite block.

The vertical angulation is placed at a "minus" and is achieved by placing the central beam of the PID perpendicular to the long axis of the premolars and the plane of the film, slightly above the border of the mandible.

The horizontal angulation is accomplished by centering the opening of the PID over the contact of the premolars. The central beam is projected in an imaginary perpendicular line down from the center of the pupil of the eye.

The premolars are centered on the radiograph, with the distal of the cuspid and the mesial of the first molar also visible.

Molars

Periapical film (size number 2) is placed *horizontally* with a slight margin (1.5 mm) showing above the occlusal surfaces (Fig. 16–14). The raised dot is *not* at the occlusal surfaces. For the maxillary molars, the raised dot is placed toward the apices of the teeth.

Cotton rolls may be used to prevent the tongue from displacing the film, or the film may be stabilized by using a disposable bite block for the patient to bite on.

The vertical angulation for the molars may be a slight plus. The PID is placed perpendicular to

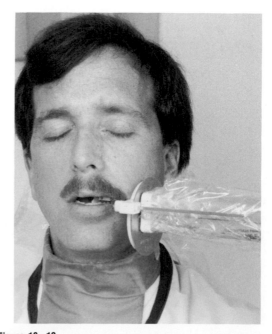

▼ **Figure 16–13**

Placement of the PID and XCP instrument for mandibular left premolar radiograph.

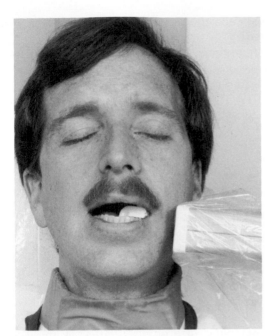

▼ **Figure 16–14**

Placement of the PID and Stabe bite block for mandibular left molar radiograph. (Stabe bite block, Rinn Corporation, Elgin, IL.)

the long axis of the film and the tooth just above the border of the mandible.

The horizontal angulation is focused on the tooth and film, on a line approximately perpendicular to the center of the eye.

The first molar is centered in the radiograph. The distal surface of the second premolar is visible on the mesial border, and the second molar is visible distally.

Retromolar Area

Periapical film (size number 2) is placed *horizontally*. The film placement is similar to that of the molar exposure; however, the horizontal angulation of the PID is moved distally.

The raised dot is *not* at the occlusal surface. For the maxillary molars, the raised dot is placed toward the apices of the teeth.

This distal-oblique projection is used for locating third molars and surveying the retromolar area. (This projection may blur the first molar by superimposing the second and third molars over it.)

Mandibular Right Quadrant

The survey of the mandibular right quadrant is accomplished in the same manner as for the mandibular left quadrant.

BITE-WING RADIOGRAPHS

Bite-wing radiographs provide views of the interproximal, coronal, and approximately one third of the cervical surface of the roots of the maxillary and mandibular teeth. They are sometimes referred to as *cavity-detecting radiographs.*

Bite-wing radiographs may be exposed of the anteriors, premolars, and molars as necessary.

To provide stability, the film is placed in a lightweight disposable bite-wing tab. The tab projects from the smooth side of the film packet. This side of the film is positioned against the lingual surfaces of the teeth. The raised dot is placed toward the apices of the mandibular teeth.

An alternative for film stabilization is the use of a positioning device, as shown in Figures 16–15 and 16–16.

Anterior Bite-Wing

The anterior bite-wing exposure provides a survey of three fourths of the long axis of each maxillary and mandibular anterior tooth. This exposure is requested to provide a closer view of the anterior interproximal surfaces, particularly if the anterior teeth are overlapped in alignment.

Periapical film (size number 0 or 1) is placed *vertically* in an anterior bite-wing tab.

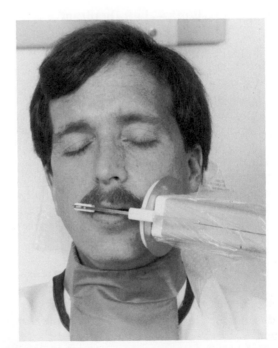

▼ **Figure 16–15**

Placement of the PID and XCP instrument for left premolar bite-wing radiograph.

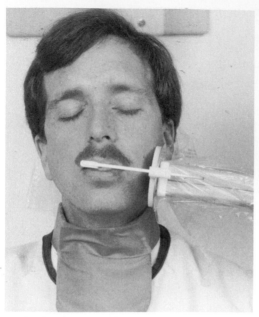

▼ **Figure 16–16**

Placement of the PID and XCP instrument for left molar bite-wing radiograph.

The tab is placed between the anterior teeth, and the teeth are closed, edge to edge, on the tab. The raised dot is placed toward the apices of the mandibular teeth.

The vertical angulation is +15 to +8 degrees. The horizontal angulation is between the contacts of the maxillary centrals.

Premolar Bite-Wing — Left Quadrant

The bite-wing tab is placed *horizontally* on a size number 1 or 2 film. The raised dot is placed toward the apices of the mandibular teeth because the mandibular molar teeth have two roots only (see Fig. 16–15).

The tab and film are moved into the mouth sideways and turned upright near the lingual surfaces of the teeth of the mandibular left quadrant.

The tab is placed on the occlusal surfaces of the mandibular premolars and moved slightly forward to the arch curvature near the cuspid. The patient is instructed to close and to hold his teeth firmly in contact with the bite-wing tab.

The tab should show facially when the cheek is retracted. For patient comfort, the extension of the tab may be folded up on the maxillary facial surface rather than permitting it to project outward, making lip closure uncomfortable for the patient.

The PID is positioned by placing the vertical angulation at +8 to +10 degrees. The horizontal angulation is placed directly over the bite-wing tab, between the premolars and toward the occlusal plane.

This projection should show the distal half of the cuspid and the contacts of the premolars and the first molar.

Molar Bite-Wing — Left Quadrant

The molar bite-wing film is prepared in the same manner, with the tab placed *horizontally* over the first and second left molars. The patient is instructed to bite firmly on the tab. The raised dot is placed toward the apices of the mandibular teeth (see Fig. 16–16).

Vertical angulation is at +8 to +10. The horizontal angulation is directed through the contacts of the first and second left molars toward the occlusal plane.

This bite-wing exposure provides an interproximal view of the distal area of the second premolar, the first and second molars, and the third molar, including some of the tuberosity and retromolar areas.

The use of the largest bite-wing film (size number 3) is advised for this projection if a survey of the retromolar area is needed.

Premolar and Molar Bite-Wings — Right Quadrant

Premolar and molar bite-wing exposures of the right half of the dentition are accomplished in the same manner as those of the left half.

OCCLUSAL RADIOGRAPHS

Film Size and Placement

Periapical film (size number 1 or 2) may be used for occlusal radiographs of small children. For the normal adult mouth, occlusal film (size number 4) is used.

The smooth side of the packet is *always* placed on the occlusal surface of the teeth in the arch to be radiographed.

The patient is seated upright and is instructed to open the mouth wide while the assistant places the film in a manner similar to that of placing a large cracker between the teeth.

The wide side of the film is inserted crosswise. For an adult with a small mouth, the narrow side of this film is inserted crosswise. The film is inserted until resistance is felt at the posterior junction of the upper and lower arches.

The patient is instructed to bite firmly on the film—but not too hard—to stabilize the packet. The patient's lips are draped around the margins of the film.

A heavy bite causes imprints that can ruin the film or pierce the film packet, resulting in artifacts on the radiograph.

Maxillary Arch—Occlusal

The patient is seated upright in the dental chair, with the maxillary occlusal plane parallel to the floor. The midsagittal plane also must be perpendicular to the floor to aid the operator in the placement of the PID (Figs. 16–17 and 16–18).

The smooth side of the film packet is placed toward the occlusal surface of the *maxillary* teeth. The patient is instructed to close firmly on the packet to stabilize the film.

With the 8-inch PID, the vertical angulation is +65 to +75 degrees. The angulation is determined by the placement of the film and the bisection of the angle of the curvature of the palatal vault and the plane of the film.

The PID is centered horizontally over the bridge of the nose and the entire occlusal film.

Mandibular Arch—Occlusal

The headrest (and the patient's head) is positioned as far back as possible. The inferior border

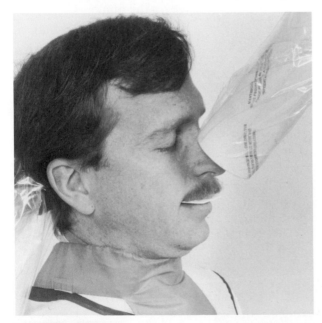

▼ **Figure 16–17**

Placement of the PID and film for maxillary occlusal radiograph. Note cylindrical PID.

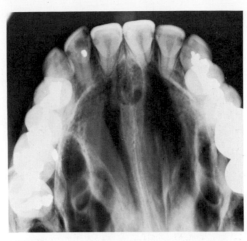

▼ **Figure 16–18**

Maxillary occlusal radiograph. The incisive canal, midpalatal suture, and the sinuses are evident. (Torres HO, Ehrlich A: Modern Dental Assisting, 4th Ed. Philadelphia, WB Saunders, 1990, p 432.)

of the mandible is aligned perpendicular to the floor as the patient opens the mouth. To provide patient comfort, the PID is brought into the proximity of the chin before the film is placed.

Placement for mandibular occlusal exposures is similar to that for maxillary occlusal exposures; however, the smooth side of the film packet must be placed toward the occlusal surface of the *mandibular* teeth. The patient is instructed to bite firmly on the packet to stabilize the film.

The 8-inch PID is placed at a right angle to the film packet. The vertical angulation is 90 degrees. For the horizontal angulation, the PID completely circles the film packet and the anterior, middle, and posterior portions of the mandible (Figs. 16–19 and 16–20).

PANORAMIC DENTAL RADIOGRAPHY

The panoramic technique is used to produce extraoral radiographs of the entire dentition and related supportive structures of the lower half of the face (Fig. 16–21).

The panoramic radiograph is approximately 12 × 5 inches in size and provides a continuous view of the tissues of the oral cavity, including the maxillary and mandibular teeth and the hard and soft supporting tissues.

It is particularly useful for survey work and in orthodontics and oral surgery. However, panoramic radiographs have limited value for the detection of caries.

The machines used for panoramic radiography are designed on the principle of curved surface laminography. These machines use an elongated

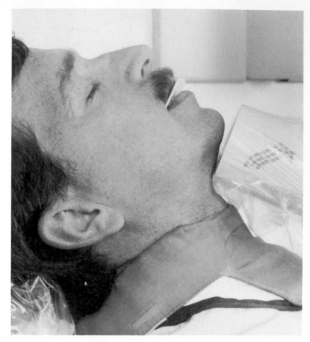

▼ Figure 16-19

Placement of the PID and film for mandibular occlusal radiograph.

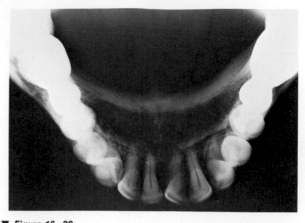

▼ Figure 16-20

Mandibular occlusal radiograph. Genial tubercles and inferior border of the mandible are visible. (Torres HO, Ehrlich A: Modern Dental Assisting, 4th Ed. Philadelphia, WB Saunders, 1990, p 432.)

single film, approximately 12 × 5 inches, in a cassette with intensifying screens. The intensifying screens aid in exposure of the film within the cassette, using as low exposure to radiation as possible.

The patient is placed in a stabilized position with the head positioned in a device holding the chin. Some units automatically shift the patient midway through the exposure; the patient should be alerted to this so that he will not be startled when it happens. Other machines may require that the patient stand during exposure.

The tube head of the machine moves slowly forward from one side of the patient as the cassette containing the film moves slowly around the opposite side of the patient. The x-radiation passes through a narrow vertical slit in the moving cassette, thus exposing the film.

PROCESSING TECHNIQUES

The Universal Precautions for infection control must be taken when handling exposed radiographs. (These are discussed in Chapter 7, "Infection Control.")

Exposed radiographs may be processed using either an automatic processor or a manual system. Both systems require the use of **developer** and **fixer** as processing solutions to bring forth and stabilize the latent image on the film.

Developer

The developer solution reacts chemically with the silver bromide salts of the film, which have been

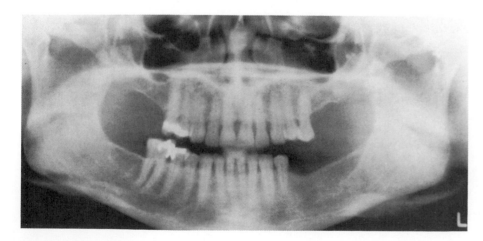

▼ Figure 16-21

A typical panoramic radiograph. (Miles DA: Radiographic Imaging for Dental Auxiliaries. Philadelphia, WB Saunders, 1989, p 150.)

partially activated by the x-radiation to produce the latent image.

The solution preserves the silver bromide compound (AgBr) on the radiograph. The nonexposed silver bromides remain on the film surface.

The developer has an alkaline base of *sodium carbonate,* which serves as an activator. *Hydroquinone,* another component, is a temperature-sensitive compound that builds up contrast on the film.

Elon brings out the image quickly but produces a low contrast. *Potassium bromide* is added as a restrainer; it controls the activity of the developing agents and prevents film fog. Oxidation of the solution is prevented by *sodium sulfite.*

Fixer

The fixer solution dissolves the light-sensitive silver bromide crystals that are not a part of the latent image and were not preserved by the developer solution.

The fixer thoroughly stops the developing action and hardens the gelatin crystals remaining on the film. This produces a permanent image of the exposed area.

The fixing solution is basically acid. A component, *sodium thiosulfate* (hyposulfite), removes the unexposed silver bromide crystals from the film emulsion.

Sodium sulfite prevents deterioration of the hyposulfite. *Potassium alum* is added to harden and shrink the soft gelatin on the film to stabilize the properties of the radiograph.

Solution Strength

Solutions are packaged in a concentrated form and must be mixed carefully following the manufacturer's instructions. Care should be taken to avoid freezing these solutions because extreme cold will reduce their effectiveness, causing film failure during processing.

The strength of the processing solutions is an important factor in developing the films:

▼ The solution tanks should be kept covered at all times to minimize evaporation of the solutions.

▼ When the solution level is low, it is *not* acceptable to add more water to raise the solution level. (Doing this weakens the solution.)

▼ The maximum effective lifetime of the processing solutions varies with use. One rule is to change the solutions every third week with routine use. However, if many x-ray films are processed, the solutions become exhausted and need to be replaced more often.

MANUAL (NONAUTOMATIC) FILM PROCESSING

The Darkroom

The darkroom serves as a laboratory for manually processing dental x-ray film. It contains a bench of working height, the processing tank, racks for drying the processed films, and possibly an electric film drier.

The darkroom must be light-proof and well ventilated. Also, because any kind of contamination can ruin a film, this work space must be kept clean and dry.

The darkroom must be free of "normal" (white) light while film is being processed. A red or orange **safe light** with a special filter and a maximum of 7 watts may be used. When placed about 4 feet above the workbench, this light will not fog the exposed film prior to processing.

Foreign substances coming into contact with unprocessed film cause artifacts (errors) on the radiographs. Therefore, the racks and clips for processing film should be free of dried processing solutions.

Racks should be rinsed and dried after each use. Soiled racks and hangers may be cleaned with a solution of sodium hypochlorite (household bleach) and rinsed thoroughly and dried prior to use.

Processing Solutions

The x-ray processing tank contains three sections. One contains the developer, and another contains the fixer. The third (central) tank holds clear running water for rinsing.

It is important to distinguish the developer tank from the fixer tank because placing the film in the fixer *prior* to developing it will ruin the radiograph.

Each solution should be stirred prior to use with a clean glass or stainless steel stirring rod. Separate rods are used to avoid contamination of one solution by the other.

Time and Temperature

The temperature of the solutions affects the length of time needed to process the exposed film. High temperatures overactivate and low temperatures underactivate the developing solution. Ideally, the temperature of the water bath and solutions should be 68°F (20°C).

If the solutions are not at this temperature, consult the chart provided by the manufacturer of the processing solutions for the recommended variations on suggested time and temperature combinations.

If the Fahrenheit temperature of the solutions is in the low 60s, it is best to wait until the temperature rises. The same is true if the temperature of the solutions is too high. An extremely high temperature also loosens the gelatinous layers of the film, thus ruining the radiograph.

The temperatures of the solutions may be gradually altered by increasing or decreasing the temperature of the rinse water. However, it is not acceptable to add anything to either the developer or the fixer except more of the same kind of solution.

Procedure

PREPARING THE FILM FOR MANUAL PROCESSING

1 Place clean paper towels on the counter and be sure the darkroom door is closed tightly.

2 Check the temperature of the solutions. Make sure film racks are clean and ready.

3 Determine whether the film packets have one or two films each.

4 With the regular light off and only the safe light on, unwrap the exposed films.

5 Open the tab on the packet and slide forward the paper liner and film. This will expose the end of the film. (As necessary, touch *only* the edges of the film. Do not touch any other part of the exposed film with the fingers.)

6 Attach the end of the film to the clip extending from the rack (hanger). The film should extend horizontally from the clip.

7 Give the film a gentle tug to make certain that it is firmly attached to the clip and to remove the packet. The films should not touch or overlap each other on the rack.

8 Identify the films with the patient's name. One way of doing this is to write the information on a piece of lead foil (from the film backing) and wrap it around the top of the hanger just above the clips.

Procedure

MANUAL PROCESSING OF THE FILM

Developing the Film

1 With only the safe light on, stir the developing solution.

2 Place the film rack gently into the solution and move up and down several times to prevent air bubbles from collecting on the dry film surface.
   Note: Air bubbles could cause artifacts on the developed radiograph.

3 Cover the developer tank tightly (the cover must be light-proof). If the temperature of the solution is at 68°F (20°C), set the timer for 5 minutes.

Rinsing the Film

1 With only the safe light on, after exactly 5 minutes uncover the developer tank.

2 Transfer the film rack to the rinse water tank and rinse for at least 30 seconds at 68°F (20°C). Rinsing stops the action of the developer.

Fixing the Film

1 With only the safe light on, transfer the film rack to the fixer solution. Gently move the rack up and down several times to remove any air bubbles.

2 Cover the tank and set the timer for 10 minutes (double the developing time). Fixing neutralizes the light-sensitive factor of the film.

3 If necessary, after at least 2 minutes in the fixer, the film may be examined under the safe light.
The film is then promptly returned to the fixer solution to complete the fixing process.

The Final Rinse and Drying

1 After the fixing process is complete, the radiographs are no longer sensitive to light and the regular white light may be used.

2 Remove the film rack from the fixer and place it in the rinse water. Rinse for at least 20 minutes at 68°F (20°C).

3 When rinsing is complete, hang the radiograph on a rack to dry.
Note: An electric dryer with a fan circulating warm air may be used for rapid drying of the radiographs. The rack is hung on a rod in the center of the dryer, and the radiographs are completely dried in 3 to 5 minutes at 120°F (44°C). (Higher temperatures will ruin the radiographs.)

AUTOMATIC FILM PROCESSING

When using an automatic film processor, unwrap the exposed film in a special light-proof recessed area of the processor.

Paddles within the unit then automatically move the film through the developer, fixer, and rinse. In only a few minutes, a dried, processed radiograph is ejected from the unit (Fig. 16–22).

The processing solutions in the machine must be fresh, and the machine itself must be kept clean. The rollers and machine parts must be thoroughly cleaned on a regular basis. (Dirty parts may cause the machine to jam or cause artifacts on the radiograph.)

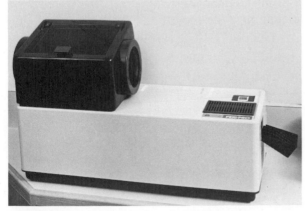

▼ Figure 16–22

Automatic film processor. Exposed film is unwrapped inside the unit by inserting left and right hands through the openings. In a few minutes, a processed and dried radiograph exits from the right side of the processor. (Torres HO, Ehrlich A: Modern Dental Assisting, 4th Ed. Philadelphia, WB Saunders, 1990, p 440.)

ERRORS IN EXPOSING AND PROCESSING FILM

The following errors, which may occur either in exposure of the film or in its processing, can cause the resulting radiographs to be of less than diagnostic quality.

Such errors must be avoided because they require that the patient be scheduled to retake the radiographs. This unnecessarily exposes the patient to additional radiation. It also causes inconvenience and delay for both patient and staff.

Foreshortened Image

A foreshortened image of a tooth is *shorter* in appearance then the actual long axis of the tooth. Foreshortening is the result of too much vertical angulation.

To correct a foreshortened image, the vertical angulation must be *reduced*.

Elongated Image

An elongated tooth image is *longer* in appearance than the actual long axis of the tooth. Elongation is an indication of too little vertical angulation.

To correct an elongated image, the vertical angulation must be *increased*.

Overlapping of Image

In overlapping of the image, the normal contacts of the teeth being radiographed are distorted on the radiograph and are superimposed on top of each other.

Overlapping is caused by incorrect horizontal angulation. Overlapping of teeth appears as white crescents at the contacts of the teeth.

If the horizontal placement is too *distal,* the tooth distal to the one being examined appears to be superimposed over the tooth intended to be radiographed.

If the horizontal placement is too *mesial,* the tooth mesial to the one being examined appears to be superimposed over the tooth intended to be radiographed.

The contacts of the teeth must be centered in the x-ray film, and the horizontal angulation of the PID should be directed on a line centered on the contacts of the teeth being examined.

Cone Cutting

Cone cutting occurs when only part of the film is exposed. The unexposed film area appears as a clear, crescent-shaped or straight-lined area. The shape of the area is determined by the shape of the PID used.

Cone cutting is caused by incorrect placement of the PID and central beam. The central beam must be directed to the center of the film and the PID must encircle the area or object to be examined and the film to be exposed.

Bending of Film

Excessive bending of the film prior to or during placement causes a distorted image or a dark line on the processed film.

Bending of film to compensate for difficulty in placement in small or irregularly shaped arches should be avoided.

When film size is a problem, a smaller film size should be selected and correctly placed to provide an accurate radiograph.

Lightness of Radiograph

Inconsistency in following a standardized exposure time causes variations in the density of the processed radiograph. However, if all other factors are constant, a film that is underexposed results in a radiograph that is too light when processed.

Consistency in the processing technique is essential. However, if insufficient exposure is the cause, the machine should be tested to be certain that all parts are working properly. (Do *not* continue to use a defective x-ray machine: Request servicing immediately.)

The radiograph may be too light if the temperature of the developing solution is too low or too cold or if the film was not left in the developer for a long enough time.

The radiograph may also be too light if the processing solutions are chemically exhausted.

Darkness of Radiograph

Dark films, showing too little contrast of the tissues, may be caused by too much exposure. Check the setting of the mA and kVp and exposure time.

Radiographs that are too dark and show little contrast may also be caused by processing in solutions that are too warm.

Fogging of Film

A fogged film lacks the sharp detail needed to be of diagnostic quality. Using old film, which has passed the manufacturer's expiration date, may result in a fogged radiograph. Exposing film to secondary radiation also causes film fogging. For this reason, films are always protected from all radiation before and after exposure.

Fogging may be caused by exposing the film to white light while the film is being unwrapped, during the time the film is in the developing solution, or prior to the recommended fixing time.

Blurred Image

A blurred image (indistinct outline of the teeth on the radiograph) is most frequently caused by movement of the patient during the film exposure.

The operator must be certain that neither the patient, the film, nor the head of the x-ray unit moves during the exposure time.

Saliva Stain

If the film packet becomes saturated with saliva, the moisture contaminates the emulsion on the film. In some instances, the emulsion may be pulled off the film as the envelope is unwrapped.

If the packet gets wet, it should be dried on removal from the mouth and the film processed as soon as possible.

To prevent saliva stains, placement and exposing techniques should be improved to avoid lengthy placement of the film in the patient's mouth.

If the patient salivates excessively, he should be instructed to swallow immediately before placement of each film.

The dentist should advise the operator what steps to take if the patient salivates heavily. (Extreme salivation can temporarily be reduced with medication, which may be prescribed by the dentist.)

Double Exposure

Exposing the same film twice results in either a dual image or a completely blackened film.

Double exposure can be avoided by establishing and following a regular routine for placement, exposure, counting, and storage of exposed film.

Herringbone Effect

A herringbone effect is produced by the pattern on the lead foil backing placed in the film packet.

A radiograph with a herringbone pattern superimposed over the teeth indicates that the film was placed *backward* in the patient's mouth (with the tab side next to the teeth being radiographed).

Always place the *smooth* side of the film packet next to the teeth to be examined.

Superimposed Objects

Images of glasses, jewelry, and hair ornaments will be superimposed on the film as artifacts if they come between the central beam, the object to be radiographed, and the film. For this reason, the patient is asked to remove any such object that will interfere with the radiographic image.

Images of orthodontic bands and partial or complete dentures will also be superimposed over the tissue (or teeth) being radiographed.

Spots or Streaks

Spots or streaks appear on film that has been exposed to crystals of dried fixing solution (or other chemicals) on the darkroom bench or on a dirty film hanger.

Incorrect rinsing of film between the developing and the fixing processes and after fixing also causes staining of the dried radiograph.

Static Electricity

In an extremely dry climate, or wherever there is very low humidity, static electricity can cause streaks on the processed radiograph.

Usually this is caused by a sudden movement while unwrapping the film. Static streaks can be avoided by using a humidifier to raise the humidity in the office and by taking care to unwrap the film slowly.

Scratches on Film

Scratches are frequently caused by the fingernails when unwrapping the film. The film packet should be opened with the edges of the paper laid back and opened carefully, with the fingers placed only on the margins of the packet.

HANDLING RADIOGRAPHS

The processed radiographs must always be handled by the *margins only* to prevent fingerprints from being superimposed on the radiographs.

Also, hands must be clean and dry. Avoid using hand lotion prior to handling because this ruins the processed radiographs.

MOUNTING RADIOGRAPHS

For ease of handling and mounting, the dry radiographs are taken from the rack and placed in anatomic order on a piece of clean white paper or on a flat, illuminated view box.

Mounts for radiographic surveys are available in various colors and materials, such as black, gray, and clear plastic and black and gray cardboard. Some operators prefer cardboard because it blocks out extraneous light when the radiographs are being viewed on the view box.

Mounts also come in a wide assortment of sizes, with different numbers and "window" sizes (openings) to accommodate the number of exposures in the patient's radiographic survey.

All the radiographs of a single series should be in the same mount, and the size of the mount selected is determined by the number of windows needed.

If there are more windows in the mount than there are radiographs in the series, the extra windows should be blocked with a black piece of paper or a cardboard blank.

This is done to keep the light from shining through the opening into the dentist's eyes when studying the radiographic series on a lighted x-ray view box.

The patient's name and age and the date on which the radiographs were taken should be placed on the mount *prior* to the mounting of the radiographs. The dentist's name and address should also be on the mount.

Raised Dot on Radiographs

The procedure for mounting radiographs should comply with the dentist's preference, and it is important that you determine the preferred method before mounting the radiographs.

It is also advisable to identify the left and right sides of the oral cavity as represented in the radiograph mount.

If radiographs are for a patient referred from another dental office, be certain to check the orientation of the raised dot to identify the patient's dentition accurately.

Convex (Outward)

If the bump of the raised dot is placed outward (convexly), toward the person mounting or reading the radiographs, it represents the facial surface of the teeth.

The left side of the radiograph corresponds to the right side of the patient's oral cavity. When radiographs are mounted this way, the upper left of the mount becomes the upper right molar area.

This system of mounting radiographs complies with the Universal Tooth Numbering System.

Concave (Inward)

If the dot is facing inward (concavely), away from the person mounting or reading the radiographs, it represents the lingual surface of the teeth.

The left side of the radiograph corresponds to the left of the patient's oral cavity. When radiographs are mounted this way, the upper left of the mount becomes the upper left molar area.

LANDMARKS FOR MOUNTING RADIOGRAPHS

Landmarks for the Maxillary Arch

The maxillary molars have *three* roots, and the maxillary first premolar has *two* roots.

The **maxillary sinus** is evident in the cuspid and premolar views of the teeth and in some instances in the area of the centrals and laterals.

The **trabeculae** of the bone are more loosely structured in the maxillary arch.

The **tuberosity** and the **hamulus** of the sphenoid bone are evident in radiographs of the third maxillary molar.

The **maxillary midsagittal suture,** the **nasal cavity,** and frequently the **incisive foramen** are evident in the central incisor area.

Landmarks for the Mandibular Arch

The **mental foramen** is visible near the apex of the first premolar, and the **mandibular canal** may be seen parallel with the apices of the molars.

In radiographs of the premolars and molars, the **mylohyoid ridge** may appear to be superimposed over the roots of these teeth. The **retromolar area** and the **ramus** of the mandible will be evident posterior to the second or third molar area.

THE RADIOGRAPHIC APPEARANCE OF ANATOMIC LANDMARKS

Dense structures that are radiopaque (RO) appear lighter (whiter) on the radiograph. Structures that are less dense are radiolucent (RL) and appear darker (grayer) on the radiograph.

Listed here are the normal anatomic landmarks, and their degree of density, as represented on dental radiographs:

1. The **lamina dura** (RO) evident on the lateral projection surrounding each tooth root of the dentition.
2. The **maxillary midsagittal suture** (RL) of the maxilla between the maxillary centrals.
3. The **maxillary sinuses** (RL) near the maxillary premolars and cuspids.
4. The **zygomatic process** (RO) on the superior border of the apices of the maxillary molars.
5. The **maxillary tuberosity** (RO) and the **hamular process** (RO) of the sphenoid bone on the distal oblique exposure of the maxillary third molar.
6. The **lateral pterygoid plate** (RO) of the sphenoid bone on the distal oblique projection of the maxillary molars.
7. The **X- or Y-shaped formation** (RO) of the anterior portion of the maxillary sinus and nasal cavity on the maxillary cuspid and premolar projections. These are particularly evident on lateral skull and face radiographs.

8. The **incisive foramen** (RL) on the projection of the anteriors of the maxillary arch. Also found on a maxillary occlusal radiograph.
9. The **nasal spine** (RO) in the area between the maxillary centrals.
10. **Nutrient canals** (RL) in some exposures of the maxillary cuspids and mandibular anteriors.
11. The **mandibular canal** (RL) in the premolar and molar projections of the mandible.
12. The **cortical plates** (RO) of the mandible on molar projections.
13. The **mental foramen** (RL) in the area of the first mandibular premolar.
14. The **external oblique ridge** (RO) and the **mylohyoid ridge** (RO) on the molar projection of the mandible.
15. The **styloid process** (RO) and the **coronoid process** (RO) of the mandible on distal oblique projections of the third molars.
16. The **inferior alveolar foramen and canal** (RL) of the mandible.

STORAGE OF RADIOGRAPHIC RECORDS

The identified radiographs are placed in the radiographic mount and may be stored with the patient's dental treatment record.

On instructions from the dentist, inactive radiographs may be removed from the mount and placed in small envelopes. The envelopes must be clearly identified with the patient's name and the date when the radiographs were taken. This is permanently filed with the patient's treatment record.

If the patient identifying information was in pencil, this may be removed from the mount, and the mount may be reused for another patient.

▼ **EXERCISES**

1. The dental radiography patient is instructed to sit upright and to _____ during exposure of the dental film.

   a. close his eyes
   b. exhale
   c. hold his breath
   d. a and c

2. The component of the developing solution that builds up contrast on the exposed film is _____ .

   a. hydroquinone
   b. potassium bromide
   c. sodium carbonate
   d. sodium sulfide

3. The tissues of the dentition that appear light on the radiograph are referred to as being _____ .

   a. dense
   b. radiolucent
   c. radiopaque
   d. translucent

4. The use of a _____ aids in controlling the patient's tendency to gag.

   a. fluoride rinse
   b. local anesthetic
   c. mouthwash
   d. topical anesthetic

5. _____ is/are worn when processing exposed dental films.

   a. Goggles
   b. Latex gloves
   c. Lead apron
   d. a, b, and c

6. A quality assurance policy in dental radiography may include the exposure and processing of a single quality film on a _____ basis.

   a. daily
   b. weekly
   c. monthly
   d. bimonthly

7. In processing exposed dental film, the fixer solution _____ the developing action and produces a permanent radiograph.

   a. advances
   b. continues
   c. reverses
   d. stops

8. In processing exposed dental film, the ideal temperature of the solutions and water bath is ——————————— °F.

   a. 60
   b. 64
   c. 68
   d. 72

9. Detail and definition in a radiograph refer to the ——————————— of the objects produced.

   a. blurring
   b. radiolucency
   c. sharpness

10. A radiographic image of a tooth that is less in size than its actual long axis is said to be ———————————.

    a. cone cut
    b. elongated
    c. foreshortened
    d. overlapped

11. A quality assurance policy on dental radiography frequently includes ——— ———————————.

    a. efficiency and safety of equipment
    b. protective barriers for patient and operator
    c. use of "C" speed film
    d. a and b

12. Cone cutting on a dental radiograph will appear as a/an ——————————— ———————.

    a. blurred image
    b. herringbone pattern
    c. overlapped image
    d. white crescent

13. A blurred image on the radiograph is caused by movement of the ——————— ——————————— during exposure of the film.

    a. film in the oral cavity
    b. head of the x-ray machine
    c. patient
    d. a, b, and c

14. The raised dot on the x-ray film is usually placed at the ——————————— of the tooth or teeth being radiographed.

    a. apical tip
    b. incisal edge
    c. occlusal surface
    d. b or c

15. When radiographing maxillary molars, the PID is positioned under the ———————————.

    a. ala of the nose
    b. border of the mandible
    c. temporomandibular joint
    d. zygomatic arch

16. A clear image of the incisive foramen is found on a/an _____ radiograph.

    a. bite-wing
    b. occlusal
    c. panoramic
    d. periapical

17. For exposure of a radiograph of the mandibular premolars, the film is placed _____ and parallel with the occlusal plane.

    a. horizontally
    b. vertically

18. Customarily, a size number _____ film is used for a periapical radiograph.

    a. 1
    b. 2
    c. 3
    d. 4

19. For a radiograph of the central and laterals, the horizontal angulation is positioned at the contacts of the _____.

    a. central and lateral
    b. centrals
    c. lateral and cuspid
    d. premolars

20. The inferior alveolar canal will appear _____ on a radiograph of the mandibular molars.

    a. radiolucent
    b. radiopaque

▼ Criterion Sheet 16–1

Student's Name _____

Procedure: *PREPARING A PATIENT FOR DENTAL RADIOGRAPHY*

Performance Objective:

The student will demonstrate preparing the operatory, making all necessary preparations prior to the arrival of the patient, and seating and preparing the patient for dental radiographs.

	SE	IE
SE = Student evaluation **C** = Criterion met **IE** = Instructor evaluation **X** = Criterion not met		
Instrumentation: Dental operatory with radiography equipment, infection control barriers, lead apron, lead thyrocervical collar, film positioning equipment, and radiographic films with appropriate storage containers.		
1. Received directions from the dentist for preparing the radiographic survey.		
2. Placed protective barriers: _____ Plastic wrap on the PID and head of the x-ray unit _____ Back and headrest of the dental chair _____ Control panel of the x-ray unit _____ Operating light switches and handles		
3. Gathered and prepared necessary equipment and films.		
4. Set dials of control panel for preselected milliamperage, kilovoltage, and exposure time as indicated by the dentist.		
5. Adjusted chair position and arm rest on side of patient entry.		
6. Received and seated the patient comfortably.		
7. Determined patient's previous exposure to x-radiation and recorded data on patient's health history.		
8. Explained the procedure to the patient. Placed lead apron and thyrocervical collar on patient. Advised patient to close eyes during each exposure.		
9. Scrubbed and dried hands. Donned latex gloves. Requested patient to remove prosthesis (if present).		
Comments:		

▼ Criterion Sheet 16–2

Student's Name _____

Procedure:	*PREPARING A DIAGNOSTIC RADIOGRAPHIC SURVEY USING THE PARALLELING TECHNIQUE*

Performance Objective:

The student will use the paralleling technique to produce a complete diagnostic-quality radiographic survey (periapical and bite-wings) on a radiographic-type manikin.

The number of radiographs in the series, the acceptable limits for chair time and exposure time, and the permissible number of retakes of radiographs are to be established by the instructor.

		SE	IE
SE = Student evaluation **IE** = Instructor evaluation	**C** = Criterion met **X** = Criterion not met		
Instrumentation: Patient, operatory, and equipment prepared in Criterion Sheet 16–1.			
1. Exposed prescribed **maxillary periapical films.**			
2. Exposed prescribed **mandibular periapical films.**			
3. Exposed prescribed **bite-wing films.**			
4. Stored films correctly before and after exposure.			
5. Checked control settings and stood behind protective barrier during each exposure.			
6. Maintained infection control procedures.			
7. Recorded number of films and amount of exposure (mAs) on patient's chart.			
Comments:			

▼ Criterion Sheet 16-3

Student's Name _____

Procedure: *PRODUCING OCCLUSAL RADIOGRAPHS*

Performance Objective:

The student will produce diagnostic-quality maxillary and mandibular occlusal radiographs.

	SE	IE
SE = Student evaluation **C** = Criterion met **IE** = Instructor evaluation **X** = Criterion not met		
Instrumentation: Patient, operatory, equipment prepared from Criterion Sheet 16–1, two size number 4 occlusal dental x-ray film packets.		
Maxillary Film:		
1. Positioned patient upright with occlusal surfaces of dentition parallel with the floor.		
2. Placed occlusal film packet with the pebbly surface next to the occlusal surfaces of the maxillary teeth.		
3. Warned patient not to bite through film packet.		
4. Positioned opening of the PID at the bridge of the nose, at a right angle and to encircle the film packet.		
5. Exposed film, removed exposed film, and stored safely.		
Mandibular Film:		
1. Positioned patient with head back so that the mandible was perpendicular with the floor.		
2. Placed occlusal film packet with the pebbly surface next to the occlusal surfaces of the mandibular teeth.		
3. Warned patient not to bite through film packet.		
4. Positioned opening of the PID encircling the tissue under the patient's chin, at a right angle and to encircle to the film packet.		
5. Exposed film, removed exposed film, and stored safely.		
Comments:		

▼ Criterion Sheet 16-4

Student's Name _____

Procedure: *DEVELOPING AND MOUNTING RADIOGRAPHS*

Performance Objective:

The student will develop a series of dental radiographs that are free of processing errors.

The student will mount this series of dental radiographs.

	SE	IE
SE = Student evaluation **C** = Criterion met **IE** = Instructor evaluation **X** = Criterion not met		
Instrumentation: Automatic developer or complete darkroom facilities. Appropriate radiographic mount, processed radiographs, view box, pen or pencil.		
1. Washed and dried hands. Donned gloves.		
2. Processed films appropriately for the method being used.		
3. Processed films were free of darkroom errors.		
4. Placed date, patient, and doctor identification information on the radiographic mount.		
5. Stated which side of the mount represented the right and left sides of the patient's mouth.		
6. Aligned radiographs on view box. Held each radiograph by margins only.		
7. Placed radiographs in the appropriate windows of the radiographic mount.		
8. Identified missing radiographs or required retakes.		
9. Blocked out any unused windows on the radiographic mount with dark paper.		
Comments:		

17 Alginate Impressions and Diagnostic Casts

▼ LEARNING OBJECTIVES

The student will be able to:

1. Describe the three major steps involved in producing accurate dental diagnostic casts.

2. Demonstrate preparing trays, mixing alginate impression material, loading trays, and assisting the operator during the taking of maxillary and mandibular impressions.

3. Describe the technique for taking a wax-bite registration.

4. Demonstrate creating maxillary and mandibular diagnostic casts from alginate impressions using the double-pour method.

5. Demonstrate trimming, finishing, and labeling maxillary and mandibular diagnostic casts.

OVERVIEW OF ALGINATE IMPRESSIONS AND DIAGNOSTIC CASTS

Diagnostic casts, which are also called *study casts* or *study models*, are exact reproductions of the teeth and surrounding structures of the maxillary and mandibular arches (Fig. 17–1).

These casts, which are important diagnostic aids, are used by the dentist in developing a treatment plan for the patient. They also serve as a permanent record of the occlusion and alignment of the teeth prior to corrective or restorative treatment. Post-treatment casts may be prepared when the dental treatment is concluded.

There are three major steps involved in the production of diagnostic casts.

1. **Alginate impressions**. These impressions must include accurate imprints of the patient's teeth and surrounding tissues. These impressions may be obtained before the patient is dismissed following the initial dental examination.

2. **Wax-bite**. A wax-bite, registering the patient's normal occlusion, may be obtained following the alginate impressions. This wax-bite aids in articulating the diagnostic casts.

   Articulation is the correct relationship of the upper and lower teeth as they occlude (come together) when the patient masticates (chews) his food.

3. **Pouring and trimming**. The impressions are poured in plaster of Paris or dental stone, trimmed, and articulated to create the diagnostic casts.

   These final steps are completed in the dental laboratory after the patient has been dismissed.

ALGINATE IMPRESSIONS

Alginate Impression Materials

Alginate is the least accurate of the impression materials used in dentistry. It is well suited for

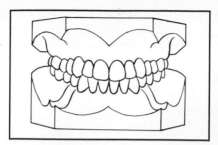

▼ **Figure 17–1**

Front view of maxillary and mandibular diagnostic casts. (Torres HO, Ehrlich A: Modern Dental Assisting, 4th Ed. Philadelphia, WB Saunders, 1990, p 486.)

making impressions for diagnostic casts; however, it is not used in situations, such as crown and bridge for final impressions, in which absolute accuracy is essential.

When the alginate powder is mixed with water, it has a pudding-like consistency. A chemical change, called *gelation* or *setting*, begins immediately, and this changes the soft mass into a firm, yet slightly elastic, consistency.

The impression material must be mixed, loaded in the tray, and positioned in the patient's mouth *before* gelation begins.

This period is referred to as **working time**. For alginate impression materials, the working time is no more than 1 minute.

Setting time refers to the length of time required for gelation to be completed. Once gelation starts, it must not be disturbed. If it is disturbed, the resulting impression will not be accurate.

Types of Alginate Impression Materials

Alginate is provided in two types: (1) **Fast set**, which gels in 1 to 2 minutes after beginning of mix, and (2) **normal set**, which gels in 2 to 4 minutes after beginning of mix.

Storing Alginate Impression Materials

Alginate impression materials deteriorate rapidly (1) at elevated temperatures, (2) in the presence of moisture, or (3) under both conditions. This deterioration causes the material either to set much too rapidly or to fail to set at all.

Premeasured foil packages ensure an accurate measure as well as protection from moisture contamination and other atmospheric conditions.

If the material is packaged in bulk in cans, these should be stored in a cool, dry location, and the lid should be tightly replaced immediately after use.

When taking alginate from the package, be careful not to inhale the powdery fumes (see Chapter 8, "Hazards Management in the Dental Office").

Measuring Alginate Impression Material

Accuracy is extremely important in measuring alginate impression material and the room-temperature water to be mixed with it. To ensure this accuracy, the powder and water measures provided by the manufacturer are used for this purpose (Fig. 17–2).

The ratio is one "scoop" of powder to one "measure" of water. The amount of material to be mixed is determined by the operator; however, the following are the amounts required for the average adult arch:

▼ 2 level scoops of powder to 2 measures of water for the mandibular arch.

▼ 3 scoops of powder to 3 measures of water for the maxillary arch.

▼ A large maxillary arch requires 3½ scoops of powder to 3½ measures of water.

If impressions are prepared of both arches, the mandibular impression is taken first. Then, when preparing the material for the maxillary tray, an extra half scoop of alginate and half measure of water is included in the mix. This extra material is used to provide tongue space in the mandibular arch impression.

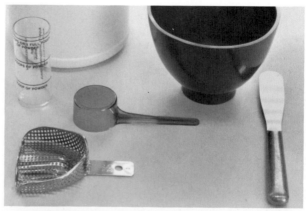

▼ **Figure 17–2**

Basic instrumentation for an alginate impression. Left to right, water measure, powder measure, mixing bowl and spatula. Lower left, maxillary impression tray.

Impression Trays

The alginate impression material is placed in the mouth using an impression tray. The most commonly used type is perforated so that the alginate oozes through these holes as it sets and is locked into place in the tray.

Impression trays are available in a range of sizes. These trays may be made of plastic (which is discarded after a single use) or of metal (which is cleaned and sterilized for reuse).

Beading wax is placed around the outer edges of the tray to protect the tissues from injury (Fig. 17–3).

This wax also aids in retaining material in the tray and prevents escaping material from entering the patient's throat and causing gagging and discomfort.

Who May Take Alginate Impressions

In states where this extended function is legal, the dentist may delegate the responsibility of obtaining alginate impressions to the qualified chairside assistant.

In other situations, the assistant mixes the impression materials, loads the trays, and aids the operator in taking the impressions.

The procedures described in the following sections describe the roles of both the assistant and the operator in obtaining the alginate impressions.

The extended function assistant who is actually taking the impressions fills both roles.

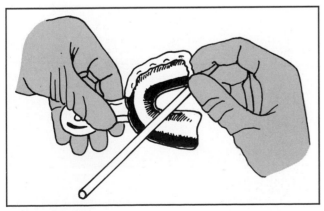

▼ **Figure 17–3**

Placing wax beading on the impression tray. (Torres HO, Ehrlich A: Modern Dental Assisting, 4th Ed. Philadelphia, WB Saunders, 1990, p 472.)

Criteria for Obtaining Alginate Impressions

1. Positioned the anterior portion of the tray over the centrals and laterals.
2. Provided adequate material in the vestibular area of the anteriors.
3. Provided depth of impression material to avoid exposure of the tray.
4. Provided detail of the labial frenum and the facial surfaces and incisal edges of the anterior teeth.
5. Provided detail of the facial, lingual, and occlusal surfaces of the posterior teeth.
6. Obtained registration of the mucobuccal attachments in the periphery of the impressions.
7. Ensured registration of the incisive papilla, tissues of the hard and soft palates, and the tuberosities on the maxillary arch.
8. Provided reproduction of the retromolar area, lingual frenum, tongue space, mylohyoid ridge, and eminence of the genial tubercle in the mandibular impression.

TAKING ALGINATE IMPRESSIONS

Instrumentation

▼ Basic setup.

▼ Alginate powder.

▼ Alginate measure (scoop provided by manufacturer).

▼ Water measure (provided by manufacturer).

▼ Water (room temperature: 70° to 72°F; 21.1° to 22.2°C).

▼ Bowl, medium size (flexible rubber).

▼ Laboratory spatula (flexible, large beavertail shape).

▼ Impression trays, maxillary and mandibular (if reusable, trays must be sterile).

▼ Beading wax (round form).

▼ Emesis basin (kidney basin).

▼ Facial tissues.

▼ Mouth rinse.

▼ Paper patient towels.

▼ Plastic drape.

▼ High volume evacuator (HVE) tip.

Procedure

PREPARING THE PATIENT

1. The mandibular impression is usually obtained first to familiarize the patient with the taste and consistency of the material prior to its placement on the palate.

2. Drape the patient and seat him in an upright position, with his head stabilized on the headrest of the dental chair.

   Draping is important to protect the patient's clothing against any spilled material.

   Seating the patient in an upright position will minimize any danger of his gagging or vomiting; however, an emesis basin is kept nearby in case of emergency.

3. Ask the patient if he has had impressions taken before. If this is his first experience, explain the procedure and the need for it.

   The patient is informed that the alginate material will have a faint flavor, taste "chalky," and feel thick and cold in the mouth.

   The patient is requested to follow the directions and cooperate during the process of obtaining the impressions.

   The patient is requested to refrain from talking during the procedure; however, he is instructed to use a hand signal if he is uncomfortable.

4. If the patient is wearing a removable dental prosthesis, request that he remove it.

   Clean the prosthesis and store it in a disinfecting solution. Return it to the patient at the end of the procedure.

5. Rinse the oral cavity with mouth rinse or water and vacuum it using the HVE. This frees the teeth and tissues of foreign substances.

6. If the patient's saliva is thick and ropy, request that the patient rinse with a suitable mouth rinse.

Procedure

SELECTING AND PREPARING THE IMPRESSION TRAYS

1. Maxillary and mandibular trays are selected by "trying" the trays in the patient's mouth.

2. Trays that have been tried in the mouth but were not selected for use must be sterilized before they are returned to storage.

3. The correct tray will meet the following criteria:

   Each tray should extend slightly beyond the facial surfaces of the teeth and approximately 2 to 3 mm beyond the third molar, retromolar, or tuberosity area of the individual arch.

   Each tray should be deep enough to provide 2 to 3 mm of impression material beyond the occlusal surface and incisal edge of the teeth.

   Each tray must be capable of retaining the impression material during insertion and withdrawal from the oral cavity.

4. Gently mold the beading wax to the outer perimeter of the trays that have been selected.

5. Place the prepared trays aside for immediate use.

Procedure

MIXING THE ALGINATE

1. Use a clean, dry flexible rubber bowl and laboratory spatula for each mix of impression material.

2. Shake the can of bulk alginate material to mix the contents. Lift the lid cautiously so that powder does not fly out into the air.

3. Use the measuring device supplied by the manufacturer to place the proper amount of alginate powder in the rubber bowl.

4. Place 1 measure of room temperature water in the bowl for each scoop of alginate powder.

5. Hold the bowl in the palm of the left hand and the spatula in the right hand. Gently mix the water and powder just until all of the powder is moist.

6. With the bowl in the left hand, vigorously *swirl* the spatula with the right hand, pressing it flat on the inside of the flexible bowl to "cream" the alginate and water.

7. During the spatulation, turn the bowl constantly in the left hand. The quick, vigorous action of the spatula is similar to spreading a mass of peanut butter on bread with the blade of a knife.

   The more rapidly and deftly the material is mixed, the more quickly the material is ready for the tray.

   Care must be taken to incorporate thoroughly all of the powder into the homogeneous mix. (**Homogeneous** means a mix with a uniform quality throughout.)

   A homogeneous mix is produced in less than 1 minute.

8. Gather the completed alginate mix into a mass in one spot on the inside edge of the bowl.

9. Mixing the alginate material and loading it in the tray must be completed within 1 minute.

Procedure

LOADING THE MANDIBULAR TRAY

1. With the right hand, load the spatula with alginate material. With the mandibular tray in the left hand, place the spatula at the lingual margin of the tray and scrape the material into the tray.

2. Use the end of the spatula to press quickly through the material down to the base of the tray. This will break any air bubbles that may be trapped as the tray is loaded with the alginate mix.

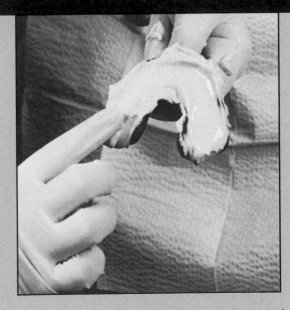

Figure 17–4 Mandibular tray loaded with alginate impression material. A moistened finger is used to smooth the surface. (Torres HO, Ehrlich A: Modern Dental Assisting, 4th Ed. Philadelphia, WB Saunders, 1990, p 473.)

Continued

3 When the tray is loaded to its periphery, put down the spatula and moisten the fingers of the right hand with room temperature water.

4 Use the wet fingers to smooth the surface of the alginate in the tray quickly (Fig. 17–4).

5 If the operator is taking the impression:
Hold the mixing bowl so that the operator can take some of the remaining alginate.
When the operator is ready, pass the filled tray with the alginate surface down

and positioned so that the operator can grasp the impression tray by the handle.

6 If the assistant is taking the impression:
Momentarily place the loaded tray on the instrument tray near the patient.
Dip the fingers of the right hand into a small bulk of the remaining alginate in the bowl.

7 The tray must be properly loaded and seated *before* the material has begun to set. If setting has already started, the impression will not be accurate.

Procedure

PLACING THE MANDIBULAR TRAY

1 Turn to the dental chair, on the right side of the patient. Ask the patient to open his mouth slightly.

2 With the left index finger and thumb, slightly retract the patient's right cheek.
Quickly place the alginate from the fingers of the right hand on the occlusal and interproximal surfaces of the patient's mandibular teeth (Fig. 17–5).
Note: This application of alginate prevents air spaces from developing in the impression when the tray is seated in the mouth.

3 Grasp the handle of the impression tray with the right hand so that the alginate and tray are facing downward.
Turn it slightly to the left and ease it into the mouth in a modified side position.
The tray is then straightened so that the handle is protruding from the oral cavity perpendicular to the anterior teeth.

4 Following the tray's insertion into the mouth, use both index fingers to position the tray evenly over the mandibular arch.

5 Use the index fingers to slightly and gently flex the patient's cheeks outward as the tray is positioned.

6 Place the index and middle fingers of each hand on top of the tray. Gently press the positioned tray firmly onto the occlusal surfaces and incisal edges of the mandibular teeth (Fig. 17–6).

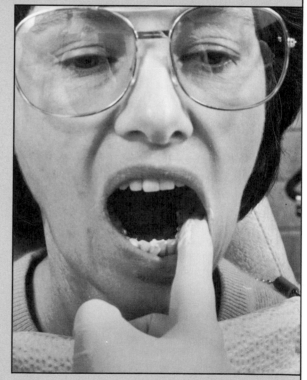

Figure 17-5 Spreading alginate impression material on the occlusal surfaces prior to placement of the mandibular tray. (Torres HO, Ehrlich A: Modern Dental Assisting, 4th Ed. Philadelphia, WB Saunders, 1990, p 473.)

7 Use the fingers of both hands to press the tray firmly down on the arch until resistance to the pressure is determined. Excess material will flow out of the perforations of the tray and around the peripheral margins.

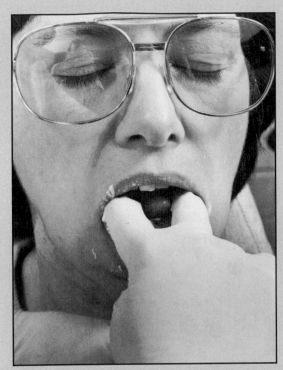

Figure 17–6 Stabilizing the mandibular impression tray on the arch. (Torres HO, Ehrlich A: Modern Dental Assisting, 4th Ed. Philadelphia, WB Saunders, 1990, p 474.)

8 Instruct the patient to raise his tongue toward the palate and then relax the tongue in the floor of the mouth. (This will avoid distortion of the impression on the mylohyoid area.)

9 Instruct the patient to breathe normally through the mouth while the tray is in place.

   If gagging occurs, the patient may be seated more upright with the head placed slightly forward.

   If the patient is in a supine position, he is instructed to turn his head to the right to ease the gagging sensation.

10 Hold the tray firmly in position while the alginate sets.

   The material has reached the set stage when the impression material does not register a dent when pressed by the finger or fingernail.

   Alginate impression material sets within 3 to 7 minutes, depending on the type of alginate (regular or fast-set), the temperature, and the consistency of the mix.

   Because of the higher body temperature, the material sets faster in the mouth than at room temperature.

Procedure

REMOVING THE MANDIBULAR TRAY

1 Place the fingers of the left hand on the top of the tray or on the edge of the maxillary teeth. This protects the incisal edge of the maxillary teeth from damage during removal of the impression tray.

2 Remove the tray very carefully by placing the thumb and index finger on the handle and exerting a firm lifting motion.

   Rough handling may cause the impression to tear during removal.

   The tray and impression should "snap up" free of the dentition.

3 If, after step 2, the tray does not snap up, it is probably "suction-sealed," and the following steps are necessary to break the suction seal.

   First, place the index finger of the right hand under the periphery of the tray at the left side of the posterior area.

   Second, place the left index finger under the periphery of the lower right side of the impression. The tray should now be easily lifted from the arch.

   If the tray still resists removal, use the air syringe to direct air under the posterior periphery of the tray to break the suction seal.

4 After the mandibular tray has been removed, instruct the patient to rinse his mouth with water or a mouth rinse. This removes any excess alginate material before the maxillary impression is taken.

5 Check the mandibular impression for accuracy. The completed impression is returned to the assistant. (See "Procedure: Caring for Alginate Impressions" later in this chapter.)

Procedure

LOADING THE MAXILLARY TRAY

1. A clean, dry bowl and spatula are used for mixing the alginate for the maxillary impression.

   If the same mixing equipment is reused, it is essential that it be clean *and* dry before beginning the next mix.

2. Fill the maxillary tray to the periphery from the posterior of the tray. This action aids in eliminating formation of air bubbles.

3. Place the bulk of the material forward in the impression tray in the anterior palatal area.

   This placement aids in preventing large amounts of material from flowing into the throat during tray placement.

   If excessive material is permitted to ooze from the back of the tray, the patient may gag as it touches the sensitive soft palate area.

   A small amount of alginate impression material remains in the laboratory bowl for use with the mandibular impression.

4. Insert the tip of the spatula down through the mass of material in the tray to avoid an airspace.

5. Moisten the fingers with tap water and smooth the surface of the alginate material.

6. Use the moistened fingers to make a slight indentation in the surface of the impression material in the tray directly over the area of the alveolar ridge (Fig. 17–7).

   Note: This indentation of the alginate material aids in the placement of the tray over the dentition and helps to prevent the formation of air bubbles.

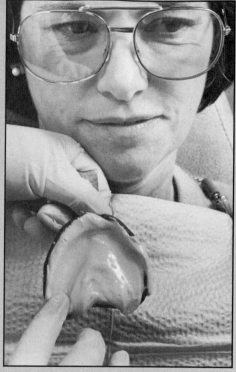

Figure 17–7 Maxillary tray loaded with alginate impression material. A moistened finger is used to make a slight indentation to prevent air bubbles. (Torres HO, Ehrlich A: Modern Dental Assisting, 4th Ed. Philadelphia, WB Saunders, 1990, p 475.)

7. If the operator is taking the impression:

   Pass the impression tray with the alginate surface up and positioned so that the operator can grasp the handle.

8. If the assistant is taking the impression:

   Momentarily place the loaded impression tray on the instrument tray where it can be reached easily.

9. Spread alginate mix on occlusal and interproximal surfaces.

Procedure

PLACING THE MAXILLARY TRAY

1. With the alginate and tray facing upward, turn the tray slightly to the left (Fig. 17–8).

2. Place the tray in the mouth with the handle of the tray positioned perpendicular to the maxillary anterior teeth.

3. Guide the tray into position by placing the posterior portion first. This ensures the distal extension of material on the maxillary tuberosity and the vestibular area in the mucobuccal and anterior vestibule.

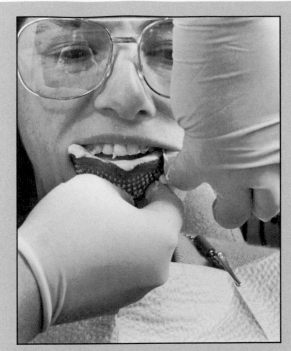

Figure 17-8 Inserting maxillary impression tray. (Torres HO, Ehrlich A: Modern Dental Assisting, 4th Ed. Philadelphia, WB Saunders, 1990, p 476.)

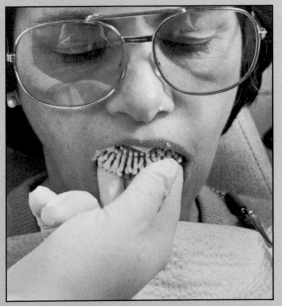

Figure 17-9 Seating maxillary impression tray. (Torres HO, Ehrlich A: Modern Dental Assisting, 4th Ed. Philadelphia, WB Saunders, 1990, p 476.)

4   Center the tray on the arch and seat it firmly in place (Fig. 17-9).

5   Tilt the patient's head forward to prevent stimulating the gag reflex.

Instruct the patient to keep his mouth open slightly and to breathe through the mouth.

Instruct the patient to hold the emesis basin under his chin in case he drools or becomes nauseated.

6   Hold the tray firmly in position while the alginate sets (within 3 to 7 minutes).

Note: The material has reached the set stage when the impression material will not register a dent when pressed by the finger or fingernail.

7   If both maxillary and mandibular impressions are being prepared, the patient may be asked to hold the tray in position. While the maxillary impression is reaching the gel stage, the mandibular impression is completed.

Procedure

REMOVING THE MAXILLARY TRAY

1   Exercise care to avoid injury to the mandibular teeth during tray removal. Use a straight, downward snapping motion to remove the maxillary impression from the mouth.

2   Examine the impression for accuracy. The completed impression is returned to the assistant. (See "Procedure: Caring for Alginate Impressions.")

3   Instruct the patient to rinse his mouth to remove any excess alginate.

4   Use an explorer and dental floss to free the interproximal spaces of impression material.

5   Before dismissing the patient, do the following:

Provide the patient with mouth rinse to rinse again.

Use a moist tissue to remove gently any alginate material from the patient's face and lips.

If the patient had to remove a dental prosthesis, rinse and return it at this time.

Procedure

COMPLETING THE MANDIBULAR IMPRESSION

1. While the maxillary impression is setting in the patient's mouth, the remaining alginate mix from the bowl is used to fill in the space in the mandibular impression that is created by the tongue.

2. With the right hand, scoop up the remaining alginate mix on the spatula.

3. Hold the mandibular impression in the left hand. Place the left thumb in the tongue void of the impression.

4. With the right hand, place the mass of alginate impression material over the left thumb.

5. Moisten the fingers of the right hand with tap water. Use the moist fingers to blend the two masses of alginate. Place and blend the surface of the new alginate about 2 mm below the lingual periphery of the mandibular impression. This ensures accurate reproduction of the dental arch or alveolar ridge.

6. The alginate mass placed in the mandibular impression will be set at the same time that the maxillary impression is set in the patient's mouth.

7. When the material is set, remove the thumb from the mandibular impression and store the impression until it is ready to be poured.

Procedure

CARING FOR ALGINATE IMPRESSIONS

1. Gently rinse the alginate impression under tap water to remove any debris. Carefully shake off any excess water.

2. Spray the impression with an iodophor disinfectant solution (see Chapter 7, "Infection Control").

3. Wrap the impression in a damp paper towel and place it in a plastic bag to be transported to the dental laboratory (Fig. 17–10).

4. Pour alginate impressions as quickly as possible because:
    When exposed to air an alginate impres-

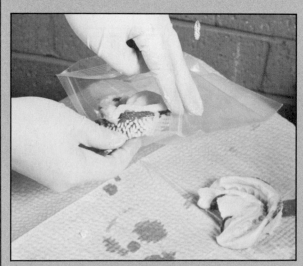

Figure 17–10 Disinfected alginate impressions are bagged for delivery to the laboratory, where they should be poured promptly. (Torres HO, Ehrlich A: Modern Dental Assisting, 4th Ed. Philadelphia, WB Saunders, 1990, p 476.)

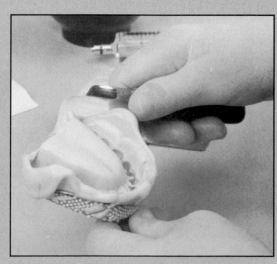

Figure 17–11 Before the model can be poured, the excess alginate must be carefully trimmed away.

sion **dehydrates** (loses water and dries out). This causes shrinkage and distortion.

If the alginate impression is stored in water, **imbibition** (soaking up water) takes place. This too causes distortion.

5 If the impression must be stored, it should be wrapped in wet towels or kept in 100 percent humidity.

An alternative is to store the impression temporarily in a 2 percent solution of po-

tassium sulfate until poured. Storage in this solution should not be for more than 20 minutes.

6 Before the impression can be poured, the excess alginate material must be trimmed away with a laboratory knife (Fig. 17–11).

Note: When trimming, take care to remove only the excess and not essential detail.

WAX-BITE REGISTRATION

A wax-bite registration is needed to show the occlusal relationship of the maxillary and mandibular teeth.

Most commonly, this is accomplished with a U-shaped wafer of baseplate wax. To add strength, a thin sheet of foil may be placed between the layers of wax.

As an alternative, a commercial wax impreg-

nated with metal filings may be used for this purpose.

Instrumentation

▼ Baseplate wax.

▼ Laboratory knife.

▼ Bowl of warm water *or* Bunsen burner and matches.

Procedure

PREPARING THE WAX

1 Warm a sheet of baseplate wax so that it can be folded without breaking.

2 Fold the wax lengthwise, as shown in Figure 17–12.

3 Repeat until a fold of three thicknesses is obtained. Trim away the excess wax (Fig. 17–13).

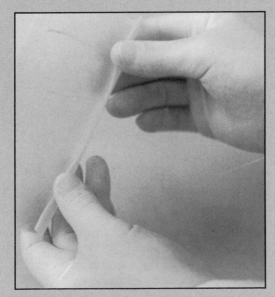

Figure 17–12 Gently warm a sheet of baseplate wax, and fold it lengthwise.

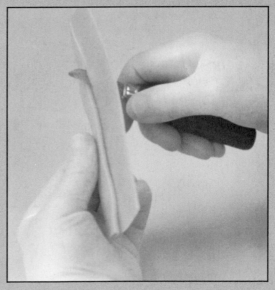

Figure 17–13 Fold the wax into three thicknesses, and trim away the excess.

Continued

4 Mold the folded wax into a **U** shape to fit in the mouth and trim away the excess (Fig. 17–14).

5 Gently warm the prepared wax.

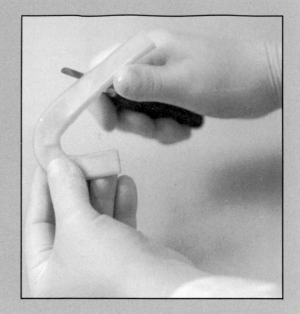

Figure 17–14 Mold the wax into a U shape to fit in the patient's mouth, and trim away the excess.

Procedure

TAKING THE BITE REGISTRATION

1 Explain the procedure to the patient, reassuring him that the wax will be warm, not hot, in his mouth.

2 Place the prepared wax over the occlusal surfaces and the anterior edge of the patient's mandibular teeth.

3 Instruct the patient to bite gently and naturally into the wax (Fig. 17–15).

4 Allow the wax to cool. (It will cool quickly and may be removed within a few minutes.)

5 Remove the wax-bite registration very carefully so as not to break or distort the wax wafer.

6 Identify the bite registration and impressions with the patient's name and place them in a laboratory tray or plastic bag for transportation to the laboratory.

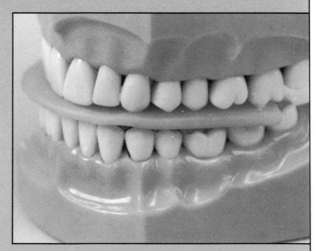

Figure 17–15 Instruct the patient to bite gently and naturally into the wax.

GYPSUM PRODUCTS

The next step is "pouring" of the alginate impression in a gypsum product such as model plaster or dental stone.

Model plaster, also known as *plaster of Paris* and *laboratory plaster*, is white and is used in preparing diagnostic casts for a case presentation.

If greater strength is required, *dental stone* may be used. Dental stone, which is usually yellow, is used most often when a stronger, more abrasion-resistant cast is needed.

The crystals that make up each type of gypsum product have a different structure and shape. The shape of these crystals determines the characteristics of the gypsum product and the appropriate water to powder ratio to be used.

When the gypsum powder is mixed with water, these particles dissolve in the water and begin to form clusters known as the **nuclei of crystallization**. It is the intermeshing of these crystals, which is part of the setting process, that gives the final gypsum product its strength and rigidity.

The greater the amount of intermeshing, the greater the strength, rigidity, and hardness of the final product. If this process is disturbed, the final product will be weakened and unsatisfactory.

Gypsum products expand as they set. Excessive expansion would distort the resulting diagnostic cast; however, carefully following the manufacturer's instructions minimizes this problem.

Water to Powder Ratio

The strength of the finished gypsum product is determined largely by the water to powder ratio. Each powder type has an optimal water to powder ratio, which has been specified by the manufacturer. These ratios should be followed carefully.

To achieve these optimal water to powder ratios, both the water and the powder must be measured accurately.

The water is measured by volume using a large syringe (Fig. 17-16). An alternative is to use a clearly marked milliliter graduate. When measuring with a graduate, always read the meniscus level of the water. (The **meniscus** is the bottom of the elliptical curve where the water touches the dry side of the container.)

Although powder can be measured by volume, measuring it by weight on a dietetic scale is more accurate and reliable (Fig. 17-17). When measuring powder in a container, it is necessary to adjust the scale first to eliminate the weight of the container.

To do this, place the empty container on the scale and manually turn the indicator dial of the scale back to zero. Add the powder only after the scale reads zero again.

Optimal Ratios

These materials should be used in keeping with the manufacturer's recommended water to powder ratio. The following are the commonly used water to powder ratios for one cast:

▼ **Model plaster.** Approximately 45 ml of water to 100 g of powder.

▼ **Dental stone.** Approximately 30 ml of water to 100 g of powder.

Too Little Water Used

If too little water is used in making the mix, the result is a dry, crumbly mass that is useless.

If the mix is too thick, and more water is added, the crystallization is abnormal and the resulting mix does not have the desired strength.

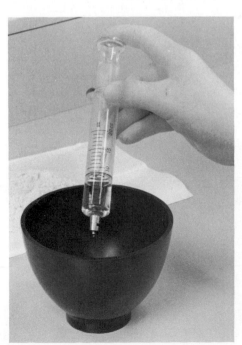

▼ **Figure 17-16**

A large glass syringe is used to measure the water accurately.

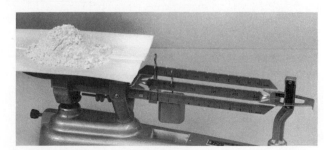

▼ **Figure 17-17**

A dietetic scale is used to measure the powder accurately.

Too Much Water Used

If too much water is used, there is a rapid change in the appearance of the material. It progresses from a stiff, putty-like mass to a thick, batter-like material and finally to a very thin, highly fluid substance.

If the mix is too thin and more powder is added after the stirring begins, the continued mixing process breaks up those crystals that have already begun to form. As a result, the final product is weak and brittle.

Setting Time

Setting time is a measure of the speed with which the mixture changes into a rigid solid. It is important to have enough working time, before the material sets, to mix and pour the material properly.

The setting of the gypsum product can be lengthened or shortened by several factors. The following are the factors that are most likely to vary during mixing.

1. **The material used**. Model plaster sets more quickly than dental stone.
2. **Water to powder ratio**. In general, the less water that is used, the shorter will be the setting time.
3. **Mixing**. The longer and more rapid the mixing, the more rapid the set.
4. **Temperature**. Higher water temperatures accelerate the setting rate, with the shortest setting time being observed at temperatures near 100°F (37.8°C).

POURING DIAGNOSTIC CASTS

The Double-Pour Method

In the double-pour method, the impressions are poured first and allowed to harden. At this time, the surfaces of the maxillary and mandibular casts are left rough.

Later, in the second pour, this roughness makes it possible to attach the second pour to create the base of the diagnostic models.

Instrumentation

▼ Maxillary and/or mandibular impressions.

▼ Model plaster (bulk or prepackaged).

▼ Glass syringe marked in milliliters.

▼ Water at room temperature (not to exceed 70°F; 21.1°C).

▼ Flexible bowl.

▼ Blunt-ended laboratory spatula.

▼ Scales (dietetic gram).

▼ Vibrator.

▼ Glass slabs (2).

▼ Laboratory knife.

▼ Beading wax (square or rope type).

▼ Boxing wax.

▼ Laboratory spatula.

▼ Bunsen burner and matches.

Procedure

MIXING MODEL PLASTER

1 Remove the impressions from storage and shake them lightly to remove excess moisture. They may also be gently blown with compressed air to remove the excess moisture.

Excess moisture on the impression causes dilution of the plaster or stone mix to be used in the pouring of the impressions.

Removing too much moisture dehydrates and distorts the alginate impression.

2 Measure 45 ml of water at 70°F (21°C). Place the measured water in the clean, flexible bowl.

3 Adjust the scale for the weight of the container, then weigh out exactly 100 g of model plaster.

4 Add the powder to the water in steady increments, permitting it to absorb the water. This prevents trapping air bubbles.

5 Hold the mixing bowl in the palm of the left hand. Place the spatula in the right hand.

To avoid spilling the powder, slowly incorporate it into the water with gentle stirring motions.

To avoid creating air bubbles, stir the mix in only one direction.

The powder and water are incorporated (mixed) in approximately 20 seconds to form a homogeneous mix.

6 Place a disposable cover over the platform of the vibrator to protect the rubber surface.

7 With the vibrator speed turned to low or medium, place the bowl of plaster mix on the vibrator platform.

Lightly press and rotate the bowl on the vibrator. This will permits any bubbles to rise to the surface (Fig. 17–18).

8 Place the bowl containing the mix near the vibrator.

9 The total time for mixing and vibration of

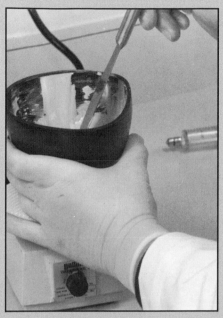

Figure 17–18 The vibrator is used to complete mixing and to eliminate air bubbles from the mix.

the model plaster mix must *not* exceed 2 minutes.

Procedure

POURING THE MAXILLARY CAST

1 Set the vibrator at low to medium speed.

Hold the maxillary alginate impression in the left hand.

Place the edge of the tray handle on the vibrator platform.

2 Dip the spatula into the bowl, picking up a small increment of the mix (Fig. 17–19).

3 Place a small mass of mix on the palatal area of the impression near the right molar area or most posterior tooth in the arch.

The material within the tray on the vibrator flows into the tooth indentations slowly, forcing the mass forward.

Place small increments of the mix frequently in the same area to provide gravitational flow.

Avoid placing large increments on top of the flowing mass because this creates bubbles by the trapping of air.

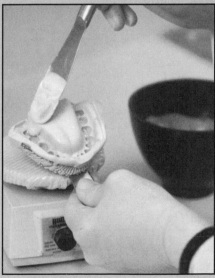

Figure 17–19 The handle of the tray is placed on the vibrator, and the mix is flowed into the posterior portion of the maxillary impression.

Continued

4 Rotate the tray slowly to its left side on the vibrator platform to provide a continuous flow of the mix throughout the maxillary impression.

At the same time, hold the tray firmly on the vibrator as increments of the mix are added.

5 Following the filling of the tooth indentations within the impression, place larger increments of mix on the vault of the palatal impression until the entire impression is filled.

6 Turn the vibrator off and pile the additional bulk of material onto the palatal area of the cast.

7 The surface of the mix should remain rough. The entire process of *mixing* and *pouring* should not take more than 5 minutes.

8 Place the poured impression and tray upright on a glass slab to permit the material to set (harden).

It may be wrapped in a damp paper towel to prevent rapid drying during the initial set.

The initial set takes place in approximately 10 to 15 minutes. In some instances, for a more dense cast the poured impression is placed in a humidor to reach a final set.

9 Clean and dry the rubber bowl, scales, water graduate, spatula, and vibrator in preparation for the mixing and pouring of the mandibular impression.

Procedure

POURING THE MANDIBULAR CAST

1 The measurements of materials for the mandibular cast are the same as for the maxillary. The mixing and vibrating technique is the same.

2 Hold the mandibular impression tray with the handle and left hand against the vibrator, with the heel of the left quadrant of the impression extended up from the vibrator, similar to the position for the maxillary impression. (The **heel** is the retromolar and lingual extension of the impression.)

3 Place the mass of mix with the spatula into the indentations of the left quadrant, third molar area. This permits the material to flow forward toward the midline as the increments of mix are added at the same posterior position.

4 Tilt the tray toward the right side as the flow reaches the anterior midline.

5 With the tooth indentation filled, place the increments of plaster mix on the peripheral margins of the impression to complete the total pour in the lingual area.

6 The surface of the mix should remain rough.

When the impression is filled to the rim, turn the vibrator off.

Place the poured impression upright on a glass slab to set.

7 Place the glass slabs containing the poured impressions away from laboratory activity and in a safe place to avoid vibration or damage from moving objects or being knocked on the floor.

Procedure

POURING THE BASE

1 The diagnostic casts are ready to receive the pour for the attachment of the base approximately 5 to 10 minutes after the initial pour.

2 Approximately one half of the formula for the cast is needed to form a base for each impression. Since a slightly thicker mix is desired, approximately 20 ml of water is used with 50 g of plaster.

3 Mix this in the same manner as for the casts.

Place the mix on the glass slab in a pile approximately 2 × 2 inches, ¾ to 1 inch thick (Fig. 17–20).

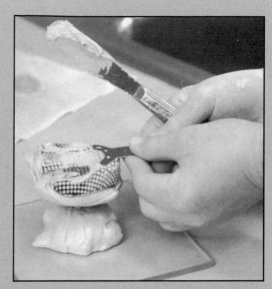

Figure 17–21 The poured cast is inverted and carefully placed on the base.

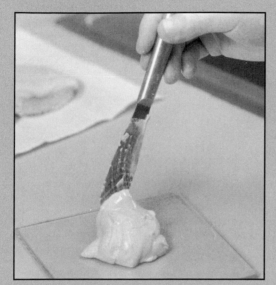

Figure 17–20 A mass of fresh plaster is placed on a glass slab to form the base of the completed model.

Commercial rubber molds may be used to form the base. These base molds provide symmetry to the casts without much trimming of the cast on the model trimmer.

4 Invert the maxillary or mandibular cast onto the base of the new mix (Fig. 17–21). Do not press down on the impression tray.

Note: As the poured cast is inverted onto the base mix, the fresh material will flow lightly. Pressure may cause the base material to flow excessively, resulting in a base that is too large and too thin.

5 With the tray held steady, use the spatula to drag the plaster base mix up onto the margins of the initial pour (Fig. 17–22).

6 Blend the old and new mix to provide continuity and to collapse any air spaces that may have formed. Care should be

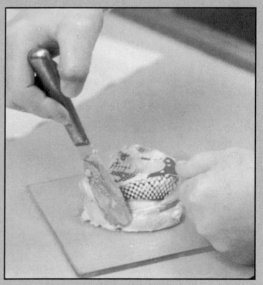

Figure 17–22 The base material is carefully dragged up over the edges of the cast without covering any of the impression tray.

taken to avoid dragging the mix up over the impression and onto the impression tray because this material may form a mechanical lock that prevents easy removal of the impression tray.

7 Position the impression tray so that the handle and the occlusal plane of the teeth of the cast are parallel with the surface of the glass slab. This alignment aids in forming a uniform thickness of base to the cast.

Procedure

SEPARATING THE CAST FROM THE IMPRESSION

1. Wait 45 to 60 minutes after the base has been poured before separating the impression from the cast.

2. Use the laboratory knife around the periphery to free the margins of the tray (Fig. 17–23).

3. Use a firm, straight, upward tug on the tray handle to free the impression from the cast (Fig. 17–24).

4. If the impression does not separate freely, determine where the tray is adhering to the cast and cautiously trim all excess material around the tray.

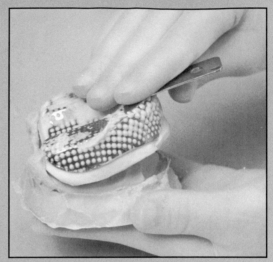

Figure 17–24 The impression and tray are lifted off with a straight up motion.

5. Again, pull the tray handle straight up from the cast with a snap. If the margins are free, the separation will occur without damaging the cast.

   Caution: Do not at any time move the tray from side to side because the motion will fracture the teeth on the cast.

6. Protruding anteriors on the cast are most difficult to separate from the impression without fracturing them.

   A slight tilt forward on the tray may accomplish separation of the impression and cast without causing fracture of the anteriors.

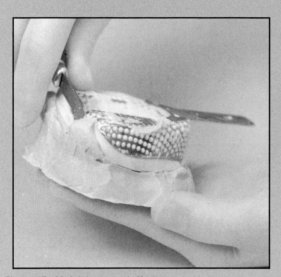

Figure 17–23 A laboratory knife is used to trim away excess carefully before separating the impression and cast.

FINISHING DIAGNOSTIC CASTS

If the casts are to be used for a case presentation, they must be trimmed geometrically for an esthetic appearance. The wax-bite registration is used to articulate these casts during the process of trimming.

Anatomic and Art Portions

The finished cast consists of two sections: the **anatomic portion**, representing the teeth and gingival attachment, and the **art portion**, which forms the base or pedestal (Figs. 17–25 through 17–27).

Generally the anatomic portion makes up two thirds and the art portion one third of the overall height of the finished cast. However, the art portion should be no more than ½ inch thick at the highest point of the impression.

The Maxillary Cast

The art portion of the maxillary cast is trimmed so that:

▼ The front (cuspid to midline) is pointed at a 30-degree angle.

▼ The sides are angled at a 65-degree angle.

▼ The heels are angled at a 115-degree angle.

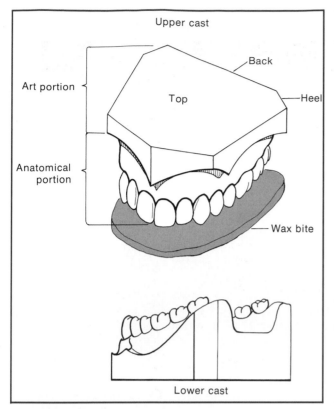

▼ **Figure 17–25**

Landmarks of diagnostic casts. (Torres HO, Ehrlich A: Modern Dental Assisting, 4th Ed. Philadelphia, WB Saunders, 1990, p 484.)

The Mandibular Cast

The art portion of the mandibular cast is trimmed so that:

▼ The front (cuspid to midline) is rounded.

▼ The sides are angled at a 55-degree angle.

▼ The heels are angled at a 115-degree angle.

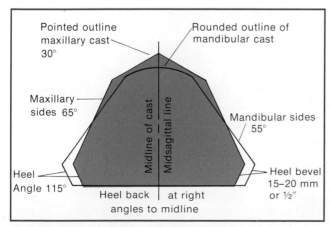

▼ **Figure 17–26**

Outline of the maxillary cast (shaded) superimposed over the outline of the mandibular cast. (Torres HO, Ehrlich A: Modern Dental Assisting, 4th Ed. Philadelphia, WB Saunders, 1990, p 486.)

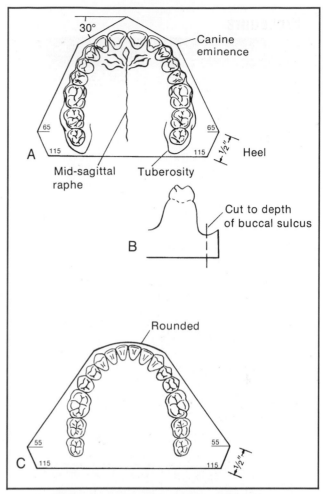

▼ **Figure 17–27**

Landmarks, angles, and cuts on art portion of casts. A. Maxillary cast. B. Cut to depth of buccal sulcus. C. Mandibular cast. (Torres HO, Ehrlich A: Modern Dental Assisting, 4th Ed. Philadelphia, WB Saunders, 1990, p. 485.)

TRIMMING DIAGNOSTIC CASTS

The casts are easier to cut on the model trimmer if they are damp. If the casts are *not* still damp from recent pouring, they should be soaked in cool water for 5 minutes before trimming.

Instrumentation

▼ Damp maxillary cast.

▼ Damp mandibular cast.

▼ Ruler.

▼ Pencil.

▼ Laboratory knife.

▼ Measuring device.

▼ Wax-bite registration.

▼ Model trimmer.

Procedure

TRIMMING THE CASTS

1 Measure the height of the overall cast. If the art portion is too high, greater than one third of the overall height of the cast, mark it to be trimmed.

2 Turn on the power and water to the model trimmer.

3 Place the base of the mandibular cast flat on the table of the model trimmer (Fig. 17–28).

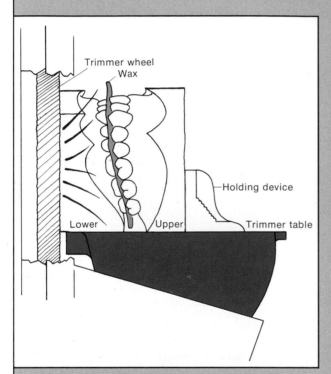

Figure 17–28 Trimming the base of the mandibular cast on the model trimmer. (Torres HO, Ehrlich A: Modern Dental Assisting, 4th Ed. Philadelphia, WB Saunders, 1990, p. 485.)

To ensure that the bases are parallel, place the other cast on the trimmer table.
Use the wax-bite to protect the teeth on the casts.
Use the holding device to hold the model firmly against the trimmer wheel and reduce the excess thickness.
If necessary, repeat these steps for the maxillary cast.
When placed on the art portion, the cast should sit flat.

4 Use a laboratory knife or the model trimmer to trim away carefully rough, bulky edges that might interfere with obtaining accurate measurements.

5 Use a laboratory knife or the model trimmer to remove excess material on the posterior area of the cast if the extensions interfere with occluding the casts.

6 Use a set divider or a rule and a pencil to draw a line on the posterior portion of the larger of the two casts.
This line should be perpendicular to the midline of the maxillary or mandibular centrals.
The line should be placed approximately 3 mm (¼ inch) in back of the third molar, retromolar, or tuberosity area.

7 Place this cast on the model trimmer, and trim it by a straight cut to that line. A minimum of 2 to 3 mm of plaster should remain in back of the last molar *after* the casts are trimmed.

8 Trim the sides of the mandibular cast by placing the heels against the angulator and the base on the platform. The angulator is set at 55 degrees (Fig. 17–29).
Avoid removing the plaster beyond the lowest portion of the mucobuccal fold on

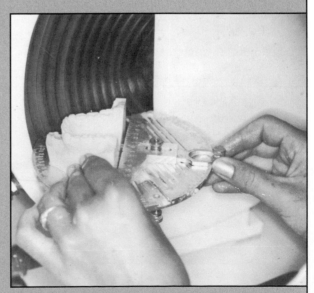

Figure 17–29 Trimming the rough edges of the cast on the model trimmer. (Courtesy of Harry W. Humphreys, DDS, MS, San Rafael, CA.)

the sides of the dental cast near the premolars and molars (the buccal frenum attachment should remain).

Trim the cast to the lowest portion of the fold only.

9 Trim the anterior area of the mandibular cast, following the curved outline of the arch, leaving the labial frenum and approximately 3 to 4 mm of the vestibular area intact (Fig. 17–30).

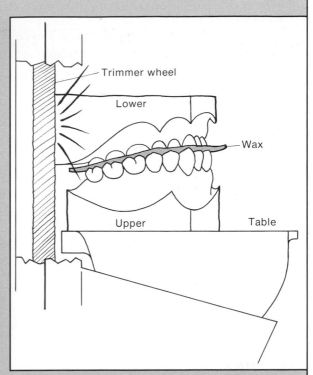

Figure 17–31 Trimming the back of the mandibular cast on the model trimmer.

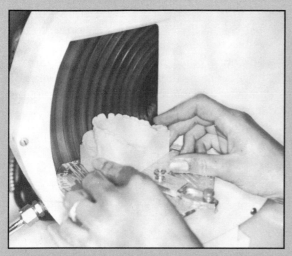

Figure 17–30 Trimming the anterior angle of a maxillary cast on the model trimmer. (Courtesy of Harry W. Humphreys, DDS, MS, San Rafael, CA.)

10 Cut the heel angles of the mandibular cast, with the angulator set at approximately 115 degrees and the base of the cast on the platform of the model trimmer.

This angle cut should align the basic heel line and the side lines of the cast.

11 Use the laboratory knife to remove carefully any beads of plaster on the occlusal surfaces of the maxillary and mandibular casts.

12 With the maxillary and mandibular casts articulated on the wax-bite, place the mandibular cast on the trimming table and trim the heels of the maxillary cast to match the trim of the mandibular cast.

13 Keep the casts together, and turn them over so that the maxillary base is on the trimming table. Trim any area of the mandibular cast that needs minor shaping (Fig. 17–31).

14 Trim the heel angles of the maxillary cast to match the heel angles of the mandibular cast.

15 With the casts still articulated and placed on their heels, trim the maxillary cast base parallel to the base of the mandibular cast.

16 Separate the casts and place the base of the maxillary cast on the trimming table.

Place the heels against the angulator, with the side cuts aligned at 65 degrees.

The side cuts on the cast are made to the lowest portion of the mucobuccal fold on the cast.

Do not remove the buccal frenum attachment.

17 With the maxillary cast base on the trimming table, place the anterior portion against the wheel at a 25-degree angle from the cuspid to the central, at the midline of the cast.

Caution: Do not remove the labial frenum attachment. These cuts provide esthetic quality to the anterior portion of the casts.

Continued

18 Place maxillary heel cuts connecting the base line and the side lines at 115 degrees.

Note: Occluded, the trimmed diagnostic casts should measure approximately 2½ to 2⅞ inches in overall height.

Optional: To provide a finished land area, a laboratory knife or sandpaper pad is used for mitering the sharp edges of the gingival and facial margins of each cast (see Fig. 17–30).

Optional: Use a thick mix of plaster and water to fill up voids or bubbles in the *moist* base or body portion of the casts.

Polishing Diagnostic Casts

Casts may be soaked for 24 hours in a warm soap solution at 160°F (71°C), or a commercial plastic model spray may be used to provide gloss to the surface of the casts.

Following soaking in the soap solution, the casts may be dried and buffed with a soft dry cloth to produce a high gloss.

The patient's name, age, and the date should be written in indelible pencil on the base or posterior of the casts.

The finished casts should be stored in absorbent paper or in a special container to avoid fracture.

The dental office may have a system of storing casts to present a "before and after" visual diagnostic aid for the patient following completion of the treatment plan.

▼█ **EXERCISES**

1. The sides of a maxillary diagnostic cast are angled to a _____ degree angle.

    a. 30
    b. 55
    c. 65
    d. 115

2. _____ requires approximately 45 ml of water to 100 g of powder.

    a. Alginate impression material
    b. Dental stone
    c. Model plaster

3. _____ time is the period when the impression material is mixed, loaded in the tray, and positioned in the patient's mouth.

    a. Gelation
    b. Setting
    c. Working

4. When taking the _____ impression, the patient is instructed to raise his tongue toward the palate.

    a. mandibular
    b. maxillary

5. The water that is used to mix the alginate for an impression should be at _____ °F.

    a. 65–68
    b. 68–70
    c. 70–72
    d. 98.6

6. For patient comfort while taking a maxillary alginate impression, the assistant should _____.

    a. be certain there is adequate material at the post dam of the tray
    b. instruct the patient to tilt his head forward
    c. tell the patient to breathe through his mouth
    d. b and c

7. When mixing dental plaster, if the mix is too thin, it _____ acceptable to add more powder.

    a. is
    b. is not

8. Reproduction of the _____ is/are included in the criteria for an acceptable mandibular alginate impression.

    a. incisive papilla
    b. mucobuccal attachment
    c. mylohyoid ridge
    d. b and c

9. Beading wax is placed on the periphery of the impression tray to _____ _____ .

    a. help retain the material in the tray
    b. protect the tissues from injury
    c. speed setting of the alginate
    d. a and b

10. The anterior area of the art portion of a mandibular cast is _____ _____ .

    a. cut at a 90-degree angle
    b. gently rounded
    c. trimmed to a 30-degree angle
    d. trimmed to a 115-degree angle

11. It is necessary to wait _____ after the base has been poured before separating the impression from the cast.

    a. 20–30 minutes
    b. 45–60 minutes
    c. 1 to 2 hours

12. A ___b___ is/are used to show the occlusal relationship of the maxillary and mandibular teeth.

    a. bilateral registration
    b. bite registration
    c. centric alignment
    d. a and c

13. When the alginate impression material has set, the mandibular tray is removed _____ .

    a. by gently rocking it back and forth
    b. laterally and upward
    c. with a firm lifting motion
    d. with a sharp upward motion

14. Each impression tray should be deep enough to provide _____ mm of impression material beyond the occlusal surfaces and incisal edges of the teeth.

    a. 1 to 2
    b. 2 to 3
    c. 3 to 4
    d. 4 to 5

15. While taking impressions, the patient should use a ___hand___ signal if he is uncomfortable.

    a. hand
    b. verbal

16. In the finished diagnostic cast, the _____ portion forms the base or pedestal.

    a. anatomic
    b. art

17. During an alginate impression, the patient should be seated in a/an _____ position.

    a. subsupine
    b. supine
    c. upright

18. Before a diagnostic cast can be trimmed, it must be _____ _____ .

    a. damp
    b. soaked in a soap solution
    c. thoroughly dry
    d. warmed to 85°F

19. ____Normal Set____ set alginate gels in 2 to 4 minutes after the beginning of the mix.

    a. Fast
    b. Normal
    c. Super

20. While taking alginate impressions, a/an _____ is kept handy just in case the patient gags or vomits.

    a. emesis basin
    b. plastic tub
    c. roll of paper towels
    d. supply of tissues

▼ Criterion Sheet 17–1

Student's Name _____

Procedure: *OBTAINING A MANDIBULAR ALGINATE IMPRESSION*

Performance Objective:

The student will obtain an acceptable alginate impression of the mandibular arch of an articulated manikin. (An acceptable impression meets the criteria outlined in the text or as specified by the instructor.)

	SE	IE
SE = Student evaluation **C** = Criterion met **IE** = Instructor evaluation **X** = Criterion not met		
Instrumentation: Mandibular typodont, alginate powder, room-temperature water, measuring devices for the water and powder, flexible rubber mixing bowl, spatula, assorted perforated mandibular trays, peripheral wax, and paper towels. (Appropriate infection control barriers will be used during all procedures actually performed on a patient.)		
1. Selected tray and modified borders with peripheral wax.		
2. Placed measured alginate powder and water in mixing bowl. Mixed to homogeneous consistency in less than 1 minute.		
3. Loaded tray. Smoothed surface of alginate with finger moistened with water.		
4. Spread alginate on occlusal and interproximal surfaces of teeth. Positioned tray so that it was centered over the teeth and arch. Pressed tray firmly into place.		
5. Allowed material to set. Removed tray in a straight upward movement without damage to the impression or discomfort to the patient.		
6. Disinfected and stored the impression until it could be poured.		
7. Cleaned bowl and spatula. Returned supplies to storage space. Left work area neat and ready for use.		
Comments:		

▼ Criterion Sheet 17–2

Student's Name _____

Procedure: *OBTAINING A WAX-BITE REGISTRATION*

Performance Objective:

The student will obtain a wax-bite registration of the patient's maxillary and mandibular dentition in centric occlusion.

	SE	IE
SE = Student evaluation **C** = Criterion met **IE** = Instructor evaluation **X** = Criterion not met		
Instrumentation: Preformed wax-bite registration wafers, pan and warm water or Bunsen burner and matches. (Appropriate infection control barriers will be used during all procedures actually performed on a patient.)		
1. Informed patient of the procedure. Examined the patient's oral cavity. Requested patient to remove prosthesis (if present). Asked patient to rinse mouth to remove debris.		
2. Selected wax wafer and warmed slightly over flame of bunsen burner or in pan of warm water.		
3. Placed wax wafer on occlusal surfaces of mandibular teeth.		
4. Directed patient to close normally (in centric occlusion).		
5. Allowed wax to cool. Asked patient to open mouth carefully.		
6. Removed wax wafer without distortion.		
7. Sprayed wax-bite registration with disinfecting solution. Placed wax-bite registration aside.		
8. Checked patient's dentition for excess wax. Asked patient to rinse mouth.		
Comments:		

▼ Criterion Sheet 17–3

Student's Name _____

Procedure: *PRODUCING DIAGNOSTIC CASTS IN DENTAL PLASTER*

Performance Objective:

Using the double-pour method, the student will produce acceptable diagnostic casts in dental plaster. (An acceptable diagnostic cast will meet the criteria specified in the text or as established by the instructor.)

		SE	IE
SE = Student evaluation **C** = Criterion met **IE** = Instructor evaluation **X** = Criterion not met			
Instrumentation: Alginate impressions, dental plaster, room-temperature water, measuring devices for water and powder, flexible mixing bowl, laboratory spatula, and a vibrator.			
1. Checked impression for acceptability. If necessary, rinsed to remove any debris, blood, or saliva.			
2. Used air syringe to remove excessive moisture from impression.			
3. Measured materials to be used.			
4. Mixed and vibrated dental plaster to homogeneous consistency within 1 minute.			
5. Used small, continuous increments to pour and complete the impression.			
6. Mixed plaster and prepared base. Placed poured impression on base. Removed excess plaster from sides of impression tray.			
7. Placed poured impression safely aside.			
8. Cleaned bowl and spatula. Returned supplies to storage space. Left work area neat and ready for use.			
Comments:			

▼ Criterion Sheet 17–4

Student's Name _____

Procedure: *TRIMMING A PLASTER DIAGNOSTIC CAST*

Performance Objective:

The student will trim a mandibular plaster diagnostic cast.

	SE	IE
SE = Student evaluation **C** = Criterion met **IE** = Instructor evaluation **X** = Criterion not met		
Instrumentation: Safety goggles, untrimmed mandibular cast (soaked in water bath), plastic ruler, pencil, laboratory knife, measuring devices (compass, gauges), and model trimmer.		
1. Donned safety goggles.		
2. Removed cast from water bath.		
3. Used a laboratory knife to remove any plaster balls from the cast.		
4. Used ruler and marked a line 3 mm down into vestibule at area parallel to the posterior teeth.		
5. Turned on model trimmer and adjusted water flow.		
6. Placed cast against trimmer wheel and cut cast to line at facial area of the posterior teeth.		
7. Marked line at long axis (midline) of each cuspid and at midsagittal. Connected lines.		
8. Placed cast against trimmer wheel and cut cast to produce a point at midsagittal (cuspid to cuspid).		
9. Placed posterior of cast against wheel and produced a line 3 mm beyond the retromolar area and perpendicular to midsagittal line. Avoided cutting into third molars or into facial surfaces of teeth.		
Comments:		

Pharmacology and Pain Control

The student will be able to:

1. Differentiate between the brand names and generic names of drugs.

2. Name five abused drugs and state why each is of concern to the dental practice.

3. Describe the placement of topical anesthetic prior to the administration of a local anesthetic.

4. Describe obtaining local anesthesia by block and infiltration injection techniques.

5. Describe the use of nitrous oxide – oxygen relative analgesia in dentistry.

6. Demonstrate the preparation of an anesthetic syringe.

7. Demonstrate passing and receiving the anesthetic syringe at chairside.

OVERVIEW OF PHARMACOLOGY AND PAIN CONTROL

Pharmacology is the study of drugs, especially as they relate to medicinal uses.

The dentist and staff are concerned with maintaining patient comfort throughout all procedures. For most patients, this is accomplished with the use of topical and local anesthetics.

PHARMACOLOGY

Prescriptions

A prescription is a written order authorizing the pharmacist to furnish a certain drug to a patient. It is made up of the components shown in Figure 18–1.

When medication is prescribed, a copy of the prescription is maintained in the patient's record.

Under no circumstances may a dental assistant prescribe medication. Medicine is dispensed *only* with the explicit instructions and under the direct supervision of the dentist.

Brand names are those drug names that are controlled by business firms and have registered trademarks. Brand names are always capitalized.

Generic names are those drug names that any business firm may use. All common and unprotected names fall into this second group. Generic names are *not* capitalized.

For example, Valium is the brand name of a drug used to treat anxiety. The generic name for Valium is diazepam.

Drug Abuse

A patient may be under the influence of drugs when he comes to the dental office. Any suspicious behavior should be called to the doctor's attention immediately.

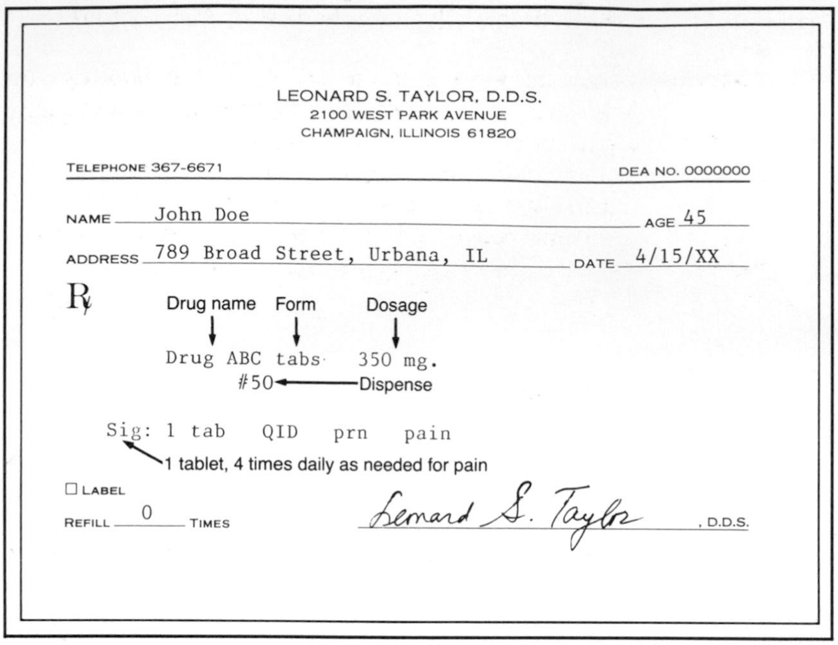

LEONARD S. TAYLOR, D.D.S.
2100 WEST PARK AVENUE
CHAMPAIGN, ILLINOIS 61820

TELEPHONE 367-6671   DEA NO. 0000000

NAME___John Doe_____ AGE _45___

ADDRESS___789 Broad Street, Urbana, IL_____ DATE _4/15/XX___

R̥

Drug name   Form   Dosage
    ↓   ↓   ↓

Drug ABC tabs·   350 mg.
    #50◄────Dispense

Sig: 1 tab   QID   prn   pain
    ↘1 tablet, 4 times daily as needed for pain
□ LABEL

REFILL ___0___ TIMES   *Leonard S. Taylor*   , D.D.S.

▼ **Figure 18–1**

Sample prescription blank. (Courtesy of Colwell Systems, Inc, Champaign, IL.)

Also, some individuals go from doctor to doctor collecting prescriptions to control a vague but severe pain that tends to "come and go" yet defies diagnosis. Alert the dentist if you suspect a patient is doing this.

Furthermore, never leave prescription pads out where they might be stolen. Instead, they should be kept in their properly locked place. The following are abused drugs of primary concern in the dental office:

▼ **Alcohol** is a depressant. Symptoms of use include impaired judgment, slurred speech, staggering, and drowsiness. It may also cause confusion and aggressive behavior. Antianxiety agents, which may be administered prior to a dental procedure, can have a deadly effect when they are combined with alcohol.

▼ **Amphetamines**, also known as *uppers*, are stimulants. They may produce excitement, increased wakefulness, talkativeness, and hallucinations.

▼ **Barbiturates**, also known as *downers*, are depressants. They may produce drowsiness, staggering, slurred speech, confusion, and aggressive behavior.

▼ **Cocaine** is a powerful central nervous system stimulant and a vasoconstrictor. It may produce extreme restlessness, excitement, tachycardia (rapid heart rate), and talkativeness.
    Caution: It is important that the dentist know whether the patient uses cocaine because cocaine may interact with the epinephrine in local anesthetic solution. This can possibly cause a dangerous increase in heart rate and blood pressure. Also, the use of cocaine can make nitrous oxide administration hazardous.

▼ **Heroin**, and other narcotics of this type, depress the central nervous system. They produce euphoria, pinpoint pupils, and drowsiness, lethargy, or stupor.

Antibiotics

Antibiotics are chemical substances that are able to inhibit the growth of or destroy bacteria and other microorganisms. (Antibiotics are *not* effective against viruses.)

The antibiotic will be selected because it is known to be particularly effective against certain bacteria. Antibiotics may be prescribed in combination to increase their effectiveness.

Patient Sensitivity

A patient may be allergic or sensitive to a specific antibiotic. A thorough medical history is therefore essential to determine that the patient has not experienced any previous allergic or adverse reactions to this agent.

Prophylactic Antibiotic Administration

As used here, the term **prophylactic** means a preventive measure. Because of the danger of a bacterial infection, prophylactic antibiotic administration is recommended for certain patients in conjunction with all dental procedures that are likely to cause bleeding.

This preventive measure is recommended for patients with a history of congenital heart disease, open heart surgery, pacemakers, and certain other forms of heart disease.

Some dentists also recommend it for patients with artificial joints, such as a hip replacement.

The antibiotic is administered *before* the patient is seen for dental treatment and is usually continued for several days after treatment.

Penicillin

Penicillin is a generic term for a group of antibiotics that are similar in chemical structure but different in their antibacterial spectrum and oral absorption rate.

Penicillin is most useful in dentistry to combat infections caused by gram-positive bacteria such as streptococci. However, it is not effective in the treatment of infections caused by many gram-negative microorganisms, viruses, or fungi.

Cephalosporins

The cephalosporin group of antibiotics is chemically related to the penicillins. They are broad-spectrum antibiotics that are active against a wide variety of both gram-positive and gram-negative organisms.

However, their dental use is limited to the treatment of infections with sensitive organisms when other agents are ineffective or cannot be used.

Erythromycin

Erythromycin closely resembles penicillin in its spectrum of antibacterial activity and may be used with penicillin-hypersensitive patients or when organisms have become penicillin-resistant.

Tetracyclines

The tetracyclines are broad-spectrum antibiotics affecting a wide range of microorganisms. However, they are not generally considered to be the drug of choice for the majority of oral infections.

The administration of tetracycline antibiotics from the second trimester of pregnancy to approximately 8 years of age may produce permanent discoloration of the teeth, which is called **tetracycline staining**.

Antianxiety Agents, Sedatives, and Hypnotics

Antianxiety agents, sedatives, and hypnotics may be used as premedication to calm an apprehensive patient prior to dental treatment.

Antianxiety agents, such as diazepam (Valium), are used to suppress mild to moderate anxiety and tension. **Sedatives** reduce excitability and create calmness. **Hypnotics** produce sleep.

Analgesics

Analgesics are drugs that dull the perception of pain without producing unconsciousness. They may be used preoperatively to relieve pain such as toothache, or they may be prescribed to relieve postoperative pain.

Mild analgesics, such as aspirin, are drugs used for the relief of low intensity pain, such as some headaches. These analgesics provide adequate pain relief for most types of dental pain, including a toothache or the discomfort that may follow the extraction of a tooth.

Strong analgesics, which include some narcotic drugs, are prescribed only for patients with severe pain such as that which follows an extensive surgical procedure.

These narcotic drugs are capable of producing physical and psychological dependence, and their extended use should be avoided. These narcotic drugs include codeine, Percodan, Demerol, morphine, and Dilaudid.

Epinephrine

Epinephrine is a vasoconstrictor. This means that it is a drug that constricts (narrows) the blood vessels. It also stimulates the heart and must be used with caution. However, epinephrine has many applications in dentistry.

Use in Local Anesthesia

Epinephrine added to the local anesthetic solution decreases blood flow in the immediate area of the injection. This decreased blood flow increases the duration of the anesthetic effect and reduces bleeding near the site of the injection.

Epinephrine is added to the local anesthetic solution in very small quantities. Usually this is in a 1:50,000 or 1:100,000 ratio of epinephrine to anesthetic solution.

Use in Gingival Retraction

Vasoconstrictors are frequently used for temporary retraction of gingival tissue from the margins of the cavity or crown preparation.

A common gingival retracting cavity agent is dry cotton cord impregnated with racemic epinephrine in a concentration of 500 to 1000 mg to the inch. (See Chapter 24, "Crown and Bridge Restorations.")

Use Following Surgical Procedures

Vasoconstrictors may be used to control diffuse bleeding following surgical procedures, such as a gingivectomy, when the surgical area is not covered by sutured tissue.

The vasoconstrictor is usually applied directly to the affected tissue on a gauze strip saturated with 1:1000 epinephrine. The strip is left in place for several minutes while surgical dressings are prepared.

Use in Severe Allergic Reactions

In the event of a severe anaphylactic allergic reaction, epinephrine may be injected subcutaneously or intramuscularly as a cardiac stimulant.

NITROUS OXIDE–OXYGEN RELATIVE ANALGESIA

The terms *analgesia*, *relative analgesia*, and *psychosedation* are all used commonly and interchangeably. In this discussion, the term relative analgesia is used.

Relative analgesia with nitrous oxide and oxygen acts primarily as a sedative to help eliminate fear and to relax the patient. Significant pain control still depends on the use of an effective local anesthesic agent.

Relative analgesia has the advantages of being a pleasant, relaxing experience for the patient with easy onset, minimal side effects, and rapid recovery (Fig. 18–2).

Although this technique has an excellent reputation for safety, it is not without danger.

1. It is a drug, and it must not be abused.
2. It should never be used for "recreational purposes" or used regularly to help one "relax."
3. Administration should always be closely monitored and properly supervised by the dentist.
4. All equipment must meet current safety standards, be kept in proper working condition, and be monitored regularly.
5. The hazards of working with nitrous oxide are discussed in Chapter 8, "Hazards Management in the Dental Office."

Contraindications for Use of Relative Analgesia

Relative analgesia is *not* recommended for patients with the following conditions:

1. An upper respiratory infection or nasal obstruction that makes breathing through the nose difficult.
2. The inability to understand what is happening.
3. Multiple sclerosis or advanced emphysema.
4. Emotional instability, such as a drug addiction or certain psychiatric conditions.

Planes of Analgesia

Analgesia is actually the first stage of general anesthesia. The analgesia stage is divided into three planes. Of these three planes, only the first two are the desired levels of relative analgesia.

Analgesia Plane 1

Respiration, blood pressure, pulse, muscle tone, and eye movements are normal. The patient is able to keep the mouth open without a mouth prop and is capable of following directions.

The patient appears to be fully conscious and relaxed. There may be a tingling in fingers, toes, lips, or tongue. There is a marked elevation of the pain reaction threshold and a diminution of fear.

Relative Analgesia Instrumentation

▼ Nitrous oxide–oxygen dispensing unit (wall installation or portable unit) with control valves and gauges (one for oxygen, one for nitrous oxide).

▼ "E" tank of oxygen (green) with a reserve tank.

▼ "E" tank of nitrous oxide (blue) with a reserve tank.

▼ Sanitized masks, adult and child sizes.

▼ Emesis basin (in case the patient vomits).

Procedure

ASSISTING DURING RELATIVE ANALGESIA INDUCTION

Note: The assistant's role in the administration of nitrous oxide–oxygen is always directly supervised by the dentist.

1. Before the patient is seated, the assistant:

   Checks each tank of nitrous oxide and oxygen to determine that the tanks are full and that the gauges are operating correctly.

   Places a clean mask on the dual tubing connection of the gas unit in readiness for the patient.

   Verifies that the air vent of the mask is closed and the exhaust valve is open.

2. The dentist talks with the patient to determine his understanding of the effects and sensations of nitrous oxide–oxygen.

3. The patient is placed in a supine position in the dental chair.

   Upon the patient's acceptance, the mask is placed over his nose and is situated comfortably.

   The patient is instructed to exhale through his mouth and to breathe deeply and naturally through his nose to receive the most effect from the nitrous oxide–oxygen.

4. The dentist signals for the assistant to begin adjustment of the knobs controlling the valves and the flow of oxygen.

   The patient is given a flow of 5 to 8 L (liters) of 100 percent oxygen for 1 minute (Fig. 18–2).

5. The patient is advised to relax and attempt to breathe as calmly and deeply as is comfortable for him.

   The assistant observes the rise and fall of the rubber bag on the gas unit, which indicates the patient's breathing volume.

   If the patient is snorting, he is breathing too deeply, causing the mask to seal at the nostrils.

   If he exhales too strongly through the mask, the vent valve makes a whistling sound.

6. The patient is introduced to nitrous oxide at the rate of 1 L per minute while the oxygen flow is decreased at a similar rate.

   A 60-second pause is made between each adjustment until the patient is

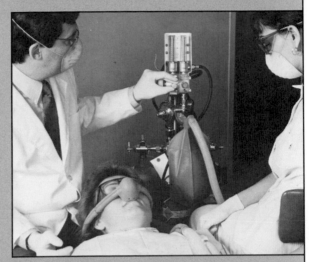

Figure 18–2 The administration of nitrous oxide–oxygen analgesia. (Torres HO, Ehrlich A: Modern Dental Assisting, 4th Ed. Philadelphia, WB Saunders, 1990, p 178.)

conscious and cooperative but pleasantly relaxed. The protective reflexes are intact and active.

The dentist or assistant, using a quiet tone, asks the patient how he feels; is he relaxed?

7. The optimal level for each patient is called the *baseline*. The oxygen–nitrous oxide gas ratio needed for this baseline varies from patient to patient.

   The least possible amount of nitrous oxide that will assure patient comfort is used.

   For most patients, 50 percent nitrous oxide *or less* is effective.

   Small children may require a lower percentage of nitrous oxide.

8. The dentist begins the procedure when the patient has reached and is maintained at the baseline level.

   For most patients, this level is a maximum of 6 to 7 total L of combined gases.

   For the patient with a 7 L per minute flow, the baseline may be 3 L of nitrous oxide and 4 L of oxygen per minute.

9. If the patient becomes nauseated, the nitrous oxide is turned off and 100 percent oxygen is administered.

   When the patient is comfortable, nitrous oxide–oxygen is again administered continuously and the procedure is continued.

Procedure

ASSISTING DURING RELATIVE ANALGESIA RECOVERY

1 When the procedure is completed:

The nitrous oxide control valve is returned to zero.

The oxygen is increased to the original 5 to 8 L flow per minute.

The patient is permitted to breathe 100 percent oxygen for about 2 minutes or until all signs of sedation are gone.

2 The patient's mask is removed and he is slowly seated upright.

The patient is questioned as to how he feels. Usually the response is a positive one, that the patient feels relaxed and comfortable.

3 Following the dismissal of the patient, the assistant records the baseline of nitrous oxide–oxygen on the patient's chart.

The patient's reaction to nitrous oxide–oxygen may vary from visit to visit according to his physical condition and degree of fatigue.

On future visits, the patient is introduced to the nitrous oxide–oxygen at the baseline recorded on his chart and adjustments are made as necessary.

Procedure

RELATIVE ANALGESIA: EQUIPMENT CARE

1 If the mask is the disposable type, discard it.

2 If the mask is the type that can be autoclaved, remove it and send it to the sterilization area.

3 If the mask cannot be autoclaved, clean it thoroughly and then disinfect it properly.

4 During operatory cleanup, clean and disinfect the tubes and equipment that were touched during treatment.

Analgesia Plane 2

Respiration, blood pressure, pulse, and muscle tone are normal. The patient appears to be relaxed and euphoric; however, he is still able to keep the mouth open and to follow directions. The patient has a pleasant feeling of lethargy. He feels safe, is less aware of his immediate surroundings, and is less concerned with activity around him.

He may feel a wave of warmth suffuse his entire body. Very often he experiences a humming or vibratory sensation throughout the body, somewhat like the soft purring of a motor.

At this time, the patient may also describe a feeling of headiness or drowsiness similar to light intoxication. His voice becomes throaty, losing its natural resonance. The patient's thoughts may wander beyond those of activity in the treatment room.

Analgesia Plane 3

If the patient becomes nauseated, vomits, or is restless, these are indications that he is in analgesia plane 3. The patient in analgesia plane 3 is no longer in relative analgesia and is moving toward the excitement stage of general anesthesia.

The patient's jaw may become rigid, and his mouth tends to close. His body may also stiffen, and the patient may appear to stare and have an angry or very sleepy look. Respiration, pulse, and blood pressure remain normal; however, the patient may have hallucinatory dreams or experience fear.

If the assistant observes the patient showing any indications of being in plane 3, the operator must be alerted immediately. A prompt increase in the oxygen supply and a decrease in nitrous oxide will return the patient to the desired plane.

TOPICAL ANESTHETICS

Topical anesthesia has a temporary effect on numbing the sensory nerve endings of the surface of the oral mucosa.

Topical anesthetics are used primarily to provide temporary numbness so that the dentist can make a "painless" local anesthetic injection through these tissues.

Ointment Topical Anesthetics

The topical anesthetic ointment is placed directly on the injection site to numb the tissue (Fig. 18–3). Because the rate of onset of topical anesthesia is slow, 2 to 5 minutes are required for optimum effectiveness.

Topical anesthetics are also used to provide temporary numbness during deep periodontal curettage. In addition, the ointment form may be used to provide temporary relief from the pain of oral injuries.

Liquid Topical Anesthetics

Liquid topical anesthetic agents are in the form of a thick liquid, containing a flavoring agent. They are applied by having the patient swish a small amount of the solution around in the mouth.

In patients who have an excessive gag reflex, liquid topical anesthetics are used to numb the surfaces of the oral tissues just prior to taking impressions or making intraoral radiographs.

They may also be used to provide temporary relief of the pain of ulcers, wounds, and other injured areas in the mouth.

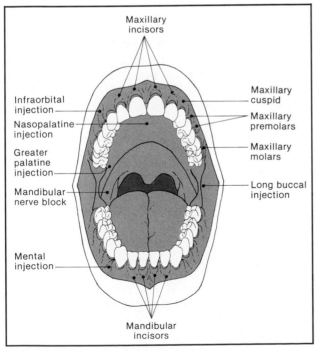

▼ **Figure 18–3**

Sites for application of topical anesthetic in preparation for injection of local anesthetic. (Torres HO, Ehrlich A: Modern Dental Assisting, 4th Ed. Philadelphia, WB Saunders, 1990, p 185.)

LOCAL ANESTHETICS

Local anesthetic agents are the most frequently used form of pain control in dentistry. These agents provide safe, effective, and dependable anesthesia of suitable duration for virtually all forms of dental surgery.

Chemical Formulation

Local anesthetic solutions for dental use may be broadly classified as **amides** or **esters**. Lidocaine (Xylocaine), mepivacaine (Carbocaine), and prilocaine (Citanest) are examples of amide solutions.

Procaine (Novocain), tetracaine (Pontocaine), and propoxycaine (Ravocaine) are examples of ester solutions.

For the rare patient who is thought to be allergic to a particular type of anesthetic, another chemical formulation may be substituted by the dentist.

Obtaining Local Anesthesia

Local anesthesia is obtained by depositing the anesthetic agent in proximity to the nerve in the area intended for dental treatment.

The local anesthetic agent then temporarily blocks the normal generation and conduction action of the nerve impulses.

Induction time is the length of time from the deposition of the anesthetic solution to complete an effective conduction blockage.

Duration is the length of time from induction until the reversal process is complete.

The action of a local anesthetic continues until the concentration is carried away by the bloodstream.

Cautions for Use

It is very important to keep the patient under observation following the injection of local anesthetic. If unusual reactions develop, supportive measures should be started promptly. (See Chapter 9, "Emergencies in the Dental Office.")

Hazards for Heart Patients

Because the action of a vasoconstrictor may cause strain on the heart, use of a local anesthetic solution **without epinephrine** is recommended for patients with a history of heart disease, hyperthyroidism, or hypertension.

Other dental uses of vasoconstrictors should also be avoided for these patients.

Administration into a Blood Vessel

Local anesthetic solution administered directly into the bloodstream can alter the function of vital organs, notably the heart. Therefore, the dentist takes precautions to ensure that the solution is not deposited directly into a blood vessel.

An aspirating type syringe is used to administer the local anesthetic so that the dentist may aspirate following insertion of the needle. (To **aspirate** means to draw back.)

If blood is aspirated, the direction of the needle is altered to avoid injecting the solution into a blood vessel.

Infected Areas

Local anesthetics are not effective when injected into an infected area. Also, with injection into an infected area, there is always the danger of spreading the infection.

Temporary Numbness

Because local anesthesia effectively blocks all pain sensation, the patient must be cautioned against biting himself while his tongue or lip is numb.

Localized Toxic Reactions

Local anesthetic solutions are, as a rule, exceptionally well tolerated by the tissues. However, they may produce a variety of local tissue changes.

In some sensitive individuals, contact with solutions containing local anesthetic agents may cause **contact dermatitis**. Anyone with a history of hypersensitivity should avoid unnecessary contact with all local anesthetics.

Paresthesia

Paresthesia, or persistent anesthesia, means that the effects of the local anesthetic do not go away within a reasonable time after the dental treatment. This is an infrequent complication of local anesthesia that may be caused by damage to the nerve or surrounding tissues.

Paresthesia is usually resolved, without treatment, in approximately 8 weeks. However, the paresthesia may be permanent if the damage to the nerve was severe.

When paresthesia occurs, the patient may call the dental office several hours after receiving local anesthesia and complain of continued numbness.

If this happens, it is important that the dental assistant let the dentist talk to the patient and not try to reassure the patient herself.

Types of Injections for Local Anesthesia

The location and innervation of the tooth, or teeth, to be anesthetized determine the topical anesthesia placement and the type of injection to be used. (See Chapter 3 for details on the innervation of the teeth.)

Infiltration Anesthesia

Infiltration anesthesia involves placement of the anesthetic solution directly into the tissues at the site of the dental procedure. This technique is most frequently used to anesthetize the maxillary teeth.

Infiltration anesthesia is possible in the maxillary teeth because of the more "porous" nature of the alveolus cancellous bone, which allows the solution to reach the apices of the teeth. (The **apices** are the tips of the roots of the teeth. It is here that the nerve enters the tooth.)

Infiltration anesthesia may also be used as a secondary injection to block gingival tissues surrounding the mandibular teeth.

Figure 18–4 shows the sites and technique for infiltration injections.

Block Anesthesia

Infiltration anesthesia is not possible for general use in the mandible because the extremely dense,

---

▼ Figure 18–4

Sites for injection of anesthetics. *A* and *B*. **Anterior superior infiltration site** (*A*, needle inserted at injection site; *B*, cross section).
C and *D*. **Posterior superior alveolar injection site** (*C*, needle inserted at injection site; *D*, cross section).
E and *F*. **Infraorbital nerve block injection site** (*E*, needle inserted at injection site; *F*, cross section).
G and *H*. **Nasopalatine nerve block injection site** (*G*, needle inserted at injection site; *H*, cross section).
I and *J*. **Anterior palatine nerve block** (*I*, needle inserted at injection site; *J*, cross section). (Torres HO, Ehrlich A: Modern Dental Assisting, 4th Ed. Philadelphia, WB Saunders, 1990, pp 189–190.)

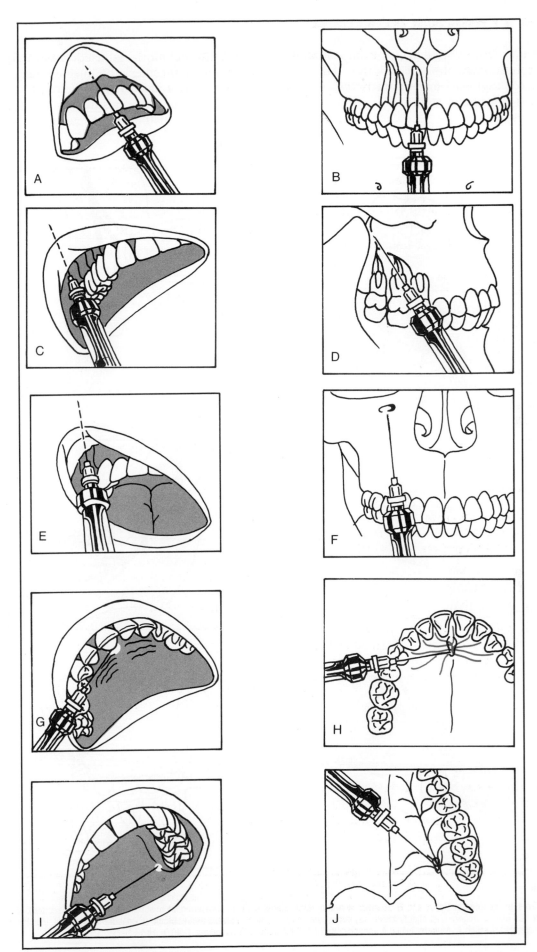

Figure 18-4 See legend on opposite page.

compact nature of the bone makes it impossible to place the solution near the apices of the teeth.

<u>Block</u> (or regional) anesthesia is obtained by injecting the anesthetic solution in the <u>proximity of the nerve trunk.</u>

This technique is used most frequently for mandibular anesthesia by injecting near the branch of the inferior alveolar nerve close to the mandibular foramen. This anesthetizes the teeth in that quadrant plus half of the tongue and lower lip.

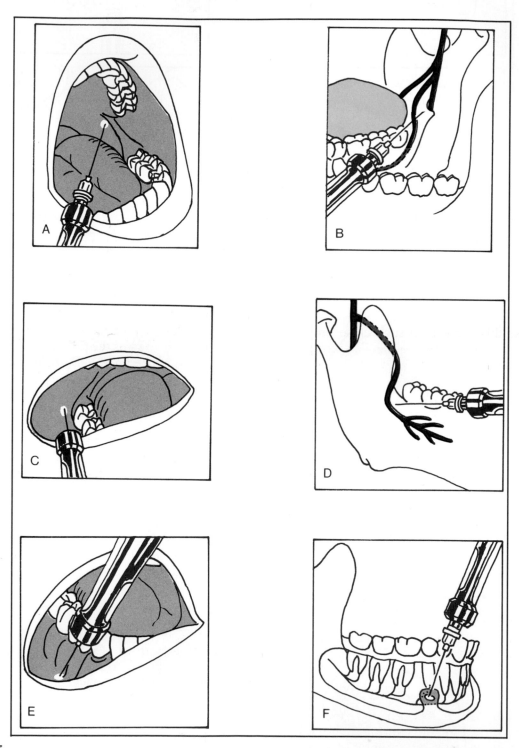

▼ **Figure 18–5**

Types of nerve block anesthesia. *A* and *B*. **Inferior alveolar nerve block** (*A*, needle inserted at injection site; *B*, cross section). *C* and *D*. **Buccal nerve block** (*C*, needle inserted at injection site; *D*, cross section). *E* and *F*. **Mental nerve block** (*E*, needle inserted at injection site; *F*, cross section). (Torres HO, Ehrlich A: Modern Dental Assisting, 4th Ed. Philadelphia, WB Saunders, 1990, p 188.)

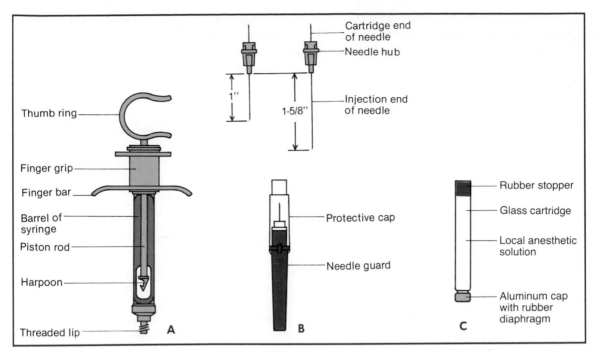

▼ **Figure 18-6**

Equipment for local anesthetic administration. *A.* Aspirating syringe. *B.* Disposable needles. *C.* Local anesthetic cartridge. (Torres HO, Ehrlich A: Modern Dental Assisting, 4th Ed. Philadelphia, WB Saunders, 1990, p 191.)

Because this nerve is in such close proximity to the blood vessels here, the dentist takes particular care in making this injection so that the solution is not deposited directly into the bloodstream.

Figure 18-5 shows the sites and technique for this and other mandibular injections.

Anesthetic Syringe

Figure 18-6*A* is a diagram of the kind of syringe used in the administration of block and infiltration local anesthesia. It is made up of the following parts.

Thumb Ring, Finger Grip, Finger Bar

These are the parts that make it possible for the dentist to control the syringe firmly and to "aspirate" effectively using one hand.

Harpoon

When the harpoon is hooked into the rubber stopper of the anesthetic cartridge, the rubber stopper can be retracted by pulling back on the piston rod. It is this action that makes aspiration possible.

To be certain that the solution is not being injected directly into the bloodstream, the dentist aspirates as he begins the injection.

To **aspirate** means to draw back, and the dentist literally draws back on the piston of the syringe to be certain the needle has not entered a blood vessel.

If the needle has entered a blood vessel, a thin line of red blood cells will be drawn into the anesthetic cartridge. Should this happen, the dentist repositions the needle before continuing.

Piston Rod

This rod pushes down the rubber stopper of the anesthetic cartridge and forces the anesthetic solution out through the needle.

Barrel of the Syringe

The barrel firmly holds the anesthetic cartridge in place. One side of the barrel is open, and the cartridge is loaded through this area. The other side has a window so that the dentist can watch for blood cells as he aspirates.

Threaded Tip

The hub of the needle is attached to the syringe on the threaded tip.

The cartridge end of the needle passes

through the small opening in the center of the threaded tip. This enables it to puncture the rubber diaphragm of the anesthetic cartridge.

Disposable Needle

The needle used for the injection is made up of the following parts (see Fig. 18–6B).

Lumen

The lumen is the hollow center of the needle through which the anesthetic solution flows.

Cartridge End of the Needle

This is the shorter end of the needle. It fits through the threaded tip of the syringe and punctures the rubber diaphragm of the anesthetic cartridge.

Needle Hub

The needle hub may be either self-threading plastic or a prethreaded metal hub. It is attached to the threaded tip of the syringe.

Needle Length

The injection end of the needle comes in two lengths. It may be either 1 inch or 1⅝ inch. Most commonly, the 1-inch "short" needle is used for infiltration anesthesia and the 1⅝-inch "long" needle is used for block anesthesia.

The tip of the needle is **beveled** (angled), and during the injection the bevel is turned toward the alveolus to deposit the solution accurately.

Needle Gage

The needle gage refers to the thickness of the needle. Gages are numbered so that the larger the gage number, the thinner the needle.

Since a longer needle needs more strength, a longer needle is commonly used in a lower gage number. The most commonly used gage numbers are 25, 27, and 30.

Anesthetic Cartridges

Local anesthetic solutions are supplied in glass cartridges with a rubber stopper at one end and an aluminum cap, with a rubber diaphragm, at the other (see Fig. 18–6C).

The rubber stopper is color-coded to indicate the epinephrine ratio of the solution. Learn to identify these and always take care to select the ratio specified by the dentist.

Also, always take the precaution of double checking the patient's chart and medical history before selecting the anesthetic solution.

Cartridges should be stored at room temperature and protected from direct sunlight.

Local Anesthetic Solution Precautions

1. Never use a cartridge that has been frozen. An extruded rubber stopper and a large air bubble are signs that the solution may have been frozen.
2. Do not use a cartridge if it is cracked, chipped,

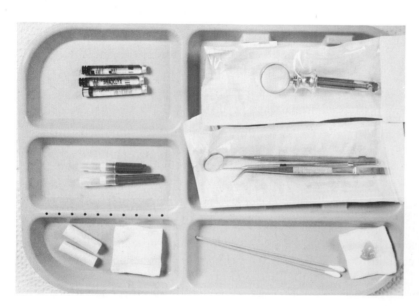

▼ **Figure 18–7**

Pre-set tray for local anesthetic administration. (Torres HO, Ehrlich A: Modern Dental Assisting, 4th Ed. Philadelphia, WB Saunders, 1990, p 193.)

or damaged in any way because it could break during pressure of the injection.

3. Never use a solution that is discolored, appears cloudy, or has passed the expiration date shown on the package.

4. Do not leave the syringe preloaded with the needle attached for an extended period of time. Doing this allows metal from the needle to contaminate the solution, and this may cause edema (swelling) following use of the solution.

Disinfecting Cartridges

Cartridges are supplied with the contents already sterilized. If necessary, the cartridge may be autoclaved once. Cartridges are *not* stored in disinfecting solution.

Just prior to use, the rubber diaphragm and cap end of the cartridge are disinfected by wiping a gauze sponge moistened with either 70 percent ethyl alcohol or undiluted isopropyl alcohol.

Discarding Used Cartridges

Never save a cartridge for reuse. Once the needle and syringe have been assembled, the cartridge must either be used or discarded.

Because of the danger of broken glass, the used cartridge is discarded in the rigid-sided sharps container in the operatory.

Administration of Local Anesthetics

The prepared local anesthetic tray and other necessary supplies are positioned at chairside. The assistant then washes her hands and dons gloves before preparing the anesthetic syringe. The syringe is prepared out of the patient's sight.

Instrumentation (Fig. 18–7)

▼ Topical anesthetic ointment.

▼ Cotton-tipped applicators.

▼ Gauze sponges and/or cotton rolls.

▼ Basic setup.

▼ Sterile syringe.

▼ Sealed disposable needle(s).

▼ Local anesthetic cartridges.

Procedure

PREPARING THE ANESTHETIC SYRINGE

1. The dentist verifies the type of anesthetic solution (brand and epinephrine content) plus the needle length and needle gage that are to be used. These choices are based on the patient's medical history and on the procedure to be performed.

2. Select the correct anesthetic cartridge. Double-check that this is the type of anesthetic specified by the dentist.
   Warning: Failure to select the correct anesthetic solution can have serious consequences for the patient.

3. Disinfect the rubber diaphragm and the cap end of the cartridge with a gauze sponge moistened with alcohol.

4. Unwrap the sterile syringe, then hold the syringe in one hand and use the thumb ring to pull back the plunger.

5. With the other hand, load the anesthetic cartridge into the syringe. The rubber

stopper end goes in first, toward the plunger.

6. Securely grasp the syringe and cartridge in one hand.
   Use the other hand to apply firm pressure (tapping the plunger handle if needed) until the harpoon is engaged (hooked) into the rubber stopper.
   To check that the harpoon is securely in place, gently pull back on the plunger.

7. Remove the protective cap from the needle, but do not remove the needle guard.

8. Screw the needle into position on the syringe. Take care to position the needle so that it is straight and firmly attached. Otherwise, the anesthetic solution may leak or not flow properly.

9. Place the prepared syringe on the tray ready for use and out of the patient's sight.

Procedure

APPLICATION OF TOPICAL ANESTHETIC

1 Place the ointment on a sterile cotton-tipped applicator.

    If taking ointment directly from a container, replace the cover immediately.

    The cotton-tipped applicator is never dipped into the ointment container a second time.

2 Dry the injection site with a sterile gauze sponge.

3 Remove the gauze sponge and position the applicator with the ointment directly on the injection site (Fig. 18–8).

4 Repeat these steps if more than one injection is to be given.

    Note: The cotton-tipped applicator is never reused.

5 Leave the applicator in place for 2 to 5 minutes. It is removed by the operator just prior to injection of the local anesthetic.

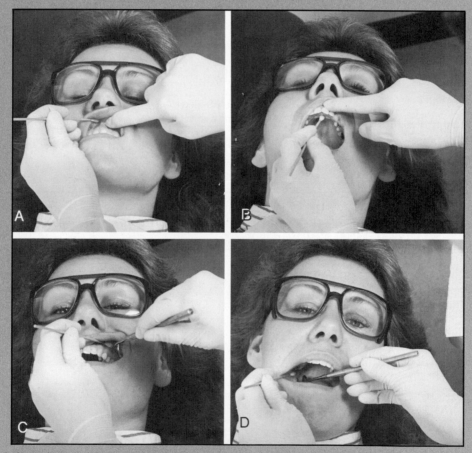

Figure 18–8 Topical anesthetic placement. *A.* Maxillary central incisor. *B.* Nasopalatine injection. *C.* Maxillary premolar. *D.* Mandibular block. (Torres HO, Ehrlich A: Modern Dental Assisting, 4th Ed. Philadelphia, WB Saunders, 1990, p 193.)

Procedure

PASSING THE SYRINGE

This exchange is made just below the patient's chin and out of the patient's line of vision.

1. The assistant loosens the needle guard but does not remove it.

2. The assistant receives the used topical anesthetic applicator with her left hand and passes the syringe to the operator with the right hand (Fig. 18–9).

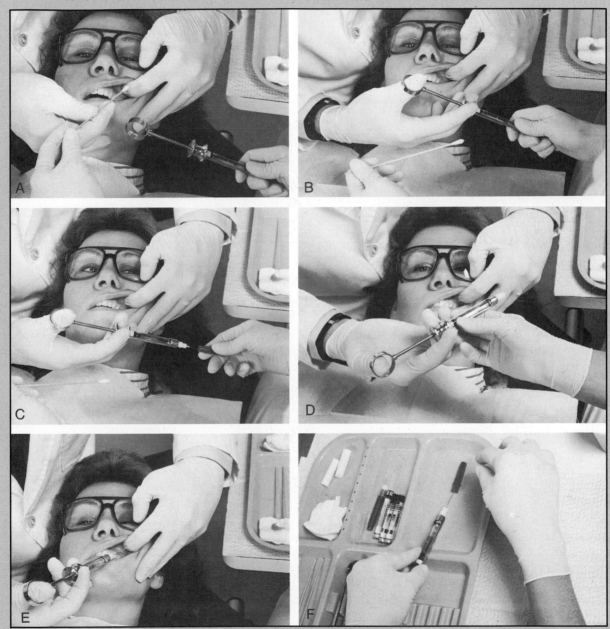

Figure 18–9 Passing and receiving the local anesthesia syringe. *A.* The assistant receives the used topical anesthetic applicator and passes the syringe to the dentist. *B.* The assistant secures the thumb ring on the dentist's finger. *C.* The assistant slips off the needle guard. *D.* The assistant rotates the syringe so that the bevel (lumen) of the needle is toward the bone. *E.* The dentist completes the injection. *F.* The assistant uses the one-handed scooping technique to recap the needle safely without touching it. (Torres HO, Ehrlich A: Modern Dental Assisting, 4th Ed. Philadelphia, WB Saunders, 1990, p 194.)

Continued

3 In passing the syringe to the operator, the assistant places the thumb ring over the operator's thumb and then the syringe is laid into the operator's open hand.

4 The assistant carefully removes the needle guard and rotates the needle bevel so that the lumen is directed toward the bone for the injection.

5 While the operator is giving the injection, the assistant guards against any sudden movement by the patient.

6 When the injection is completed, the assistant carefully receives the used syringe and hands the operator the air-water syringe. The air-water syringe and high volume evacuator (HVE) tip are used to rinse the patient's mouth.

7 Replace the needle guard over the needle before the used syringe is returned to the tray.

Recapping the Needle

Needle-stick injuries are serious, and Occupational Safety and Health Adminstration (OSHA) regulations state the needle *must not* be recapped unless the employee can demonstrate that no alternative is feasible or that such action is required by a special medical procedure.

If recapping is required, an acceptable method is the one-handed scoop technique, which is shown in Figure 18–9F. This involves the following steps.

1. Place the needle guard on the tray. Do *not* hold it.
2. Gently "tease" the end of the used needle into the open end of the guard.
3. Keep fingers off the guard until the end of the needle is covered.
4. Once the end of the needle is covered, it is safe to pick up the guard and slip it into position.

Care of a Needle-Stick Injury   Pg 139

All needle-stick injuries must be treated as being potentially infectious and very serious. They must also be reported to the dentist. See Chapter 9 for details on the treatment of a needle-stick injury.

Syringe Care

Do *not* bend or break the needle by hand before discarding it. During cleanup, discard the used needle (with the needle guard still in place) in a suitable "sharps" container. (See Chapter 8, "Hazards Management in the Dental Office.")

The used syringe is returned to the sterilization area to be cleaned and sterilized for use again.

▼ EXERCISES

1. The used needle is discarded in the _____.

   a. operatory
   b. sharps container ✓
   c. sterilization area
   d. a and b

2. The local anesthetic syringe transfer is made _____.

   a. just below the patient's chin ✓
   b. level with the patient's eyes
   c. over the patient's chest
   d. a, b, or c

3. _Hypnotics_ _____ produce sleep.

   a. Antianxiety agents *lessens anxiety & tension*
   b. Hypnotics *induces sleep.* ✓
   c. Sedatives – *calms & reduces excitability*
   d. b and c

4. Epinephrine is usually added to local anesthetic solution in a _____ ratio.

   a. 1:25,000
   b. 1:50,000
   c. 1:100,000
   d. b or c ✓

5. The prophylactic administration of _____ is indicated for patients with a history of certain types of heart disease, pacemakers, and artificial joints.

   a. antibiotics ✓
   b. mild analgesics
   c. premedication
   d. sedatives

6. The tank of _O₂_ gas is always green.

   a. nitrous oxide ✓
   b. oxygen

7. In analgesia plane _____, the patient is nauseated or restless.

   a. 1
   b. 2
   c. 3

8. If administered from the second trimester of pregnancy to approximately 8 years of age, _d_ may produce permanent discoloration of the developing teeth.

   a. cephalosporin
   b. erythromycin
   c. penicillin
   d. tetracycline ✓

9. A vasoconstrictor _____ b _____ the blood vessels.

    a. expands
    b. narrows

10. If the patient becomes nauseated during the adminstration of nitrous oxide–oxygen, _____.

    a. all gases are discontinued
    b. 100 percent oxygen is adminstered
    c. the flow of nitrous oxide is decreased
    d. the flow of nitrous oxide is increased

11. Antianxiety agents, which may be administered prior to a dental procedure, may have a deadly effect when combined with _____ a _____.

    a. alcohol *is a depressant, confusion, aggression, slurred speech*
    b. amphetamines
    c. barbiturates
    d. epinephrine

12. _____ a _____ anesthesia is achieved by injecting the anesthetic solution in the proximity of the nerve trunk.

    a. Block
    b. Infiltration

13. A needle-stick injury is _____ a _____.

    a. always potentially dangerous
    b. not dangerous if the needle has not been used yet
    c. potentially dangerous only if the needle was used for a high-risk patient

14. In the event of a severe anaphylactic allergic reaction, _____ a _____ may be injected as a cardiac stimulant.

    a. cephalosporin
    b. diazepam
    c. epinephrine
    d. erythromycin

15. A _____ a. 1" _____-inch needle is used for administering infiltration anesthesia.

    a. 1
    b. 1½
    c. 2
    d. a or b

16. _____ Cocaine _____ combined with local anesthetic solution may cause a dangerous increase in heart rate and blood pressure.

    a. Alcohol
    b. Cocaine *stimulant CNS? + vasoconstriction*
    c. Morphine
    d. Penicillin

17. _____ Aspirin _____ is an example of a mild analgesic that may be recommended for any discomfort that may follow the extraction of a tooth.

a. Aspirin
b. Codeine
c. Dilaudid
d. Morphine

18. Antibiotics _____ *b* _____ effective against viruses.

a. are
b. are not

19. The needle guard is removed _____ .

a. after the syringe is placed in the operator's hand
b. by the operator just prior to the injection
c. prior to passing the syringe
d. when the syringe is prepared

20. If the patient moves beyond the second plane of nitrous oxide–oxygen relative analgesia, _____ oxygen will help return the patient to the desired plane.

a. decreased
b. increased

21. The _____ *d* _____ on the local anesthetic syringe makes it possible to aspirate to be certain that the needle has not entered a blood vessel.

a. barrel
b. harpoon
c. hub
d. piston rod

22. Local anesthetic with epinephrine _____ *b* _____ recommended for patients with a history of heart disease.

a. is
b. is not

23. When applying topical anesthetics, _____ *c* _____ minutes are required for optimum effectiveness.

a. 1 to 2
b. 2 to 3
c. 2 to 5   *319*
d. 3 to 6

24. _____ *a* _____ names are controlled by business firms, have registered trademarks, and are always capitalized.

a. Brand
b. Generic
c. Prescription
d. Trade

25. _____ *e* _____ anesthesia numbs all of the teeth in the affected quadrant.

a. Block
b. Infiltration

▼ Criterion Sheet 18–1

Student's Name _____

Procedure: *PREPARING A LOCAL ANESTHETIC SYRINGE*

Performance Objective:

The student will demonstrate the preparation of a local anesthetic syringe for a mandibular block local anesthetic injection.

	SE	IE
SE = Student evaluation **C** = Criterion met **IE** = Instructor evaluation **X** = Criterion not met		
Instrumentation: Sterile local anesthetic syringe, disposable needle of appropriate length, cartridge of local anesthetic solution, gauze sponges, disinfecting solution. (Appropriate infection control barriers will be used during all procedures actually performed on a patient.)		
1. Washed hands and donned gloves.		
2. Disinfected needle end of anesthetic cartridge.		
3. Placed cartridge in syringe and engaged harpoon.		
4. Opened disposable needle packet without touching or contaminating the needle.		
5. Attached the needle to the syringe.		
6. Loosened needle guard and left it on the needle.		
7. Placed prepared syringe on the instrument tray.		
Comments:		

▼ **Criterion Sheet 18 – 2**

Student's Name _____

Procedure: *ANESTHETIC SYRINGE TRANSFER*

Performance Objective:

The student will demonstrate the transfer of the local anesthetic syringe to the operator while seated at chairside.

		SE	IE
SE = Student evaluation **C** = Criterion met **IE** = Instructor evaluation **X** = Criterion not met			
Instrumentation: Prepared local anesthetic syringe, cotton-tipped applicator for topical anesthetic. (Appropriate infection control barriers will be used during all procedures actually performed on a patient.)			
1. If not already gloved, washed hands and donned gloves.			
2. Loosened needle guard.			
3. Received used topical anesthetic applicator with left hand.			
4. Transferred the syringe with the right hand.			
5. Positioned syringe in operator's right hand.			
6. Removed the needle guard.			
7. Rotated the bevel toward the bone.			
8. Guarded against sudden patient movement during the injection.			
Comments:			

19 Rubber Dam

▼ LEARNING OBJECTIVES

The student will be able to:

1. State eight indications for the use of rubber dam.
2. Describe the specialized types of rubber dam and rubber dam clamps.
3. Demonstrate punching rubber dam for placement on single or multiple maxillary or mandibular teeth.
4. Demonstrate assisting in the placement, inversion, and removal of rubber dam.

OVERVIEW OF RUBBER DAM

The use of rubber dam is an important part of quality dental treatment and infection control. A coordinated team of operator and assistant can place the rubber dam in 1½ to 2 minutes.

Indications for Use of Rubber Dam

1. It prevents the patient from accidentally swallowing debris, small fragments of a tooth, a piece of a dental bur, scraps of restorative material, or the broken point of a dental instrument.
2. It serves as a protective barrier and is an important part of the infection control program.
3. It improves visibility for either direct or indirect approach dental procedures.
4. It maintains the dry operating field needed for the placement of restorative material and for the cementation of cast restorations.
5. It provides contrast of tooth tissues with the dark field of the dam and reduces glare from the moist surfaces of tissues of the oral cavity.
6. It protects the remainder of the oral cavity from exposure to infectious material when an infected tooth is opened during endodontic treatment.
7. It catches excess solution that may drip from the syringe in irrigation of the canal during endodontic treatment.
8. It protects the tooth from contamination by saliva and plaque if pulpal exposure accidentally occurs.
9. It catches bits of material in the carving of an amalgam restoration or the direct wax carving of an inlay pattern.
10. It retracts the interdental papilla to provide accessibility in preparing and placing a restoration in the gingival third of a tooth.
11. It retracts the lips and tongue from the field of operation and discourages patient conversation.

RUBBER DAM EQUIPMENT

Figure 19–1 shows a pre-set tray with all of the equipment needed for the placement and removal of rubber dam.

335

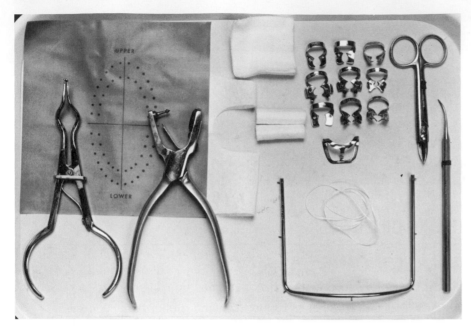

▼ Figure 19-1

Tray setup for rubber dam placement and removal. Major items from left to right: stamped rubber dam, rubber dam clamp forceps, rubber dam punch, rubber dam frame (lower right), rubber dam clamps (upper right), scissors and beavertail burnisher (far right). (Torres HO, Ehrlich A: Modern Dental Assisting, 4th Ed. Philadelphia, WB Saunders, 1990, p 507.)

Rubber Dam Material

Rubber dam is a thin, flexible sheet of rubber that may be purchased in precut pieces indicated by size, color, and weight (Fig. 19-2).

The size of the rubber dam is 6 × 6 inches for the posterior and 5 × 6 inches for the anterior application on adult dentition and 5 × 5 inches for children's teeth.

Rubber dam is available in colors ranging from light to dark gray-brown, green, and blue. The darkest shade is preferred by most operators because the color provides the desired contrast between the dam and the tissues of the tooth.

The weights are light, medium, and heavy. Some operators prefer the dark, heavyweight dam, as it withstands abuse when placed over crowns, fixed bridges, or teeth with close contacts. Also, the heavier rubber dam rarely tears from contact with the dental instruments during the cavity preparation.

The manufacturer prepares the material with a powdered surface to prevent the surfaces from adhering to each other while packed in the box.

The manufacturer suggests that the rubber dam be washed, dried, sterilized, and repowdered before use.

Rubber Dam Stamp and Template

The rubber dam stamp, used with an ink pad, is used to mark the rubber dam with predetermined markings for an "average arch" (see Fig. 19-2).

An alternative is the use of a rubber dam template. This is a sample plate with measurements of the primary and permanent dentition. The template is placed under the rubber dam, and a pen is used to mark the punch holes.

Rubber Dam Holders

A holder is necessary to keep the rubber dam stretched so that it fits tightly around the teeth and is not in the operator's way.

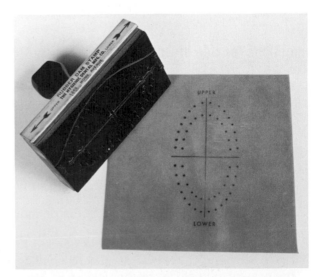

▼ Figure 19-2

Rubber dam and stamped rubber dam. (Torres HO, Ehrlich A: Modern Dental Assisting, 4th Ed. Philadelphia, WB Saunders, 1990, p 502.)

The holder most commonly used is Young's frame. This is a U-shaped holder, of stainless steel or plastic, with sharp projections on its outer margin. The rubber dam is stretched over the projections of the frame to provide stabilization.

The frame shown in Figure 19–3 is plastic. The frame shown in the figures demonstrating rubber dam application is a metal Young's frame (see Figs. 19–13 through 19–22). These frames may be sterilized by autoclaving.

Young's frame is always placed on the outside of the dam away from the face. Because the frame holds the rubber dam lightly away from the face, it may be placed with or without a rubber dam napkin.

Rubber Dam Napkin

A rubber dam napkin is a disposable piece of fabric that may be placed under the rubber dam next to the patient's skin.

A napkin is used to increase patient comfort by absorbing water, saliva, and perspiration. It is a necessity for patients who are sensitive to latex rubber.

Rubber Dam Punch

The rubber dam punch has an adjustable **stylus** (cutting tip) that strikes a hole in the **punch plate**. It is used to punch the holes in the rubber dam.

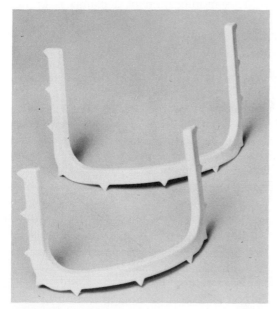

▼ Figure 19–3

Plastic rubber dam frame. (Courtesy of The Hygenic Corporation, Akron, OH.)

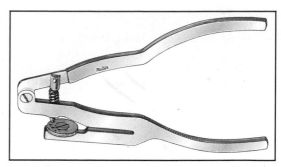

▼ Figure 19–4

Lightweight rubber dam punch. (Courtesy of Miltex Instrument Co., Lake Success, NY.)

One type of rubber dam punch is shown in Figure 19–4. A slightly different type is shown in Figure 19–1. Both types of punches are used in the same manner.

The punch plate contains holes in varying sizes. By adjusting the position of the punch plate under the stylus, you can produce holes of the different sizes as needed.

Holes must be punched firmly and cleanly because a ragged hole will tear easily as the dam is placed over the crown of the tooth. A ragged hole may also cause the rough margin to irritate the gingiva and may cause leakage of moisture around the tooth.

It is also important to prevent nicking, breaking, or dulling of the stylus on the punch plate. To accomplish this, the stylus must be placed directly over the hole in the punch plate.

Positioning the Punch Plate

When the punch plate is moved, a slight click may be heard as the plate falls into the correct position. Always check that the position is correct by slowly lowering the stylus point over the hole in the punch plate.

It is also advisable to place a mark on the extension in back of the punch plate to indicate 1 inch. This mark automatically designates the margin of rubber dam for the first punch hole for the maxillary anterior teeth at the midline of the dam.

Size of Holes on Rubber Dam Punch Plate

▼ Number 1—upper lateral, lower central, and lateral.

▼ Number 2—upper central, upper and lower cuspids, and premolars.

▼ Number 3—upper and lower molars.

▼ Number 4—large molars and bridge abutments.

▼ Number 5—long-span fixed bridge.

Rubber Dam Clamp Forceps

Rubber dam clamp forceps are used in the placement and removal of the rubber dam clamp. The beaks of the forceps fit into holes in the clamp.

One type of rubber dam clamp forceps is shown in Figure 19–5. A slightly different type is shown in Figure 19–1. Both types of forceps are used in the same manner.

The handles of the forceps work with a spring action. A sliding bar keeps the handles of the forceps in a fixed position while the clamp is being held. The handles are squeezed to release the clamp.

Ligatures

A length of dental floss is *always* attached to a rubber dam clamp before it is tried in the mouth or placed. The purpose of this ligature is to make it possible to retrieve a clamp should it accidentally be dislodged and swallowed or aspirated by the patient.

Also, a length of dental floss or dental tape may be used as a ligature to hold the other end of the dam in place.

Rubber Dam Clamps

The rubber dam clamp is the primary means of anchoring and stabilizing the rubber dam. These clamps are made of chrome or nickel-plated steel and may be sterilized by autoclaving.

They are tension-designed with four jaws that firmly contact the cervical area of the tooth to be clamped. Normally, the clamp should fit near or slightly below the cementoenamel junction.

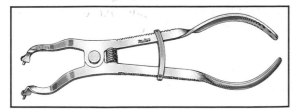

▼ **Figure 19–5**

Lightweight rubber dam clamp forceps. (Courtesy of Miltex Instrument Co, Lake Success, NY.)

All prongs of the jaws must be in contact with the tooth. This contact establishes a facial lingual balance that stabilizes the clamp.

If the caries is low on the gingival third of the tooth surface, it is necessary to place the clamp lightly on the cementum of the tooth.

If the clamp is not placed properly, it may spring off the tooth and injure the tissues. Also, displacement of the clamp may injure the patient, operator, or assistant.

Caution is advised to stabilize the clamp firmly on the tooth before the clamp forceps is loosened.

A basic assortment of rubber dam clamps is shown in Figure 19–6. Notice that each clamp has a specific use.

▼ The term **universal** means the same clamp may be placed on the same type of tooth on the upper right or lower left quadrants.

▼ A **winged** clamp is designed with extra projections to help retain the rubber dam.

▼ A **wingless** clamp does not have extra projections to engage the dam.

Clamp Modification

It is essential that the clamp be placed on sound tooth structure. If necessary, a standard clamp can be modified to compensate for a malposed or misshapen tooth or a malposed carious lesion.

The operator may use a carbide bur, a disc, or a stone to modify the jaws or contour of the clamp. This modification of a clamp is known as **festooning** the clamp.

PUNCHING THE RUBBER DAM

Each application of the rubber dam is planned keeping in mind the tooth or teeth involved in the procedure to be performed.

The Key Punch Hole

The tooth holding the rubber dam clamp is known as the **anchor tooth**. The key punch hole is the hole in the rubber dam that is to be placed over the anchor tooth.

The key punch hole is the single most important consideration in the application of the rubber dam. The diagrams in Figures 19–7 through 19–10 may be used as a guide to establish the key punch hole.

▼ **Figure 19-6**

Basic assortment of rubber dam clamps. *Clamp number and use.*

00—Small maxillary or mandibular premolars and incisors (winged).
W00—Small maxillary or mandibular premolars and incisors (wingless).
2—General clamp for larger mandibular premolars (winged).
W2—General clamp for larger mandibular premolars (wingless).
7—Universal mandibular molar clamp (winged).
W7— Universal mandibular molar clamp (wingless).
8—Universal maxillary molar clamp (winged).
W8—Universal maxillary molar clamp (wingless).
8A—Partially erupted or irregularly shaped smaller primary molars (winged).
W8A—Partially erupted or irregularly shaped smaller primary molars (wingless).
14A—Partially erupted or irregularly shaped larger molars (winged).
W14A—Partially erupted or irregularly shaped larger molars (wingless).
W2A—Premolar clamp (wingless).
9—Universal double-bowed anterior clamp (winged).
W9—Universal double-bowed anterior clamp (wingless).
W14—Molar clamp (wingless).
W56—Molar clamp (wingless).
W3—Primary molars (wingless).
(Courtesy of The Hygenic Corporation, Akron, OH.)

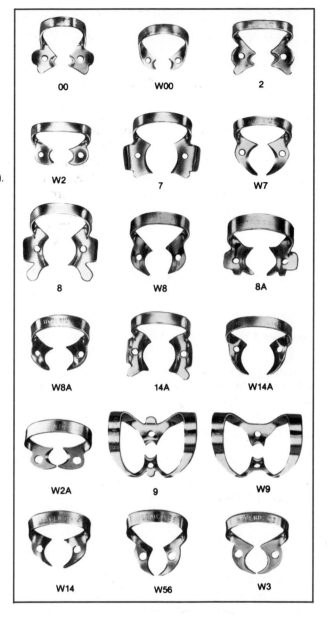

The Teeth to Be Exposed

For stability of the dam and for convenience, if possible, eight to 10 teeth are exposed through the dam. Exceptions are exposure of one or two teeth for root canal therapy or when a single tooth is being treated.

At least one tooth posterior to the tooth being operated on should be exposed; having two posterior teeth exposed is preferable.

The Septum

The rubber dam between the holes of the punched dam is called the septum. When the dam is placed, this septum must slip between the teeth without tearing.

Generally, from 3 to 3.5 mm of rubber dam are allowed between the edges of the holes in the dam (not between the centers of the holes).

Because of the small size of the mandibular anteriors, these holes are punched closer together than those for posterior teeth.

Maxillary and Mandibular Applications

When the dam is punched for maxillary application, the dam is divided vertically into imaginary halves. Holes for the maxillary anterior teeth are

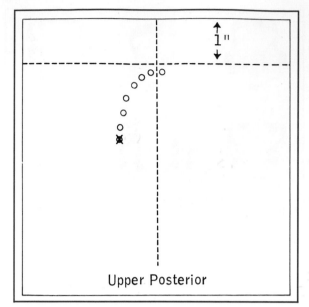

▼ **Figure 19–7**

Punching 6 × 6 inch rubber dam for maxillary posterior placement. Key punch hole on maxillary second molar. Holes for anterior teeth are punched 1 inch from the upper edge of the rubber dam. (Torres HO, Ehrlich A: Modern Dental Assisting, 4th Ed. Philadelphia, WB Saunders, 1990, p 505.)

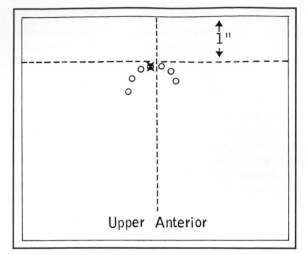

▼ **Figure 19–9**

Punching 5 × 6 inch rubber dam for maxillary anterior placement. Key punch hole on maxillary central incisor is placed 1 inch from the upper edge of the rubber dam. (Torres HO, Ehrlich A: Modern Dental Assisting, 4th Ed. Philadelphia, WB Saunders, 1990, p 505.)

punched 1 inch from the upper edge of the dam, as shown in Figure 19–11A.

When the dam is punched for mandibular application, the dam is divided vertically into imaginary thirds and horizontally into halves. Holes for the mandibular anterior teeth are punched 2 inches from the edge of the dam as shown in Figure 19–11B.

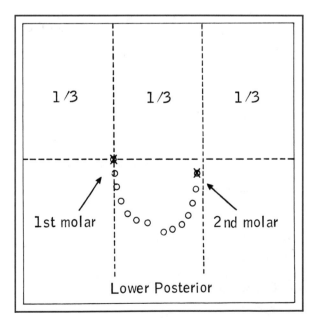

▼ **Figure 19–8**

Punching 6 × 6 inch rubber dam for mandibular posterior placement. On the left of the diagram, the key punch hole is placed for a mandibular first molar. On the right of the diagram, the key punch hole is placed for a mandibular second molar. Notice how placement of holes differs from the lower edge of the rubber dam. (Torres HO, Ehrlich A: Modern Dental Assisting, 4th Ed. Philadelphia, WB Saunders, 1990, p 505.)

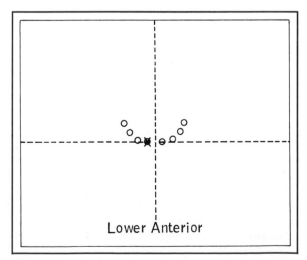

▼ **Figure 19–10**

Punching 5 × 6 inch rubber dam for mandibular anterior placement. Key punch hole on mandibular central incisor. An equal number of teeth on either side aids in stabilizing the rubber dam. (Torres HO, Ehrlich A: Modern Dental Assisting, 4th Ed. Philadelphia, WB Saunders, 1990, p 505.)

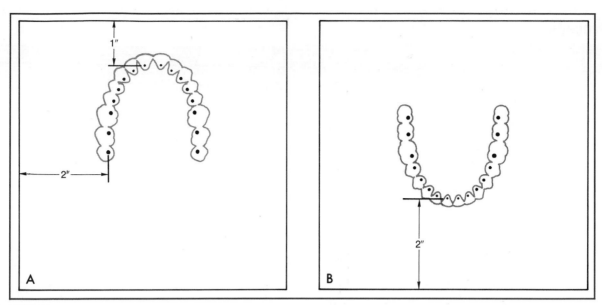

▼ **Figure 19-11**

Diagram of rubber dam. Dots represent punch holes. *A.* Maxillary arch. *B.* Mandibular arch. (Torres HO, Ehrlich A: Modern Dental Assisting, 4th Ed. Philadelphia, WB Saunders, 1990, p 506.)

Important Considerations

Other considerations for punching the remaining holes in the dam are as follows.

Shape of the Arch and Alignment of the Teeth

1. Punching the curve of the arch too flat results in folds and stretching of the rubber dam on the lingual surface.
2. Punching the arch too curved results in folds and stretching of the dam. It also increases the difficulty in inverting the edges of the rubber dam under the gingival margin.
3. Adjustments must be made for malaligned teeth.

Appropriate Hole Sizes and Placement

1. The correct size of the holes for the specific tooth to be exposed must be selected.
2. A larger hole is necessary for the key punch hole.
3. The holes for the incisors should be located near the midline of the rubber dam.
4. The hole for the last molar to be included in the dam application should be placed on the imaginary one third horizontal line of the rubber dam.

Holes for Class V Restorations

1. The holes for the tooth to be restored with a Class V restoration should be punched 1 mm facially from the normal location.

2. One millimeter of extra rubber should be allowed between the neighboring teeth in the arch.

PLACING RUBBER DAM

Local anesthetic solution is administered, and the teeth to be exposed for placement of the rubber dam are cleaned of calculus and plaque.

Instrumentation (see Fig. 19-1)

▼ Basic setup.

▼ Precut rubber dam, 6 × 6 or 6 × 5 inches.

▼ Rubber dam stamp or template and pen.

▼ Rubber dam punch.

▼ Rubber dam clamps (2).

▼ Rubber dam clamp forceps.

▼ Young's frame.

▼ Dental floss or dental tape for ligatures.

▼ Cotton rolls.

▼ Lubricant for lips—zinc oxide ointment.

▼ Lubricant for dam—petroleum jelly or shaving cream.

▼ Beavertail burnisher, number 2 or 34.

▼ High volume evacuator (HVE) tip.

Procedure

PATIENT PREPARATION FOR RUBBER DAM PLACEMENT

1. The assistant rinses the patient's mouth with water. Excess water is removed with the HVE tip.

2. The operator receives the mouth mirror and explorer from the assistant and checks tissue surfaces for debris.

3. The operator receives a ligature to check the contact areas of the teeth to be isolated.

4. If the contacts are too snug, the operator may use a lightning strip to reduce contact slightly. (A **lightning strip** is a thin metal strip with serrations on one or both sides, used to reduce metallic or tight contacts on adjacent teeth.)

5. The operator notes any irregularity of teeth in the alignment of the arch.

Procedure

PUNCHING THE RUBBER DAM

1. The assistant hands the rubber dam punch to the operator and holds the dam without stretching it as the operator punches holes (Fig. 19–12).

   If the anterior teeth are to be clamped, the superior (upper) border of the dam is held toward the operator.

   If the posterior teeth are to be clamped, the inferior (lower) border of the dam is held toward the operator.

   Alternative option: The assistant may be given the task of punching the dam.

2. *Optional*: For patient comfort, the assistant may apply zinc oxide ointment to the patient's lip with a cotton roll.

3. The assistant uses petroleum jelly or shaving cream placed on a cotton roll to lubricate lightly the holes on the tooth surface (undersurface) of the dam. This eases

placement of the dam over the contact area.

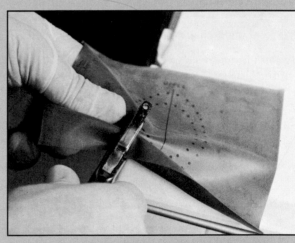

Figure 19–12 Punching the rubber dam. (Torres HO, Ehrlich A: Modern Dental Assisting, 4th Ed. Philadelphia, WB Saunders, 1990, p 507.)

Procedure

PLACING THE RUBBER DAM CLAMP

1. The assistant attaches a ligature to the bow of the clamp and then places the clamp in the rubber dam forceps.

2. The assistant transfers the rubber dam clamp forceps with the clamp pointed in position toward placement on the tooth to the operator (Figs. 19–13 and 19–14).

3. The operator checks the clamp for fit on the key tooth. The clamp is removed, and the forceps and clamp are returned to the assistant (Fig. 19–15).

4. The assistant passes the bow of the clamp through the keyhole of the dam for the tooth to be clamped.

5. The ligature attached to the clamp bow is kept free of the dam to ensure a quick retrieval in case of accidental displacement.

6. The length of the ligature is placed to the opposite side of the arch, away from the field of operation.

7. The assistant passes the rubber dam clamp forceps to the operator, with handles in forward position and beaks pointed correctly for placement of the clamp on the upper or lower arch.

   For placement of the clamp on the mandibular teeth, the operator receives forceps in the right hand with a palm grasp.

   For placement of the clamp on the maxillary teeth, a reverse palm grasp is used.

8. The operator gathers the excess rubber

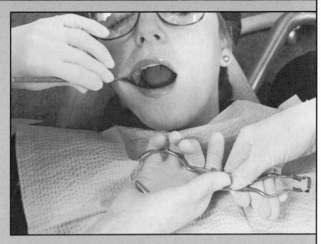

Figure 19–14 The operator receives the rubber dam forceps and clamp with a palm grasp. (Torres HO, Ehrlich A: Modern Dental Assisting, 4th Ed. Philadelphia, WB Saunders, 1990, p 508.)

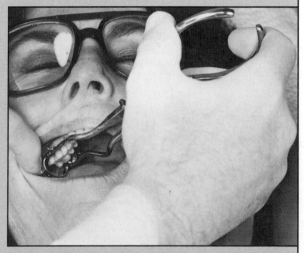

Figure 19–15 The operator tries the clamp on the maxillary molar to check proper fit. (Torres HO, Ehrlich A: Modern Dental Assisting, 4th Ed. Philadelphia, WB Saunders, 1990, p 509.)

dam edges and ligature in the left hand. This permits visibility into the mouth for placement of the clamp.

The lingual jaw is placed first on the lingual surface of the tooth. This serves as a fulcrum for placement of the facial jaw.

This is followed by placement of the facial jaw on the facial surface of the tooth.

9. Once stability is achieved, with both jaws touching the gingival line of the tooth, the operator releases the forceps from the clamp.

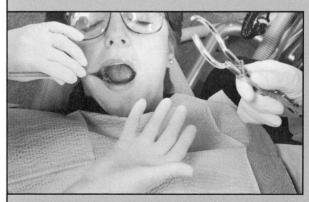

Figure 19–13 The assistant passes the rubber dam forceps and clamp. (Torres HO, Ehrlich A: Modern Dental Assisting, 4th Ed. Philadelphia, WB Saunders, 1990, p 508.)

Procedure

PLACING THE RUBBER DAM AND FRAME

1. The dam is placed over the bow of the clamp on the anchor tooth and is eased under the clamp.

   Caution: The assistant must be alert to protect the patient's face in case the clamp accidentally slips from its position on the tooth.

2. The operator holds the edges of the dam and hands the forceps to the assistant.

3. *Optional:* If the rubber dam napkin is used, the assistant holds the napkin over the fingers of the left hand and receives the edges of the dam from the operator.

   The assistant and operator spread the dam out over the surface of the napkin and over the lower section of the face.

4. Young's frame is placed on the outside of the dam away from the face. The dam is engaged on the projections of the frame to ensure a smooth and stable fit.

Procedure

LIGATING THE RUBBER DAM

1. The assistant hands a length of dental floss to the operator, who uses it to pass each portion of the rubber dam septum between proximal contacts of the teeth to be exposed (Figs. 19–16 and 19–17).

2. The assistant places the index fingers of both hands on lingual and facial surfaces of the tooth to aid the operator in slipping the dam septum through the contact areas.

3. If the contacts are extremely tight, the operator may use floss or the beavertail burnisher to wedge slightly between the teeth at the interproximal area. This slight ac-

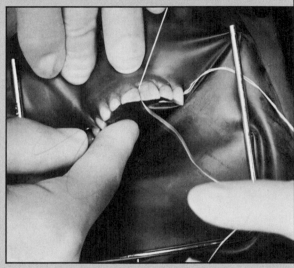

Figure 19–17 Passing rubber dam septum through contacts using dental floss. (Torres HO, Ehrlich A: Modern Dental Assisting, 4th Ed. Philadelphia, WB Saunders, 1990, p 510.)

tion encourages the septum to slip through the tight contacts.

4. A secondary clamp, a dental floss ligature, or a small piece of rubber dam may be used to stabilize the dam on the tooth exposed at the opposite end of the quadrant to be operated on.

5. *Optional:* The assistant may place a saliva ejector under the dam in the floor of the mouth for patient comfort.

   The saliva ejector is placed on the side opposite of the key tooth so that it is out of the way during the operative procedure.

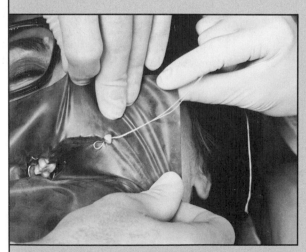

Figure 19–16 The operator ligates the rubber dam with dental floss. (Torres HO, Ehrlich A: Modern Dental Assisting, 4th Ed. Philadelphia, WB Saunders, 1990, p 509.)

Procedure

INVERTING THE RUBBER DAM

1. The operator receives the beavertail burnisher or explorer to proceed with inverting the edges of the dam around the lingual and facial surfaces of the teeth to be exposed. (**Invert** means to turn inward or to turn under.)

2. Just before the operator inverts the dam, the assistant <u>dries</u> the tooth with soft blasts of air from the air syringe (Fig. 19–18).

   When the tooth surface is dry, the margin of the stretched dam usually inverts into the gingival sulcus as the dam is released.

   If the dam is punched correctly and is not strained or wrinkled, the inversion may be accomplished quite easily by gen-

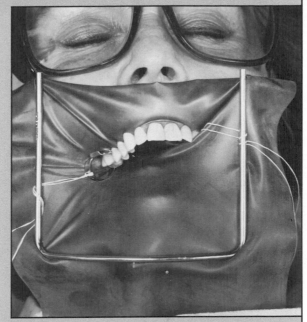

Figure 19–19 **Completed rubber dam application.** (Torres HO, Ehrlich A: Modern Dental Assisting, 4th Ed. Philadelphia, WB Saunders, 1990, p 511.)

tly stretching and relaxing the dam near the cervix of each tooth.

3. To aid in the inversion of the dam under the free gingival margin, the assistant may use a length of dental floss, passing it gently through each contact.

4. The operator may place softened compound under the bows of the clamp to ensure its stabilization.

5. The field is now prepared for the operative procedure (Fig. 19–19).

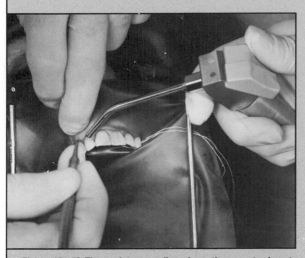

Figure 19–18 **The assistant applies air as the operator inverts the rubber dam using a beavertail burnisher.** (Torres HO, Ehrlich A: Modern Dental Assisting, 4th Ed. Philadelphia, WB Saunders, 1990, p 510.)

REMOVAL OF RUBBER DAM

Instrumentation

When the procedure has been completed, the dam may be removed with the patient still in a full reclining position. Some operators prefer to have the patient positioned upright for removal of the rubber dam.

▼ Basic setup.

▼ Rubber dam clamp forceps.

▼ Dental floss, 14 to 16 inches in length.

▼ Suture scissors.

▼ Finishing knife.

▼ Mouth rinse.

▼ HVE tip.

Procedure

REMOVING A RUBBER DAM

1. The assistant uses the HVE tip to remove any debris from the surface of the rubber dam.

2. If the dam was stabilized by a ligature, the assistant hands the operator a finishing knife to cut the ligature.

   The ligature is cut by placing the knife edge under the knot at the interproximal space and severing the knot, using a pull toward the occlusal surface.

3. The cut ligature is removed by holding the knot and pulling the ligature through the interproximal area with the cotton pliers.

4. If a saliva ejector was used, the assistant removes it.

5. The assistant hands suture scissors to the operator with the right hand and holds the margin of the dam with the left hand.

6. The operator places the index finger and thumb over and under the superior edge of the dam and follows the scissors from posterior to anterior as each septum is stretched and severed (Fig. 19–20).

   When all septa are cut, the dam is pulled lingually to free the rubber from the interproximal space. The scissors are returned to the assistant.

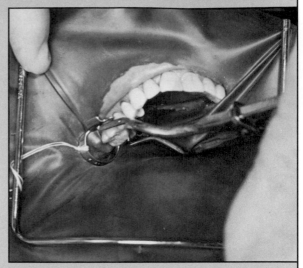

Figure 19–21 The operator removes the clamp. (Torres HO, Ehrlich A: Modern Dental Assisting, 4th Ed. Philadelphia, WB Saunders, 1990, p 511.)

7. The assistant passes the operator rubber dam clamp forceps in position for the right hand (handles forward).

   The operator removes the clamp and returns forceps and clamps to the assistant (Fig. 19–21).

8. The operator removes both dam and frame. The patient's mouth, lips, and chin are wiped free of moisture.

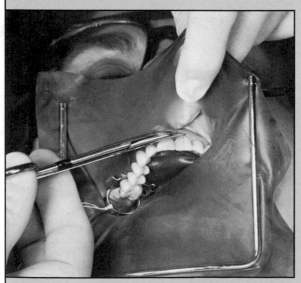

Figure 19–20 Cutting the rubber dam septum prior to the removal of the dam. (Torres HO, Ehrlich A: Modern Dental Assisting, 4th Ed. Philadelphia, WB Saunders, 1990, p 511.)

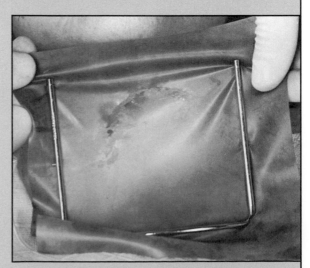

Figure 19–22 The used dam is inspected to detect any tears or missing pieces. (Torres HO, Ehrlich A: Modern Dental Assisting, 4th Ed. Philadelphia, WB Saunders, 1990, p 512.)

9 The used dam is placed over a light-colored surface and inspected to detect that the total pattern of the torn rubber dam has been removed (Fig. 19–22).

10 If a fragment of the rubber dam is missing, the operator is alerted to check the corresponding interproximal area of the oral cavity.

   Caution: Fragments of rubber dam left under the free gingiva can cause gingival irritation.

11 The operator massages the gingiva of the area covered by the dam to increase circulation, especially to the tissue supporting the anchor clamp.

12 The assistant rinses the patient's mouth with warm water and mouth rinse and uses the HVE tip to remove the debris and excess water.

13 The operator checks all areas of the mouth with an explorer and mouth mirror.

14 Dental floss is placed through each contact to be certain that all interproximal areas are free of rubber dam and compound.

15 If a restoration has been placed, the patient's occlusion is checked following removal of the rubber dam.

▼ **EXERCISES**

1. A _____ frame is placed on the outside of the dam away from the face.

   a. Ferrier
   b. Hollenback
   c. Woodbury
   d. Young's

2. Manufacturers recommend that rubber dam be _____ before use.

   a. washed and dried
   b. repowdered
   c. sterilized
   d. a, b, and c

3. _____ rubber dam clamps have extra projections to aid in holding the dam.

   a. Modified
   b. Posterior
   c. Winged
   d. Wingless

4. Just prior to placement, the holes on the tooth surface side of the rubber dam are lubricated lightly with _____.

   a. petroleum jelly
   b. shaving cream
   c. zinc oxide ointment
   d. a or b

5. A _____ inch rubber dam is used for children's teeth.

   a. 4×5
   b. 5×5
   c. 5×6
   d. 6×6

6. A length of dental floss is attached to a rubber dam clamp before _____
   _____.

   a. it is tried in the mouth
   b. the rubber dam is placed over the clamp

7. When punching the rubber dam, a number _____ hole is used to go over upper and lower molars.

   a. 1
   b. 2
   c. 3
   d. 4

8. Some operators prefer _____ rubber dam because it withstands abuse when placed over crowns, fixed bridges, or teeth with close contacts.

    a. dark heavyweight
    b. dark lightweight
    c. gray lightweight
    d. green heavyweight

9. When the dam is punched for _____ application, the dam is divided vertically into imaginary halves.

    a. mandibular
    b. maxillary

10. When punching the rubber dam, _____ mm of rubber dam are allowed between the edges of the holes.

    a. 2.0 to 2.5
    b. 2.5 to 3.0
    c. 3.0 to 3.5
    d. 3.5 to 4.0

11. The _____ hole in the rubber dam is placed over the tooth holding the rubber dam clamp.

    a. anchor
    b. clamp
    c. key punch
    d. a or c

12. The patient's lips may be lubricated with _____ prior to placement of the rubber dam.

    a. petroleum jelly
    b. shaving cream
    c. topical anesthetic ointment
    d. zinc oxide ointment

13. Punching the arch of the rubber dam too _____ will result in folds and stretching of the rubber dam on the lingual surface.

    a. curved
    b. flat

14. Just before the operator inverts the rubber dam, the assistant _____
    _____.

    a. dries the tooth
    b. places vaseline on the tooth to lubricate it
    c. sprays the tooth with water to clean it
    d. c then a

15. When preparing to punch the rubber dam to clamp the posterior teeth, the dam is held with the _____ border toward the operator.

    a. inferior
    b. superior

16. When trying the clamp on for size, the rubber dam forceps and clamp are passed to the operator _____ the rubber dam.

    a. with
    b. without

17. The operator uses a _____ to invert the edges of the rubber dam around the lingual and facial surfaces of the teeth to be exposed.

    a. beavertail burnisher
    b. finishing knife
    c. separator wrench
    d. spoon excavator

18. To assure that the rubber dam holes are punched cleanly, the _____ _____ must be placed directly over the hole in the punch plate.

    a. forceps
    b. extension
    c. nib
    d. stylus

19. Following removal, the rubber dam is reassembled to _____ _____.

    a. check the extent of the restoration
    b. determine that the entire rubber dam was removed
    c. determine the condition of the gingiva
    d. prepare for the sterilization procedure

20. A length of dental floss is _____.

    a. attached to the rubber dam clamp
    b. used to pass the rubber dam between the teeth
    c. used as a ligature to secure the rubber dam
    d. a, b, and c

▼ Criterion Sheet 19–1

Student's Name _____

Procedure: *PUNCHING RUBBER DAM*

Performance Objective:

The student will punch rubber dam for placement over teeth as specified by the operator or instructor.

		SE	IE
SE = Student evaluation **C** = Criterion met **IE** = Instructor evaluation **X** = Criterion not met			
Instrumentation: Rubber dam, rubber dam punch, rubber dam stamp and ink pad *or* a rubber dam template and a pen or pencil. (Appropriate infection control barriers will be used during all procedures actually performed on a patient.)			
1. Marked rubber dam indicating where holes were to be punched.			
2. Positioned holes away from the edges of the dam according to the teeth to be included in the dam application.			
3. Positioned stylus of the rubber dam punch carefully. The rubber dam punch stylus was not dulled or nicked.			
4. Punched the correct number of holes for the teeth being exposed.			
5. Punched holes of the correct size for the teeth being exposed. Holes were clean and round.			
6. Distance between holes and curvature of the arch permitted smooth application of the dam.			
Comments:			

▼ Criterion Sheet 19-2

Student's Name _____

Procedure: *ASSISTING IN PLACING RUBBER DAM*

Performance Objective:

The student will assist the operator in placing a rubber dam on a manikin or patient.

SE = Student evaluation **C** = Criterion met **IE** = Instructor evaluation **X** = Criterion not met	**SE**	**IE**
Instrumentation: Basic setup, previously punched rubber dam, rubber dam setup. (Appropriate infection control barriers will be used during all procedures actually performed on a patient.)		
1. Prepared clamp with a dental floss ligature. Placed clamp in rubber dam clamp forceps. Passed forceps and clamp to operator.		
2. Received clamp and forceps. Passed the clamp bow through the keyhole of the rubber dam. Returned clamp, forceps, and rubber dam to operator.		
3. Received forceps. Passed rubber dam frame to operator.		
4. Aided operator in passing rubber dam between proximal contacts.		
5. Aided operator in inverting rubber dam.		
6. Aided operator in ligating and stabilizing rubber dam.		
Comments:		

▼ **Criterion Sheet 19–3**

Student's Name _____

Procedure: *ASSISTING IN REMOVING RUBBER DAM*

Performance Objective:

The student will assist the operator in removing the rubber dam.

SE = Student evaluation **C** = Criterion met **IE** = Instructor evaluation **X** = Criterion not met	**SE**	**IE**
Instrumentation: Basic setup, rubber dam clamp forceps, suture scissors, finishing knife, dental floss, warm water syringe, mouth rinse, HVE tip, and cleansing tissues. (Appropriate infection control barriers will be used during all procedures actually performed on a patient.)		
1. Passed finishing knife to sever ligature.		
2. Received finishing knife. Passed suture scissors to cut each rubber dam septum.		
3. Received suture scissors. Passed rubber dam clamp forceps.		
4. Received rubber dam clamp forceps and clamp.		
5. Received rubber dam frame.		
6. Checked rubber dam for tears or missing pieces.		
7. Reported status of used rubber dam to the operator.		
8. Used tissue to wipe patient's face clean gently. Rinsed the patient's oral cavity.		
Comments:		

20 Dental Cements

▼ LEARNING OBJECTIVES

The student will be able to:

1. List at least five of the cements most commonly used in dentistry and state the primary uses of each.
2. Describe the types and functions of cavity liners and varnishes.
3. Describe the manipulation and uses of polycarboxylate, intermediate restorative material (IRM), ortho-ethoxybenzoic acid (EBA), and glass ionomer cements.
4. Demonstrate mixing zinc phosphate cement for the cementation.
5. Demonstrate mixing zinc oxide–eugenol cement for use as a sedative base.
6. Demonstrate mixing calcium hydroxide liner.

OVERVIEW OF DENTAL CEMENTS

Cements play many important roles in dentistry. These include roles as **cementation agents** for cast restorations, **protective bases,** and **temporary restorations.**

Cementation of Cast Restorations

When used for the cementation of a cast restoration, dental cements are called **luting agents.** (A **luting agent** is the cement that holds something in place.)

These cements are used for the cementation of cast restorations such as inlays, onlays, crowns, and bridges. (This role is discussed in Chapter 24, "Crown and Bridge Restorations.") They are also used to hold orthodontic bands and appliances in place. (This role is discussed in Chapter 27, "Orthodontics.")

Different types of cement are used as luting agents to hold a temporary coverage in place. (**Temporary coverage** is placed between visits: After the tooth has been prepared for the cast restoration and before that restoration is ready to be cemented into place.)

Protective Bases

Protective bases, frequently referred to as *cement bases,* are placed to protect the pulp.

Cements are used under a restoration as **insulating bases** to protect the pulp from thermal shock due to a sudden temperature change in the tooth.

Other cements are used as **sedative bases** to soothe the pulp, which has been irritated by decay, injury, or the trauma of the cavity preparation.

355

Temporary Restorations

Temporary restorations are also referred to as *intermediate restorations*. As the name implies, these are placed in situations in which, for some reason, the tooth is not ready to receive a permanent restoration.

Types and Uses of Dental Cements, Liners, and Varnishes

To fill these varied roles, many different types of cements are used. Also, one type of cement may be used for several different purposes.

▼ **Zinc phosphate cement** is used for the cementation of cast restorations and fixed orthodontic appliances. It is also used as an insulating base and as a temporary restoration.

▼ **Zinc oxide–eugenol (ZOE) cement** is used for the cementation of temporary coverage and as a sedative base.

▼ **Intermediate restoration material (IRM)** is used as an intermediate restoration, which will last up to 1 year.

▼ **Ortho-ethoxybenzoic acid (EBA) cement** is used as a cementation of cast restorations.

▼ **Polycarboxylate (polyacrylate) cement** is used for the cementation of cast restorations and in the direct bonding of orthodontic appliances. It may also function as an insulating base.

▼ **Glass ionomer cement** is used for the cementation of cast restorations and as an insulating base. It also serves as a restorative material for Class V cavities and cervical eroded areas.

▼ **Cavity liner** is used in direct and indirect pulp capping and as a protective liner for the cavity preparation.

▼ **Cavity varnish** is used to seal the dentin and margins of the cavity preparation.

Special Precautions

Each type of cement has its own special characteristics and must be mixed and used according to the manufacturer's instructions. However, the following special precautions apply to all cements:

▼ The liquid and powder must be prepared by the same manufacturer. *Do not substitute a different brand of powder or liquid.*

▼ The powder to liquid ratio recommended by the manufacturer is critical. Follow these recommendations and take care to measure precisely.

▼ The powder to liquid ratio also depends on the intended use of the mix. The mix for an insulating base is thicker than one for cementation. A thicker mix requires more powder to less liquid.

▼ Exposure to the air causes deterioration of the cement components. Always replace the caps on the bottles of liquid and powder immediately.

▼ Eugenol, which is the liquid for some cements, causes the deterioration of rubber. To prevent this, never place the dropper in a horizontal position. Always empty the dropper and return it to its place after use.

▼ Some cements are mixed on a glass slab. Others are mixed on a lightweight or heavyweight paper mixing pad (waxed or plain). Always use the appropriate mixing surface.

▼ The goal is to achieve a homogeneous mix within the permissible mixing time. (**Homogeneous** means that the resulting mix of material is evenly distributed and uniform in texture throughout.)

▼ Once set, cement is difficult to remove. Clean the equipment used in mixing and placing the cement as soon as possible.

ZINC PHOSPHATE CEMENT

Zinc phosphate cement is most frequently used for the cementation of cast restorations. It may also be used as an insulating base in deep cavity preparations.

Because the liquid of this cement is acid and irritating to the pulp, it is necessary to protect the pulp by placing a cavity liner under the cement base.

Types of Zinc Phosphate Cement

Zinc phosphate cements are classified into two types.

Type I, fine grain, is designed for the accurate seating of precision appliances and for other uses.

Type II, medium grain, is recommended for all uses *except* the cementing of precision appliances. This includes use as an insulating base.

Exothermic Action

Zinc phosphate cement is exothermic in action. (**Exothermic** means giving off heat.)

In order to dissipate this heat prior to placement in the cavity preparation, the cement must be spatulated thoroughly on the cool, dry glass slab.

The temperature of the glass slab is an important variable in the mixing of zinc phosphate cement. The ideal slab temperature is 68°F.

A higher temperature causes acceleration of the set of the cement. A lower slab temperature may cause moisture to condense on the slab, and this moisture adversely affects the set of the mix. (The temperature at which this condensation occurs is known as the **dew point**.)

It is critical that the powder be added to the liquid in very small increments and spatulated thoroughly after each addition. This procedure also dissipates the heat of the chemical action and retards the set of the cement.

Mixing and Setting Times

The maximum mixing time for zinc phosphate cement is 2 minutes, and the setting time in the mouth is 5 to 7 minutes.

Prolonging the setting time allows the operator more working time. This is particularly important during cementation and may be accomplished by:

▼ Using a cool, dry slab.

▼ Decreasing the rate at which the powder increment is incorporated into the liquid at each increment.

▼ Allowing a pause after the *initial* incorporating of a pinhead amount of powder into the liquid. Allow this to stand for 2 or 3 minutes. (Check manufacturer's directions for exact time.)

▼ Decreasing the powder to liquid ratio.

Mixing Zinc Phosphate for Cementation

All brands of zinc phosphate cement are mixed in basically the same manner. This includes:

▼ Dividing the powder into progressively smaller sections

▼ Incorporating the sections into the liquid in a specific sequence based on their size.

▼ Mixing each increment for a specific time.

However, each manufacturer uses a slightly different system for sectioning the powder and for the mixing time for each increment. Prior to actually mixing a cement, always read and follow the manufacturer's directions for the brand being mixed.

The following procedure gives general, not brand specific, instructions for mixing zinc phosphate cement.

Instrumentation

▼ Glass slab (cool and dry) $1 \times 3 \times 6$ inches.

▼ Spatula (flexible stainless steel).

▼ Powder and liquid.

▼ Powder dispenser.

▼ Liquid dispenser.

Procedure

MIXING ZINC PHOSPHATE FOR CEMENTATION

1. Place the measured powder on the right two thirds of the glass slab. Immediately replace the cap on the powder bottle.

2. Use the spatula to flatten the powder and divide it into sections according to the manufacturer's instructions.

3. Pick up and swirl the bottle of liquid. Use the dropper to dispense the drops of liquid on the left portion of the slab. Expel excess liquid back into the bottle and replace the cap immediately (Fig. 20–1).

4. Incorporate each increment in the sequence and for the length of time specified by the manufacturer (Fig. 20–2).

Continued on following page

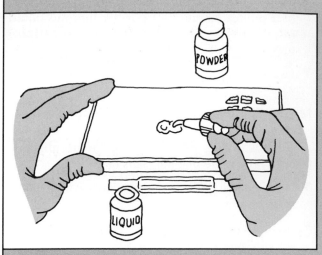

Figure 20-1 Dispensing zinc phosphate cement liquid on the slab. Notice how the powder is divided into sections. (Torres HO, Ehrlich A: Modern Dental Assisting, 4th Ed. Philadelphia, WB Saunders, 1990, p 524.)

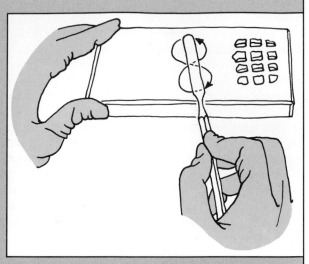

Figure 20-3 Mixing the zinc phosphate cement, using a figure-eight motion. (Torres HO, Ehrlich A: Modern Dental Assisting, 4th Ed. Philadelphia, WB Saunders, 1990, p 525.)

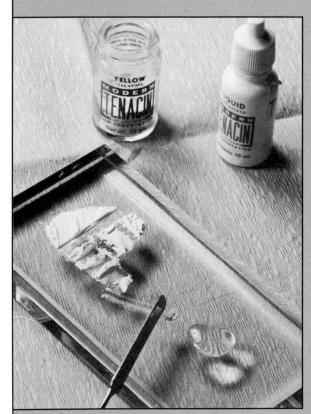

Figure 20-2 Incorporating a very small amount of zinc phosphate powder into the liquid. (Torres HO, Ehrlich A: Modern Dental Assisting, 4th Ed. Philadelphia, WB Saunders, 1990, p 524.)

5 Mix the powder and liquid using a figure-eight rotary motion over an area that is approximately the size of a silver dollar (Fig. 20-3).

6 To avoid wasting material, do not allow the mix to cover more than one third of the slab.

7 Complete the mix within 2 minutes.

8 Test the consistency for cementation by placing the flat blade of the spatula into the mix and lifting the spatula vertically.

9 The consistency is correct when the mix adhering to the spatula elongates into a strand when held about 1 inch from the slab (Fig. 20-4).

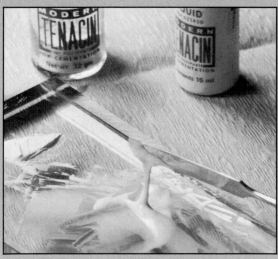

Figure 20-4 Testing the mix of zinc phosphate cement for cementation. (Torres HO, Ehrlich A: Modern Dental Assisting, 4th Ed. Philadelphia, WB Saunders, 1990, p 525.)

Mixing Zinc Phosphate Cement for an Insulating Base

A thicker mix is needed for an insulating base. This is obtained by using a larger portion of powder with the same mixing procedure. The resulting mix has a thick, putty-like consistency (Fig. 20-5).

An explorer, plastic instrument, or spoon excavator is used to place the mix in the cavity preparation. The base is gently packed into place using smooth amalgam condensers of graduated sizes.

To prevent the mix from sticking to the instruments, the tips of the condensers are treated with alcohol or cement powder.

Care of Slab and Instruments

To prevent the hardening of the cement mix on the spatula and the glass slab, they should be cleaned immediately after placement of the cement in the tooth.

If they are cleaned immediately, the cement mix disintegrates when rinsed with tap water. The slab and spatula are dried with a clean paper towel and stored.

Avoid scratching the glass slab because any rough areas on the slab will retain particles of the previous mix. If incorporated into a new mix, these particles cause a faster set of the zinc phosphate cement. Also, if the glass slab is chipped, bits of glass may be incorporated into the cement mix.

If the mix has hardened on the slab and spatula, it can be loosened by permitting a solution of bicarbonate of soda and water to stand on the slab and spatula.

This solution dissolves the cement compound. The slab and spatula are then rinsed with tap water, dried with a clean towel, and stored.

ZINC OXIDE–EUGENOL CEMENT

Zinc oxide–eugenol (ZOE) cement is used as a sedative dressing for sensitive teeth and as an insulating base for deep, permanent restorations (Fig. 20-6).

It is also used for the cementation of temporary coverage; however, it is *not* used for the cementation of permanent cast restorations.

ZOE is also *not* used under composite resin restorations because the eugenol in the liquid retards the setting of the resin materials.

To prevent other materials from being contaminated by the pungent odor of the eugenol, the eugenol liquid and zinc oxide powder are stored away from other dental materials.

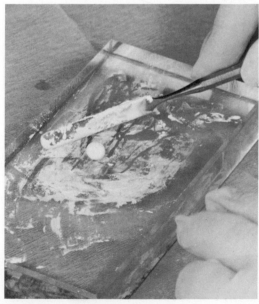

▼ **Figure 20-5**

Testing the mix of zinc phosphate cement for an insulating base. (Torres HO, Ehrlich A: Modern Dental Assisting, 4th Ed. Philadelphia, WB Saunders, 1990, p 525.)

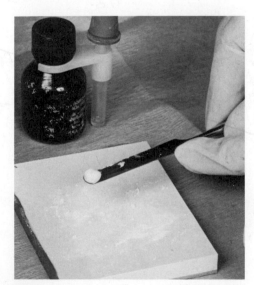

▼ **Figure 20-6**

Zinc oxide–eugenol mixed for a sedative base. (Torres HO, Ehrlich A: Modern Dental Assisting, 4th Ed. Philadelphia, WB Saunders, 1990, p 528.)

Mixing and Setting Times

ZOE is usually mixed on an oil-resistant (parchment) paper pad. However, a glass slab is used if a slower set is required. (If a glass slab is used, it is reserved *only* for mixing ZOE and is not used for mixing other cements.)

The normal mixing time is 45 to 60 seconds, and normal setting time is 4 to 5 minutes.

Mixing ZOE Cement for Cementation of Temporary Coverage

The following procedure gives general, not brand specific, instructions for mixing ZOE cement.

Instrumentation

▼ Parchment paper pad.

▼ Spatula (small and flexible).

▼ Zinc oxide powder and dispenser.

▼ Eugenol liquid and dropper.

▼ Isopropyl alcohol or oil of orange solvent.

Care of Mixing Pad and Instruments

The top sheet of the mixing pad is carefully removed and discarded. The spatula is wiped free of the mix with a clean tissue.

Procedure

MIXING ZOE CEMENT FOR CEMENTATION OF TEMPORARY COVERAGE

[1] Measure 1 scoop of powder and place it on the mixing pad. Replace the cap on the powder container immediately (Fig. 20–7).

[2] Dispense 3 drops of liquid near the powder on the mixing pad. Replace the cap on the liquid container immediately.

[3] Incorporate the powder and liquid in one or two increments.

[4] Mix and then for 5 seconds strop (wipe vigorously) the material over a large area of the mixing pad (Fig. 20–8).

[5] The mix should be smooth and creamy and completed within 45–60 seconds.

[6] Use the edge of the spatula to place the mix on the edge of the temporary coverage.

[7] Take care not to trap air bubbles while letting the mix flow into the interior of the temporary coverage.

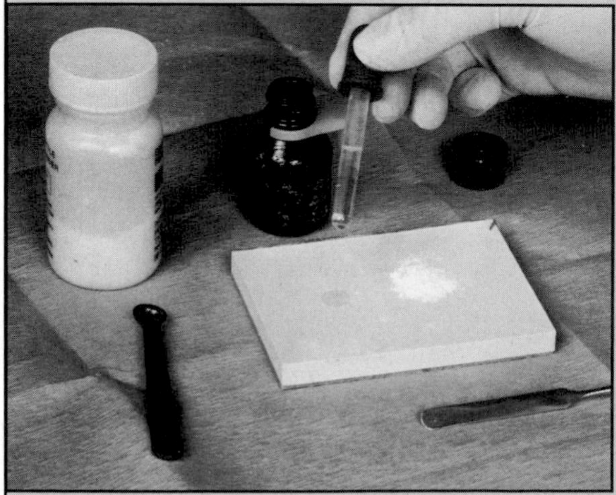

Figure 20–7 Dispensing zinc oxide–eugenol powder and liquid. (Torres HO, Ehrlich A: Modern Dental Assisting, 4th Ed. Philadelphia, WB Saunders, 1990, p 527.)

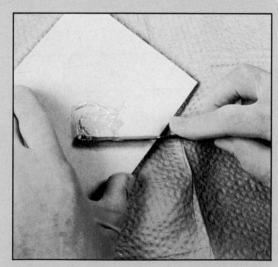

Figure 20–8 Mixing zinc oxide–eugenol cement. (Torres HO, Ehrlich A: Modern Dental Assisting, 4th Ed. Philadelphia, WB Saunders, 1990, p 527.)

If ZOE cement has hardened, the instruments may be wiped with alcohol or oil of orange solvent to soften and loosen the cement.

INTERMEDIATE RESTORATIVE MATERIAL

Intermediate restorative material (IRM) is a reinforced zinc oxide–eugenol composition that is used for intermediate (temporary) restorations that last up to 1 year.

Instrumentation (Fig. 20–9)

▼ Parchment paper pad.

▼ Spatula (small and flexible).

▼ Powder and dispenser.

▼ Liquid and dropper.

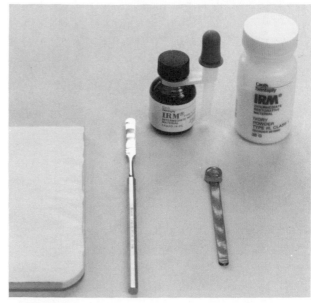

▼ **Figure 20–9**

IRM cement instrumentation. Left to right, paper mixing pad, small spatula, liquid and dropper, measure for powder, and powder.

Procedure

MIXING INTERMEDIATE RESTORATIVE MATERIAL

1. Dispense 1 large scoop of powder and 1 drop of liquid on the mixing pad.

2. Bring in one half of the powder and mix quickly.

3. Bring the remaining powder into the mix in two to three increments and spatulate thoroughly. The mix appears quite stiff.

4. Strop (wipe vigorously) the mix for 5 to 10 seconds. The resulting mix should be smooth and adaptable. The mix is completed in 1 minute.

EBA (Fortified ZOE)

ORTHO-ETHOXYBENZOIC ACID CEMENT

The addition of *ortho-ethoxybenzoic acid* (EBA) to the eugenol liquid and of fillers to the zinc oxide powder results in a composition referred to as EBA cement.

Quartz or AL

The resulting product is stronger than ZOE cement and is used for permanent cementation of inlays, crowns, and bridges.

The procedure for measuring and mixing EBA cement is similar to that for ZOE cement. An acceptable homogeneous mix is accomplished within 30 seconds.

POLYCARBOXYLATE (POLYACRYLATE) CEMENT

Polycarboxylate cement, also referred to as *carboxylate cement*, is frequently used for the cementation of cast restorations and for the direct bonding of orthodontic brackets.

It may also be used as a nonirritating base under either amalgam or composite restorations.

Measuring the Powder and Liquid

Use the powder measure supplied by the manufacturer. Press this firmly down into the powder in the bottle. As the measure is removed from the bottle, use the spatula to scrape excess powder so that the powder is flush with the top of measuring cup.

The liquid may be measured using either the plastic squeeze bottle, as shown in Figure 20–10, or by the calibrated syringe type liquid dispenser supplied by the manufacturer. (Of the two, the syringe calibrated dispenser is more accurate.)

When using a calibrated syringe type liquid dispenser, 1 full calibration of liquid is obtained by moving the plunger from one full calibration mark to the next full calibration mark.

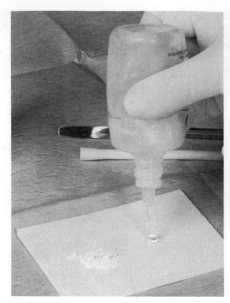

▼ Figure 20-10

Dispensing liquid for polycarboxylate cement.

If using the plastic squeeze bottle, hold the bottle in a vertical position and squeeze. Release pressure when the drop separates from the nozzle.

Powder to Liquid Ratios

For cementation, use 1 scoop of powder to 3 drops of liquid, or 1 scoop of powder to 1 full calibration of liquid from the calibrated liquid dispenser.

For an insulating base, the ratio is 1 scoop of powder to 2 drops of liquid, or use 1 scoop of powder to ⅔ calibrations of liquid from the calibrated liquid dispenser.

For a heavier consistency, use 2 scoops of powder to 1 full calibration of liquid from the calibrated liquid dispenser.

Mixing and Setting Times

The mix is spatulated until the desired glossy consistency is obtained. This *must* be completed within 30 seconds.

Do not use the mix if it has lost its glossy appearance or reached the stringy (tacky) stage on the slab.

When used as a base, the cement is permitted to set for approximately 5 minutes prior to the placement of the permanent restoration.

Mixing Polycarboxylate Cement for Cementation

The following are general, not brand specific, instructions for polycarboxylate cement.

Instrumentation

▼ Heavy paper pad or cool and dry (68°F) glass slab.

▼ Spatula (flexible steel).

▼ Polycarboxylate powder and measure.

▼ Polycarboxylate liquid and measure.

▼ Spoon excavator (small) or plastic instrument.

Procedure

MIXING POLYCARBOXYLATE CEMENT FOR CEMENTATION

1. Dispense 1 scoop of powder onto the mixing pad.

2. Dispense 3 drops of liquid immediately prior to mixing.

3. Use the spatula to incorporate all of the powder into the liquid at one time.

4. Complete mix to a glossy consistency within 30 seconds (Fig. 20-11).
   Do not overspatulate.
   Do not use the mix if it has lost its glossy appearance or reached the stringy (tacky) stage on the mixing pad.

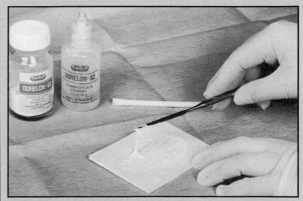

Figure 20-11 Mixing polycarboxylate cement mixed for cementation. (Torres HO, Ehrlich A: Modern Dental Assisting, 4th Ed. Philadelphia, WB Saunders, 1990, p 529.)

Care of Mixing Pad and Instruments

Carefully tear off the top sheet of the mixing pad. If a glass slab was used, clean it and the spatula immediately after use and before the material has set. To do this, wipe the slab and instruments with a wet tissue under running water.

Once the material has set, it can be removed with a 10 percent sodium hydroxide solution.

GLASS IONOMER CEMENT

Glass ionomer cement, also known as *alumino-si-licate-polyacrylate* (ASPA), is created by combining very fine glass powder with a solution of polymeric organic acid.

This material is radiopaque and has a fluoride-releasing base that is beneficial under composite and amalgam restorations.

It chemically bonds to enamel and dentin and can be acid-etched with the surrounding enamel to accept a composite restoration.

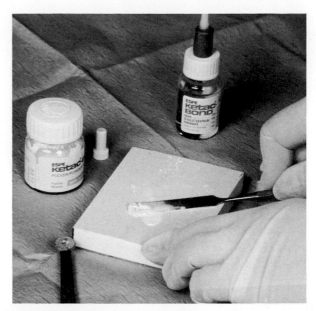

▼ **Figure 20-12**

Mixing glass ionomer cement. (Torres HO, Ehrlich A: Modern Dental Assisting, 4th Ed. Philadelphia, WB Saunders, 1990, p 530.)

Specific Formulations

Unlike the cements previously discussed, glass ionomer cements come in special formulations for each specific application. For example, one type is used for cementation; another is used as a protective base; and another type is used to restore Class V cavities, abraded areas, and erosion root caries.

Because there are many varieties of the glass ionomer cements, it is particularly important to read and follow the directions for the specific type of cement being used.

Powder to Liquid Ratios

The powder to liquid ratio may be 1 scoop of powder to 1 drop of liquid or 1 scoop of powder to 2 drops of liquid.

Mixing and Setting Times

Working time for glass ionomer cements ranges from 30 seconds to 2 minutes (Fig. 20-12).

The cement must be placed while still glossy and before it loses its shiny appearance. The setting time ranges from 3 to 6 minutes.

Glass Ionomer Capsules

Some glass ionomer cements are supplied in a premeasured capsule, which contains both the powder and the liquid. The following are general, not brand specific, instructions for using glass ionomer capsules.

Procedure

MIXING GLASS IONOMER CEMENT FROM CAPSULES

1 Activate the capsule using the "activator" provided by the manufacturer (Fig. 20-13).

2 Place the activated capsule in a high-speed amalgamator and triturate (mix) for 10

seconds. (The use of an amalgamator is described in Chapter 21, "Amalgam Restorations.")

Continued on following page

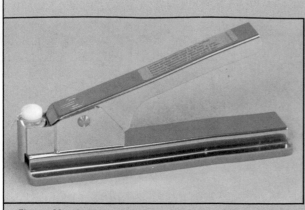

Figure 20-13 An "activator" is used to activate the glass ionomer cement capsule.

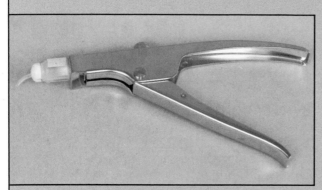

Figure 20-14 After the glass ionomer cement capsule has been triturated, it is placed in the dispenser.

3 Insert the capsule into the "applier" supplied by the manufacturer and immediately release the sealing pin (Fig. 20-14).

4 Dispense the material by squeezing the applier (Fig. 20-15).

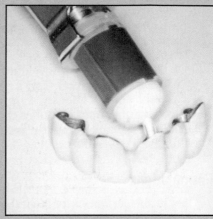

Figure 20-15 Glass ionomer cement being dispensed for the cementation of a maxillary anterior fixed bridge. (Photo courtesy of ESPE-Premier Sales Corp, Norristown, PA.)

CAVITY LINERS

Cavity liners are used to provide a barrier for the protection of pulpal tissue from chemical irritation caused by cements and composites. They also help to reduce the sensitivity of fresh cut dentin.

Calcium hydroxide is the most widely used cavity liner because it is protective of the pulp and is compatible with *all* restorative materials.

ZOE is occasionally used as a cavity liner; however, it cannot be used under composites because the eugenol retards the set of these restorative materials.

When both a liner and an insulating base are required, the liner is placed first. Once it is set, the insulating base is placed over the lining agent (Fig. 20-16).

Calcium hydroxide is supplied in a two-paste

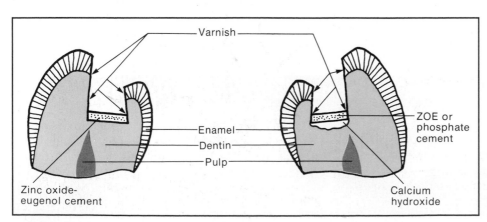

Varnish

Enamel
Dentin
Pulp

Zinc oxide-eugenol cement

ZOE or phosphate cement

Calcium hydroxide

▼ **Figure 20-16**

The use of dental cements as pulpal protective material and sedative base in cavity preparation. (Torres HO, Ehrlich A: Modern Dental Assisting, 4th Ed. Philadelphia, WB Saunders, 1990, p 522.)

(base and catalyst) system. The catalyst and base pastes *must* be from the same manufacturer.

Calcium hydroxide may be self-cured, or it may require light-curing. The description that follows is of a self-cured, two-paste mix.

Instrumentation

▼ Parchment paper pad (small).

▼ Spatula (small) or ball-point type mixer-applicator.

▼ Calcium hydroxide base and catalyst.

Care of Mixing Pad and Instruments

The used sheet is removed from the mixing pad and discarded. The used instruments are wiped clean before the material has set.

CAVITY VARNISHES

Copal Cavity Varnish

Copal cavity varnishes are a thin liquid consisting of one or more resins in an organic solvent. They are used primarily to seal the dentinal tubules and may be used under an amalgam restoration. This

---

Procedure

MIXING CALCIUM HYDROXIDE

1. Dispense equal amounts of catalyst and base onto the paper pad (Fig. 20–17). Approximately 1 to 2 mm are used, depending on the size of the cavity preparation.

2. Use the small spatula or ball-shaped mixer-applicator in a circular motion to mix the two materials quickly. Working within a small area of the pad, obtain a homogeneous mix in 10 seconds (Fig. 20–18).

   Note: Do not spread the material out on the pad. It wastes the material.

3. The mix is applied using the ball-shaped mixer-applicator.

4. The small spoon excavator, or explorer point, is used to remove any irregular areas of calcium hydroxide.

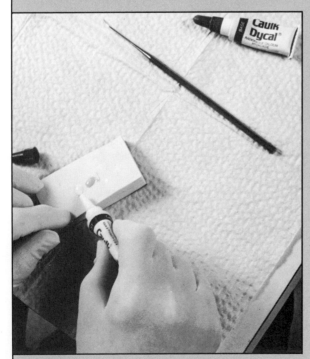

Figure 20–17 Dispensing calcium hydroxide catalyst and base. (Torres HO, Ehrlich A: Modern Dental Assisting, 4th Ed. Philadelphia, WB Saunders, 1990, p 531.)

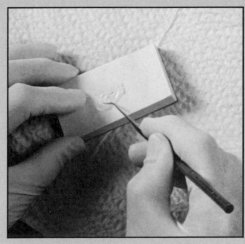

Figure 20–18 Mixing calcium hydroxide catalyst and base. (Torres HO, Ehrlich A: Modern Dental Assisting, 4th Ed. Philadelphia, WB Saunders, 1990, p 532.)

material is *not* compatible with composite resin restorative materials.

A thin coating of cavity varnish may be applied over the cavity liner and/or insulating base. A second application may also be placed to coat the surfaces of the dentin thoroughly and to fill any voids from bubbles created when the first application dries.

Copal cavity varnish has an organic solvent that quickly evaporates, leaving the resin as a thin film over the preparation. It dries within a few seconds.

For proper use, this varnish should be just a little thicker than water. If it becomes slightly thickened, it is thinned very cautiously with solvent. If the liquid becomes very thick, it is discarded.

Because varnishes do not provide adequate insulation against the thermal conduction of metal restorations, it may be necessary to add an insulating base for this purpose. If so, the varnish is applied before the base is placed.

Universal Cavity Varnish

Universal varnishes, also known as *dentin sealants*, are formulated for use under *all* types of restorative materials including cement bases and amalgam and composite restorations.

Instrumentation

▼ Copal cavity varnish.

▼ Solvent (if needed).

▼ Applicator (brush or flexible wire loop).

▼ Cotton pellets.

▼ Cotton pliers.

Procedure

PROCEDURE FOR PREPARING CAVITY VARNISH

1. Open the bottle and dip the applicator tip into the fluid. An alternative applicator is a *small* sterile cotton pellet held in cotton pliers (Fig. 20–19).

2. To prevent evaporation, replace the cap on the bottle immediately.

3. Pass the prepared applicator to the operator.

4. If necessary, the operator removes any excess varnish from the enamel with a fresh cotton pellet.

5. If a second application of cavity varnish is to be placed, repeat the previous steps.

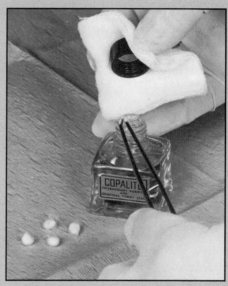

Figure 20–19 Dispensing cavity varnish. (Torres HO, Ehrlich A: Modern Dental Assisting, 4th Ed. Philadelphia, WB Saunders, 1990, p 533.)

▼ EXERCISES

1. Type _____ zinc phosphate cement is designed for the accurate seating of precision castings.

   a. I
   b. II

2. A/An _____ base is placed to soothe the pulp that has been irritated by decay, injury, or the trauma of the cavity preparation.

   a. insulating
   b. intermediate
   c. sedative
   d. temporary

3. A restoration of intermediate restorative material will last up to _____ _____ .

   a. 3 months
   b. 6 months
   c. 1 year
   d. 5 years

4. Polycarboxylate cement _____ inserted after it has lost its glossy appearance.

   a. is
   b. is not

5. When mixing cements, the powder to liquid ratio depends on the _____ _____ .

   a. intended use
   b. manufacturer's instructions
   c. mixing technique used
   d. a and b

6. Zinc oxide–eugenol cement is used for a _____ .

   a. base under composite restorations
   b. cement for temporary crowns
   c. sedative base
   d. b and c

7. A solution of _____ is used to remove a mix of zinc phosphate cement that has hardened on a glass slab and spatula.

   a. bicarbonate of soda
   b. citric acid
   c. eugenol
   d. oil of orange

8. Copal varnish _____ acceptable for placement under an amalgam restoration.

   a. is
   b. is not

9. A calibrated syringe type liquid dispenser may be used when dispensing the liquid for _____ cement.

   a. EBA
   b. IRM
   c. glass ionomer
   d. polycarboxylate

10. _____ may be used under all types of restorative materials.

    a. Calcium hydroxide
    b. Copal varnish
    c. Zinc oxide–eugenol
    d. a and b

11. Exothermic means to _____ heat.

    a. give off
    b. take in

12. Ortho-ethoxybenzoic acid (EBA) cement is used for _____ _____ .

    a. a base under a composite restoration
    b. a temporary restoration
    c. cementation of cast restorations
    d. b or c

13. _____ bonds directly with enamel, dentin, and cementum.

    a. Cavity liner
    b. EBA cement
    c. Glass ionomer cement
    d. Universal varnish

14. When mixing zinc phosphate cement, a cool dry slab will _____ _____ the setting time.

    a. prolong
    b. shorten

15. The zinc phosphate cement is correct for _____ when the mix drops from the spatula in an elongated droplet when held 1 inch from the slab.

    a. an insulating base
    b. cementation

16. _____ is used to soften and loosen zinc oxide–eugenol cement that has hardened on an instrument.

    a. Alcohol
    b. Baking soda
    c. Oil of orange solvent
    d. a or c

17. It _____ acceptable to mix powder and liquid from different manufacturers as long as they are for the same type of cement.

    a. is
    b. is not

18. Glass ionomer capsules are mixed _____.

    a. by mechanical trituration
    b. on a ceramic slab
    c. on a chilled glass slab
    d. on a paper pad

19. Zinc phosphate cement is used _____.

    a. as a surgical dressing
    b. for the cementation of permanent restorations
    c. for the cementation of temporary crowns
    d. in place of a cavity liner

20. Cavity varnish is placed _____ the cavity liner or insulating base.

    a. over
    b. under

▼ Criterion Sheet 20-1

Student's Name _____

Procedure: *MIXING ZINC PHOSPHATE CEMENT FOR CEMENTATION*

Performance Objective:

The student will state the brand name and the manufacturer's recommended powder to liquid ratio for cementation.

The student will demonstrate preparing a mix of zinc phosphate cement for the cementation of a cast restoration.

	SE	IE
SE = Student evaluation **C** = Criterion met **IE** = Instructor evaluation **X** = Criterion not met		
Instrumentation: Glass slab (68°F), flexible spatula, and cement powder and liquid with manufacturer's dispensers. (Appropriate infection control barriers will be used during all procedures actually performed on a patient.)		
1. Brand name: _____. Powder to liquid ratio for cementation: _____.		
2. Dispensed appropriate amounts of powder on the right two thirds of the slab and divided this into sections.		
3. Dispensed appropriate amount of liquid on left side of slab. Expelled excess liquid into bottle and tightly replaced cap.		
4. Used a figure-eight rotary motion to incorporate slowly a very small amount of powder into the liquid.		
5. Paused for 15 to 20 seconds.		
6. Completed additional powder increments. Achieved homogeneous mix of cement within specified time.		
7. Tested mass for droplet break 1 inch from slab.		
8. Cleaned slab and spatula and put materials away.		
Comments:		

▼ Criterion Sheet 20–2

Student's Name _____

Procedure: *MIXING ZINC OXIDE–EUGENOL CEMENT FOR A SEDATIVE BASE*

Performance Objective:

The student will state the brand name and the manufacturer's recommended powder to liquid ratio for a sedative base.

The student will then demonstrate preparing a mix of zinc oxide–eugenol cement for a sedative base.

		SE	IE
SE = Student evaluation **C** = Criterion met			
IE = Instructor evaluation **X** = Criterion not met			
Instrumentation: Paper pad, flexible spatula, and cement powder and liquid with manufacturer's dispensers. (Appropriate infection control barriers will be used during all procedures actually performed on a patient.)			
1. Brand name: _____. Powder to liquid ratio for cementation: _____.			
2. Dispensed appropriate amounts of powder and liquid onto the paper pad. Expelled excess liquid into bottle and tightly replaced cap.			
3. Used the spatula flat on its side to incorporate a medium amount (½ scoop) of powder into liquid.			
4. Spatulated mass together in a small area.			
5. Incorporated more powder and spatulated in a small area.			
6. Completed homogeneous mix within 45 seconds.			
7. Completed mix was of a putty-like consistency.			
8. Removed used materials, cleaned spatula, and put materials away.			
Comments:			

▼ Criterion Sheet 20-3

Student's Name _____

Procedure: *MIXING CALCIUM HYDROXIDE LINER*

Performance Objective:

The student will demonstrate mixing calcium hydroxide for use as a cavity liner.

	SE	IE
SE = Student evaluation **C** = Criterion met **IE** = Instructor evaluation **X** = Criterion not met		
Instrumentation: Small paper pad, ball-shaped mixer-applicator, and calcium hydroxide base and catalyst. (Appropriate infection control barriers will be used during all procedures actually performed on a patient.)		
1. Dispensed equal amounts of catalyst and base onto paper pad.		
2. Used mixer-applicator in a circular motion to mix the materials.		
3. Obtained a homogeneous mix within 10 seconds.		
Comments:		

21 Amalgam Restorations

▼ LEARNING OBJECTIVES

The student will be able to:

1. State one major advantage and one disadvantage of amalgam restorations.

2. Define these terms related to amalgam restorations: mechanical retention, microleakage, pulpal floor, and the names of the cavity walls (buccal, dentinal, distal, facial, gingival, incisal, labial, lingual, mesial, proximal).

3. List the six steps in cavity preparation.

4. Define these terms related to the structure of amalgam: alloy, mercury, high-copper alloy, mercury to alloy ratios, and trituration.

5. Identify the parts of a Tofflemire retainer and demonstrate the assembly of a Tofflemire retainer.

6. Demonstrate preparing a pre-set tray for the placement of an amalgam restoration.

7. Demonstrate assisting during the preparation and placement of an amalgam restoration.

OVERVIEW OF AMALGAM RESTORATIONS

Amalgam restorations, also known as *silver fillings*, are one of the most common type of dental restoration for placement in the posterior teeth (Fig. 21–1).

The major advantages of amalgam as a restorative material are its strength and durability. These characteristics make it capable of withstanding the great pressure brought against it during mastication (chewing).

Another advantage is the plasticity of freshly mixed amalgam. This means that before it hardens, the material can be placed into a prepared cavity and carved to restore the normal contours of the tooth.

The major disadvantage of amalgam as a restorative material is that it does not match the tooth color. For this reason, amalgam is used primarily on the surfaces of the posterior teeth, which are not visible when the patient smiles.

TERMINOLOGY RELATED TO AMALGAM RESTORATIONS

Mechanical Retention

Mechanical retention is the process of holding together materials that will *not* adhere (stick) to each other. Because amalgam does not adhere to the tooth structure, it must be held in place by mechanical retention.

Therefore, the cavity preparation for an amal-

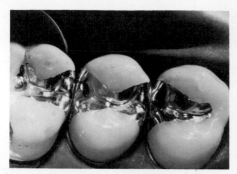

▼ **Figure 21-1**

Finished amalgam restorations. (Baum L, Phillips RW, Lund MR: Operative Dentistry, 2nd Ed. Philadelphia, WB Saunders, 1985, p 337.)

gam restoration must be shaped to provide the mechanical retention that will hold the restoration in place.

In a composite restoration, the tooth and restorative material are **bonded.** Because the tooth and restorative material actually adhere to each other, it is not necessary to rely on mechanical retention to hold the restoration in place. (Composite restorations are discussed in Chapter 22, "Cosmetic Dentistry.")

Microleakage

With mechanical retention, there is usually a microscopic space between the tooth and a restoration. This space permits the microleakage of fluids, microorganisms, and debris from the mouth down the walls of the cavity preparation and into the pulp.

If the microleakage is severe, it may cause the tooth to remain sensitive following placement of the restoration.

Cavity Classifications

Cavity classifications are discussed in Chapter 14, "The Dental Examination."

Cavity Walls

A cavity wall is a side of the cavity preparation that aids in enclosing restorative material. Each wall is named for the surface of the tooth toward which it is placed.

The **mesial wall** is nearest the mesial surface of the tooth; the **distal wall** is nearest the distal surface of the tooth. These two are also referred to as **proximal walls.**

The **buccal wall** is nearest the cheek; the **labial wall** is nearest the lips. Together they are also known as the **facial wall.**

The **lingual wall** is located toward the lingual surface. The **incisal wall** is located toward the incisal edge of an anterior tooth.

The **axial wall** is that portion of the prepared tooth located near the pulpal area and parallel with the long axis of the tooth.

The **dentinal wall** is the portion of the cavity wall that consists of dentin. The **pulpal floor,** which is actually the *pulpal wall*, is the floor of the cavity preparation overlying the pulp. It is at a right angle to the other cavity walls.

The **gingival wall** is the wall of the preparation that is nearest the gingiva. Like the pulpal floor, it is at a right angle to the other cavity walls.

THE PRINCIPLES OF CAVITY PREPARATION

A cavity preparation is a surgical operation that removes caries and a limited amount of healthy tooth structure to prepare the tooth to receive and retain the restoration. The principles of cavity preparation describe the steps that the dentist follows in order to prepare a tooth for an amalgam restoration.

The type of cavity being prepared and the operator's personal preference influence which rotary and hand instruments are used in each step.

The steps are described here separately for teaching purposes. Actually, the dentist performs several at the same time.

Step 1: Outline Form

The outline form is the curved shape and border of the proposed restoration and of the tooth surface.

This step is usually performed with a high-speed handpiece and a number 245 bur.

Step 2: Resistance and Retention Form

The **resistance form** is the shape and relationship of the cavity walls that protect the tooth structure and restorative material against fracture. (Enamel that is not properly supported will fracture.)

This step is usually performed with a high-speed handpiece and a number 245 bur.

The **retention form** is the shape and relationship of the cavity walls that provide the mechanical retention necessary to hold the restoration in place.

This step is usually performed with a high-speed handpiece and a number 169-L taper fissure or ¼ round bur.

Step 3: Convenience Form

The convenience form is the amount of cavity opening that is necessary so that the operator can gain access to the cavity preparation for the insertion and finishing of the restorative material.

This step, which is generally done in conjunction with the outline form, is usually performed with a high-speed handpiece and a number 245 bur.

Step 4: Removal of Caries

The removal of caries is the process of removing the decayed and decalcified enamel and dentin. Active decay left under a restoration may cause further damage to the tooth because of recurrent caries.

This is usually performed with a number 4 or 6 round bur in a low-speed handpiece or with a spoon excavator.

Step 5: Refinement of the Cavity Walls and Margins

The refinement of the cavity walls and margins is also referred to as *finishing the enamel walls and margins*. This is the process of angling, beveling, and smoothing the walls of the cavity preparation.

This step is usually performed with a plain cut fissure bur in a high-speed handpiece. Finishing of the proximal surfaces may also require the use of hand instruments, such as enamel hatchets and margin trimmers.

Step 6: Debridement of the Cavity

Debridement of the cavity is the process of removing all of the debris from the preparation to ensure a clean, dry surface for the placement of the restoration.

This step is performed by thoroughly rinsing the preparation with warm water.

After debridement, the cavity is gently dried with warm air and cotton pellets. This must be done very carefully so that the dentin is not damaged by being dried out in the process.

THE STRUCTURE OF AMALGAM

An **amalgam** is an alloy in which mercury is one of the metals. (An **alloy** is the production of the fusion of two or more metals.)

In dentistry, amalgam restorative material is formed by mixing mercury with an alloy that contains silver, tin, copper, and sometimes zinc.

High-Copper Alloys

High-copper alloys, which are currently used in dentistry, are so called because they contain a higher percentage of copper than was used in earlier low-copper alloys.

High-copper alloys can be classified according to particle shape as **spherical** (round particles) and **admixed** (a combination of lathe-cut and spherical particles).

These particle shapes influence the trituration and working characteristics (condensing and carving) of the resulting amalgam mixture.

Mercury

Pure mercury is a metal that is liquid at room temperature, has a mirror-like appearance, and pours cleanly from its container. Mercury is a hazardous substance and must be handled with proper care. (See under "Special Mercury Considerations" in Chapter 8.)

Mercury to Alloy Ratios

The mercury to alloy ratio is important in that this ratio influences the ease of trituration as well as the plasticity (workability) of the amalgam mass.

This is expressed as an alloy to mercury ratio. A 1:1 ratio is widely used. This is 1 portion of amalgam to 1 portion of mercury by weight.

Preloaded capsules, such as those shown in the upper right corner of Figures 21–2 and 21–3 contain the mercury and alloy already measured in the proper ratios.

Trituration

Trituration, also known as *amalgamation*, is the process by which the mercury and alloy are mixed

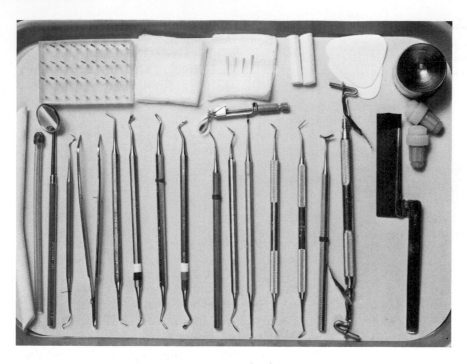

▼ **Figure 21-2**

Pre-set tray for an amalgam restoration.
(Torres HO, Ehrlich A: Modern Dental Assisting, 4th Ed. Philadelphia, WB Saunders, 1990, p 547.)

together to form the "plastic" mass of amalgam needed to create the dental restoration.

The preloaded capsule of amalgam alloy and liquid mercury contains a **pestle,** which aids in the mixing process. Within the capsule, a thin membrane also separates the mercury and alloy until they are ready to be mixed.

Just prior to placing the capsule in the amalgamator it must be activated to break the separating membrane (see Fig. 21-3).

The activated capsule is placed in the amalgamator and the cover is closed to prevent mercury vapors from escaping during trituration. (An **amalgamator** is a mechanical device used to triturate amalgam. See Fig. 8-2.)

The amalgamator is set for and operated for the length of time specified by the manufacturer's directions.

An amalgam well, a glass dappen dish, or an amalgam squeeze cloth is used to receive the freshly mixed amalgam. (An amalgam well is shown in the upper right-hand corner of Figure 21-2.)

In a proper mix, the plastic mass of amalgam is free of dry alloy particles and does not stick to the sides of the capsule.

The fresh mix is dumped from the capsule into the receptacle, the pestle is removed, and the mix is loaded directly into the amalgam carrier. Amalgam is never touched with the hands and must not be allowed to be contaminated with moisture.

At the end of the procedure, any remaining amalgam scrap is discarded into a sealed container, where it is covered with radiographic film processing fixer. (This precaution prevents mercury vapors from escaping.)

Condensation of Amalgam

The freshly mixed amalgam is placed by increments into the cavity preparation, starting with the small end of the amalgam carrier and later switching to the larger end of the amalgam carrier.

After each increment, the operator condenses the amalgam, beginning with a small condenser and gradually working up to a larger size.

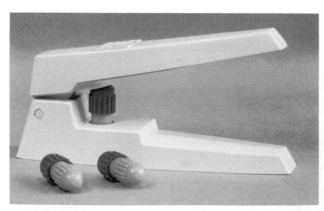

▼ **Figure 21-3**

Just prior to placing the capsule in the amalgamator, it is activated to break the separating membrane.

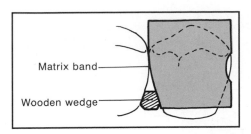

▼ **Figure 21–4**

Cross section of a modified wooden wedge in place. Note adaptation of band at gingival embrasure (lingual view). (Torres HO, Ehrlich A: Modern Dental Assisting, 4th Ed. Philadelphia, WB Saunders, 1990, p 543.)

Condensation firmly packs the amalgam into all areas of the preparation and brings any excess mercury to the surface.

The cavity is "overfilled" so that the excess mercury-rich material can be carved away and then removed with the high volume evacuator (HVE) tip.

MATRIX BANDS, RETAINERS, AND WEDGES

A **matrix** is a metal or plastic band used to replace the missing wall of a tooth during placement of the restorative material. (The plural of matrix is *matrices*.)

A **retainer**, or holder, is necessary to secure the matrix in position around the tooth. The Tofflemire matrix retainer is the one most commonly used for amalgam restorations, and it is described here.

A **wedge**, made of either plastic or wood, is used to adapt the matrix band to the gingival contours of the tooth. If necessary, a knife is used to shape the wedge for a better fit (Fig. 21–4).

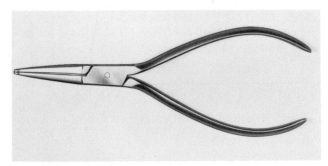

▼ **Figure 21–5**

A number 110 (How) pliers may be used to aid in placing and removing the wedge. (Courtesy of Rocky Mountain Orthodontics, Denver, CO.)

A number 110 (How) **pliers**, hemostat, or the operator's fingers are used as an aid in placing and removing the wedge (Fig. 21–5).

Matrix Bands

The stainless steel matrix bands that are used with the Tofflemire retainer are available in **premolar**, **molar**, and **universal** sizes.

When the ends of the curved band are brought together, they form a slightly modified **V** shape.

▼ The **larger** circumference of the band is the *occlusal edge* and is always placed toward the occlusal of the tooth.

▼ The **smaller** circumference of the band is the *gingival edge* and is always placed toward the gingiva.

In preparation for use, the matrix band must be contoured (shaped) in the interproximal area so that it properly contacts the tooth next to it.

THE TOFFLEMIRE MATRIX RETAINER

When a Class II (two- or three-surface) amalgam restoration is placed, a matrix band, retainer, and wedge are used to replace temporarily the missing walls of the prepared tooth and to provide the contours of the tooth.

The assistant is responsible for assembling the matrix band in the retainer. This should be done before the procedure is started or while the operator is completing the placement of the base and cavity liner.

An assembled retainer is shown in the upper middle portion of Figure 21–2.

The retainer is assembled so that it can be positioned at the facial surface of the tooth with handle extending out of the mouth at the corner of the lips.

Parts of the Tofflemire Retainer

Outer Guide Slots

The outer guide slots, also known as *guide channels*, at the end of the retainer serve as channels to guide the loop of the matrix band. The channel selected is determined by the quadrant being treated (Fig. 21–6).

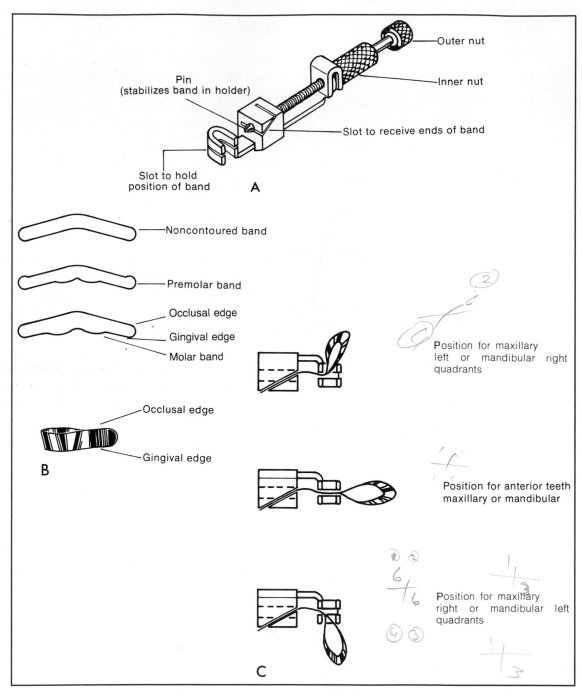

▼ **Figure 21-6**

Tofflemire matrix band and holder. *A.* Slot placed toward the gingivae in all positions. *B.* Assorted sizes and shapes of matrix bands and a matrix band with ends positioned for placement. *C.* Matrix band positions for use in different areas of the mouth. (Torres HO, Ehrlich A: Modern Dental Assisting, 4th Ed. Philadelphia, WB Saunders, 1990, p 542.)

- The **left** guide channel is used for the maxillary left and the mandibular right quadrants.

- The **straight** guide channel is used for anterior maxillary or mandibular teeth.

- The **right** guide channel is used for the maxillary right and the mandibular left quadrants

Diagonal Slot Vise

The diagonal slot vise is a box-like structure used to position the ends of the matrix band within the retainer.

The ends of the matrix band slip into the diagonal slot that runs all the way across the slot vise. This surface of the retainer is always positioned toward the gingiva.

Spindle

The spindle, also known as a *pin* or *rod*, is a screw that fits into the diagonal slot vise to hold the ends of the matrix band. When placing the matrix band into the diagonal slot vice, the spindle point must be clear of the slot.

Outer Nut

The outer nut is used to tighten or loosen the spindle within the diagonal slot vise. To tighten the spindle, turn the outer nut away from you. To loosen the spindle, turn the outer nut toward you.

Be careful not to turn it too far or the diagonal slot vise will fall off the spindle. If this happens, insert the end of the spindle into the diagonal slot vise and turn the outer nut away from you.

Inner Nut

The inner nut is used to adjust the size of the matrix band loop. The size of the loop formed depends on the tooth to be restored.

To make the loop smaller, turn the inner nut away from you. To make the loop larger, turn the inner nut toward you.

Instrumentation for Assembly

- Tofflemire matrix retainer.
- Matrix bands (premolar and molar).
- Burnisher (egg and ball).

Procedure

ASSEMBLING THE TOFFLEMIRE RETAINER

1. Determine the tooth to be treated and select the appropriate matrix band.

2. To contour the matrix band:
   Place the outer surface of the band on a semi-hard surface (such as the back of a mixing pad).
   Use the "egg end" of the burnisher to press against the inner surface of the band so that it is bulging outward at the contact area.

3. Bring the ends of the band evenly together. With ends touching, place the occlusal edge (larger circumference) of the band into the diagonal slot vise.

4. Turn the outer knob clockwise to secure the spindle on the matrix band.

5. Guide the loop through the appropriate guide channel. If necessary, use the handle of an instrument to "open" the loop of the band.

6. Turn the inner knob slightly to close the band. If necessary, use the handle of an instrument to open (fully extend) the loop of the band.

7. Return the assembled matrix and retainer to the instrument tray until it is needed.

THE AMALGAM RESTORATION

The following steps are performed in the preparation and placement of a Class II MO (mesio-occlusal) amalgam restoration. The exact choice of instruments depends on the operator's preferences.

Instrumentation

- Basic setup.
- Local anesthetic setup.
- Rubber dam setup (optional).
- Burs (operator's choice).
- Spoon excavators (small and medium).
- Enamel hatchets (mesial and distal).
- Other hand cutting instruments (operator's choice).
- Calcium hydroxide base and catalyst.

- ▼ Ball applicator (small).
- ▼ Cavity varnish.
- ▼ Cotton pellets.
- ▼ Tofflemire retainer, matrix band, and burnisher.
- ▼ Number 110 pliers.
- ▼ Wooden wedges.
- ▼ Premeasured capsules of alloy and mercury.
- ▼ Amalgam well.

- ▼ Amalgam carrier.
- ▼ Amalgam condensers (large and small, smooth and serrated).
- ▼ Carvers (discoid-cleoid, Hollenback).
- ▼ Holder for articulating paper.
- ▼ Articulating paper.
- ▼ Cotton rolls.
- ▼ HVE tip.

Procedure

THE CAVITY PREPARATION

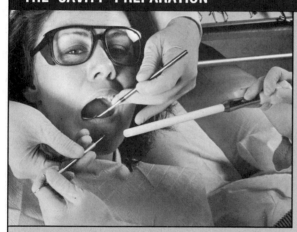

Figure 21–7 The operator receives the explorer to examine the tooth prior to beginning the preparation. (Torres HO, Ehrlich A: Modern Dental Assisting, 4th Ed. Philadelphia, WB Saunders, 1990, p 367.)

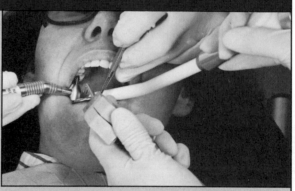

Figure 21–8 During the preparation, the operator uses the handpiece, and the assistant maintains a clear operating field. (Torres HO, Ehrlich A: Modern Dental Assisting, 4th Ed. Philadelphia, WB Saunders, 1990, p 367.)

1. A local anesthetic is administered. (Review this in Chapter 18, "Pharmacology and Pain Control.")

2. Rubber dam may be placed. (Review this in Chapter 19, "Rubber Dam.")

3. The assistant transfers the mouth mirror and explorer to the operator (Fig. 21–7).

4. The assistant prepares the high-speed handpiece with the number 245 bur. The assistant receives the used explorer and transfers the handpiece.

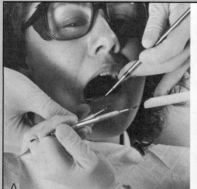
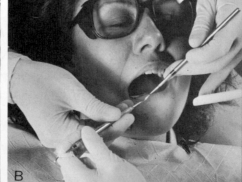

Figure 21–9 Instrument exchange during the cavity preparation. *A.* The assistant holds the next instrument parallel to the "used" instrument that he or she will receive. *B.* The assistant palms the used instrument and places the next instrument into the operator's hand in the position of use. (Torres HO, Ehrlich A: Modern Dental Assisting, 4th Ed. Philadelphia, WB Saunders, 1990, p 367.)

5 The assistant uses the HVE to maintain a clear operating field (Fig. 21–8).

6 As necessary, the assistant:
Changes the bur in the high-speed handpiece.
Prepares the low-speed handpiece ready with a large round bur.
Transfers and receives hand instruments

(such as spoon excavator, enamel chisel, or gingival margin trimmer) (Fig. 21–9).

7 Upon completion of the cavity preparation, the assistant uses the water syringe to remove all debris from the cavity preparation.

8 Warm air or cotton pellets are used to gently dry the tooth preparation.

Procedure

PLACING THE SEDATIVE BASE AND CAVITY LINER (Fig. 21–10)

1 At a signal from the operator, the assistant mixes and transfers the calcium hydroxide and applicator.

2 The assistant receives the used applicator

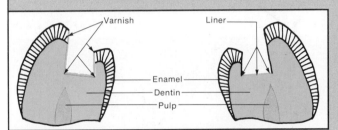

Figure 21–10 Placement of cavity liner and varnish in cavity preparation. (Torres HO, Ehrlich A: Modern Dental Assisting, 4th Ed. Philadelphia, WB Saunders, 1990, p 533.)

and transfers a spoon excavator or explorer.

3 The assistant:
Places a small cotton pellet in the cotton pliers.
Dips the cotton pellet into the cavity varnish and immediately closes the varnish container.
Passes the cotton pliers and pellet to the operator.
Repeats the previous step for the placement of a second layer of varnish. (This fills any voids created as the first application dries and reduces the possibility of microleakage.)

Procedure

PLACING THE MATRIX AND WEDGE

1 With the left hand, the assistant passes the assembled matrix and matrix holder to the operator.

2 The operator passes the mirror back to the assistant, receives the matrix and holder, and places the matrix around the prepared tooth.

3 The assistant places the broad end of the matrix wedge in the number 110 pliers at right angles to the beaks and grips the handles to hold the wedge securely.

4 With the left hand, the assistant holds the number 110 pliers by the points with the handles extended toward the operator's

right hand and passes it to the operator.

5 The operator places the wedge (usually from the lingual of the preparation) and returns the number 110 pliers to the assistant. With the right hand, the assistant uses the air syringe to keep the area dry.

6 With the left hand, the assistant receives the number 110 pliers and transfers an explorer, which the operator uses to check the preparation.

7 The assistant receives the explorer and transfers a spoon excavator, which the operator uses to burnish the band to the adjacent tooth.

Procedure

MIXING THE AMALGAM

1. The assistant activates the capsule, places it in the amalgamator, and closes the cover.

2. The amalgamator is set for the number of seconds recommended by the manufacturer.

3. At a signal from the operator, the amalgamator is turned on to triturate the amalgam.

4. Immediately after amalgamator stops, the assistant opens the cover and removes the capsule.

5. The amalgam is emptied directly into a dry amalgam well and the pestle is removed.

Procedure

PLACING AND CONDENSING THE AMALGAM

1. During this process, the operator condenses each increment of amalgam after it has been placed in the preparation.

   With the left hand, the assistant passes the smallest condenser to the operator.

   With the right hand, the assistant loads amalgam into the small end of the amalgam carrier.

   The assistant dispenses the amalgam firmly into the cavity preparation as directed by the operator (Fig. 21–11).

2. *Alternative:* Some operators prefer to have the assistant transfer the loaded amalgam carrier. In this situation:

   The assistant loads the carrier and transfers it to the operator, who then dispenses the amalgam into the cavity preparation.

   The assistant receives the empty carrier, transfers the appropriate condenser, and refills the carrier.

3. The process is repeated as the operator condenses the amalgam mass into the cavity preparation.

4. When placement and condensation are complete, the assistant:

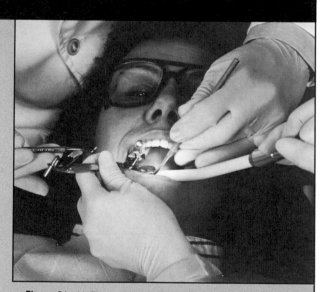

Figure 21–11 The assistant places amalgam in the preparation as directed by the operator. (Torres HO, Ehrlich A: Modern Dental Assisting, 4th Ed. Philadelphia, WB Saunders, 1990, p 549.)

Uses the left hand to receive the last condenser and transfers the explorer to the operator.

Uses the right hand to empty the amalgam carrier and replaces it on the instrument tray in its original position.

Procedure

CARVING THE AMALGAM RESTORATION

1. Throughout the carving process, the assistant uses the HVE tip to remove all amalgam scraps and debris.

2. The assistant receives the used explorer and transfers the large discoid-cleoid carver to the operator.

3. The assistant receives the used carver and transfers the number 110 pliers for the removal of the band and wedge.

4. The assistant receives the used retainer, band, wedge, and number 110 pliers and

transfers the explorer to the operator.

5. The assistant receives the explorer and transfers carvers (progressing from large to smaller) as specified by the operator.

6. *Optional:* The operator may use dental tape or floss to check the interproximal gingival margin. If necessary, a finishing knife or file is used to reduce any excess on the facial and lingual surfaces.

7. If rubber dam was placed, it is removed at this time.

Procedure

ADJUSTING THE OCCLUSION

1. The assistant places articulating paper in the articulating paper holder and passes the prepared holder to the operator in the position of use.

2. The operator places the articulating paper on the teeth to be checked and instructs the patient to close his teeth together very cautiously (Fig. 21–12). Sudden closure on a high amalgam restoration will fracture the restoration.

3. The assistant hands a carving instrument to the operator for use in reducing any high spots (which are indicated by blue marks) on the amalgam restoration.

4. The surface of the new restoration is again checked with articulating paper and carved until no blue marks appear when in light occlusion.

5. The assistant places a large cotton pellet in the cotton pliers and moistens the cotton with water.

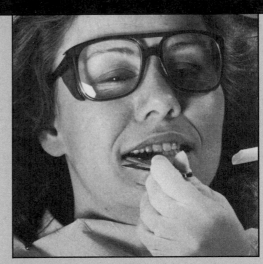

Figure 21–12 Articulating paper is placed and the patient is instructed to close very gently. (Torres HO, Ehrlich A: Modern Dental Assisting, 4th Ed. Philadelphia, WB Saunders, 1990, p 550.)

This is passed to the operator, who gently rubs it on the surface of the amalgam to dull the finish.

Procedure

FINAL STEPS

1. Following the final carving, the water syringe and HVE are used to rinse the oral cavity.

2. The patient is cautioned not to chew on the restoration for a few hours until it reaches full strength. (This takes approximately 6 to 7 hours.)

3. The patient is dismissed.

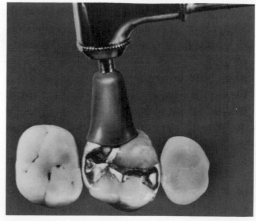

▼ **Figure 21–13**

Amalgam polishing cup. The cup, which is impregnated silicone, is dampened and applied under low speed. (Courtesy of Shofu Dental Corp, Menlo Park, CA.)

FINISHING AND POLISHING OF THE AMALGAM RESTORATION

The amalgam restoration may receive additional polishing at the patient's next visit (Figs. 21–13 and 21–14).

At this time the operator uses a series of rubber cups and points in the right-angle handpiece to polish the surface and margins of the restoration.

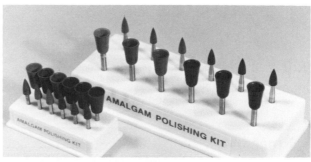

▼ **Figure 21–14**

Amalgam polishing kit showing assorted mounted cups and points. (Courtesy of Shofu Dental Corporation, Menlo Park, CA.)

▼ EXERCISES

1. Scrap amalgam is discarded so that it is covered with _____ ____.

   a. disinfecting solution
   b. radiographic film processing developer
   c. radiographic film processing fixer
   d. water

2. When starting to place amalgam, the _____ end of the carrier is used first.

   a. larger
   b. smaller

3. Amalgam restorations are held in place by _____.

   a. adhesion
   b. bonding
   c. cementation
   d. mechanical retention

4. The _____ circumference of the matrix band is the occlusal edge.

   a. larger
   b. smaller

5. The _____ form is the shape and relationship of the cavity walls that protect the tooth structure and restorative material against fracture.

   a. convenience
   b. outline
   c. resistance
   d. retention

6. A/An _____ is a mechanical device used to triturate amalgam.

   a. amalgamator
   b. pestle
   c. triturator

7. The _____ of the Tofflemire retainer adjusts the size of the matrix band loop.

   a. diagonal slot vise
   b. inner nut
   c. outer nut
   d. spindle

8. A _____ is used to adapt the matrix band to the gingival contours of the tooth.

   a. ball burnisher
   b. number 110 How pliers
   c. retainer
   d. wedge

9. The purpose of overfilling a cavity is so that the _____.

    a. matrix band may be removed without fracturing the restoration
    a. mercury-rich excess material can be carved away
    c. occlusion may be carved without exposing the pulp

10. If a rubber dam was placed, this is removed _____ the occlusion is checked.

    a. before
    b. after

11. The _____ wall of a cavity preparation is nearest the cheek.

    a. buccal
    b. distal
    c. lingual
    d. mesial

12. The diagonal slot on the box of the Tofflemire matrix retainer is placed _____ the gingiva.

    a. away from
    b. toward

13. Caries removal is usually performed with a _____.

    a. enamel hatchet
    b. round bur in a low-speed handpiece
    c. spoon excavator
    d. b or c

14. Amalgam is an alloy in which one of the metals is _____.

    a. copper
    b. mercury
    c. silver
    d. tin

15. The wedge is removed _____ the matrix band and holder are removed.

    a. before
    b. after

16. _____ firmly packs the amalgam into all areas of the preparation and brings any excess mercury to the surface.

    a. Amalgamation
    b. Condensation
    c. Trituration
    d. a or c

17. The matrix band is contoured _____.

    a. after the band and retainer are positioned in the mouth
    b. after the band is placed in the retainer
    c. before the band is placed in the retainer

18. When finished with the last condenser, the operator receives the _____ _____.

   a. explorer
   b. first carver
   c. pliers to remove the wedge and band

19. _____ is/are used in placing and removing the wedge.

   a. A cotton pliers
   b. A How (110) pliers
   c. The operator's fingers
   d. b or c

20. A _____ is a metal or plastic band used to replace the missing wall of a tooth during placement of the restorative material.

   a. matrix
   b. retainer
   c. wedge

▼ Criterion Sheet 21–1

Student's Name _____

Procedure: *PREPARING A TOFFLEMIRE RETAINER*

Performance Objective:

The student will prepare a Tofflemire matrix for placement on the mandibular first molar.

SE = Student evaluation C = Criterion met IE = Instructor evaluation X = Criterion not met	SE	IE
Instrumentation: Tofflemire matrix retainer, assorted molar matrix bands, ball burnisher, and paper pad. (Appropriate infection control barriers will be used during all procedures actually performed on a patient.)		
1. Selected and fitted matrix band.		
2. Contoured the matrix band.		
3. Placed band in retainer through the correct guide slot.		
4. Tightened the spindle and adjusted the size of the loop.		
5. Used an instrument handle to open the loop of the band fully.		
6. Returned the prepared retainer to the instrument tray.		
Comments:		

▼ Criterion Sheet 21–2

Student's Name _____

Procedure: *ASSISTING DURING THE PREPARATION AND PLACEMENT OF AN AMALGAM RESTORATION*

Performance Objective:

The student will prepare the necessary instruments and assist the operator at chairside during the preparation and placement of an amalgam restoration.

SE = Student evaluation **IE** = Instructor evaluation	**C** = Criterion met **X** = Criterion not met	**SE**	**IE**
Instrumentation: Amalgam pre-set tray containing instruments specified by the operator, including a prepared Tofflemire matrix band and retainer and a fully equipped dental operatory. (Appropriate infection control barriers will be used during all procedures actually performed on a patient.)			
1. Procured all of the necessary instruments and supplies.			
2. Washed hands, donned gloves, and placed mask.			
3. Assisted the operator during the cavity preparation.			
4. Mixed and passed the calcium hydroxide cavity liner.			
5. Assisted in the placement of the matrix and wedge.			
6. At a signal from the operator, mixed the amalgam.			
7. Transferred the loaded amalgam carrier and condensers.			
8. Assisted during the removal of the wedge and matrix band.			
9. Assisted during carving and adjusting the occlusion.			
Comments:			

22 Cosmetic Dentistry

▼ LEARNING OBJECTIVES

The student will be able to:

1. Describe cosmetic dentistry and define these related terms: bonding, enamel bonding, dentin bonding, veneer, direct-bonded resin veneer, indirect-bonded resin veneer, porcelain veneer.

2. State four patient responsibilities in maintaining cosmetic restorations.

3. Describe the major characteristics of the three forms of composites.

4. Differentiate between self-cured and light-cured polymerizing resins.

5. List the special precautions to be taken while placing a cosmetic restoration.

6. Describe the steps in preparation and placement of a direct-bonded resin veneer.

7. Describe the steps in preparation and placement of an indirect-bonded veneer.

8. Describe the steps in preparation and placement of a Class II posterior composite restoration.

9. Demonstrate assisting during the preparation and placement of a Class III anterior composite restoration.

OVERVIEW OF COSMETIC DENTISTRY

The term cosmetic dentistry, also known as *esthetic dentistry*, primarily describes the placement of tooth-colored composite restorations, veneers, and other restorations to improve the appearance of the anterior teeth.

This term also includes the use of composites to:

▼ Narrow or close the diastema between widely spaced teeth. (A **diastema** is an abnormal space that is usually found between the maxillary central incisors.)

▼ Repair surfaces that are broken, chipped, or worn.

▼ Cover badly stained teeth.

▼ Place tooth-colored restorations in the posterior teeth.

Because extensive tooth preparation is not usually necessary, many cosmetic dentistry restorations can be comfortably placed without a local anesthetic.

Veneers

A veneer is a thin layer of tooth-colored material that is bonded to the surface of a prepared tooth. Veneers are most frequently placed on the facial surfaces of the anterior teeth and may be used to mask chips, gaps, and discoloration.

Direct-Bonded Resin Veneers

A direct resin veneer is formed of composite material that is applied and bonded directly to the tooth surface.

Indirect-Bonded Resin Veneers

An indirect resin veneer is fabricated in the dental laboratory from an impression taken by the dentist. The completed veneer is returned to the dental office and is bonded to the etched tooth at a second patient visit.

Bonded Porcelain Veneers

A porcelain veneer is fabricated of porcelain material, in the dental laboratory, from an impression taken by the dentist.

The completed veneer is returned to the dental office and is bonded to the etched tooth at a second patient visit.

Prior to cementation, the inner surface of the porcelain veneer must be etched. This is usually etched by the laboratory before the veneer is returned to the dental office. An alternative is to etch the veneer at chairside just prior to placement.

Patient Responsibilities

The patient must be aware of his responsibilities in maintaining cosmetic restorations. The patient must:

1. Use a soft toothbrush, with a nonabrasive toothpaste, to maintain excellent oral hygiene.
2. Avoid mouthwashes with a high alcohol content. (Alcohol weakens the bond of the porcelain.)
3. Avoid chewing ice and biting hard foods with the treated teeth.
4. Recognize that a veneer may have to be replaced as a result of wear, discoloration, or fracture. However, a veneer restoration that is properly cared for will provide excellent service.

COMPOSITE RESTORATIVE MATERIALS

Forms of Composites

Composite restorative materials, which are also called *resins*, consist of an organic polymeric matrix reinforced with an inorganic filler. (Compos-

organic matrix
inorganic filler

ites are just one form of resin that is used in dentistry. Other types of resin are used to create dentures and removable orthodontic appliances.)

Composites are classified according to the size of the filler. The amount of filler, the particle size, and the type of filler are all important factors in determining the strength and wear resistance characteristics of the material. They also influence the polished finish of the restoration.

Macrofilled Composites

The macrofilled composites contain the largest of filler particles, providing greater strength, but a duller, rougher surface when finished.

Macrofilled composites are used in areas where greater strength is required to resist fracture.

Microfilled Composites

As the name implies, the inorganic filler in microfilled composites is much smaller in size than that of a macrofilled composite.

Microfilled composite resins are capable of producing a highly polished finished restoration and are used primarily in anterior restorations, where smoothness is the primary concern.

Hybrid Composites

Hybrid composites contain both macrofill and microfill particles. The hybrids are more polishable than the macrofilled composites and have more strength than the microfilled composites. They also have good wear resistance and excellent shading characteristics.

Polymerization

Polymerization is the process whereby a resin material is changed from a plastic state (in which it can be molded or shaped) into a hardened restoration. There are two forms of polymerization used in curing resins.

Self-Cured Composites   *2 pastes. Mix before 1~1½ wt*

In self-cured composites, polymerization is brought about by a chemical reaction. Self-cured composites are supplied as two pastes: initiator (catalyst) and accelerator.

These pastes are mixed together, placed, and allowed to cure. When the cure is complete, the restoration is polished.

Depending on the manufacturer, the working time for self-cured composites is approximately 1 to 1½ minutes, and setting time is about 4 to 5 minutes from the start of the mix.

Light-Cured Composites

Light-cured composites are polymerized by exposure to a special curing light. These composites are supplied as a single paste in a light-proof syringe (Fig. 22–1).

After the composite has been inserted into the preparation, the visible light source is used to cure the material. Curing time varies between 20 and 60 seconds.

The exact curing time depends on the manufacturer's instructions, the thickness and size of the restoration, and the shade of the restorative material used. (The darker the shade, the longer the curing time required.)

When using a curing light, the operator must wear special protective glasses or use a curing paddle (see Fig. 8–3; Fig. 22–2.) (Also review Chapter 8, "Hazards Management in the Dental Office.")

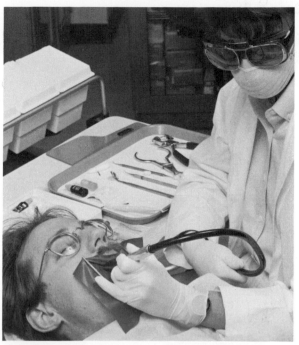

▼ **Figure 22–2**

The operator must either wear special protective glasses or use a protective paddle when light-curing composite materials. The patient must close his or her eyes and/or use protective eyewear. (Torres HO, Ehrlich A: Modern Dental Assisting, 4th Ed. Philadelphia, WB Saunders, 1990, p 150.)

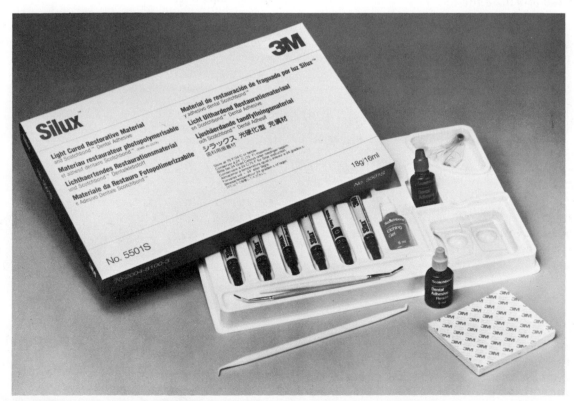

▼ **Figure 22–1**

Light-cured restorative composite resin material. (Courtesy of Dental Products Division, 3M Health Care Group, St. Paul, Minnesota.)

Special Precautions

The following precautions are important in determining the success of composite restorations.

1. The health of the gingival tissues is essential. If the patient's oral hygiene is poor, the dentist may postpone treatment until the health of the gingival tissues has improved.
2. Prior to bonding and placement of a composite, the tooth must be cleaned of all calculus, plaque, and debris.

> An unflavored pumice slurry should be used for this purpose. (**Pumice slurry** is a thin mixture of pumice and water.)

> If a prophy paste is used, it must be free of fluoride. (Fluoride interferes with the etching process.)

> If a prophy paste is used, it must be free of flavoring oils. (Oil interferes with the bonding process.)

3. The tooth being treated must be isolated to keep it free of contamination such as blood, moisture, or debris.

> Rubber dam may be placed.

> If rubber dam is not placed, cotton rolls are used to isolate the tooth.

> Retraction cord is also used to control bleeding and to retract the gingival tissue temporarily away from the preparation. (Retraction cord is discussed in Chapter 24, "Crown and Bridge Resorations.")

4. The air and water supply used to dry an etched tooth must be free of oil or debris. (Oil and debris interfere with the bonding process.)
5. When indicated, a calcium hydroxide cavity liner is applied. A liner containing eugenol is *not* used because it would interfere with the polymerization of the composite.

Pulpal protection

BONDING

Bonding, which is also known as *acid etch technique*, is the physical adherence (sticking together) of one substance to another. This technique makes it possible to bond composite restorative materials directly to the enamel and dentin of the tooth.

Because bonded restorations do not depend on mechanical retention, it is possible to restore the tooth with a less invasive preparation than is

Advantages
1) Less extensive preps
2) Microleakage is less (∴ of interlocking) around margins

required for a restoration, which must depend on mechanical retention.

Enamel Bonding

Enamel bonding is accomplished by etching the enamel to create a surface of microscopic undercuts. These are also referred to as *enamel tags* (Fig. 22–3). (Review the structure of enamel in Chapter 4, "Dental Anatomy and Tooth Morphology.")

The restorative material penetrates into these undercuts and forms resin tags that mechanically interlock with the enamel surface.

▼ Only the enamel surface to be bonded to a restorative material is etched.

▼ The etching solution is 35 to 50 percent phosphoric acid. Also known as an *etchant*, this solution is provided in the form of a liquid or a gel.

▼ The etching solution is applied directly from a syringe type applicator or is dabbed on the enamel surface to be treated. It is *not* wiped or rubbed on, for this would destroy the enamel undercuts that are formed.

▼ The amount of time required to etch a surface is usually about 45 to 60 seconds. (The exact etching time depends on the manufacturer's instructions.)

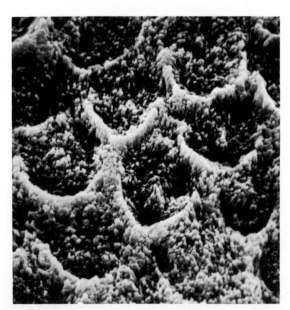

▼ **Figure 22–3**

Microscopic appearance of etched enamel surface. (Phillips RW: Elements of Dental Materials, 4th Ed. Philadelphia, WB Saunders, 1984, p 170.)

▼ After the enamel has been etched, it is rinsed thoroughly with water for 20 to 30 seconds. (The exact rinsing time depends upon the manufacturer's instructions.)

▼ Successfully etched enamel has a frosty white, or ground glass, look.

▼ When bonding both enamel and dentin, the enamel is prepared first.

Dentin Bonding

Depending on the type of restoration, it may also be necessary to create a direct bond to the dentin. This is *not* the same as enamel bonding.

Enamel bonding is based on the undercuts formed when the enamel is etched. In dentin bonding, these undercuts are not formed. Therefore, dentin bonding is based on chemical rather than micromechanical bonds to dentin surfaces.

▼ When using dentin bonding and enamel bonding systems, they must be compatible. To be certain, it is recommended that both systems be from the same manufacturer.

▼ The solution used in dentin bonding is called the **primer.**

▼ The primer is brushed on the dentin surface for approximately 30 to 60 seconds. (The exact time depends on the manufacturer's instructions.)

▼ The primer on the dentin of the tooth is agitated with a slight scrubbing motion the entire time.

▼ The primer is *not* rinsed off.

▼ The preparation is air dried for 15 seconds or until the dentin appears dull and dry. (The exact drying time depends on the manufacturer's instructions.)

Adhesive Application

After the enamel has been etched and the dentin has been primed, an adhesive is placed.

▼ One or 2 drops of adhesive are dispensed into a clean well of a mixing tray or onto a dispensing pad.

▼ A brush is used to apply a uniform coating of the adhesive immediately to the dried, primed dentin and etched enamel surfaces.

▼ If necessary, the adhesive is thinned slightly with a gentle stream of air.

▼ The adhesive is light-cured.

▼ The tooth is now ready to receive the composite restoration.

CLASS III COMPOSITE RESTORATIONS

The following procedure describes the placement of a Class III restoration in using a light-cured composite that is supplied in a prepackaged syringe.

Shade Selection

It is possible to select a shade of composite that will very closely match the natural tooth. In order to get an accurate match, this shade must be selected in excellent light, with the natural tooth wet, before the rubber dam is placed, and prior to the tooth preparation.

The manufacturer provides a shade guide to aid in the selection of exactly the right color to match the patient's natural dentition. This guide is a holder with a removable piece for each color.

During the shade selection process, the individual shade piece is removed from the holder, moistened, and placed next to the natural tooth.

Any shade guide piece that was tried next to a natural tooth must be disinfected before it is returned to the holder.

Matrix Strips

When a proximal wall is being replaced, it is necessary to use a matrix to replace the missing wall temporarily. For a Class III composite restoration, a strip matrix is used. This may be clear plastic (Mylar) or metal.

Unlike the matrices for posterior restorations, strips are not placed in a retainer. Instead they are positioned between the teeth. Prior to placement, a Mylar strip may be contoured by drawing it over the rounded back end of the cotton pliers.

After the restorative material has been placed, the matrix strip is pulled tightly over the cavity preparation and held securely in place until the restorative has been cured.

Wedges

A round or triangular wooden wedge may be placed prior to the preparation to protect the gingival tissues.

After the matrix is in position, a wedge is placed to separate the teeth slightly and to ensure proper proximal contact. The wedge also prevents gingival excess (overhangs) of restorative material.

Wedges are placed and removed with a number 110 pliers.

Finishing and Polishing the Restoration

Finishing and polishing are an essential part of creating a successful composite restoration.

Finishing burs, 12- and 30-fluted, are used in contouring and refining the restoration (Fig. 22–4).

A number 12 scalpel blade, in a Bard-Parker handle, may be used to remove excess flash from edges of the restoration. (**Flash** is excess material that has escaped during placement of the restorative material.)

Abrasive strips and/or interproximal knives may be used to smooth the interproximal area (Fig. 22–5).

Assorted mounted points, stones, wheels, and discs, such as those shown in Figures 22–6 and 22–7, are used in the final finishing and polishing of the restoration.

Instrumentation

▼ Basic setup.

▼ Local anesthetic (if indicated).

▼ Manufacturer's shade guide.

▼ Rubber dam.

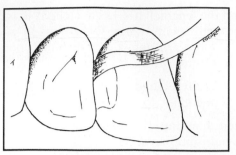

▼ **Figure 22–5**

Finishing strips are used for interproximal finish. (Baum L, Phillips RW, Lund MR: Operative Dentistry, 2nd Ed. Philadelphia, WB Saunders, 1985, p 235.)

▼ Instruments for cavity preparation (operator's choice).

▼ High volume evacuator (HVE) tip.

▼ Etching gel or solution and applicator.

▼ Bonding resin and brush.

▼ Calcium hydroxide base and catalyst.

▼ Applicator for calcium hydroxide.

▼ Wedges.

▼ Plastic matrix strips.

▼ Number 110 pliers.

▼ Prepackaged syringe of composite resin.

▼ Curing light.

▼ Shield *or* polarized glasses for use with curing light.

▼ Finishing kit.

▼ Abrasive strips.

▼ Articulating paper.

▼ Polishing kit.

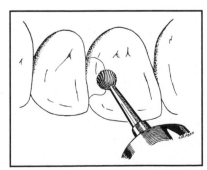

▼ **Figure 22–4**

Carbide finishing burs are used to provide the desired contour. (Baum L, Phillips RW, Lund MR: Operative Dentistry, 2nd Ed. Philadelphia, WB Saunders, 1985, p 235.)

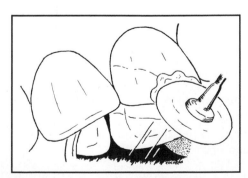

▼ **Figure 22–6**

A polishing disc is used for the final finish. (Baum L, Phillips RW, Lund MR: Operative Dentistry, 2nd Ed. Philadelphia, WB Saunders, 1985, p 236.)

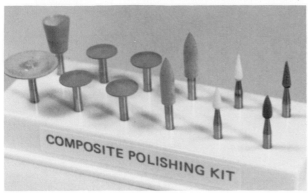

▼ **Figure 22-7**

Composite polishing kit. (Courtesy of Shofu Dental Corp, Menlo Park, CA.)

CLASS II POSTERIOR COMPOSITE RESTORATION

This Class II composite restoration is placed using a dentin and enamel bonding system with two types of light-activated hybrid composites.

Instrumentation

▼ Basic setup.

▼ Instruments for cavity preparation (operator's choice).

▼ HVE tip.

▼ Etchant gel.

▼ Mixing wells (provided by manufacturer).

▼ Bonding agent and applicator.

▼ Syringeable composite (supplied in a preloaded syringe).

▼ Condensable composite (supplied in cartridges).

▼ Matrix, retainer, wedges, and number 110 pliers.

▼ Plastic amalgam carrier.

▼ Condensers (smooth).

▼ Ball burnisher.

▼ Finishing burs.

▼ Polishing discs, points, and cups.

▼ Low speed handpiece.

Procedure

PLACING A CLASS III RESTORATION

1 If indicated, local anesthetic is administered.
   The tooth is cleaned.
   The shade is selected.
   Optional: A rubber dam may be placed.

2 The tooth is prepared, and, when indicated, a calcium hydroxide cavity liner is place.

3 The enamel is etched, rinsed and dried.

4 The contoured matrix strip is placed and wedged.

5 The bonding resin is applied and light-cured.

6 The syringe type composite is dispensed directly into the preparation and allow it to light-cure on the lingual and facial surfaces.

7 The matrix and wedge is removed.

8 12- and 30-fluted finishing burs are used in the high speed handpiece for contouring.

9 The interproximal surface is smoothed with abrasive strips.

10 Articulating paper is used to check the occlusion and the required adjustments are made.

11 Polishing discs, points, and cups are used in the low speed handpiece to polish the restoration.

12 A final coating of the sealant material is placed over the finished restoration.

Curing time 4-5 wks

Procedure

PLACING A CLASS II POSTERIOR COMPOSITE RESTORATION

Tooth Preparation

1. If indicated, a local anesthetic is administered and the rubber dam is placed.

2. The cavity preparation is completed.

3. A calcium hydroxide cavity liner is placed to protect the pulp.

Etching the Enamel

4. The gel etchant is placed and the tooth is etched.

5. The tooth is thoroughly rinsed to remove all traces of acid. It is dried with oil-free and moisture-free air.

6. The matrix band is placed and wedged.

Bonding

7. One drop each of activator and resin is dispensed into one of the mixing wells.

8. The bonding agent is applied with a brush to all of the dentin and etched enamel surfaces.

9. A gentle air stream is used to spread the bonding agent.

10. A second coat of the bonding agent is applied and then spread with a stream of air.

11. The entire bonding agent surface is light-cured.

Placement of the Restorative Material

12. The tip of syringeable material is used to place the restorative material into the deepest portion of the cavity. This layer is light-cured.

13. The condensable material is placed with either a plastic amalgam carrier or a plastic placement instrument. This is condensed with a smooth surface condenser.

14. Prior to curing, the occlusal anatomy is formed by using a ball burnisher or waxing instrument.

15. After the occlusal layer has been cured, the matrix band is removed and the restoration is light-cured buccally and lingually.

16. The restoration is contoured and finished with a 12- and 30-bladed finishing bur in a high speed handpiece with air-water spray.

17. The rubber dam is removed and the occlusion is adjusted.

Finishing and Polishing the Restoration

18. Polishing discs, stones, and points are used in a low speed handpiece with water spray.

19. The polishing paste is applied with a webbed prophy cup in a low speed handpiece and the surface is polished for 60 seconds.

OVERVIEW OF A DIRECT COMPOSITE VENEER

The procedure described here is direct composite veneer using a hybrid composite material in different shades to simulate the natural color variations of the dentin, enamel, and incisal edge of the tooth.

Procedure

APPLYING A DIRECT COMPOSITE VENEER

Shade Selection

1. The tooth is cleaned with a pumice slurry.

2. The shades are selected.

3. The rubber dam is placed.

Tooth Preparation

4 A diamond bur, in the high speed handpiece, is used to prepare the facial surface of the tooth.

5 The prepared tooth is etched, rinsed, and air-dried.

6 A coat of bonding agent is applied to all etched enamel surfaces and light-cured.
   Optional: Some operators apply two coats of bonding agent.

Placement of the Layers and Incisal Shades

7 The dentin shade is applied and cured.

8 The enamel shade is applied to the labial surface.

9 A waxing instrument is used to place de-

velopmental grooves in the labial surface. This is light-cured.

10 The translucent incisal shade is applied next and is light-cured.

Finishing and Polishing

11 Finishing burs, 12- and 30-fluted, are used for gross reduction, contouring, and finishing.

12 A finishing strip is used to smooth the interproximal area to create a smooth margin.

13 If necessary, a scalpel or interproximal knife is used to remove excess flash from edges of the restoration.

14 The finishing kit is used to polish the veneer to create a high shine.

OVERVIEW OF AN INDIRECT-BONDED VENEER

Preparation Visit

1. Immediately prior to the preparation, the teeth are cleaned with a pumice slurry.
2. The shade is selected, and the tooth is isolated with cotton rolls.
3. Using a high speed handpiece, the operator removes approximately half the thickness of the enamel from the gingival and incisal portions of the tooth.
4. An impression is taken of the prepared teeth.
5. An opposing arch impression and bite registration are also taken.
6. Because veneer preparations do not normally expose the dentin, temporary coverage is usually not necessary.
7. The patient is dismissed and rescheduled for cementation after the veneer has been returned by the laboratory.

Cementation Visit

1. The shade is selected for the resin cement to be used. The cement shade is important because it will have impact on the color of the veneer.
2. The cement is mixed, and the restoration is cemented in place.
3. The operator checks the occlusion and makes adjustments as necessary.

▼ EXERCISES

1. Successfully etched enamel has a _____d._____ look.

   a. frosty white
   b. ground glass
   c. shiny
   d. a and b

2. A/An _____d b_____ is used to trim excess flash from the edges of the restoration.

   a. 12-fluted bur
   b. interproximal knife
   c. scalpel
   d. b or c

3. When bonding both enamel and dentin, the _____(b)_____ is prepared first.

   a. dentin
   b. enamel

4. When preparing a tooth for acid etching, a prophy paste with flavoring oils _____(b)_____ be used.

   a. may
   b. may not

5. An indirect-bonded veneer is placed in _____two visits_____.

   a. one visit
   b. two visits

6. When dentin primer is placed, it is _____b._____.

   a. gently dabbed on the surface
   b. not rinsed off
   c. rinsed off
   d. a and c

7. A shade selection is made _____ the rubber dam is placed.

   a. after
   b. before

8. When placing a Class II composite restoration, the occlusal anatomy is placed _____before_____ the material is cured.

   a. after
   b. before

9. In _____Enamel_____ bonding, microscopic undercuts are formed.

   a. dentin
   b. enamel

10. _Polymerization_ is the process whereby a resin material is changed from a plastic state into a hardened restoration.

    a. Acid etching
    b. Bonding
    c. Polymerization
    d. None of the above

11. When placing a Class III anterior composite restoration, a matrix _____ _band_ is/are necessary

    a. band
    b. band and retainer

12. In light-curing a composite, the _darker_ the shade, the longer the curing time.

    a. darker
    b. lighter

13. A/an _Veneer_ is a thin layer of tooth-colored material that is bonded to the surface of a prepared tooth.

    a. acid etch
    b. diastema
    c. etchant
    d. veneer

14. _Self cured_ composites are supplied as two pastes: initiator (catalyst) and accelerator.

    a. Light-cured
    b. Self-cured

15. Patients with cosmetic restorations must avoid mouthwashes with a high alcohol content because alcohol _____.

    a. erodes the restoration
    b. irritates the gingival tissues
    c. stains the restoration
    d. weakens the bond of the porcelain

16. A liner with eugenol _is not_ placed under a composite restoration.

    a. is
    b. is not

17. A _Macrofilled_ composite, with large filler particles, provides greater strength but a duller, rougher surface.

    a. hybrid
    b. macrofilled
    c. microfilled
    d. self-curing

18. When preparing a tooth for acid etching, the polishing paste must be free of
_____ *fluoride* _____ because it interferes with the etching process.

    a. air
    b. fluoride
    c. oil
    d. pumice

19. A/An _____ *c* _____ may be contoured by drawing it over the rounded back end of the cotton pliers.

    a. abrasive strip
    b. metal matrix band
    c. mylar strip

20. Placement of a Class II posterior composite restoration involves the use of a
_____ *d* _____ composite.

    a. condensable
    b. self-curing
    c. syringeable
    d. a and c

---

23 Custom Trays and Elastomeric Impressions

▼ LEARNING OBJECTIVES

The student will be able to:

1. Describe the uses of custom trays and elastomeric impression materials.
2. Describe taking a paste bite registration.
3. Demonstrate the construction and finishing of a custom impression tray.
4. Demonstrate preparing polysulfide impression materials.
5. Demonstrate preparing silicone impression materials.
6. Demonstrate preparing polysiloxane impression materials.

OVERVIEW OF CUSTOM TRAYS AND ELASTOMERIC IMPRESSION MATERIALS

Elastomeric impression materials are extremely accurate and are frequently used when creating fixed restorations such as a cast inlay, crown, or bridge. (These procedures are discussed in Chapter 24, "Crown and Bridge Restorations.")

Several different types of elastomeric impression materials are used in dentistry. Each material has its own special characteristics and uses. However, all of these materials are rubber-like in nature, and as a group they are frequently referred to as **rubber base impression materials**.

To ensure an accurate impression, some elastomeric impression materials are used in custom trays that fit closely over the teeth and area being treated.

Other impression materials require a two-step impression technique, which is used with a disposable commercial tray.

Custom trays are constructed on a diagnostic cast that was made from an impression of the arch *before* the teeth were prepared. The production of diagnostic casts is discussed in Chapter 17, "Alginate Impressions and Diagnostic Casts."

Custom trays may be constructed to cover edentulous arches, as shown in Figure 23–1, or to cover only a quadrant. (See Figs. 23–2 through 23–6 for the construction of a quadrant tray.)

Custom trays are commonly constructed in the dental office using one of the following materials or techniques.

▼ A **vacuum molding** machine, which heats and shapes the material.

▼ A **light-cured resin,** which is hardened in a light-curing unit.

▼ A **thermoplastic material,** which is softened in warm water, shaped, and allowed to cool.

▼ An **acrylic resin,** which is mixed, shaped, and allowed to self-cure.

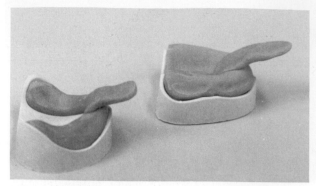

▼ **Figure 23-1**

Custom impression tray for edentulous arches. The mandibular tray is on the left, the maxillary tray is to the right.

BASIC TRAY CONSTRUCTION

No matter what type of tray material is used, there are certain basic steps that are taken in preparing a custom tray.

Cast Preparation

Before the tray can be constructed, the cast must be checked for undercuts. **Undercuts** are areas in the cast that might create problems in removing the tray. These may be caused by malpositioned teeth, bubbles, or indentations. If undercuts are present, they are "filled" with utility wax.

Next the **outline of the finished tray** is marked in pencil on the cast. This must provide adequate coverage without extending into the undercuts beyond the last tooth in the quadrant. (When this happens, it is difficult to remove the tray and impression from the mouth.)

Spacers and Stops

During the construction of the tray, a spacer is used to create room in the tray for the impression material. Depending on the tray material being used, the spacer may be made of **wax, asbestos substitute, aluminum foil**, or **paper**. In Figure 23-2, wax has been used as a spacer.

Stops are placed to prevent the tray from seating too deep in the arch or quadrant. They also allow for an adequate quantity of impression material around the preparations.

In a custom tray, the stops are created by making several small triangular-shaped holes in the spacer material. These stops are placed on the occlusal surfaces of the nonprepared teeth in the quadrant.

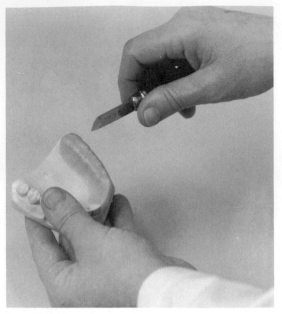

▼ **Figure 23-2**

The wax spacer for a quadrant tray is shaped to cover the area under the tray. A laboratory knife is used to cut stops into the spacer.

Separating Medium

The prepared cast, spacer, and immediate surrounding area are painted with a separating medium so that the tray can readily be separated from the cast (Fig. 23-3).

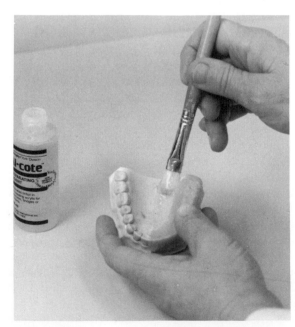

▼ **Figure 23-3**

The spacer and cast are painted with a separating medium.

Tray Construction

The tray material is prepared so that it is pliable. The material is then flattened into a patty or roll and shaped to fit the tray area indicated on the diagnostic cast.

The excess material is trimmed away while it is still soft (Fig. 23–4). (The more carefully the material is trimmed, the less finishing will have to be done.)

Tray Handle

A handle is placed on the anterior portion of the tray to facilitate placement and removal (Fig. 23–5). The handle must:

▼ Be long enough to be grasped firmly when placing and removing the tray.

▼ Extend out of the opening of the mouth.

▼ Be parallel to the occlusal surfaces of the teeth.

▼ Be at a right angle to the incisal edges of the anterior teeth.

Removing the Spacer and Finishing the Tray

After the tray has hardened, it is taken from the cast and the spacer material is removed (Fig. 23–6). As necessary, the edges of the tray are

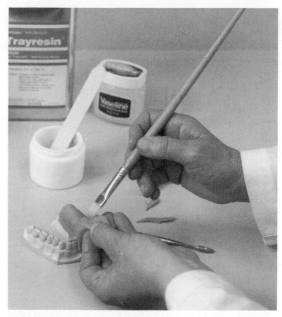

▼ **Figure 23–5**
A handle is shaped and fitted to the tray.

trimmed or smoothed so that there are no rough edges to harm the tissues of the oral cavity.

Tray Adhesive

Elastomeric impression material is held in place in the tray with a tray adhesive that is painted on the inner surface of the custom tray. This adhesive is

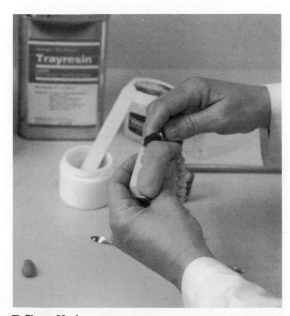

▼ **Figure 23–4**
A laboratory knife is used to cut away excess tray material.

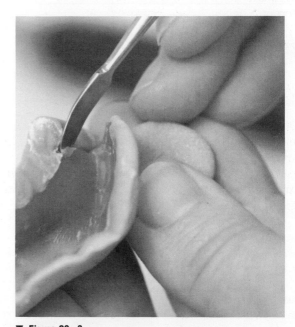

▼ **Figure 23–6**
The spacer is removed from the completed tray.

specified by the manufacturer of the impression material.

Usually a tray receives two coats of adhesive. The first coat may be applied so that it has time to dry. This may be in the laboratory or at chairside just prior to the preparation of the teeth.

A second coat may be applied shortly before the tray is to be used, usually while the operator is placing the retraction cord around the prepared tooth.

Acrylic Resin Custom Trays

Custom trays may be constructed using a self-polymerizing (cold-cure) acrylic tray resin. The potential hazards of working with this material are discussed in Chapter 8, "Hazards Management in the Dental Office."

Tray resins are supplied as a powder (polymer) and liquid (monomer). The powder and liquid must be from the same manufacturer. Also, they must be measured and mixed according to the manufacturer's instructions.

Either a sheet of baseplate wax or an asbestos substitute is used as a spacer for an acrylic resin tray. (In the following procedure description, wax is used.)

Because the heat given off as the tray resin hardens melts the wax and makes it difficult to remove, a wax spacer should be removed before the tray reaches its final set.

To do this, wait until the acrylic is firm but not yet cool. Carefully lift the tray off the diagnostic cast and remove most of the wax spacer. Return the tray to the diagnostic cast until it has finished setting and complete the cleaning out of the inside of the tray after it has set.

The used spacer material may be saved to serve as a guide to determine how much tray type impression material should be dispensed.

The following is a description of the preparation of custom trays for an edentulous arch.

Preparing Custom Trays for Edentulous Arches

Instrumentation

▼ Diagnostic cast (full arch).

▼ Tray resin (monomer and polymer).

▼ Measures (liquid and powder).

▼ Baseplate wax.

▼ Laboratory knife.

▼ Wooden tongue blade.

▼ Wax spatula number 7.

▼ Glass jar and lid, or paper cup.

▼ Petroleum jelly.

▼ Tray adhesive and brush.

Procedure

PREPARING THE CAST

1. If undercuts are present, fill them with utility wax.

2. Outline the tray on the cast.

3. Cut a length of wax, warm it, and place it on the cast over the area of the tray (Fig. 23–7).

4. Use a warm plastic instrument to lute (secure) the wax to the cast (Fig. 23–8).

5. If indicated, use the wax spatula to place stops (small triangular holes) in the spacer.

6. Paint the prepared cast and wax with separating medium (Fig. 23–9).

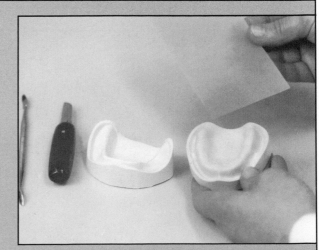

Figure 23–7 A sheet of wax is warmed prior to shaping it to fit the cast.

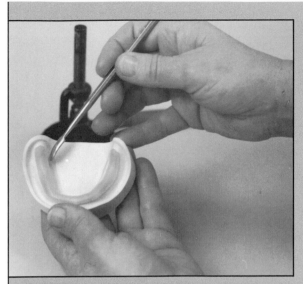

Figure 23–8 After the spacer has been fitted and trimmed, a warm instrument is used to lute the edges to the cast. (This is an edentulous mandibular arch.)

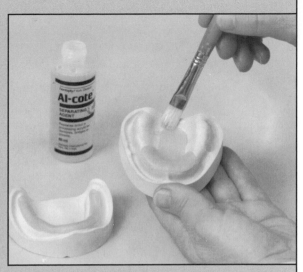

Figure 23–9 The completed spacer and the cast are painted with separating medium. (Note that the spacer is mushroom shaped on this edentulous maxillary arch.)

Procedure

MIXING THE MATERIAL

1 Following the manufacturer's instructions, measure the powder and liquid for the tray into the paper cup or glass container (Fig. 23–10).

2 Use the small wooden tongue blade to mix the powder and liquid (Fig. 23–11). A homogeneous mix should be obtained within 30 seconds. The mix will be thin and sticky.

3 Set the mix aside for 2 to 3 minutes to allow polymerization. (Self-polymerizing material may be placed in a covered jar during this stage.)

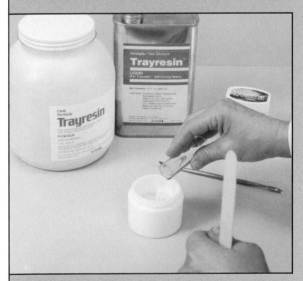

Figure 23–10 The tray resin is measured using the measuring devices provided by the manufacturer.

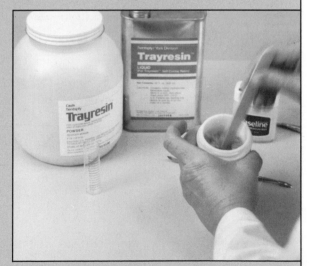

Figure 23–11 The tray resin is mixed according to the manufacturer's directions.

Procedure

FORMING THE TRAY

1. When the mix has reached a doughy (not sticky) stage, remove it from the container with the spatula.

2. Lubricate the palms of the hands with petroleum jelly and knead the resin to form a thick patty.

3. Mold the resin dough into a flattened form approximately the size of the wax spacer.

4. Place the resin dough on the cast to cover the wax spacer (Fig. 23–12). Adapt it to extend 1 to 1.5 mm beyond the edges of the wax spacer.

5. Use a plastic instrument or laboratory knife to trim away the excess tray material (Fig. 23–13).

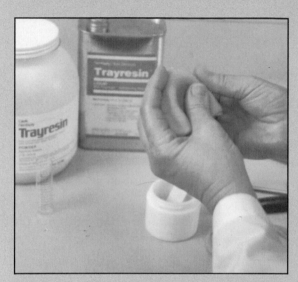

Figure 23–12 When the tray resin has reached the doughy stage, it is removed from the container. The palms of the hands are coated with petroleum jelly, and the material is shaped to the cast.

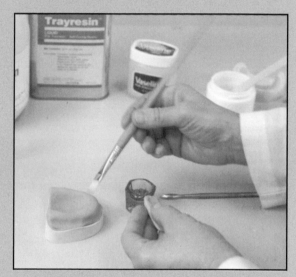

Figure 23–14 A handle is formed and placed on the tray.

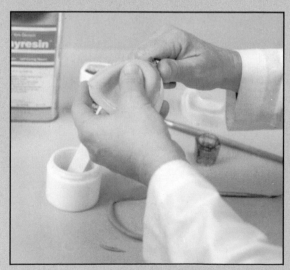

Figure 23–13 While the material is still soft, a laboratory knife is used to trim away the excess.

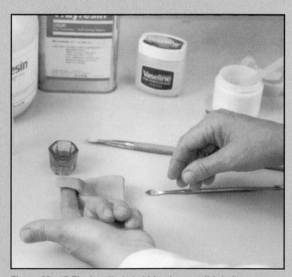

Figure 23–15 The handle is held in place until it is firm.

6 Use a piece of the scrap material to form the handle.

Moisten both the handle and the area where it is to be attached with tray resin liquid (Fig. 23–14).

Press the handle in place and gently hold it in place until the material has hardened (Fig. 23–15).

7 After 7 to 10 minutes, when the resin reaches the initial set, remove the tray from the cast and remove the wax spacer from the inside of the tray (Fig. 23–16).

8 If necessary, use a small stiff brush to clean all traces of the spacer material from the inner surface of the tray.

9 Return the tray to the diagnostic cast until it has reached final cure.

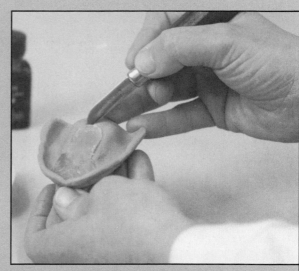

Figure 23–16 The wax spacer is removed from the palate of the maxillary tray before it reaches its final set.

Procedure

FINISHING THE TRAY

1 If the edges of the tray are rough, it is necessary to smooth them.

With an acrylic tray, this may be accomplished using an acrylic bur in the straight handpiece in the laboratory. An alternative is to trim the edges on the laboratory bench lathe.

Always wear protective goggles when grinding acrylic.

2 Paint the inner surface of the completed tray with tray adhesive for the impression material to be used (Fig. 23–17).

Figure 23–17 The prepared tray, including the edges, is painted with tray adhesive provided by the manufacturer of the impression material to be used.

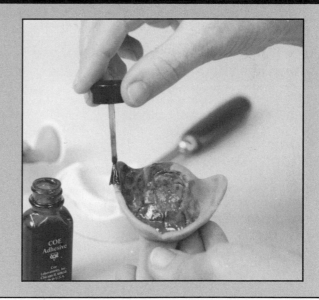

OVERVIEW OF VACUUM-FORMED CUSTOM TRAYS

Procedure

PREPARING THE CAST

1. Soak the prepared master cast in warm water for 20 minutes. (This avoids having air in the cast cause spaces under the acrylic sheet.)

2. Place paper strips over the teeth of the cast. (These strips serve as the first layer of spacers.)

3. Place the cast on the platform of the molding unit.

4. Place a moistened styrofoam layer over the entire cast. (This forms the remainder of the spacer.)

Procedure

FORMING THE TRAY

1. Check the controls of the vacuum molding unit, and adjust to heat the electric element in the unit. (Follow the manufacturer's directions.)

2. Select the thickness of the acrylic sheet to be used:
   For a maxillary tray, a 2-mm thickness.
   For a mandibular tray, a 3-mm thickness.

3. Adjust the controls of the unit, according to the manufacturer's instructions, for the amount of vacuum pressure to be used. (The setting for a tray is usually 2 to 3 psi.)

4. Heat the acrylic on the heating element.

5. Swing the heated acrylic over the cast and apply the selected pressure.

6. Allow the acrylic to cool for approximately 2 minutes. Release the pressure and remove the cast with the tray.

Procedure

ADDING A HANDLE

1. Mix cold-cure acrylic monomer and polymer to construct a handle for the tray.

2. Moisten the anterior section of the tray, near the incisal area, with monomer.

3. Shape and attach the resin handle. The handle must be parallel with the occlusal surfaces, at a right angle to the anterior teeth so that it will extend out of the mouth.

4. Allow the resin to reach final set.

Procedure

FINISHING THE TRAY

1. Separate the cast and tray.

2. Trim away excess acrylic from the periphery of the tray with acrylic burs in the straight handpiece.

3. If desired, polish the exterior surface of the tray.

4. Paint the interior surface of the completed tray with adhesive for the impression material to be used.

ELASTOMERIC IMPRESSION MATERIALS

Types of Elastomeric Impression Materials

Four types of elastomeric impression materials are commonly used in dental practices: **polysulfide**, **silicone**, **polysiloxane**, and **polyether.**

Elastomeric impression materials, which are self-curing, are provided as a base and catalyst. The curing reaction, as they change from a paste into a rubber-like material, begins as soon as the base and catalyst materials are brought together. The change occurs in a two-stage process.

The first stage (**initial set**) results in a stiffening of the paste without the appearance of elastic properties.

The material may be manipulated only during this first stage, and a homogeneous mix must be completed within the limited working time specified by the manufacturer.

The second stage (**final set**) begins with the appearance of elasticity and proceeds through a gradual change to a solid rubber-like mass.

The material must be in place in the mouth before the elastic properties of the final set start to develop.

Forms of Elastomeric Impression Materials

These impression materials are generally supplied in three types: **light-bodied** (syringe type), **regular**, and **heavy-bodied** (tray type). These materials are also described by their viscosity—light viscosity, medium viscosity, and heavy viscosity. (**Viscosity** is the characteristic of a material that causes it *not* to flow.)

The syringe type and tray type may be used together to obtain an accurate impression of the details of a preparation. A special syringe, or extruder gun, is used to place the light-bodied material into the preparation (Fig. 23–18).

Then a custom tray, loaded with heavy-bodied material, is immediately placed in the mouth *over* the light-bodied material.

When using these materials, first the assistant mixes the light-bodied material and loads the syringe. Then, while the operator is using the syringe, the assistant mixes the heavy-bodied material and loads the tray.

Putty = Extremely heavy bodied 'poor flow'

Special Precautions

▼ Elastomeric impression materials stain clothing. Handle them with care.

▼ The patient's clothing is usually covered with a plastic drape prior to taking an impression.

▼ Each type of elastomeric impression material must be manipulated following the manufacturer's instructions for that type of material.

▼ The catalyst and base come packaged together. Do *not* mix tubes from another package or from another manufacturer.

▼ When dispensing these materials from a tube, place the opening of the tube on the clean surface of the mixing pad. With a wiping motion, clean the opening of the tube and replace the cap immediately.

▼ Do not interchange caps of the base and accelerator tubes. If this happens, the contents of the tubes will be ruined.

Cleanup

The impression supplies should be cleaned up and returned to storage as quickly as possible.

Spatula. When finished using a spatula, wipe it clean with a tissue and then carefully discard the tissue. If it is not possible to clean the spatula immediately, wait until the material has set and then peel it off the spatula surface.

Mixing Pads. Carefully peel off the top sheet of each mixing pad and discard it. Return the mixing pad to the correct box.

Impression Material. If any material is found on the side of the tube, wipe it clean with a tissue. Check that the tops are tight and then return the correct pair of tubes to the same box.

Impression Syringe or Extruder Gun. Once the impression material has set, clean the syringe or

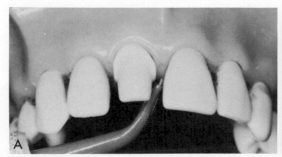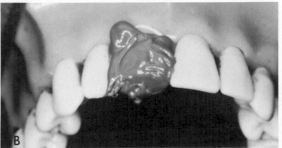

▼ **Figure 23–18**

The injection of rubber impression material begins at the most remote or difficult margin (**A**) and continues until the preparations are fully covered (**B**). (Baum L, Phillips RW, Lund MR: Operative Dentistry, 2nd Ed. Philadelphia, WB Saunders, 1985, p 457.)

extruder gun by peeling away the set material. Wipe gun free of smudges and store for future use.

POLYSULFIDE IMPRESSIONS

base – mercaptan

Polysulfide impression materials are available as three types: **light-bodied** (syringe type), **regular**, and **heavy-bodied** (tray type). Each type is supplied as two pastes: The base and the catalyst.

Described here is the use of the syringe and tray types of polysulfides to take a quadrant impression.

Instrumentation

▼ Custom tray painted with adhesive.

▼ Paper pads (2) (manufacturer's specifications).

▼ Large tapered spatulas (2).

▼ Polysulfide syringe type impression material (base and accelerator).

▼ Polysulfide heavy-bodied impression material (base and accelerator).

▼ Impression material syringe.

Procedure

PREPARATION OF SYRINGE TYPE MATERIAL

1. Extrude approximately 1¼ to 2 inches of the **syringe type base material** onto a clean paper pad. Wipe the tube opening clean and recap immediately.

2. Extrude an equal length of **syringe type accelerator** onto the paper pad below the base material. Wipe the tube opening clean and recap immediately.

3. Place the spatula tip into the accelerator and stir the material into the base with a circular motion.

4. Fully spatulate and incorporate the base and accelerator to produce a homogeneous mix within the 45 to 60 seconds of mixing time (Fig. 23–19A).

5. Follow the manufacturer's instructions for loading the syringe.

6. Pass the prepared syringe to the operator. Loading and assembly time should not exceed 30 seconds.

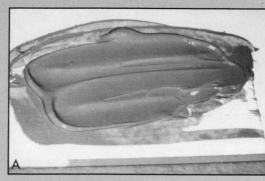

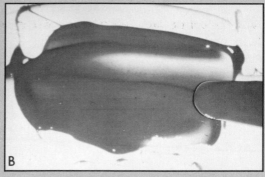

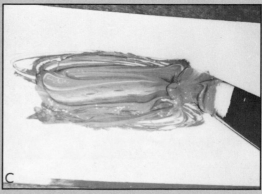

Figure 23-19 Any rubber material must be mixed to be smooth and homogeneous in color whether it is a polysulfide (*A*) or silicone material (*B*). Streaks must not be left in (*C*). (Baum L, Phillips RW, Lund MR: Operative Dentistry, 2nd Ed. Philadelphia, WB Saunders, 1985, p 456.)

Procedure

PREPARING TRAY TYPE MATERIAL

1. Use a clean mixing pad and clean spatula.

2. Extrude the **tray type base material** to the appropriate length. Wipe the tube opening clean and recap immediately.

3. Extrude the same length of **tray type accelerator**. This is placed approximately 1 inch from the base paste on the pad. Wipe the tube opening clean and recap immediately.

4. Use a clean spatula to complete a homogeneous mix within 45 seconds to 1 minute.

5. Pick up the bulk of the tray mix with the spatula and load the material into the tray.

6. The assistant receives the syringe from the operator and passes the loaded tray.

7. The approximate setting time for the impression material is 8 to 12 minutes from the beginning of the mix of the syringe material.

SILICONE IMPRESSIONS

Silicone impression materials, also known as *condensation silicones*, are available as two pastes: The base and the catalyst. The catalyst is also supplied in liquid form.

Silicones are available as light-bodied, regular, and heavy-bodied (silicone putty) material.

Silicone putties may be dispensed and mixed with the gloved hands. These materials are *not* affected by handling with latex gloves.

Mixing Silicone Impression Materials

1. The instrumentation is the same as that used for manipulating polysulfide materials.
2. The base and accelerator are dispensed on a paper pad as directed by the manufacturer.
3. If the accelerator is supplied as a liquid, it is measured in drops. Place these drops on or near the base material.
4. The base paste is mixed into the liquid with a circular motion (Fig. 23–19*B*).

POLYSILOXANE IMPRESSIONS

Polysiloxane, also known as *addition type silicone* or *polyvinylsiloxane,* is available as light-bodied (wash), regular (medium), and heavy-bodied (putty) materials. These are supplied as a two-paste system.

The light-bodied and regular materials are mixed using an **extruder gun,** which automatically mixes the catalyst and base (Fig. 23–20).

The light-bodied material is extruded directly from the gun into the preparation.

The regular (medium) weight material is loaded from the mixing tip into the custom tray.

The extruder gun is loaded, used, and cared for according to the manufacturer's directions. After use, the empty gun is disinfected.

The heavy-bodied putty may be dispensed and mixed with the hands. However, contact with latex gloves may severely retard the setting of the putty.

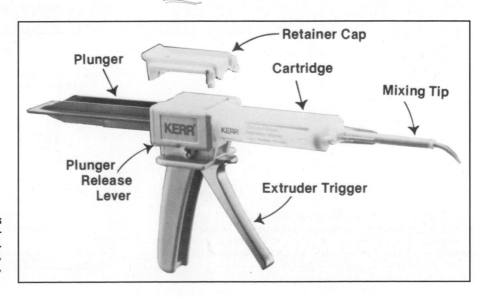

▼ Figure 23–20

Extruder gun used to mix and express polysiloxane syringe material simultaneously onto tooth preparations. (Courtesy of Kerr Manufacturing Co, subsidiary of Sybron Corp, Romulus, MI.)

Plastic (vinyl) overgloves *must* be worn when handling and mixing these materials.

Two-Step Impression Technique

The following is a description of the use of polysiloxane material in a two-step impression technique.

The heavy-bodied putty material is used to take a **preliminary impression** before the teeth are prepared. A stock tray, or a custom tray, may be painted with adhesive and used for this initial impression.

The **final impression** is taken after the teeth have been prepared. This time syringe material is extruded around the prepared tooth, and the preliminary impression is again seated firmly in the mouth. The two impression materials bond together to form an extremely accurate impression.

Taking Polysiloxane Impressions

Instrumentation

▼ Stock tray.

▼ Mixing pad.

▼ Light-bodied (wash) (base and catalyst) polysiloxane.

▼ Heavy-bodied (putty) (base and catalyst) polysiloxane.

▼ Measuring scoops.

▼ Extruder gun and accessories (tips).

▼ Plastic sheet spacers.

▼ Plastic overgloves.

▼ Spatula.

Procedure

ASSEMBLING THE EXTRUDER GUN

1. Follow the manufacturer's directions for assembling the extruder gun.

2. Insert the cartridges into the gun and engage the plunger.

3. Check cartridge to be certain plunger and cartridge are engaged.

4. Twist off sealing cap on cartridge.

5. Squeeze trigger of gun and extrude ½ inch of base and catalyst from the cartridge. Wipe end of cartridge.

6. Engage fresh disposable mixing tip on cartridge and twist to lock with a one quarter turn.

7. The syringe assembly is set aside for later use.

Procedure

PREPARING THE PUTTY MATERIAL FOR PRELIMINARY IMPRESSION

1. Scoop up equal portions of **putty base** and **catalyst** and place them on the mixing pad.

2. Don plastic overgloves; then use the spatula to incorporate the base and catalyst.

3. Scoop up the mix and knead it with the hands. Complete a homogeneous mix in 30 seconds.

4. Load the tray with the putty mix. Use a gloved finger to place a slight indentation in tray material where the teeth will be.

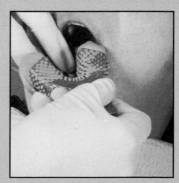

Figure 23–21 Placement of the mandibular tray with polysiloxane material for the preliminary impression. (Torres HO, Ehrlich A: Modern Dental Assisting, 4th Ed. Philadelphia, WB Saunders, 1990, p 717.)

5 Cover the tray material with a plastic sheet spacer. Hand the prepared tray to the operator. (The spacer creates room in the preliminary impression so that additional impression material can be added for the final impression.)

6 The operator positions the tray in the patient's mouth over the teeth to be prepared (Fig. 23–21). The tray remains in place for 4 minutes and is then removed.

7 Remove the spacer and check the impression for accuracy and freedom from wrinkles and bubbles.

8 Set this preliminary impression aside for later use after the teeth are prepared.

Procedure

PREPARING THE FINAL IMPRESSION

1 The prepared extruder gun is passed to the operator. The wash material is extruded over, into, and around the prepared teeth (Fig. 23–22).

2 A generous amount of wash mix is then extruded into the putty mix in the preliminary impression until the putty material in the tray is filled.

3 The operator receives the tray and immediately seats it over the prepared teeth.

4 The tray is held in place on the dental arch for 4 minutes and then removed (Fig. 23–23).

5 The impression is rinsed, inspected for detail, and sprayed with a disinfectant.

6 The impression may be poured (without distortion) within 10 minutes *or* after 12 to 24 hours.

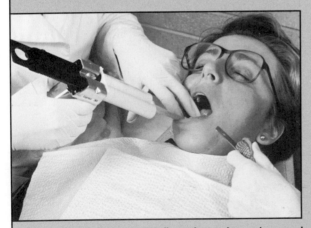

Figure 23–22 Extruder gun dispensing syringe mix around tooth preparations. The assistant holds the preliminary impression ready to be seated over the syringe material. (Torres HO, Ehrlich A: Modern Dental Assisting, 4th Ed. Philadelphia, WB Saunders, 1990, p 718.)

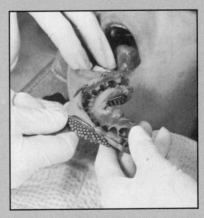

Figure 23–23 The completed polysiloxane impression of the mandibular arch. (Torres HO, Ehrlich A: Modern Dental Assisting, 4th Ed. Philadelphia, WB Saunders, 1990, p 718.)

POLYETHER IMPRESSIONS

Polyether impression materials are supplied as two pastes: the base and catalyst. A thinner, or body modifier, is also included (Fig. 23–24).

The body modifier is added to the mix to reduce the thickness of the mix and/or to extend the working time.

The mixing technique is very similar to that for polysulfide materials. These impressions must be stored in a dry place until poured.

THE OPPOSING ARCH

An impression of the opposing arch is also necessary for use by the dental laboratory. An alginate

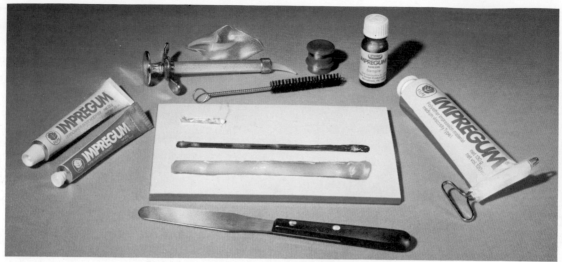

▼ Figure 23–24

Polyether impression material. (Courtesy of Premier Dental Products Co, Norristown, PA.)

impression is commonly used for this purpose. (Alginate impressions are discussed in Chapter 17, "Alginate Impressions and Diagnostic Casts.")

BITE REGISTRATION PASTE IMPRESSION

An accurate bite registration is necessary to establish the proper occlusal relationship when mounting the casts on the articulator. (An **articulator** is a device that simulates the movements of the mandible and the temporomandibular joint.)

Elastomeric impression material, applied from an extruder gun, may be used for this purpose. An alternative is the use of a zinc oxide–eugenol (ZOE) bite registration paste.

These pastes are supplied in two tubes (Fig. 23–25). The base is usually brown, and the accelerator is a different color (blue or pink).

The ZOE registration paste reaches an initial set in a few minutes when mixed and placed in the warmth of the patient's mouth.

Instrumentation

▼ Base registration paste and accelerator.

▼ Spatula.

▼ Paper mixing pad.

▼ Disposable plastic bite frame with gauze.

▼ Utility wax.

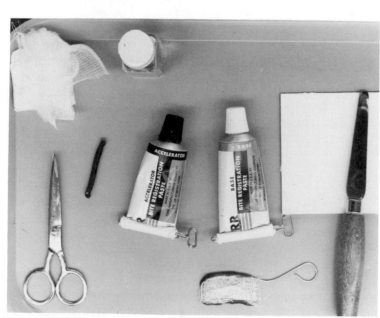

▼ Figure 23–25

Instrumentation for paste bite registration. (Torres HO, Ehrlich A: Modern Dental Assisting, 4th Ed. Philadelphia, WB Saunders, 1990, p 722).

Procedure

PREPARING BITE REGISTRATION PASTE

1 Assemble the disposable bite frame and gauze.

2 For a quadrant impression, extrude 1¼ inches of each material onto the mixing pad. Place the base and accelerator so that they are 1 inch from each other.

3 At a signal from the operator, combine the accelerator and base. Spatulate until a homogeneous mix is obtained (approximately 30 seconds).

4 Spread the mix to a depth of approximately 2 mm on both sides of the gauze.

5 Hand the frame to the operator. Use tissues to wipe the spatula clean immediately. Remove and discard the used sheet from the mixing pad.

6 In the patient's mouth, the paste will set in approximately 3 minutes to a semi-hard consistency.

▼◣ **EXERCISES**

1. When mixing elastomeric impression materials, the elastic properties of the material develop during the ___b___ set.

   a. initial
   b. final

2. When working with syringe type and tray type impression materials, the _____ material is mixed first.

   a. syringe type
   b. tray type
   c. doesn't matter which is mixed first

3. The spacer is removed from the custom tray just _____.

   a. after the tray material has hardened
   b. before painting the tray with adhesive
   c. prior to use

4. The accelerator for silicone impression material is supplied as a _____
   _____.

   a. gel
   b. liquid
   c. paste
   d. putty

5. If the edges of an acrylic tray are rough, they may be smoothed by _____
   _____.

   a. coating them with wax
   b. heating them
   c. trimming with an acrylic bur

6. A custom tray is constructed on a cast that was made from an impression of the arch _____ the teeth were prepared.

   a. after
   b. before

7. Tray acrylic is mixed with a _____.

   a. laboratory knife
   b. wax spatula
   c. wooden tongue blade

8. _____ are placed to prevent the tray from seating too deep in the arch or quadrant.

   a. Spacers
   b. Stops
   c. Undercuts
   d. a, b, and c

9. When mixing elastomeric materials, it _____ is not _____ acceptable to mix tubes from another package as long as they are from the same manufacturer.

   a. is
   b. is not

10. Vinyl overgloves must be worn when mixing heavy-bodied polysiloxane putty.

    a. true
    b. false

11. Elastomeric impression materials are mixed on a _____.

    a. chilled glass slab
    b. paper pad
    c. room temperature glass slab

12. The handle of a custom tray is placed on the _____ portion of the tray.

    a. anterior
    b. buccal
    c. occlusal
    d. posterior

13. When constructing a custom tray using the vacuum technique, _____ sheets are placed over the cast to form a spacer.

    a. acrylic
    b. styrofoam
    c. wax
    d. b or c

14. The tray adhesive is specified by the manufacturer of the _____ material.

    a. impression
    b. tray

15. The mixing time for polysulfide impression syringe material should not exceed _____.

    a. 30 to 45 seconds
    b. 45 to 60 seconds
    c. 1 to 2 minutes
    d. 2 to 3 minutes

16. Silicone impression materials _____ are not _____ affected by handling with latex gloves.

    a. are
    b. are not

17. ZOE bite registration paste will set in the patient's mouth in approximately _____ 3 _____ minute(s).

    a. 1
    b. 2
    c. 3
    d. 5

18. The spatula used for mixing elastomeric impression material may be cleaned by _____.

    a. wiping it immediately clean with a tissue
    b. peeling off the material after it has set
    c. soaking it in hot water
    d. a and b

19. Before constructing the tray, the cast and spacer are painted with _____
    _____.

    a. separating medium
    b. solvent
    c. tray adhesive

20. Light-bodied _____ impression materials are mixed using an extruder gun.

    a. polysiloxane
    b. polysulfide
    c. silicone
    d. a and c

Criterion Sheet 23-1

Student's Name _____

Procedure: *CONSTRUCTING A CUSTOM ACRYLIC IMPRESSION TRAY*

Performance Objective:

The student will demonstrate the construction of a custom acrylic impression tray for the mandibular left quadrant.

	SE	IE
SE = Student evaluation **C** = Criterion met **IE** = Instructor evaluation **X** = Criterion not met		
Instrumentation: Cast of mandibular left quadrant with a bridge preparation, pencil, laboratory knife, utility wax, wax for spacer, warm water or a bunsen burner, wax spatula, tray resin and measuring devices, glass jar with lid or a paper cup, small spatula or wooden tongue blade, and petroleum jelly.		
1. Filled undercuts on cast with utility wax.		
2. Marked cast at line for extension of custom tray.		
3. Shaped spacer over cast to extension line.		
4. Used wax spatula to cut stops in the spacer on nonprepared teeth.		
5. Mixed tray resin according to manufacturer's directions. Allowed mix to reach doughy stage (2 to 3 minutes).		
6. Lubricated palms of hands with petroleum jelly. Kneaded resin to form a thick patty.		
7. Shaped resin dough on cast to form tray and handle. The handle extended out of the mouth from the front of the arch. The handle was at a right angle. The handle was parallel with the occlusal surfaces of the teeth.		
8. Removed tray from cast after resin reached initial set. Removed spacer material from tray.		
9. Reseated tray on cast until acrylic was fully set.		
Comments:		

▼ Criterion Sheet 23–2

Student's Name _____

Procedure:	*MIXING POLYSULFIDE (RUBBER BASE)* *LIGHT-BODY (SYRINGE) IMPRESSION MATERIAL*

Performance Objective:

The student will mix the impression material and load the syringe within the accept-able time limit.

			SE	IE
SE = Student evaluation	**C** = Criterion met			
IE = Instructor evaluation	**X** = Criterion not met			

	SE	IE
Instrumentation: Paper pad, stiff spatula, polysulfide syringe material (base and acceler-ator), syringe and disposable tip, dappen dish and tissues. (Appropri-ate infection control barriers will be used during all procedures actually performed on a patient.)		
1. Extruded equal lengths (1¼ to 2 inches) of base and accelerator on mixing pad. Replaced caps on tubes immediately.		
2. Placed tip of spatula in the accelerator. Stirred accelerator into the base with a circular motion. Spatulated mass of material on mixing pad. Achieved homogeneous mix within 60 seconds.		
3. Used spatula to place bulk of material into dappen dish.		
4. Dipped sleeve of syringe into material. Used plunger to draw the material up into the sleeve.		
5. Used tissues to clean end of sleeve. Placed tip device on end of syringe sleeve. Loading and assembly completed within 30 seconds.		
6. Cleaned up all materials and work space. Returned supplies to storage.		
Comments:		

▼ Criterion Sheet 23-3

Student's Name _____

Procedure: *MIXING POLYSILOXANE HEAVY-BODY (PUTTY) IMPRESSION MATERIAL*

Performance Objective:

The student will mix the impression material and load the tray within the acceptable time limit.

		SE	IE
SE = Student evaluation **IE** = Instructor evaluation	**C** = Criterion met **X** = Criterion not met		
Instrumentation: Paper pad, stiff spatula, polysiloxane heavy-bodied (putty) material (base and catalyst), measuring scoop, plastic sheet spacer, custom tray (painted with adhesive), and vinyl overgloves. (Appropriate infection control barriers will be used during all procedures actually performed on a patient.)			
1. Measured 1½ scoops of putty (base material). Placed putty on mixing pad. Scored putty with spatula.			
2. Dispensed accelerator onto scored area of putty. Mixed putty and accelerator on pad with spatula.			
3. Donned vinyl overgloves. Picked up mass of impression material and kneaded it in hands. Achieved homogeneous mix within 30 seconds.			
4. Loaded mix into prepared tray. Used gloved finger to place a slight indentation in tray material.			
5. Covered tray material with plastic sheet spacer. Tray ready for use within time specified by manufacturer.			
6. Cleaned up all materials and work space. Returned supplies to storage.			
Comments:			

24 Crown and Bridge Restoration

▼ LEARNING OBJECTIVES

The student will be able to:

1. Differentiate between inlays, onlays, and full crowns.
2. Describe the components of a fixed bridge and state the functions of each.
3. Describe the steps in the preparation and cementation of a single crown.
4. Describe the steps in the preparation and cementation of a fixed bridge.
5. Describe the use of gingival retraction cord.
6. Describe the use of temporary coverage between crown and bridge visits.

OVERVIEW OF CROWN AND BRIDGE RESTORATIONS

The construction of crown and bridge restorations is part of the specialty of *fixed prosthetics.*

A **fixed prosthesis** is a precision cast replacement for missing teeth that is cemented into place. (A **prosthesis** is a replacement for a body part. In this instance, a lost tooth or teeth.)

A **removable prosthesis** is a replacement for missing teeth or tissues that may be placed and removed by the patient. (Removable prosthodontics is discussed in Chapter 25, "Complete and Partial Removable Dentures.")

These cast restorations are fabricated by the dental laboratory based on the exact instructions as found in the **written prescription** from the dentist.

The laboratory may *not* proceed without a written prescription. A copy of the prescription is retained with the patient's records.

The metal used for these cast restorations is usually a gold alloy in which gold is a primary ingredient. However, other **high noble alloys** are also used. These alloys are so named because the main ingredients are referred to as noble metals. (The noble metals used in dentistry are **gold, palladium,** and **platinum**.)

Inlays and Onlays

Cast inlays and onlays may be used to restore a tooth that has been severely damaged by fracture, caries, or wear. These castings have the advantage of being stronger and longer lasting than an amalgam restoration.

An **inlay** is a cast restoration to restore one, two, or three surfaces of a single tooth: For example, the occlusal, mesio-occlusal, or mesio-occlusodistal surfaces where the remaining tooth margins are intact (Fig. 24-1). Inlays are also used for some Class V restorations.

An inlay may be made of gold, composite, porcelain, or composite resin. The material selected depends on the surfaces to be restored.

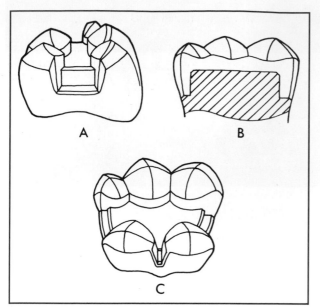

▼ Figure 24–1

Class II MOD gold inlay preparation of a mandibular first molar. *A.* Proximal view of the preparation. *B.* Cross section of the preparation. *C.* Occlusal view of the preparation. (Torres HO, Ehrlich A: Modern Dental Assisting, 4th Ed. Philadelphia, WB Saunders, 1990, p 556.)

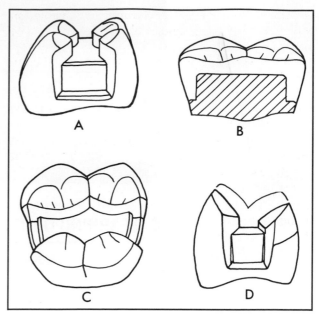

▼ Figure 24–2

Class II MOD gold onlay preparation of a mandibular premolar. *A.* Proximal view of the preparation. *B.* Cross section of the preparation. *C.* Occlusal view of the preparation. *D.* Proximal view indicating height of the restoration. (Torres HO, Ehrlich A: Modern Dental Assisting, 4th Ed. Philadelphia, WB Saunders, 1990, p 555.)

In an anterior tooth, a tooth-colored material is important because it will show as the patient talks or smiles.

In a posterior tooth, the greater strength of a metallic restoration may be required to withstand the forces of mastication (chewing).

An **onlay**, which is usually constructed of a gold alloy, is a cast restoration to restore the occlusal surface, margins, and frequently two or more cusps of the occlusal surface of a posterior tooth (Figs. 24–2 and 24–3).

Full Crowns

A **full crown** is a cast restoration that covers the entire anatomic crown of the tooth. (The anatomic crown of the tooth is discussed in Chapter 4, "Dental Anatomy and Tooth Morphology.")

This may be a single crown placed on an anterior or posterior tooth, or it may be joined with other bridge parts to serve as the abutment for a fixed bridge.

A **veneer crown** is also referred to as a *porcelain-fused-to-metal (PFM) crown.* A PFM crown is a full crown constructed of a high noble alloy with a thin veneer of porcelain fused to the exterior surface. This creates a strong, yet esthetically pleasing, tooth-colored restoration.

The porcelain may cover only the facial surface of the crown, with the occlusal surface or incisal edge and other tooth surfaces in gold.

Components of a Fixed Bridge

A **fixed bridge** replaces one or more adjoining missing teeth in the dental arch. This is referred to

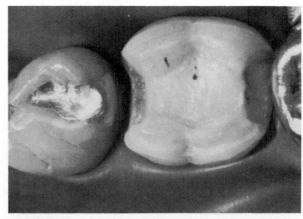

▼ Figure 24–3

A clinical MOD onlay preparation. (Baum L, Phillips RW, Lund MR: Operative Dentistry, 2nd Ed. Philadelphia, WB Saunders, 1985, p 424.)

as a fixed bridge because the finished restoration is cemented in place and may not be removed by the patient.

Each fixed bridge consists of a series of components, or units, that are attached together.

An **abutment,** or *retainer,* is a natural tooth (or an implant) that becomes the support for the replacement tooth or teeth.

An abutment tooth may be prepared with an onlay or cast crown. A bridge usually has one or two abutments to support it at both ends.

A **pontic** is an artificial tooth that replaces a missing natural tooth. The occlusal or incisal edge of the pontic is fabricated of cast gold to provide biting and chewing strength. However, like a crown, the pontic may have a porcelain facing so that it resembles natural tooth structure.

There is a pontic for each missing tooth. The span of a single bridge does not usually exceed replacing more than two missing teeth that are next to each other.

A **three-unit bridge** consists of two abutments (one on either end) and a pontic in the middle to replace a missing tooth.

FULL CROWN PREPARATION

Some of the steps in the preparation and cementation of a single crown are described in greater detail in separate sections later in this chapter or in other chapters.

Instrumentation (First Visit)

▼ Basic setup.

▼ Alginate impression setup.

▼ Local anesthetic setup.

▼ High-speed and low-speed handpieces.

▼ Diamond stones and burs (operator's choice).

▼ Gingival retraction cord setup.

▼ Elastomeric-type impression setup.

▼ Bite registration setup.

▼ Temporary coverage setup.

▼ High volume evacuator (HVE) tip.

Procedure

CROWN PREPARATION: FIRST VISIT

1. Preliminary impressions are obtained, disinfected, and put aside. (See under "Preliminary Alginate Impressions," later in this chapter.)

2. Local anesthetic solution is administered. (See Chapter 18, "Pharmacology and Pain Control.")

3. The operator uses the high-speed handpiece to:
   Reduce slightly the crown height and bulk of the tooth.
   Remove any caries.
   Taper the gingival third of the crown to prepare the chamfer, or shoulder (Fig. 24–4).

4. During the preparation, the assistant retracts the tongue, lips, and cheek and uses the HVE to provide a clear operating field.

5. The next step is gingival retraction. (See under "Gingival Retraction.")

6. The final impression and bite registration are taken. (See Chapter 23, "Custom Trays and Elastomeric Impressions.")

7. Temporary coverage is placed. (See under "Temporary Coverage.")

8. The patient is reappointed to return for placement of the completed prosthesis.

9. The written prescription, impressions, and bite registration are sent to the laboratory for construction of the casting and finishing of the crown.

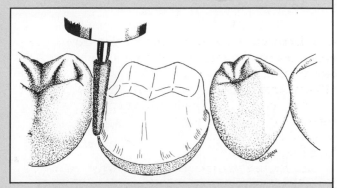

Figure 24–4 A crown preparation involves reducing the height and bulk of the tooth. (Baum L, Phillips RW, Lund MR: Operative Dentistry, 2nd Ed. Philadelphia, WB Saunders, 1985, p 433.)

Instrumentation (Second Visit)

▼ Basic setup.

▼ Local anesthetic setup.

▼ Isopropyl alcohol.

▼ Cotton-tipped applicator.

▼ Tongue blades or crown seater.

▼ Cavity varnish.

▼ Cement setup (operator's choice).

▼ Articulating paper and holder.

▼ Crown remover.

▼ Scaler.

▼ Finishing stones and points.

▼ Low-speed handpiece.

Procedure

CROWN PREPARATION: SECOND VISIT

1   Before the appointment, the assistant determines that the cast crown is ready and has been returned to the office.

2   Local anesthetic solution is administered if necessary.

3   The temporary coverage is removed from the tooth. The operator removes any temporary cement that may be remaining on the tooth. (Isopropyl alcohol on a cotton-tipped applicator may be used sparingly for this purpose.)

4   The operator uses an explorer to check all margins of the prepared tooth to be certain that they are intact and are free of temporary cement.

5   The operator seats the crown and determines that it is fitted properly.

6   A wooden tongue blade is placed on the incisal edges or the occlusal surfaces, and the patient is instructed to bite on the blade to seat the crown fully.

7   The occlusal surface of the crown is adjusted as necessary. The crown is removed from the tooth and repolished (Fig. 24–5).

8   The tooth is dried and prepared for cementation. This step may include two thin coats of cavity varnish applied to protect the pulp from reacting negatively to the acid in the cement.

9   Upon a signal from the operator, the assistant mixes the cement, distributes it evenly over the inner surface of the crown, and hands the crown to the oper-

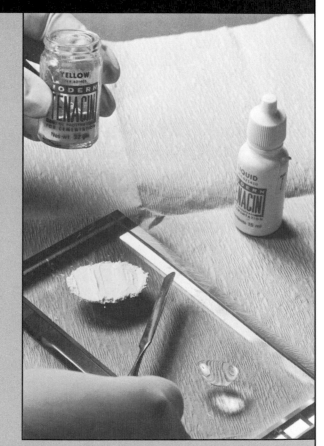

Figure 24–5 Zinc phosphate cement is one choice for the permanent cementation of a cast restoration. (Torres HO, Ehrlich A: Modern Dental Assisting, 4th Ed. Philadelphia, WB Saunders, 1990, p 222.)

ator (Fig. 24–6). (Cements are discussed in Chapter 20, "Dental Cements.")

10   The operator forces the crown onto the tooth preparation and has the patient bite again on the tongue blade or crown

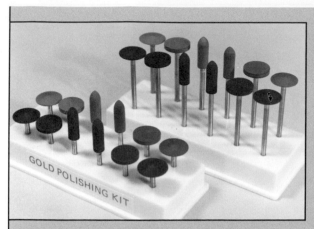

Figure 24-6 Kit for polishing gold restorations. The kit contains six Brownie points for finishing, three Greenie points for polishing, and three Supergreenie points for superpolishing. (Courtesy of Shofu Dental Corp, Menlo Park, CA.)

seater to seat the crown completely. The cement is permitted to harden (usually 7 to 10 minutes).

11 Using an explorer, small spoon excavator, or scaler, the operator gently removes the excess cement from the gingival margin and surface of the crown.

12 The operator passes knotted dental floss through the interproximal areas to remove any remaining cement.

13 The patient's mouth is rinsed and vacuumed.

14 The patient's occlusion is checked again with articulating paper.

15 If necessary, the occlusion is adjusted and the crown is polished again.

16 The patient is dismissed.

FIXED BRIDGE PREPARATION

Instrumentation (First Visit)

▼ Basic setup.

▼ Local anesthetic setup.

▼ Alginate impression setup.

▼ High-speed and low-speed handpieces.

▼ Diamond stones and burs, mandrels, and discs (operator's choice).

▼ Retraction cord setup.

▼ Bite registration setup.

▼ Temporary coverage setup.

▼ HVE tip.

Instrumentation (Second Visit)

▼ Basic setup.

▼ Local anesthetic setup.

▼ Crown remover.

▼ Crown seater.

▼ Mallet.

▼ Tongue blade (wood).

▼ Temporary cement setup.

▼ Cotton rolls.

▼ Elastomeric impression setup.

Procedure

FIXED BRIDGE: FIRST VISIT

1. A local anesthetic solution is administered.

2. Preliminary alginate impressions of both arches are made for study casts.

3. The bite registration is obtained.

4. As with a single crown, the operator uses the high-speed handpiece to prepare the crown of the tooth.

5. Gingival retraction is the next step. (See under "Gingival Retraction.")

6. Temporary coverage is prepared and placed. (See under "Temporary Coverage.")

7. The patient is scheduled for a second visit and dismissed.

8. The written prescription, impressions, and bite registration are sent to the laboratory for casting and finishing of the crown (Fig. 24–7).

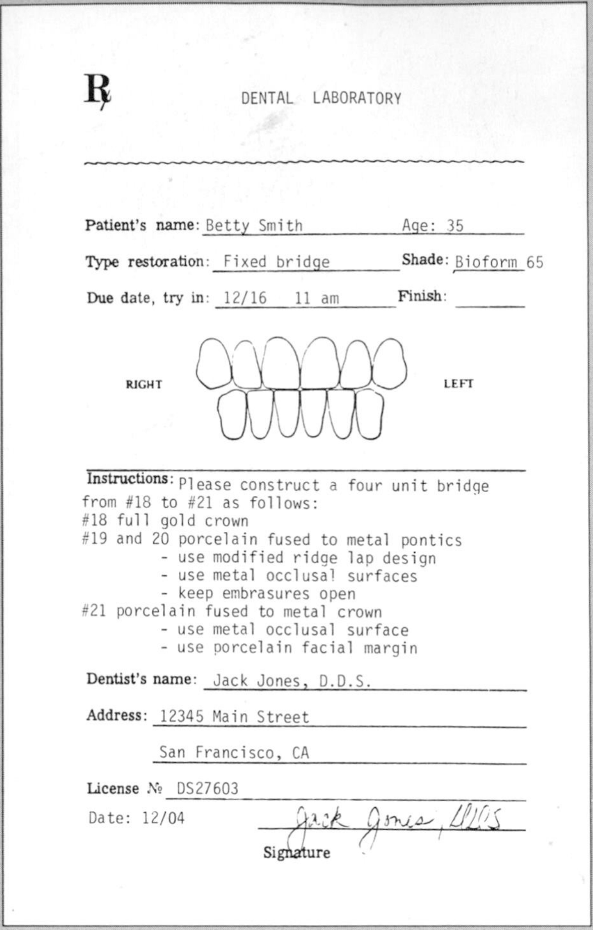

R̸   DENTAL LABORATORY

Patient's name: Betty Smith   Age: 35

Type restoration: Fixed bridge   Shade: Bioform 65

Due date, try in: 12/16   11 am   Finish:

RIGHT   LEFT

Instructions: Please construct a four unit bridge
from #18 to #21 as follows:
#18 full gold crown
#19 and 20 porcelain fused to metal pontics
      - use modified ridge lap design
      - use metal occlusal surfaces
      - keep embrasures open
#21 porcelain fused to metal crown
      - use metal occlusal surface
      - use porcelain facial margin

Dentist's name: Jack Jones, D.D.S.

Address: 12345 Main Street

San Francisco, CA

License № DS27603

Date: 12/04   Jack Jones, DDS
                   Signature

Figure 24–7 Written prescription for a four-unit fixed bridge with two abutments and two pontics. (Torres HO, Ehrlich A: Modern Dental Assisting, 4th Ed. Philadelphia, WB Saunders, 1990, p 734.)

Procedure

FIXED BRIDGE: SECOND VISIT

1. Before the appointment, the assistant determines that the castings are ready and have been returned to the office.

2. A local anesthetic is administered.

3. The temporary coverage is removed carefully, so as not to fracture the margins of the preparation. This is cleaned and set aside for future use.

4. The gold casting abutments are tried on the individual abutment teeth.
   The teeth carefully to determine the accurate fit of the crowns.

If the abutments do not fit, impressions must be retaken and the temporary coverage replaced.

5. If the castings fit, they are left in place and an elastomeric impression is taken.

6. The tray is removed gently. The castings may be removed with the impression.

7. The temporary coverage is replaced.

8. The patient is scheduled for a third visit and dismissed.

Instrumentation (Third Visit)

▼ Basic setup.

▼ Local anesthetic setup (optional).

▼ Rubber dam setup (optional).

▼ Crown remover.

▼ Crown seater.

▼ Mallet.

▼ Tongue blade (wood).

▼ Cementation setup (operator's choice of cement).

▼ Articulating paper and holder.

▼ Scaler.

▼ Finishing stones and points.

▼ Rubber cup (prophylaxis).

▼ Right-angle (prophy) handpiece (RAHP).

▼ Polishing pastes.

Procedure

FIXED BRIDGE: THIRD VISIT

1 Before the appointment, the assistant determines that the bridge is ready and has been returned to the office.

2 A local anesthetic is administered if necessary. If the patient can tolerate the slight discomfort of drying the teeth, a local anesthetic solution is *not* administered. (Proceeding without anesthesia permits more accurate adjustments when checking the patient's occlusion.)

3 Placement of a rubber dam is optional for a maxillary bridge; however, it is advised for seating of a mandibular bridge.

    The rubber dam helps to control saliva, moisture contamination, and the patient's tongue.

4 The temporary bridge coverage is removed, cleaned, and set aside (for future use in case the bridge does not fit).

5 The completed bridge (with the units soldered and polished) is tried on the prepared teeth.

6 A wooden tongue blade is placed over the incisal edges or occlusal surfaces, and the patient is advised to bite firmly on the blade. The margins and occlusion are checked.

7 A crown remover is used to remove the bridge carefully from the teeth. If there is any roughness on the bridge, this is buffed away.

8 Upon a signal from the operator, the assistant mixes the cement, fills the abutments with cement and hands the completed bridge to the operator, who seats the bridge.

9 The assistant hands a crown seater to the operator.

    The operator positions the crown seater.

    The assistant may be asked to use the mallet to tap on the extreme end of the crown seating instrument.

10 The patient is instructed to close firmly on the bridge and quickly reopen his mouth to prevent saliva from touching the cement.

    Note: If a rubber dam is in place, this step is omitted.

11 Any excess cement is removed from the exterior of the crown or abutments. If a rubber dam was used, it is removed at this time.

12 The assistant places articulating paper in the holder and passes it to the operator or places it on the occlusal surfaces of the mandibular teeth. The patient is requested to close and simulate chewing.

13 The operator uses a stone or point in the low-speed handpiece to reduce the high spots on the bridge.

14 Polishing paste (on a rubber cup attach-

Continued on following page

ment of the low-speed handpiece) may be used to produce a final polish.

15 The assistant instructs the patient about oral hygiene procedures needed to care for the new fixed bridgework, and the patient is dismissed.

16 The patient may be advised to return to the dental office in 72 hours to allow the operator to check the occlusion and function of the fixed bridge.

BASIC STEPS

Preliminary Alginate Impressions

Preliminary alginate impressions are usually taken of both arches *before* the teeth are prepared. (Alginate impressions and creating diagnostic casts are discussed in Chapter 17, "Alginate Impressions and Diagnostic Costs.")

A preliminary impression of the arch being treated is used to create a custom tray for the elastomeric impression, which is taken *after* the teeth have been prepared. (Custom trays and elastomeric impressions are discussed in Chapter 23, "Custom Trays and Elastomeric Impressions.")

The impression of the opposing arch is used to create the opposing arch cast, which is used in articulating the casts.

An alginate impression taken before the teeth are prepared may be used in creating temporary coverage to protect the teeth between visits.

Gingival Retraction

Prior to taking the final impression, it is necessary to force the gingival tissue temporarily away from the margins of the preparation.

This step, which is called gingival retraction, is necessary so that the final impression includes the finish line of the completed preparation. This finish line, which is also known as the *margin*, extends into the gingival sulcus at the cervix of the tooth.

The method most frequently used for gingival retraction utilizes **gingival retraction cords**. These cords are available as **plain** or **braided** cord and as **impregnated** cord, which contains medicaments, or as **nonimpregnated** cord, which does not contain medicaments.

The impregnated forms usually contain epinephrine, which is a vasoconstrictor. Epinephrine causes blood vessels to constrict and the tissues to contract temporarily. This keeps the area free of hemorrhage (bleeding) and permits the operator to obtain a clear impression.

However, a high epinephrine content is potentially hazardous to the patient with cardiovascular diseases. Therefore, impregnated retraction cord is applied sparingly. If the patient is sensitive to epinephrine, other medicaments are substituted.

Instrumentation

▼ Basic setup.

▼ Gingival retraction cord.

▼ Scissors.

▼ Blunt packing instrument.

▼ Saliva ejector.

Procedure

GINGIVAL RETRACTION

1 When the preparation is complete, the area is rinsed and gently dried.

2 The assistant cuts a length of cord (1 to 1½ inches) and transfers it to the operator in cotton pliers.

3 The assistant transfers the blunt packing instrument to the operator for use in very gently displacing the gingiva temporarily and forcing the cord into the gingival sulcus (Fig. 24–8).

4 The cord is left in place for 5 to 7 minutes, depending on the type of chemical retraction used.

⁵ The retraction cord is removed just prior to the use of the syringe type elastomeric impression material.

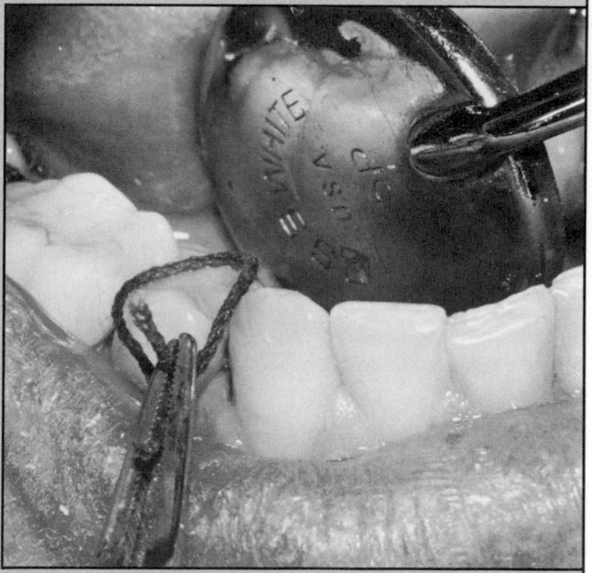

Figure 24–8 A loop of retraction cord is placed around the tooth and gently tamped into the gingival sulcus. (Torres HO, Ehrlich A: Modern Dental Assisting, 4th Ed. Philadelphia, WB Saunders, 1990, p 705.)

Temporary Coverage

The patient wears the temporary covering to protect the prepared teeth between appointments prior to the delivery of the fixed prosthesis. The construction and seating of temporary coverage may be delegated to the expanded function dental assistant.

Properly constructed temporary coverage further protects the tooth by keeping it slightly out of occlusion. This reduces the possibility of further trauma to the recently prepared tooth (Fig. 24–9).

The following is a description of the construction of acrylic temporary coverage for a single crown.

Instrumentation

▼ Alginate impression (prior to preparation of the teeth).

▼ Self-curing monomer and polymer (in shades to match the natural teeth).

▼ Separating medium.

▼ Pipette.

▼ Spatula (small cement).

▼ Small glass jar with lid.

▼ Scissors.

▼ Surgical knife (optional).

▼ Beavertail burnisher.

▼ Articulating paper and holder.

▼ Mandrel and discs (garnet and sandpaper).

▼ Greenstone acrylic trimming bur.

▼ Assorted burs (operator's choice).

▼ Low-speed handpiece.

▼ Pumice.

▼ Lathe.

▼ Rag wheels.

▼ Safety goggles.

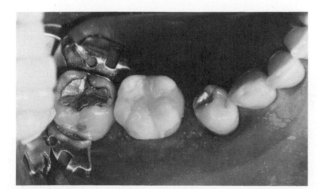

▼ **Figure 24–9**

Acrylic temporary coverage cemented in place. (Baum L, Phillips RW, Lund MR: Operative Dentistry, 2nd Ed. Philadelphia, WB Saunders, 1985, p 474.)

Procedure

FABRICATING TEMPORARY COVERAGE

1 Place a small amount of the selected shade of polymer resin in a clean jar. With a pipette draw up a few drops of monomer and dispense them into the jar, saturating the polymer.

2 Use the small spatula to blend the acrylic resin to a homogeneous mix.
   Place the lid on the jar, and set the jar aside for 2 to 3 minutes.
   Permit the resin to reach a "doughy" stage, as specified by the manufacturer.

3 Remove the lid and take the resin dough out of the jar with the spatula or beaver-tail burnisher.

4 Coat the prepared teeth with petroleum jelly or a liquid separating medium to facilitate separating the acrylic dough from the preparation.

5 Remove the alginate impression from the humidor and gently dry the area of the prepared teeth.

6 Place the resin dough within the impression, in the area of the prepared teeth. Replace the impression tray in the patient's mouth.

7 Following the initial set of resin (approximately 3 minutes), carefully remove the impression tray from the patient's mouth.

8 Remove the temporary covering from the impression. Rinse the temporary covering with lukewarm water and then dry it.

9 Remove any "flash" from the temporary covering with scissors, a bur, or a sandpaper disc in the low-speed handpiece. The covering is trimmed down to within 1 mm of the gingival shoulder of each tooth.

10 Try the temporary covering on the teeth for fit and occlusion.

11 Remove the temporary covering from the mouth. As the resin reaches the final set, it may be taken to the laboratory, where it is polished with a garnet disc and a clean, white rag wheel on the laboratory lathe.
   Note: Caution is necessary in this process, as the rag wheel could remove a large bulk or overheat and warp the temporary covering. Safety goggles must be worn throughout the polishing procedure.

Cementation of Temporary Coverage

The temporary coverage is held in place with a cement that is *not* permanent, but that can be easily removed at the next visit.

Zinc oxide–eugenol (ZOE) cement may be used for this purpose (Fig. 24–10). However, other cements may be selected because the ZOE does not interact with the acrylic of the temporary coverage.

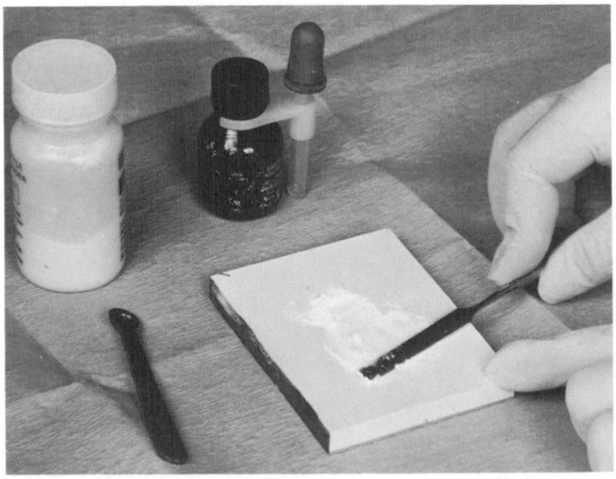

▼ Figure 24–10

Mixing zinc oxide–eugenol cement for the placement of temporary coverage. (Torres HO, Ehrlich A: Modern Dental Assisting, 4th Ed. Philadelphia, WB Saunders, 1990, p 223.)

Procedure

CEMENTATION OF TEMPORARY COVERAGE

1. Thoroughly dry the tooth preparation to receive and retain the temporary coverage.

2. Mix the cement and fill the temporary coverage.

3. Place the filled temporary coverage on the prepared tooth and pass it to the operator.

4. To aid in pushing the temporary crown into place, the operator may place a blunt crown pusher or cotton roll on the occlusal surface or incisal edge and request that the patient bite down.

5. The cement is allowed to set (approximately 5 to 7 minutes).

6. An explorer is used to remove excess material carefully from the gingival margins and interproximal areas of the temporary coverage.

7. As necessary, the occlusion is adjusted and the coverage is given a final polishing. This may be accomplished with a fine-grit polishing agent in the low-speed handpiece.

8. The patient is instructed to bite and chew carefully with the temporary covering and is scheduled for the delivery of the permanent crown or bridge.

Preformed Crowns

Instead of constructing custom coverage, a preformed crown may be used. These are available in a variety of materials, sizes, and tooth shapes (Fig. 24–11).

The appropriate tooth shape and size are selected, fitted to the tooth, and cemented temporarily in place.

Tooth-colored acrylic is preferred for anterior teeth. Prepared posterior teeth may be protected by the placement of a preformed aluminum or a stainless steel temporary crown.

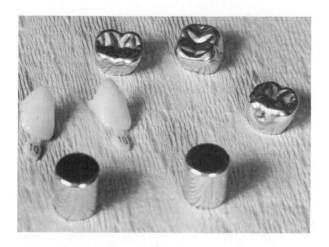

▼ **Figure 24–11**

Types of preformed temporary coverage. At the top are preformed posterior crowns with anatomic features. In the center are acrylic anterior temporary crowns. At the bottom are preformed crowns without anatomic features. (Torres HO, Ehrlich A: Modern Dental Assisting, 4th Ed. Philadelphia, WB Saunders, 1990, p 578.)

▼ EXERCISES

1. A fixed prosthesis is a precision cast replacement that _____ ____ .

   a. can be removed by the dentist for cleaning
   b. can be removed by the patient for cleaning
   c. is permanently cemented on the prepared teeth

2. Before the teeth are prepared, an alginate impression is taken of _____ _____ .

   a. both arches
   b. the arch being treated
   c. the opposing arch

3. Gingival retraction is essential to expose the _____ near the gingival margin.

   a. cementum
   b. dentin
   c. preparation
   d. retention grooves

4. Between visits, the prepared tooth is protected by _____ .

   a. an onlay
   b. a sedative filling
   c. a veneer
   d. temporary coverage

5. In a fixed bridge, the replacement for a missing tooth is a/an _____ _____ .

   a. abutment
   b. pontic
   c. retainer
   d. veneer

6. An _____ may be used as a Class V restoration.

   a. inlay
   b. onlay

7. _____ is a noble metal.

   a. Gold
   b. Palladium
   c. Platinum
   d. a, b, and c

8. A/An _____ holds each end of a fixed bridge in place.

   a. abutment
   b. pontic
   c. retainer
   d. a and c

9. Custom acrylic temporary coverage is constructed using an alginate impression that was taken _____ the teeth were prepared.

   a. after
   b. before

10. Excess cement between the teeth may be removed by using _____ _____ .

    a. a beavertail burnisher
    b. a rubber prophy cup
    c. a separating strip
    d. knotted dental floss

11. Zinc oxide–eugenol cement may be used to _____ .

    a. cement the temporary coverage
    b. permanently cement the cast restoration
    c. protect the pulp from heat

12. The abbreviation PFM stands for _____ .

    a. partial-facing-metal
    b. porcelain-facing-on-mesial
    c. porcelain-fused-to-metal
    d. protect-facial-and-mesial

13. A fixed bridge replaces _____ .

    a. one or more adjoining missing teeth in the dental arch
    b. two or more missing teeth anywhere in the same dental arch

14. Articulating paper is used to detect _____ .

    a. defects in the margin of the restoration
    b. high spots on the occlusal surface
    c. rough edges on the restoration

15. At the second crown and bridge appointment, the _____ .

    a. bridge is temporarily cemented in place
    b. components of the bridge are tried in the mouth
    c. crown preparations are refined

16. When temporary coverage is removed at the cementation visit, it is _____ .

    a. discarded immediately
    b. saved until the permanent crown has been cemented

17. If using zinc phosphate cement, the prepared tooth may be protected with _____ .

    a. separating medium
    b. two coats of cavity varnish
    c. petroleum jelly
    d. either a or c

18. Custom temporary coverage should _____ .

    a. free the tooth from contact with the neighboring teeth
    b. maintain the tooth in occlusion
    c. take the tooth slightly out of occlusion
    d. a and b

19. The final impression for a cast restoration is taken using _____ impression material.

    a. alginate
    b. elastomeric

20. When using a rag wheel to polish temporary coverage, _____ _____ .

    a. care must be taken to avoid overheating
    b. care must be taken to avoid warping
    c. safety goggles must be worn
    d. a, b, and c

25 Complete and Partial Removable Dentures

▼ LEARNING OBJECTIVES

The student will be able to:

1. Differentiate between complete and partial removable dentures.

2. Identify these components of a partial removable denture: saddle, clasps, framework, rests, and bars.

3. Identify these components of a complete removable denture: base, flange, border, and post dam.

4. Describe the steps in the construction of a partial removable denture.

5. Describe the steps in the construction of a complete removable denture.

6. Describe the care of complete and partial removable dentures.

OVERVIEW OF COMPLETE AND PARTIAL REMOVABLE DENTURES

Removable prosthodontics is the specialty limited to the fabrication and fitting of complete and partial removable dentures to replace missing teeth. Each of these appliances is called a **removable prosthesis**.

The prompt replacement of missing teeth is important because without adequate replacements, the patient cannot speak or chew properly. The contour of the face and the function of the temporomandibular joint are also affected.

The primary application of a removable prosthesis is to replace missing dentition and restore occlusion. A removable prosthesis must:

▼ Fit snugly and comfortably.

▼ Not be displaced during chewing.

▼ Be removed for cleaning.

▼ Be replaced easily after cleaning.

There are two major groupings of these appliances: Partial removable dentures and complete removable dentures.

A **partial removable denture** replaces one or more teeth in one arch and receives its support and retention from the underlying tissues and some of the remaining teeth.

A **complete removable denture** replaces all of the teeth in one arch. A complete denture receives all its retention and support from the underlying tissues of the alveolar ridges, hard and soft palate, and oral mucosa.

PARTIAL DENTURES

Partial Denture Components

The basic components in the design of the appliance are the **framework, connector, saddle, clasps, rests,** and **artificial teeth** (Figs. 25–1 and 25–2).

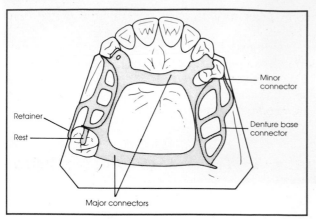

▼ **Figure 25–1**

The parts of a maxillary removable partial denture. (Kratochvil FJ: Partial Removable Prosthodontics. Philadelphia, WB Saunders, 1988, p 8.)

Framework

The framework is the cast metal skeleton that provides a basic support and rigidity for the saddle and the connectors of the partial denture.

Instead of a metal framework, some partials are made with an acrylic base.

Connector

The connector, which is also known as a *bar*, joins the right and left quadrant framework of the partial denture.

The maxillary partial denture has a **palatal connector**. The mandibular partial denture has a **lingual connector**.

The connector also helps to form support for the remaining teeth so that the stress on the teeth is evenly distributed.

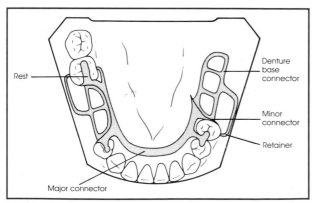

▼ **Figure 25–2**

The parts of a mandibular removable partial denture. (Kratochvil FJ: Partial Removable Prosthodontics. Philadelphia, WB Saunders, 1988, p 8.)

Saddle

The saddle is the portion of the appliance that rests on the oral mucosa covering the alveolar ridge. It also retains the artificial teeth.

The saddle is usually constructed of acrylic. However, to provide stability a metal mesh framework as an extension of the connector is usually embedded in the acrylic.

The **flange** of the saddle extends to the area of retention on the natural landmarks of the arches. In the **mandibular arch,** the flange extends from the retromolar area lingually to the mylohyoid ridge and facially to the oblique ridge.

In the **maxillary arch,** the flange extends from the curvature of the residual ridge into the buccal vestibule and partially into the palate.

Clasps

The metal clasps help support and provide stability to the partial denture. The clasp is designed to encircle the abutment tooth just below the extent of the convexity and the undercut area of the tooth. (An **undercut** is the portion of a tooth that lies between the height of contour and the gingivae.)

Rests

The rest is the metal projection on, or near, the clasp. The rest is precision designed to control the extent of the "seating" of the prosthesis as it is inserted into the oral cavity and placed on the teeth.

The most commonly used rests are designed to lie in a prepared recess on the occlusal or lingual surface of a tooth.

It is important that the **occlusal rest** not interfere with the patient's normal occlusion. A **lingual rest** is placed on the cingulum of the tooth.

In some instances, an amalgam or a cast restoration may be used to protect the tooth structure from wear by providing a stable receptacle for a rest.

Precision Attachments

A precision attachment is a **retainer**. It may be used to increase the stability of a partial denture. A precision attachment consists of two parts.

▼ The **receptacle** (the female portion) is contained in a cast restoration in the abutment tooth.

▼ The **fitted part** (the male portion) is attached to the framework of the partial denture.

Artificial Teeth

Slot teeth are porcelain tooth facings that fit onto a metal backing that has been soldered to the metal framework or connector of the partial denture.

Tube teeth are artificial posterior teeth prepared with a recessed hole in the base of the crown. A tube tooth is fixed in position by cementing it onto a cast projection of the saddle.

Abutment Teeth

A portion of the support for a partial denture comes from the abutment teeth, which receive and hold the clasps and rests.

Because they have strong roots, the cuspids and the molars are the teeth best suited for use as abutments.

Individually the maxillary and mandibular anterior teeth are the least acceptable as abutments. However, when they are splinted together, the anterior teeth may be used as abutments. This is because splinting distributes the stress of serving as an abutment evenly over several teeth.

Preparation of Abutment Teeth

Preparation of abutment teeth is determined by the type of rest selected. A recessed area may be prepared to receive the rest on the clasp of the partial denture. This preparation may involve:

1. A slight modification of the tooth itself.
2. The modification of an amalgam restoration if present.
3. The construction of a special cast restoration with a recessed area to receive a precision attachment.

First Appointment for a Partial Denture

At the first appointment the dentist examines the patient to determine that a partial removable denture is the most desirable treatment plan. This examination includes a thorough clinical examination, medical history, complete radiographic survey, photographs of the face, and impressions for diagnostic casts.

At this time the dentist also determines whether the patient requires other dental treat-ment *prior* to the construction of the partial denture.

This may include operative dentistry or periodontal, endodontic, or surgical treatment. If so, this treatment must be completed so that the healing of these tissues has taken place before the prosthodontic treatment begins.

Second Appointment—Secondary Impressions

Prior to the second appointment, custom impression trays are made on the diagnostic casts (see Chapter 23, "Custom Trays and Elastomeric Impressions").

The secondary impression is required to provide the dentist and the laboratory technician with the *exact* replica of the dental arch and the musculature attachments.

The **working casts,** also known as *refractory casts,* are made from the secondary impression. The working casts are used in the construction of the baseplates, bite rims, wax setup, and finished partial denture.

Essentials of the Maxillary Secondary Impression

1. The palatal rugae and the post dam of the hard and soft palatal junction should be evident.
2. The tuberosities, the hamular notches, and the peripheral muscle attachments at the frenula must be noted.
3. If a cleft palate exists, the perforation must be presented.
4. If a torus palatinus is evident in the palatal vault, it must be presented in the impression. If the torus interferes with the design of the appliance, it may be necessary to remove it surgically. (A **torus palatinus** is a benign bony growth on the surface of the hard palate at the midpalatal suture.)

Essentials of the Mandibular Secondary Impression

1. The configuration of the mylohyoid ridge and the retromolar pads must be represented.
2. Peripheral muscle and tongue attachments are represented.
3. If a torus mandibularus is evident, it must be presented in the impression. If the torus interferes with the design of the appliance, it may be necessary to remove it surgically. (A **torus mandibularus** is a benign bony growth on the inner (lingual) surface of the mandible that is usually located near the cuspids and premolars.)

Instrumentation for Secondary Impression

▼ Basic setup.

▼ Custom tray(s) (mandibular and/or maxillary).

▼ Stick compound and plasticized beading wax.

▼ Wax spatula to adapt materials.

▼ Elastomeric (syringe and tray) impression setup.

▼ Bite registration setup.

▼ Shade guide.

Bite Registration

A bite registration is needed to provide an accurate duplication of the relationship of the patient's jaws in centric occlusion. (**Centric** refers to the way the mandibular teeth occlude with the maxillary teeth when the patient closes the teeth together in a natural bite. See Chapter 23, "Custom Trays and Elastomeric Impressions.")

Selecting Shade and Mold of the Artificial Teeth

After the secondary impression, the shade and mold of the teeth are selected. The goal in selecting the shade (color) and mold (shape) of the artificial teeth is to match the patient's natural teeth as closely as possible.

When choosing the tooth shade and mold, the dentist considers the age, the body size of the patient, the length of the lip, and the space to be occupied by the artificial tooth.

The shade and mold are selected using a shade guide provided by the tooth manufacturer. To identify the teeth, the mold and shade number

---

Procedure

SECONDARY IMPRESSION

1. The custom tray is either the perforated type or coated with tray adhesive for the elastomeric impression material.

2. The periphery of the tray is beaded either with the plasticized wax or with stick compound. This prevents the rough margins of the tray from touching the patient's tissue, and it aids in retaining the impression material in the tray.

3. The tray is handed to the operator.

   If stick compound was used, the operator softens it over a flame. When warm, the tray is quickly placed in the patient's mouth.

   If plasticized wax was used, the tray is placed in the patient's mouth without the heating step.

4. The patient is directed to make facial, speaking, and swallowing movements to develop the base and extensions at the margins of the impression tray.

   This step is called **muscle trimming**, and the purpose is to adapt the peripheral compound or wax to the area of muscle attachments.

5. The tray is removed from the patient's mouth, dried, and recoated with adhesive.

6. The syringe elastomeric impression material is prepared and passed to the operator.

   The operator places the material in the recessed rest preparations and the undercut areas of the teeth.

7. The tray impression material is prepared.

   The assistant receives the used syringe and hands the loaded tray to the operator.

   The operator seats the tray over the syringe mix. The syringe and tray material blend together to produce a smooth impression without voids.

8. Following the set of the impression material, the tray is removed.

   The impression is rinsed, dried with warm air, and inspected for defects or missing details.

   If there are discrepancies in the critical areas of the impression, the procedure must be repeated.

9. An additional impression of the opposing arch is taken in alginate.

10. A bite registration is obtained, and the shade and mold of the artificial teeth are selected.

Procedure

SELECTING THE SHADE AND MOLD OF THE ARTIFICIAL TEETH

1 A sample tooth is removed from the shade guide holder. It is moistened with saliva or water to represent the moist surface of the natural tooth in the oral cavity.

2 The shade of the artificial tooth is checked by natural light (preferably north light) to determine an accurate shade.

3 The mold and shade of the artificial teeth selected are written on the patient's chart.

4 This information, plus the name of the manufacturer and the material of the teeth, is also noted on the written laboratory prescription, which is sent to the dental laboratory with the impressions (Fig. 25–3).

5 The sample teeth are returned to the shade guide. The entire shade guide is disinfected after each use.

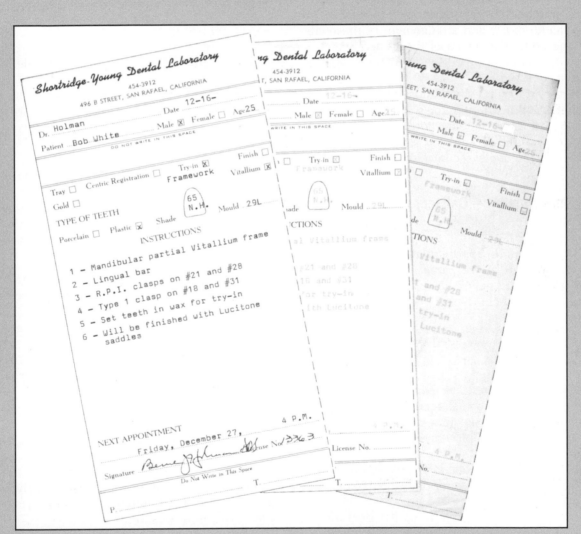

Figure 25–3 Prescription for a mandibular removable partial denture. (Courtesy of B. J. Holman, DDS, and Shortridge-Young Dental Laboratory, San Rafael, CA.)

are imprinted by the manufacturer on the back of each sample tooth.

Third Appointment—Try-In of the Wax Setup

Prior to the appointment time, the assistant checks to determine that the case has been returned to the office.

At the "try-in" appointment, the appliance consists of the framework and the artificial teeth set in wax. At this visit the following areas are checked:

1. The fit of the framework and the occlusion against the opposing arch are checked. If indicated, another bite registration will be taken.
2. The shade, mold, and arrangement of the teeth are checked. Acceptance of the esthetics of the prosthesis is determined by the dentist and the patient.
3. During the try-in, the dentist may alter the alignment of the teeth in the wax.
4. Changes of the design are noted in writing. The written prescription and the wax setup are forwarded to the dental technician to be finished.

Fourth Appointment—Delivery of the Partial Denture

A 20- to 30-minute appointment is usually adequate for delivery of the partial denture. The day before the appointment, the assistant determines that the case has been completed and returned to the dental office (Fig. 25-4).

1. The operatory is prepared with a pre-set tray with the materials and instruments for adjustment of the denture.
2. The new prosthesis has been scrubbed with soap and water and disinfected. It is stored in water or a moist container and is rinsed with water just prior to placement in the patient's mouth.
3. After the patient is seated, he is asked to remove the original or temporary appliance that he may be wearing.
4. The dentist places the new partial denture in the patient's mouth and makes adjustments as necessary.
5. Following the adjustments, the partial denture may be polished on the laboratory lathe, using the appropriate pastes and sterile buffing wheels.
6. The partial denture is scrubbed with soap, water, and a brush; is rinsed and disinfected;

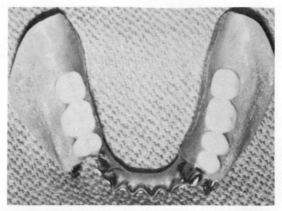

▼ **Figure 25-4**

A finished mandibular removable partial denture. (Kratochvil FJ: Partial Removable Prosthodontics. Philadelphia, WB Saunders, 1988, p 155.)

and is returned to the operatory for delivery to the patient.

7. The patient is given instructions on the placement and removal and care of the partial denture.

Care of Abutment Teeth and Partial Denture

It is essential that the patient with a partial denture maintain good oral hygiene. The importance of this cannot be overemphasized. The patient is instructed to:

1. After eating remove the partial denture and brush or rinse it so that the clasps, rests, and saddles are clean.
2. Carefully brush and floss all remaining natural teeth.
3. When not wearing it, store the prosthesis in water. (The acrylic saddle will warp if it is allowed to dry.)

Post-Delivery Check

The patient is given an appointment to return within 2 to 3 days after the delivery of the partial denture. A 10- to 20-minute appointment is usually adequate for this post-delivery visit.

At this time the dentist removes the partial denture and checks the mucosa for pressure areas, and, if warranted, minor adjustments may be made.

When the dentist is satisfied that the prosthesis is functioning correctly, the patient is given a recall appointment (usually several months later).

It is important that the patient return regularly for these recall visits, so that the dentist may evaluate the fit and function of the prosthesis and the patient's oral hygiene.

COMPLETE DENTURES

Components of a Complete Denture

A complete denture consists of the **base** and **artificial teeth** (Fig. 25–5).

Base

The base of the denture is designed to fit over and beyond the residual alveolar ridge so that it can securely support the artificial teeth.

To provide strength, the base may be constructed of acrylic or may be reinforced with metal mesh embedded in the acrylic.

The **flange** is that part of the denture base that extends over the attached mucosa from the cervical margin of the teeth to the border of the denture. The **border** is the circumferential margin of the denture.

The maxillary denture base must cover the entire hard palate to form the **posterior palatal seal.** This seal serves an essential function in holding the denture in place.

The posterior palatal seal, which is also known as the **post dam,** takes place as the denture rests on the junction of the hard and soft palates.

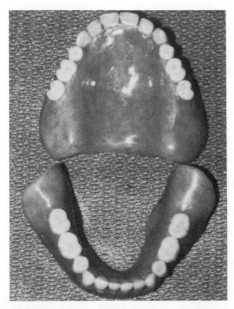

▼ **Figure 25–5**

Maxillary and mandibular complete removable dentures. (Morris AC, Bohannan HM, Casullo DP: The Dental Specialties in General Practice. Philadelphia, WB Saunders, 1983, p 578.)

Artificial Teeth

The denture teeth are composed of acrylic or porcelain and are designed to be retained in the acrylic base of the denture.

The **anterior denture teeth** simulate the form and landmarks of the natural tooth crown. Small gold pins extending from the back of the tooth in the cingulum area help retain the anterior tooth in the acrylic of the denture base.

The design of the **posterior denture teeth** is modified to reduce the effects and pressures of occlusion that are transmitted through the denture to the oral mucosa and the residual alveolar ridge.

Third molars are excluded on dentures to provide an accurate fit of the denture and to provide space in the posterior region for the patient to close, swallow, speak, and chew.

A natural tooth functions as an individual unit, whereas 14 artificial teeth attached to each denture base constitute a single unit. For this reason, the posterior teeth are designed in two mold types: anatomic and nonanatomic.

Anatomic posterior teeth are designed with "normal" cusps and ridges reproduced on the occlusal surface to aid in the mastication of food. Each anatomic posterior tooth has a hole in the base, which permits the acrylic to flow into the hole to hold the tooth in place on the denture.

Nonanatomic posterior teeth, also known as *geometric teeth* or *tube teeth,* are so named because they do not have extensive anatomic detail. Instead they are rounded and somewhat concave or flat on the occlusal surface. The nonanatomic tooth has a hole in the bottom that permits it to be set on a metal peg extending up from the saddle of the denture.

First Appointment for Complete Dentures

A preliminary appointment, similar to that for a partial denture, is necessary for the complete examination, radiographs, photographs, diagnostic casts, and case planning.

Second Appointment—Secondary Impression

The secondary impression must be accurate because the resulting master or working casts are used in the construction of the baseplates and bite rims (Figs. 25–6 and 25–7).

The secondary impression is obtained in a custom tray, using an elastomeric impression material.

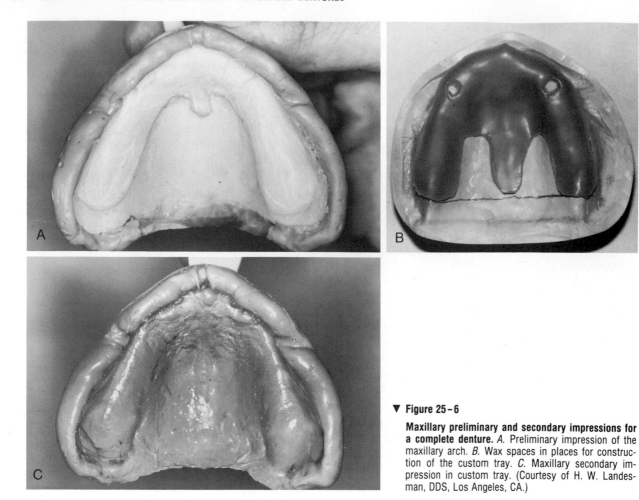

▼ **Figure 25–6**

Maxillary preliminary and secondary impressions for a complete denture. *A.* Preliminary impression of the maxillary arch. *B.* Wax spaces in places for construction of the custom tray. *C.* Maxillary secondary impression in custom tray. (Courtesy of H. W. Landesman, DDS, Los Angeles, CA.)

Essentials of the Secondary Impression

1. The material should be distributed evenly over the tray and should extend beyond the tray margins.
2. The impression must be free of bubbles and show an adequate flow of material into all the key areas.
3. The landmarks of the dental arches should be accurately reproduced in the impression.
4. The **maxillary impression** should include the hamular notches, post dam, tuberosities, and frenum attachments.
5. The **mandibular impression** should include the retromolar pads, oblique ridge, outline of the mylohyoid ridge, and the genial tubercles, plus the lingual, labial, and buccal frena.

Third Appointment — Baseplates and Bite Rims

A **baseplate**, which is constructed by the labora-tory technician on the master casts, temporarily represents the base of a denture.

Baseplates, which are usually made of wax or acrylic resin, are used for:

▼ Making bite relationship records.

▼ The articulation of casts.

▼ Arranging artificial teeth in bite rims.

▼ Trial placement in the mouth.

The **bite rims**, which are also known as *occlusal bite rims*, are built on the baseplate from several layers of wax molded together or from preformed wax rim forms.

The bite rims register vertical dimension and the occlusal relationship of the mandibular and maxillary arches. (**Vertical dimension** is the space provided by the height of the teeth in normal occlusion.)

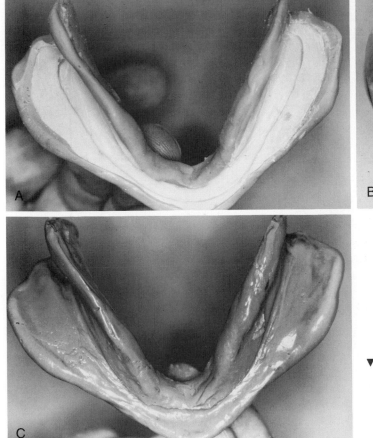
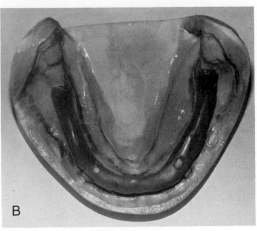

▼ **Figure 25-7**

Mandibular preliminary and secondary impressions for a complete denture. *A.* Preliminary impression of the mandibular arch. *B.* Wax spaces in places for construction of the custom tray. *C.* Mandibular secondary impression in custom tray. (Courtesy of H. W. Landesman, DDS, Los Angeles, CA.)

Try-In of Baseplate–Bite Rim Assembly

The baseplate–bite rim assembly is tried in the patient's mouth by the dentist. The primary vertical and centric relationships of the dental arches are recorded on the occlusal rims.

The dentist establishes the correct closure and the maxillary-mandibular relationship of the patient's dental arches. The height of the patient's natural "smile line" may be recorded on the wax of the baseplate–bite rim assembly.

Final Impression

To obtain the detail of the soft tissue and the alveolar ridges, zinc oxide–eugenol (ZOE) impression paste is mixed and flowed into the baseplates (Fig. 25-8).

ZOE paste tends to fracture easily, and this impression in the acrylic resin baseplates must be removed very carefully from the mouth.

After marking the centric occlusion, the high lip line (smile line), and the vertical cuspid eminence on the wax rims, the dentist may lute the occlusal rims together while they are in place in the patient's mouth. To do this, quick-setting plas-

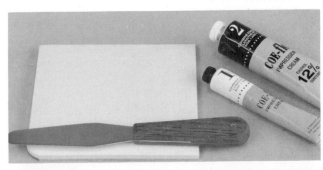

▼ **Figure 25-8**

Zinc oxide–eugenol impression paste may be used for the final impression. (Courtesy of Coe Laboratories, Inc, Chicago, IL.)

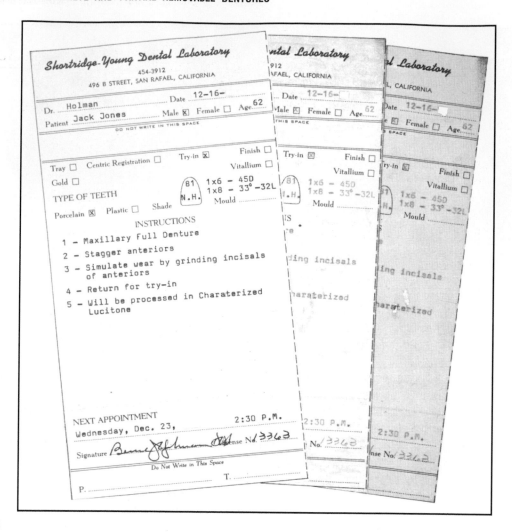

▼ **Figure 25-9**

Prescription for a maxillary removable complete denture. (Courtesy of B. J. Holman, DDS, and Shortridge-Young Dental Laboratory, San Rafael, CA.)

ter may be placed on the posterior facial areas of the wax rims on the occlusal line.

The luted occlusal rims are carefully removed from the oral cavity and placed on the laboratory **articulator**. (An **articulator** is a laboratory device that simulates the movements of the mandible and the temporomandibular joints.)

Selecting the Artificial Teeth

At this appointment, the mold, shade, and material of the artificial teeth to be placed in the denture are selected. These are determined in the same way as for the teeth of a partial denture.

After the impressions, bite registration, and tooth selection have been completed, the dentist writes and signs the written prescription and returns the case to the laboratory technician for completion of the wax setup (Fig. 25-9).

Fourth Appointment—Try-In of the Wax Setup

The patient is scheduled to try the temporary wax setup of the complete denture. This procedure is referred to as the "try-in" of the wax setup.

The complete denture try-in consists of the appliance constructed of the acrylic baseplates, the bite rims, and the artificial teeth set in wax to resemble gingival tissue.

The teeth are articulated according to the bite registration of the patient's occlusion, established on the articulator through a Gothic arch tracing.

The complete denture try-in, which has been constructed by the laboratory technician on an articulator, is returned to the dental office prior to the patient's appointment. The complete denture try-in is disinfected prior to placement in the patient's oral cavity.

Procedure

TRY-IN OF THE WAX SET-UP

1 The shade and mold of the teeth and the simulated alignment of the teeth on the alveolar ridge are checked for adaptation with the lips and face.

2 The extension of the flanges of the denture is checked for comfort to the patient and retention of the prosthesis in the mouth during facial and tongue movements.

3 The retention of the denture setup is checked as the patient verbalizes the *f, v, s,* and *th* sounds, and swallows and yawns.

4 The muscle attachments of the dental arch are checked with the spaces provided in the design of the baseplate.

5 The amount of fullness provided by the wax in the anterior and lateral facial areas is checked to make sure that it represents a natural configuration.

6 The patient's reaction to his appearance and the comfort of the denture wax setup are determined.

7 The occlusion of the denture is checked with the teeth of the opposing arch.

8 The adaptation of the lips and the ability of the lips to cover the teeth and form a smile are checked while the wax setup is in place.

9 Following the check of all these factors to the satisfaction of the dentist and the patient, the patient is scheduled for an appointment for delivery of the denture.

10 The dentist prepares a written prescription for the laboratory technician to finish the construction of the complete denture.

Fifth Appointment—Delivery of the Complete Denture

1. The day before the appointment, the assistant verifies that the denture has been completed and returned to the dental office.
2. The patient is seated, and the previously worn denture is removed.
3. The new denture, which has been disinfected and rinsed, is inserted into the patient's mouth. The shade and mold of the artificial teeth are checked for natural appearance.
4. The patient is requested to perform the facial expressions and the actions of swallowing, chewing, and speaking, using *s* and *th* sounds. These sounds also are appropriate for exercises to help the patient learn to speak normally with the new denture.
5. The occlusal contacts are checked by using carbon articulating paper. Cusps that are too high in contact will be marked with the color of the articulating paper.
6. If the cusps are too high, the denture is removed from the mouth and the cusps are carefully reduced by using a heatless stone mounted on a straight handpiece (SHP).

   The denture is replaced in the mouth, and the procedure is repeated until the cusps appear to be in occlusion with the opposing arch.
7. When the patient is pleased with the esthetics, function, and comfort of the denture, another appointment is made for the post-delivery checkup. (This visit is similar to a post-delivery checkup for a partial denture.)
8. Before dismissal, the patient should be warned that full adjustment to wearing the new denture will take several days or weeks.

   Wearing the denture constantly will speed the adjustment.

   A temporary modification of eating habits may be necessary during this period (see Chapter 5, "Preventive Dentistry and Nutrition").

Oral Hygiene and Care of the Complete Denture

The patient is instructed in the home care of the oral tissues and the new denture.

1. Remove the denture and thoroughly cleanse all surfaces at least once each day. A special den-

ture brush may be recommended for this purpose.

2. When cleaning the denture, hold it carefully over a sink half filled with water. This precaution will minimize damage if the denture is dropped.

3. While the denture is out of the mouth, thoroughly rinse the oral tissues.

4. When not being worn, the denture must be kept moist to avoid warpage of the acrylic.

RELINING COMPLETE AND PARTIAL DENTURES

At some time in the future, following resorption of the tissues (alveolar ridge and mucosa), a denture may need to be relined to ensure a proper fit.

Relining is the process of placing permanent base material into the area covering the gingival tissue. Relining may be accomplished either as a temporary chairside procedure in the office or as a more permanent procedure that is completed in the dental laboratory.

With a laboratory relining, the current prosthesis may be used as an impression tray. The impression in the prosthesis is sent to the dental laboratory for completion of the relining process.

When this is returned to the dental office, it is tried in the patient's mouth and minor adjustments are made as necessary.

▼ EXERCISES

1. A _____ removable denture is one that is retained in the oral cavity using clasps.

   a. complete
   b. partial

2. A mandibular partial denture has a _____ connector.

   a. buccal
   b. facial
   c. lingual
   d. palatal

3. Master casts are created from the _____.

   a. bite registration
   b. diagnostic casts
   c. secondary impression

4. The _____ of a precision attachment is contained in a cast restoration in the abutment tooth.

   a. extension
   b. fitted part
   c. flange
   d. receptacle

5. Individual anterior teeth _____ desirable as abutments for a partial denture.

   a. are
   b. are not

6. Prior to delivery to the patient, the new prosthesis is _____.

   a. autoclaved
   b. disinfected
   c. scrubbed with soap and water
   d. b and c

7. Complete dentures _____ include the third molars.

   a. do
   b. do not

8. To retain the elastomeric material, the impression tray may be _____ with wax.

   a. beaded
   b. contoured
   c. extended

9. A secondary impression is taken in a _____ impression tray.

   a. custom
   b. stock

10. As a result of changes in the mouth, after several months it may be necessary to _____ a dental prosthesis.

    a. rebuild
    b. reline
    c. repair
    d. replace

11. A lingual rest is placed on the _____ of the tooth.

    a. cementoenamel junction
    b. cervix
    c. cingulum
    d. incisal edge

12. _____ teeth are artificial posterior teeth with a recessed hole in the base of the crown.

    a. Pin
    b. Slot
    c. Tube

13. If other dental treatment is necessary, it is completed _____ the partial denture is constructed.

    a. after
    b. before

14. A _____ is a benign bony growth on the surface of the hard palate.

    a. rugae
    b. torus palatinus
    c. torus mandibularus
    d. tuberosity

15. The mold describes the _____ of an artificial tooth.

    a. shade
    b. shape
    c. size
    d. b and c

16. A _____ minute appointment is usually adequate for the delivery of a partial denture.

    a. 10–20
    b. 20–30
    c. 30–40
    d. 40–50

17. When an acrylic prosthesis is not being worn, it should be _____ .

    a. kept moist
    b. stored in a cool dry place
    c. stored in a warm dry place

18. _____ light is preferred when selecting a tooth shade.

    a. East
    b. North
    c. South
    d. West

19. The _____ is the circumferential margin of a denture.

    a. border
    b. flange
    c. saddle

20. The _____ register vertical dimension and the occlusal relationship of the mandibular and maxillary arches.

    a. baseplates
    b. bite rims
    c. diagnostic casts
    d. secondary impressions

26 Pediatric Dentistry

▼ LEARNING OBJECTIVES

The student will be able to:

1. State the patient population served by pediatric dentistry and describe the special concerns of the pediatric dentist.
2. Describe the steps in the application of pit and fissure sealants.
3. Describe the use of fixed and removable space maintainers.
4. Describe the steps in making a vacuum formed custom mouth guard.
5. Describe the application of topical fluoride using a commercial fluoride gel and trays.

OVERVIEW OF PEDIATRIC DENTISTRY

The practice of a pediatric dentist is usually limited to the treatment of a patient from birth through the stage of mixed dentition (13 to 14 years).

Although many of the procedures performed for children are similar to those for other patients, children also have special needs. Of special concern to the pediatric dentist is:

▼ Early detection and prevention of developmental abnormalities.

▼ Preventive care so that the child will never experience dental pain or come to fear dental treatment.

▼ Teaching good oral hygiene habits that the child will maintain throughout his lifetime.

INSTRUMENTATION FOR PEDIATRIC DENTISTRY

Most of the procedures performed in providing dental care for children are similar to those for adults. For example, amalgam and composite restorations are prepared and placed in the same manner.

However, in some situations, a special size or modification of an instrument is required in order to fit the size and shape of the primary tooth or to accommodate the smaller size of a child's mouth. For example:

▼ When placing rubber dam, a special size rubber dam material and clamp may be needed (see Chapter 19, "Rubber Dam").

▼ In oral surgery, specifically designed forceps may be needed to grasp the primary tooth so that it can be extracted (see Chapter 30, "Oral Surgery").

THE EXAMINATION

The examination for the pediatric patient includes all of the elements that are part of a thorough examination of an adult.

Radiographs are taken only as needed to detect decay, disease, or potential developmental abnormalities.

Coronal Polishing or Dental Prophylaxis

After the examination, if only a limited amount of plaque is present, a coronal polishing procedure may be performed for the child. In some states this may be performed by a qualified extended function dental assistant (EFDA).

If calculus and heavy plaque are present, a dental prophylaxis is performed by the dentist or hygienist (see Chapter 28, "Periodontics").

TOPICAL FLUORIDE APPLICATION

If the child has a high decay rate or lives in an area where the water is not fluoridated, the dentist may prescribe topical fluoride applications. Depending on the type of fluoride and the needs of the child, these treatments may be repeated every 6 months.

Topical fluoride applications may also be recommended for adults with a high decay rate or with exposed root structure that is prone to decay.

Caution: Prior to treatment the parent or patient should be warned that decalcified areas and carious lesions may turn dark with stain from the stannous fluoride.

Topical Fluoride Trays

The goal of the fluoride treatment is to saturate all of the tooth surfaces thoroughly with the solution. This is accomplished using a tray that closely fits around the teeth and forces the solution onto all of the tooth surfaces.

Fluoride trays are available in several sizes, including child, small, medium, and large. They are designed, as shown in Figure 26–1, to treat a single arch at one time. A two-part tray is designed to treat both arches at once.

These trays are disposable and are discarded after a single use.

Instrumentation

▼ Basic setup.

▼ Preformed commercial trays.

▼ Commercial fluoride gel.

▼ High volume evacuator (HVE) tip.

▼ Cotton rolls.

▼ Saliva ejector tip.

Procedure

APPLYING A TOPICAL FLUORIDE TREATMENT

1 The teeth are thoroughly cleaned, rinsed, and dried. A fluoride polishing agent may be used for this purpose.
Note: The teeth *must* be free of all plaque and debris prior to the application of the topical fluoride.

2 The size and type of tray for the treatment to be performed are selected.

3 The fluoride gel is dispensed into the tray.

4 The patient is informed of the procedure.
The child is warned *not* to swallow the fluoride gel. (To do so may cause nausea.)
The child is instructed to sit upright and to relax but not to talk or swallow while the tray is in place. (Tongue movement would displace the tray.)

5 The tray is placed on the mandibular arch. Touching the tongue or cheeks with the solution during placement of the trays should be avoided.

6 The saliva ejector is placed to remove the excess fluids from the mouth and to pre-

vent the patient from swallowing the solution.

7 The mandibular tray is left in place for a maximum of 4 to 5 minutes and then removed.

8 The maxillary tray is placed in the same manner. The saliva ejector is placed to remove the excess fluids from the mouth and to prevent the patient from swallowing the solution.

9 The maxillary tray is left in place for a maximum of 4 to 5 minutes and then removed.
Alternative: Both arches may be treated at the same time by using trays. If so, the total treatment time is a maximum of 4 to 5 minutes.

10 The HVE is used to remove the excess saliva so that the patient does not need to swallow. Do *not* rinse the oral cavity when the procedure is completed.

11 The patient is advised not to eat, drink, or rinse his mouth for approximately 30 minutes.

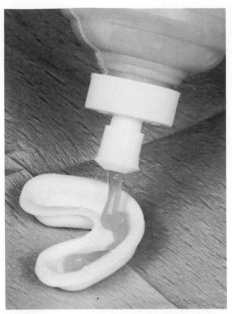

▼ **Figure 26–1**

Dispensing topical fluoride solution into the disposable tray. (Torres HO, Ehrlich A: Modern Dental Assisting, 4th Ed. Philadelphia, WB Saunders, 1990, p 567.)

PIT AND FISSURE SEALANTS

Pit and fissure sealants are used to prevent decay in the hard-to-clean, naturally occurring deep pits and narrow fissures on the occlusal surfaces of the molars and premolars.

Sealants are indicated if the patient's teeth already show a high incidence of caries but have not decayed in these areas.

Sealants are *not* indicated if decalcification or decay has already begun in these areas. If this has happened, a restoration should be placed.

When indicated, sealants may be applied to the occlusal surfaces of the primary molars soon after these teeth have erupted. Sealants are also applied to the occlusal surfaces of the permanent molars and premolars soon after they have erupted.

Types of Sealants

A **self-curing** sealant reaches a cure by chemical reaction. These sealants require mixing a base and catalyst. They have a limited working time of 1 to 2 minutes, and then time must be allowed for the material to cure.

Follow the manufacturer's instructions for the mixing procedure and exact curing time.

A **light-cured sealant** is cured by exposure to a special visible white light for approximately 10 to 20 seconds per tooth. (Follow the manufacturer's instructions for exact curing times.)

When using the curing light, the operator and patient must wear special protective glasses. An alternative is to use a protective paddle (see Chapter 8, "Hazards Management in the Dental Office").

Preparation of the Teeth

Before the application of the sealant, a coronal polish is performed on the teeth with a *nonfluoride, oil-free abrasive* (Fig. 26–2).

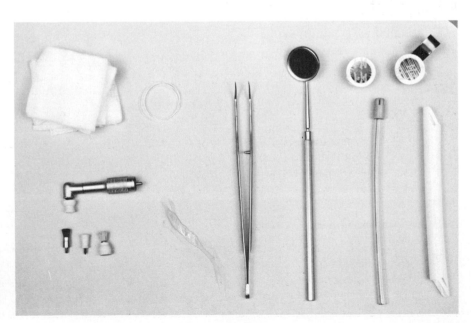

▼ **Figure 26–2**

Coronal polish instrumentation prior to placement of sealants. Note that a nonfluoride and oil-free abrasive is used. (Torres HO, Ehrlich A: Modern Dental Assisting, 4th Ed. Philadelphia, WB Saunders, 1990, p 571.)

The tooth surfaces must be fluoride-free because the etching solution and sealant do *not* readily adhere to enamel that is fluoride-treated. Also, the fluoride neutralizes the effectiveness of the phosphoric acid in the etching solution.

Any oil in the prophy paste, such as a flavoring oil, will also interfere with bonding and adherence of the sealant.

Application of Sealants

During the application of the sealants, it is essential that the teeth remain dry and not be contaminated with saliva. The application of rubber dam prior to treatment is the best means of protecting the working area.

If rubber dam is not applied, cotton rolls are used to isolate the teeth being treated. A saliva ejector and HVE may also be necessary to make certain that the teeth are not contaminated.

The application described here is a light-cured sealant (Fig. 26–3).

Instrumentation

▼ Basic setup.

▼ Coronal polishing setup.

▼ Rubber dam setup.

▼ Etching (conditioner) liquid or gel (35 to 50 percent phosphoric acid).

▼ Sealant.

▼ Dappen dishes or receptacle supplied by the manufacturer.

▼ Cotton rolls.

▼ Cotton pellets, small to medium size.

▼ Applicator for sealant (brush, mini-sponge, or disposable cartridge as provided by manufacturer).

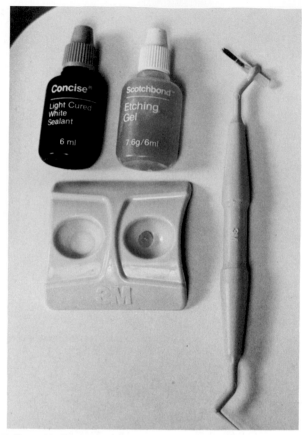

▼ **Figure 26–3**

Sealant materials and instrumentation. (Courtesy of 3M Products, St. Paul, MN.)

▼ Curing paddle or protective glasses.

▼ Visible curing light.

▼ Articulating paper.

▼ Slow-speed handpiece.

▼ Small, round, white stone.

Procedure

ETCHING THE TEETH

1. The operator cleans the teeth with a mixture of fine pumice and water. The assistant thoroughly rinses the mouth for at least 10 seconds using clear water.

2. The assistant or operator uses the air syringe to dry thoroughly each tooth to be sealed for a minimum of 30 seconds.

3 The assistant and operator place and stabilize the rubber dam (Fig. 26–4).

4 The assistant:

Places a few drops of the enamel etching (conditioner) solution in a dappen dish.

Places a small cotton pellet in the cotton pliers.

Dips the cotton pellet into the conditioning solution.

Hands the cotton pellet, in the cotton pliers, to the operator.

5 The operator gently dabs, but does not rub, the occlusal surfaces of the teeth to be treated.

Each tooth is etched for a full 60 seconds.

The teeth are dabbed continuously for approximately 5 seconds after the initial application of the conditioner.

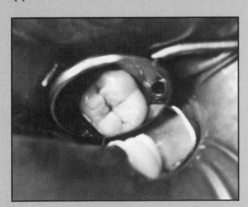

Figure 26–4 Examination of the tooth after the rubber dam application and prior to the sealant placement. (Torres HO, Ehrlich A: Modern Dental Assisting, 4th Ed. Philadelphia, WB Saunders, 1990, p 572.)

6 After the allotted etching time:

The teeth are sprayed with water for at least 30 seconds to stop the etching action.

The assistant uses the HVE to remove the water and solution from the oral cavity.

The assistant uses warm air to dry thoroughly the etched tooth surfaces.

7 The etched surfaces of the dried teeth should appear dull, whitish, satiny, and frosted (Fig. 26–5). If these surfaces do not have this appearance, the etching solution is applied again for another 60 seconds.

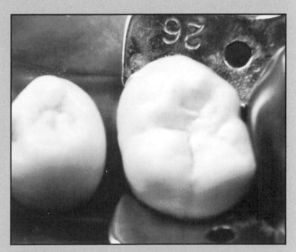

Figure 26–5 The etched surfaces of the dried teeth appear dull, whitish, satiny, and frosted in appearance. (Torres HO, Ehrlich A: Modern Dental Assisting, 4th Ed. Philadelphia, WB Saunders, 1990, p 572.)

Procedure

APPLYING THE SEALANT

1 The assistant places the sealant material in a second receptacle.

2 If necessary, the operator or assistant uses the air syringe to dry the teeth thoroughly.

Note: The teeth *must* be dry before and during the application of the sealant.

3 With the left hand, the assistant passes the applicator (camel hair brush, mini-sponge, or applicator tip) to the operator's right hand.

With the right hand, the assistant holds the dappen dish (with sealant) near the patient's chin.

4 The operator dips the applicator into the sealant and paints the occlusal surfaces of the teeth that have been conditioned by etching (Figs. 26–6 and 26–7).

5 When finished, the operator returns the applicator to the assistant.

Continued on following page

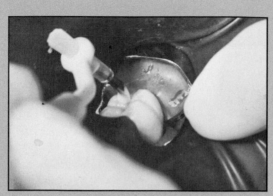

Figure 26-6 The sealant is painted onto the occlusal surfaces of the teeth. (Torres HO, Ehrlich A: Modern Dental Assisting, 4th Ed. Philadelphia, WB Saunders, 1990, p 572.)

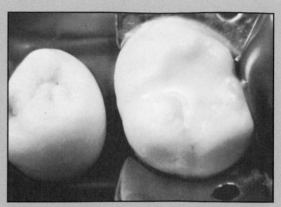

Figure 26-7 Surface of the tooth with the freshly applied sealant. (Torres HO, Ehrlich A: Modern Dental Assisting, 4th Ed. Philadelphia, WB Saunders, 1990, p 573.)

Procedure

CURING THE SEALANT

1. The operator exposes the sealant to the curing light as specified by the manufacturer (Fig. 26-8).

    This is usually for 20 seconds per tooth.

    The tip of the light is held 1 to 2 mm from the surface being cured.

2. The operator checks for cure of the sealant by passing an explorer over the surface.

    If the sealant is hard and the surface is intact, finishing may begin.

    If there are discrepancies in the sealant surface, it is re-etched for 30 seconds and resealed.

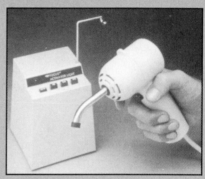

Figure 26-8 Demonstration of an activator light for curing the sealant. In actual use, the operator would be wearing gloves. The operator must also wear special glasses or use a protective paddle while operating the activator light. (Courtesy of Teledyne Getz, Elk Grove Village, IL.)

Procedure

FINISHING THE SEALANT

1. The rubber dam is removed.

2. The assistant places a piece of articulating paper in the cotton pliers and hands them to the operator.

3. The operator uses the articulating paper to check the height of the occlusal surface of each tooth.

4. If the sealant is too high in occlusion, the assistant places a small round stone into the handpiece and passes the handpiece to the operator.

5. The operator adjusts the occlusion and returns the handpiece to the assistant.

6. Prior to dismissal, the patient is informed that the pit and fissure sealant is intact and no precautions are necessary. The adult accompanying the child is advised that the sealants should be examined at 6-month intervals to determine that they are still intact.

SPACE MAINTAINERS

Following premature loss of a primary tooth, a space maintainer is designed to maintain the space until the normal eruption of the subsequent permanent tooth.

A **removable space maintainer** may be taken in and out by the patient. A **fixed space maintainer** is cemented in place and may not be removed by the patient. Examples of fixed space maintainers are shown in Figure 26–9.

MOUTH GUARDS

A mouth guard fits over the maxillary dentition to protect the teeth from accidental injury. Mouth guards should be used by *all* athletes involved in contact sports.

Commercial mouth guards may be purchased in assorted mold sizes to approximate the arch size of the patient. However, the best protection is achieved with a custom mouth guard, which is constructed to fit the patient's dentition precisely (Fig. 26–10).

The first step in constructing a custom mouth guard is to take an alginate impression of the maxillary arch. This is then poured to form a study cast (see Chapter 17, "Alginate Impressions and Diagnostic Casts").

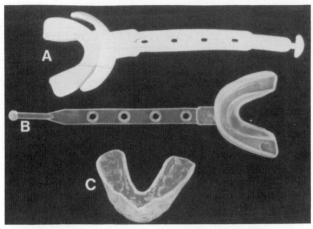

▼ **Figure 26–10**

Three types of mouth guards. *A.* Stock mouth guard. *B.* Mouth-formed protector. *C.* Custom-fit mouth guard. (Pinkham JR: Pediatric Dentistry: Infancy Through Adolescence. Philadelphia, WB Saunders, 1988, p 499.)

The steps in the construction of a vacuum formed mouth guard are shown and described in Figure 26–11.

Upon delivery, the patient is advised to keep the mouth guard clean and, when it is not placed in the mouth, to keep it in a box or closed container of water. If it is not stored properly, the mouth guard will warp and not fit correctly.

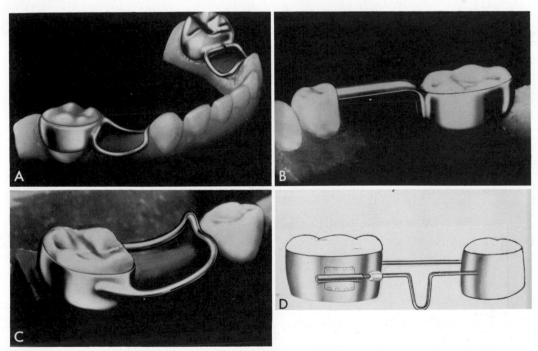

▼ **Figure 26–9**

Types of fixed space maintainers. *A.* Space maintainer with rectangular loop soldered at mesial of band and cemented in place. *B.* Occlusal bar space maintainer. *C.* Open-ended maintainer soldered at facial/lingual of stainless steel band. *D.* Jack screw maintainer, adjustable type. (Courtesy of Rocky Mountain Orthodontics, Denver, CO.)

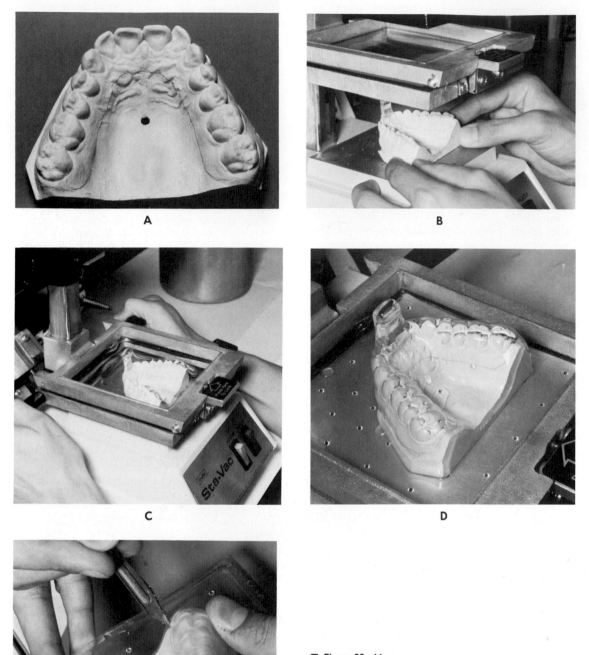

▼ **Figure 26-11**

Construction of a custom mouth guard. *A.* The finish (trim) line is marked on the maxillary cast in indelible pencil. A hole has been placed in the cast to allow air to escape during the vacuum process. *B.* Plastic mouth guard material is placed in adapter and heated until it sags. Note vinyl strap attachment tab already in place on anterior of the cast. *C.* Frame is placed in lowest position, and vacuum is turned on for 5 to 10 seconds. *D.* Material is adapted to the forms of the cast. *E.* While it is still warm, excess material around margin is trimmed with a scalpel or sharp laboratory knife. The next step is to heat gently the strap attachment tab and bend it forward in a 45-degree angle.

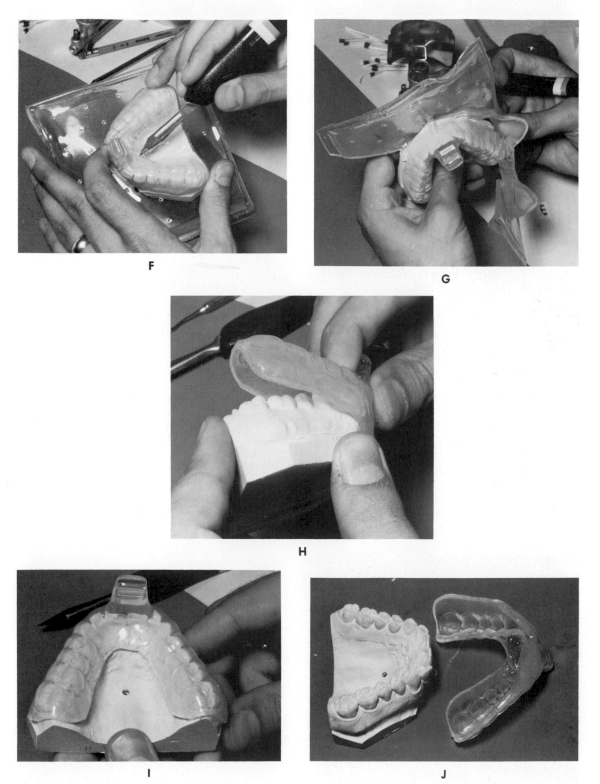

▼ **Figure 26–11** *Continued*

F. The scalpel blade is heated and used to trim through material to the finish line marked on the case. *G.* Excess material is carefully trimmed from the cast. *H.* The mouth guard is carefully removed from the cast and checked for rough margins. *I.* The margins are trimmed to remove rough edges, and the mouth guard is reinserted on the cast. *J.* The finished mouth guard. Note that the maxillary guard does not cover the palate. (Courtesy of Regina Dreyer Thomas, RDH, MPH, Holmdel, NJ.)

▼ EXERCISES

1. Topical fluoride applications may be recommended for _____ _____ .

   a. adults with a high decay rate
   b. children living in areas where the water is not fluoridated
   c. children with a high decay rate
   d. a, b, and c

2. If only a limited amount of plaque is present, a/an _____ _____ may be performed for the child.

   a. coronal polishing
   b. dental prophylaxis
   c. oral hygiene procedure

3. The trays of topical fluoride solution are left in place for _____ minutes.

   a. 1 to 2
   b. 3 to 4
   c. 4 to 5
   d. 5 to 6

4. Immediately prior to the application of the etching solution, the teeth are _____ .

   a. thoroughly dried
   b. thoroughly rinsed
   c. treated with topical fluoride
   d. b, then a

5. After use, a topical fluoride tray is _____ .

   a. autoclaved
   b. discarded
   c. disinfected
   d. dry heat sterilized

6. _____ are fabricated for all participants in contact sports.

   a. Bite planes
   b. Mouth guards
   c. Splints
   d. Retainers

7. Sealants _____ indicated in areas where decay has already begun.

   a. are
   b. are not

8. When not in use, a mouth guard should be stored _____ .

   a. in a closed container of water
   b. where it will stay dry

9. Following a topical fluoride treatment, the patient is advised _____.

   a. to brush teeth as soon as he gets home
   b. not to eat, drink, or rinse his mouth for approximately 30 minutes
   c. to rinse his mouth immediately
   d. a and c

10. A custom mouth guard is usually constructed to fit the _____ _____ arch.

    a. mandibular
    b. maxillary
    c. a and b

11. The etching solution is applied with a scrubbing motion.

    a. true
    b. false

12. A mouth guard _____ cover the entire palatal area.

    a. does
    b. does not

13. Radiographs are taken on children _____.

    a. only as needed
    b. to detect decay
    c. to detect developmental abnormalities
    d. a, b, and c

14. Before the application of the sealant, the teeth are cleaned and polished with _____.

    a. a fluoride-free abrasive
    b. an oil-free abrasive
    c. topical fluoride
    d. a and b

15. Following premature loss of a primary tooth, a _____ is designed to save the space until the normal eruption of the subsequent permanent tooth.

    a. bite block
    b. bite plane
    c. mouth guard
    d. space maintainer

16. When constructing a custom mouth guard, the strap attachment is placed on the _____ of the cast.

    a. anterior
    b. posterior

17. The practice of pediatric dentistry is usually limited to patients from birth through _____.

    a. high school
    b. the mixed dentition stage
    c. when the child reaches grade-school age

18. During the application of topical fluorides, the child should be encouraged to _____.

   a. hold his breath
   b. not swallow any of the solution
   c. rinse his mouth thoroughly
   d. swish the excess solution around his mouth

19. If indicated, sealants are applied to the occlusal surfaces of the _____ _____ teeth.

   a. anterior
   b. permanent
   c. primary
   d. b and c

20. A self-curing sealant has a working time of _____ minutes.

   a. 1 to 2
   b. 2 to 3
   c. 3 to 4
   d. 4 to 5

27 Orthodontics

▼ LEARNING OBJECTIVES

The student will be able to:

1. Describe preventive, interceptive, and corrective orthodontics.
2. Identify the specialized instrumentation used in orthodontics.
3. Describe the role of orthodontic separators.
4. Describe the steps in the selection, cementation, and removal of orthodontic bands.
5. Describe the steps in the placement, ligation, and removal of the arch wire.
6. Describe the steps in the direct bonding of orthodontic brackets.

OVERVIEW OF ORTHODONTICS

Orthodontics is that specialty of dentistry concerned with the supervision, guidance, and correction of all forms of malocclusion of the growing or mature dentofacial structures. (The classifications of malocclusion are described in Chapter 4, "Dental Anatomy and Tooth Morphology.")

Orthodontic treatment may be divided into three broad categories: preventive, interceptive, and corrective.

Preventive Orthodontics

Preventive orthodontics includes:

1. Early detection of developmental abnormalities and harmful oral habits, which might create orthodontic problems.
2. The control of caries to prevent premature loss of primary teeth.
3. If a primary tooth is lost prematurely, preventive orthodontics includes the placement of a space maintainer appliance to save sufficient space to allow the permanent tooth to erupt into normal position. (Space maintainers are discussed in Chapter 26, "Pediatric Dentistry.")

Interceptive Orthodontics

Interceptive orthodontics consists of steps taken to prevent or correct problems as they are developing. This may include:

1. Removal of primary teeth that may be contributing to malalignment of the permanent dentition.
2. The serial extraction of teeth to correct overcrowding in the arch. This treatment is used only when more conservative methods of treatment will not be effective.

Corrective Orthodontics

Corrective orthodontics refers to the use of appliances to restore the dental apparatus to full functional and esthetic condition.

Most frequently, these are **fixed appliances** that are cemented in place.

An alternative is the use of **removable appliances.** These may be placed and removed by the patient under the direction of the orthodontist.

INSTRUMENTATION FOR ORTHODONTICS

Some of the specialized instruments used in orthodontics are shown in Figure 27–1 and throughout this chapter.

THE CONSULTATION VISIT

The patient's first visit is for a consultation, which includes obtaining a comprehensive medical history, photographs, and a radiographic series and taking impressions for diagnostic casts.

There is usually a separate fee for the consultation, and this should be quoted to the parent or responsible party making the appointment.

At the end of the consultation visit, the patient and parents, if the patient is a minor, are given an appointment to return for the presentation of the diagnosis and treatment plan.

ORTHODONTIC APPOINTMENTS

Banding Appointment

The appointment for the placement of bands and arch wires may require an hour. This visit starts with a coronal polishing procedure, a check for caries, and oral hygiene instruction. After this the dentist proceeds with the banding process.

Treatment Appointments

Appointments of shorter duration, usually 10 to 20 minutes, are needed to check the progress of

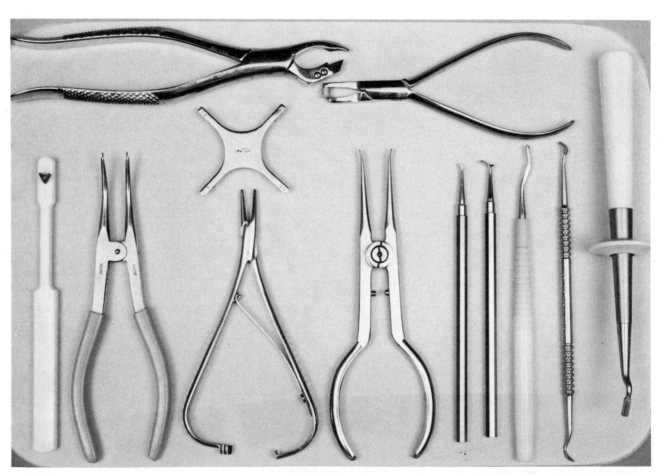

▼ **Figure 27–1**

Assorted orthodontic instruments. *Top left:* band cutter; *top middle:* Boone gauge; *top right:* band remover. *Lower portion (left to right):* band seater, separator forceps, ligature instrument with lock on handles, ligature-tying pliers, band-seating instrument, band-seating and bracket-seating instrument, maxillary band-seating instrument, Schure instrument, band-seating instrument. (Torres HO, Ehrlich A: Modern Dental Assisting, 4th Ed. Philadelphia, WB Saunders, 1990, p 623.)

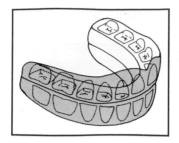

▼ **Figure 27-2**

A removable orthodontic positioner. This type of appliance is used at the completion of treatment to stabilize the position of the recently treated teeth. (Torres HO, Ehrlich A: Modern Dental Assisting, 4th Ed. Philadelphia, WB Saunders, 1990, p 644.)

treatment, to maintain and adjust bands and arch wires, and to take care of accidental damage to appliances.

Post-Treatment Appointments

The bands or bonded brackets are removed at the completion of the treatment. Usually at this time a removable retainer appliance is provided to the patient to stabilize the new alignment (Fig. 27-2).

Post-treatment appointments of approximately 15 minutes are necessary to determine that the realignment of the dentition is being maintained.

PREPARATION FOR ORTHODONTIC BANDING

Orthodontic Bands

Bands are preformed stainless steel rings that are fitted around the teeth and cemented in place. Each orthodontic band has a bracket welded on the facial side that serves as an attachment for the arch wire (Fig. 27-3).

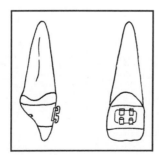

▼ **Figure 27-3**

Distal and facial views of a banded tooth. Note the bracket on the facial surface and the seating lug on the lingual surface. (Torres HO, Ehrlich A: Modern Dental Assisting, 4th Ed. Philadelphia, WB Saunders, 1990, p 634.)

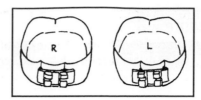

▼ **Figure 27-4**

Right and left mandibular first molar bands. (Torres HO, Ehrlich A: Modern Dental Assisting, 4th Ed. Philadelphia, WB Saunders, 1990, p 632.)

Bands usually have a **seating lug** that is placed on the lingual side. This lug aids in seating the band properly on the tooth.

The bands placed on the last molars in each arch generally have **buccal tubes** on the facial side. The ends of the arch wire fit into the buccal tube.

Sizes and Shapes of Bands

Bands are made in specific shapes for individual teeth: Centrals, laterals, cuspids, premolars, and molars. They also come in a wide range of sizes to accommodate the great variations among individual teeth.

Bands are divided into upper (maxillary) and lower (mandibular) and, in many cases, right and left to compensate for individual tooth differences (Fig. 27-4).

The incisal or occlusal edge of the band is slightly rolled or contoured, whereas the gingival edge is straight (Fig. 27-5). When placing the band, the gingival edge goes over the tooth first.

Orthodontic Separators

Prior to the cementation visit, orthodontic separators are placed to create temporary space between the teeth so that full orthodontic bands may be fitted and cemented.

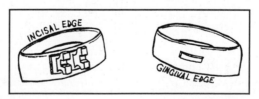

▼ **Figure 27-5**

The incisal or occlusal edge of the band is rolled or slightly contoured. The gingival edge is smooth. (Torres HO, Ehrlich A: Modern Dental Assisting, 4th Ed. Philadelphia, WB Saunders, 1990, p 626.)

Procedure

SELECTING AND FITTING BANDS

1. Prior to the banding visit, the bands are selected and fitted on the patient's diagnostic cast.

   Finger pressure, a Schure instrument, band driver, or condenser may be used to seat the band (Figs. 27–6 through 27–8).

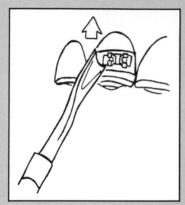

Figure 27–6 A band driver placed on bracket flange to position an anterior bracket. (Torres HO, Ehrlich A: Modern Dental Assisting, 4th Ed. Philadelphia, WB Saunders, 1990, p 627.)

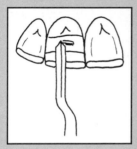

Figure 27–7 A band driver placed on lingual seating lug to position an anterior bracket. (Torres HO, Ehrlich A: Modern Dental Assisting, 4th Ed. Philadelphia, WB Saunders, 1990, p 628.)

A Boone gauge is used to measure that the bracket slot is in the appropriate place (Figs. 27–9 and 27–10).

A band sizer (stretcher) may be required to expand a band gently.

Contour pliers may be needed to shape the gingival margins of the band.

2. The bands are removed from the diagnostic cast and are placed in a tray in proper sequence for cementation on the patient's teeth.

   Incisor, cuspid, and premolar bands may be removed with the scaler end of the Schure instrument.

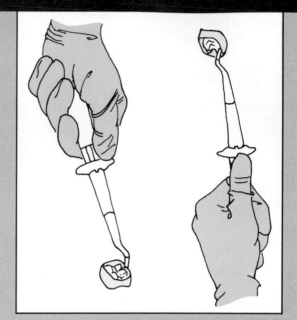

Figure 27–8 A Schure band driver used to seat posterior mandibular and maxillary bands. (Torres HO, Ehrlich A: Modern Dental Assisting, 4th Ed. Philadelphia, WB Saunders, 1990, p 633.)

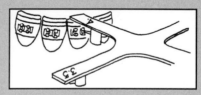

Figure 27–9 A Boone gauge used for measuring the height of bands. (Torres HO, Ehrlich A: Modern Dental Assisting, 4th Ed. Philadelphia, WB Saunders, 1990, p 628.)

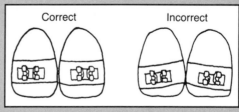

Figure 27–10 Correct and incorrect placement of bands. (Torres HO, Ehrlich A: Modern Dental Assisting, 4th Ed. Philadelphia, WB Saunders, 1990, p 628.)

Molar bands are removed with the band-removing pliers.

3. Bands that were tried on a patient's cast *but not used* are recontoured and put aside for sterilization and reuse.

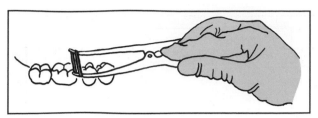

▼ **Figure 27–11**

Using elastic separating pliers for the placement of a posterior elastic separator. (Torres HO, Ehrlich A: Modern Dental Assisting, 4th Ed. Philadelphia, WB Saunders, 1990, p 624.)

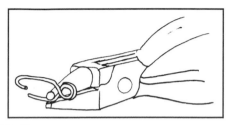

▼ **Figure 27–12**

Using a long-beak pliers to hold and place a steel spring separator. (Torres HO, Ehrlich A: Modern Dental Assisting, 4th Ed. Philadelphia, WB Saunders, 1990, p 624.)

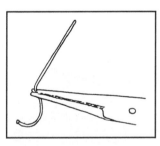

▼ **Figure 27–13**

Using a hemostat to grasp and place a brass wire separator. (Torres HO, Ehrlich A: Modern Dental Assisting, 4th Ed. Philadelphia, WB Saunders, 1990, p 625.)

There are three types of separators:

▼ **Elastic** ring posterior separators and dumbbell anterior separators (Fig. 27–11).

▼ **Steel spring** (Fig. 27–12).

▼ **Brass wire** (Fig. 27–13).

Mixing Cements for Orthodontic Bands

Just prior to the cementation of the bands, the separators are removed and the teeth are given a thorough coronal polishing.

In mixing cements for the cementation of orthodontic bands, a very cold dry slab and a chilled spatula are used.

This shortens the mixing time, lengthens the setting time, and makes it possible to cement several bands from the same mix. (Mixing cements for the cementation is discussed in Chapter 20, "Dental Cements.")

Instrumentation

▼ Orthodontic bands (selected and fitted).

▼ Masking tape.

▼ Chilled cement slab, aluminum or porcelain coated with polytef (Teflon).

▼ Chilled stainless steel spatula.

▼ Gauze squares, 2 × 2 inches.

▼ Alcohol (isopropyl).

▼ Cement, powder, and liquid.

▼ Band seater.

▼ Band driver and mallet.

▼ Scaler and explorer.

Procedure

CEMENTATION OF ORTHODONTIC BANDS

1 Preselected orthodontic bands are placed on small squares of masking tape with the gingival margin of the band upright.

2 Immediately prior to cementation, the slab and spatula are removed from the refrigerator and brought to the operatory.

3 A gauze square saturated with alcohol is used to wipe the surface of the slab. A dry gauze square is used to dry the slab.
Optional: The bands are placed on the surface of the cold slab to chill them.

4 At a signal from the orthodontist, the ce-

Continued on following page

ment is mixed quickly to obtain a homogeneous mix within 30 seconds.

5 The orthodontic band is held by the margin of the masking tape so that the gingival surface is upright, and the cement spatula is scraped over the margin. This allows the cement to flow into the circumference of the band (Fig. 27–14).

6 The cement-filled band is transferred to the orthodontist.

7 For posterior bands, the band seater is picked up by the tip and the handle is placed into the operator's hand.

8 For anterior bands, the band driver and a mallet are passed to the operator.

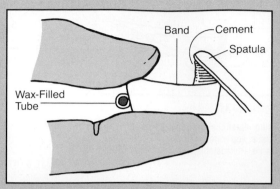

Figure 27–14 Placing cement in the orthodontic band. (Torres HO, Ehrlich A: Modern Dental Assisting, 4th Ed. Philadelphia, WB Saunders, 1990, p 633.)

9 After the cement has set, a scaler or explorer is used to remove the excess cement on the enamel surfaces.

PLACEMENT AND LIGATION OF ARCH WIRES

Instrumentation

▼ Preformed arch wires.

▼ Preformed ligature tie wires.

▼ Ligature-tying pliers.

▼ Ligature wire-cutting pliers.

▼ Schure instrument.

▼ How pliers.

Procedure

PLACING THE ARCH WIRE AND LIGATURE TIE WIRES

1 The preformed arch wire is inserted from the anterior portion of the mouth so that both ends are placed into the tube slot on the banded posterior molar in both the right and the left quadrants.

2 The anterior portion of the arch wire is first eased into the anterior brackets and then into the premolar brackets on each side of the arch.

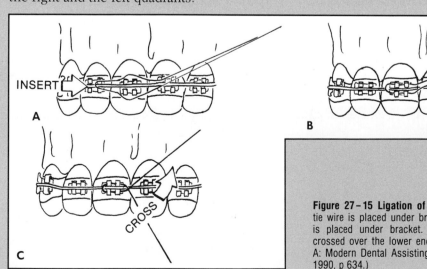

Figure 27–15 Ligation of wires. A. Preformed loop of ligature tie wire is placed under bracket projections. B. Ligature tie wire is placed under bracket. C. Top end of ligature tie wire is crossed over the lower end and pulled taut. (Torres HO, Ehrlich A: Modern Dental Assisting, 4th Ed. Philadelphia, WB Saunders, 1990, p 634.)

3 A preformed tie wire is selected. The loop end is bent into a 45-degree angle.

4 The loop of the tie wire is placed around the four extensions of the bracket on the band. The wire is guided behind the brackets and over the arch wire, securing the arch wire in place (Fig. 27–15).

5 The ends of the tie wire are pulled taut by hand with the top wire pulled down over the arch wire and across the bottom wire. The bottom wire is pulled up.

6 Ligature-tying pliers are used to wind wires together so that the top wire is turned under first (Fig. 27–16).

7 The wire is twisted to approximately 4 to 5 mm in length and is laid down toward the side of the arch.

8 After all ligature wires are tied, they are cut with the ligature wire-cutting pliers to leave 3- to 5-mm pigtails extending.

9 The Schure instrument or Gross ligature wire tucker instrument is used to tuck the cut ligature wire pigtails into the space around the brackets and under the arch wire toward the gingiva.

10 The patient is requested to close his mouth and run his tongue around the brackets. If a sharp area is noted, it is necessary to recheck the tucking of all cut ligatures.

11 The distal ends of the arch wire are crimped with How pliers to prevent their dislodgment from the slot.

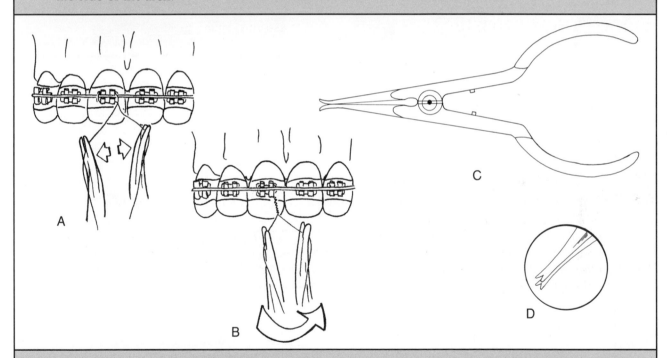

Figure 27–16 Technique for tightening ligature tie wire. *A.* Ends of the tie wire are secured on the tie pliers. *B.* Loose ends of the wire are wrapped around the hub of the pliers. The pliers are twirled and the wire is tied. *C.* Coon ligature-tying pliers. *D.* Close-up of beaks of ligature-tying pliers. (Torres HO, Ehrlich A: Modern Dental Assisting, 4th Ed. Philadelphia, WB Saunders, 1990, p 635.)

Removal of Ligature Tie Wires and Arch Wire

The patient wears protective eyewear and is requested to keep his eyes closed during the process to avoid having a piece of wire injure the eye.

The assistant and the orthodontist wear glasses for protection of their eyes, as for other procedures in dentistry.

Procedure

REMOVING LIGATURE TIE WIRES AND ARCH WIRE

1. A Schure instrument or scaler is used to pull the pigtail of the tie wire free of the arch wire and bracket.

2. The ligature wire is held in the left hand with a hemostat. The ligature wire-cutting pliers are held in the right hand.

3. The ligature wire-cutting pliers are placed on the wire next to the pigtail and the wire is snipped, pulled free with the hemostat, and placed on the instrument tray.

4. These steps are repeated until all ligature wires have been removed.

5. The arch wire is removed by straightening the crimp in the posterior end of the wire placed in the tube on a posterior tooth in each quadrant.

6. The arch wire is pulled forward, free of the brackets.

Procedure

REMOVING ORTHODONTIC BANDS

1. Band-removal pliers are used to remove posterior bands (Fig. 27-17). If necessary, a crown cutter may be used to cut the band free from the tooth surface.

2. Anterior bands are removed by applying the Schure instrument, a heavy scaler, or band-removal pliers to the gingival and incisal margins and pulling toward the incisal edge of the tooth.

3. After the bands have been removed, the teeth are scaled free of cement and given a coronal polishing to remove all fragments of cement.

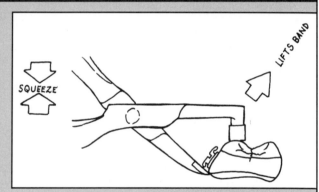

Figure 27-17 Use of a band-removal pliers in the removal of a posterior band. (Torres HO, Ehrlich A: Modern Dental Assisting, 4th Ed. Philadelphia, WB Saunders, 1990, p 633.)

DIRECT BONDING OF BRACKETS

As an alternative to full bands, which completely surround the tooth, orthodontic brackets may be bonded directly to the surface of the teeth.

A self-polymerizing composite or a polycarboxylate cement, such as Durelon, is used for this purpose. (Review cements in Chapter 20, "Dental Cements.")

Procedure

BONDING THE BRACKETS

1. The brackets to be used are selected and, if necessary, are adapted and contoured to fit on the tooth surface (Figs. 27-18 and 27-19).

2. The brackets are placed in sequence in a bracket tray for quick identification during cementation.

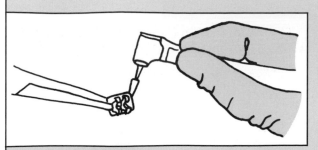

Figure 27–18 Modifying bracket to fit the tooth surface. (Torres HO, Ehrlich A: Modern Dental Assisting, 4th Ed. Philadelphia, WB Saunders, 1990, p 615.)

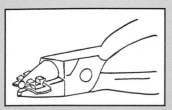

Figure 27–19 Contouring the bracket with bird-beak pliers. (Torres HO, Ehrlich A: Modern Dental Assisting, 4th Ed. Philadelphia, WB Saunders, 1990, p 616.)

3 The teeth to be treated are cleaned with a pumice and water slurry (Fig. 27–20).

4 The teeth are rinsed, dried, and isolated with cotton rolls.

5 The facial tooth surface to receive the bracket is etched, rinsed, and dried (Figs. 27–21 and 27–22).

6 If not previously treated, the inner surface of the bracket is etched, rinsed, and dried.

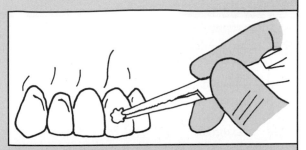

Figure 27–21 Etching the tooth surface. (Torres HO, Ehrlich A: Modern Dental Assisting, 4th Ed. Philadelphia, WB Saunders, 1990, p 616.)

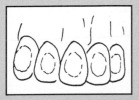

Figure 27–22 The etched surface appears dull and chalky. (Torres HO, Ehrlich A: Modern Dental Assisting, 4th Ed. Philadelphia, WB Saunders, 1990, p 616.)

7 Freshly mixed cement (which is still glossy) is placed on the prepared tooth surface *and* on the inner surface of the bracket (Fig. 27–23).

8 The band is positioned on the tooth and held in place with firm hand pressure (Fig. 27–24).

9 The cement is allowed to set for 15 minutes before attaching any wires or springs.

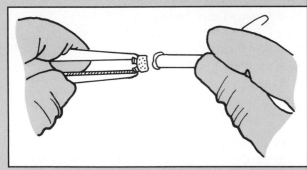

Figure 27–23 Placing cement on the back of the bracket. (Torres HO, Ehrlich A: Modern Dental Assisting, 4th Ed. Philadelphia, WB Saunders, 1990, p 617.)

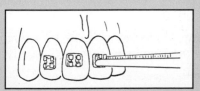

Figure 27–24 Placing the bracket on the tooth. (Torres HO, Ehrlich A: Modern Dental Assisting, 4th Ed. Philadelphia, WB Saunders, 1990, p 617.)

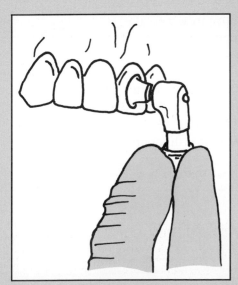

Figure 27–20 Polishing the tooth surface. (Torres HO, Ehrlich A: Modern Dental Assisting, 4th Ed. Philadelphia, WB Saunders, 1990, p 616.)

▼ **EXERCISES**

1. _____ orthodontic treatment consists of steps taken to prevent or correct problems as they are developing.

   a. Adjustive
   b. Corrective
   c. Interceptive
   d. Preventive

2. A _____ on the lingual side of the band is used to help position the band.

   a. buccal tube
   b. hook
   c. seating lug

3. A Schure instrument is used to _____.

   a. crimp an arch wire
   b. remove an anterior band
   c. seat a band
   d. b or c

4. A polycarboxylate cement _____ be used in the direct bonding of orthodontic brackets.

   a. may
   b. may not

5. When preparing for the cementation of bands, the slab and spatula should be _____.

   a. chilled
   b. moistened
   c. warmed to 80°F
   d. none of the above

6. When applying the acid etching solution in a direct bonding procedure, the operator continuously _____ the enamel surface.

   a. dabs
   b. dries
   c. rubs
   d. smooths

7. A Boone gauge is a measuring device used in the placement of orthodontic bands.

   a. true
   b. false

8. A comprehensive medical history, photographs, radiographs, and impressions for diagnostic casts are usually taken at the _____ visit.

   a. banding
   b. consultation
   c. treatment

9. Orthodontic bands are selected _____.

   a. at the banding visit
   b. prior to the banding visit

10. When placing a band, the _____ edge goes over the tooth first.

    a. incisal
    b. gingival
    c. occlusal
    d. a or c

11. After the bands are removed, the teeth are _____.

    a. given a coronal polish
    b. scaled free of cement
    c. treated with topical fluoride
    d. a and b

12. The ends of the arch wire are placed in the _____ on the banded posterior molars.

    a. bonded brackets
    b. "S" hooks
    c. seating lugs
    d. tube slots

13. Orthodontic bands are divided into _____ to compensate for individual tooth differences.

    a. left and right
    b. sizes
    c. upper and lower
    d. a, b, and c

14. Prior to the direct bonding of brackets, the teeth are cleaned using a fluoride paste.

    a. true
    b. false

15. Prior to initial placement, the tie wire is bent into a _____ degree angle.

    a. 25
    b. 35
    c. 45
    d. 90

16. Ligature-tying pliers are twisted so that the _____ wire is turned under first.

    a. bottom
    b. top

17. Orthodontic treatment visits are usually scheduled for _____ minutes.

    a. 5 to 10
    b. 10 to 20
    c. 20 to 30
    d. 30 to 60

18. The _____ edge of an orthodontic band is rolled or contoured.

    a. gingival
    b. incisal
    c. occlusal
    d. b or c

19. _____ separators are placed between anterior teeth.

    a. Brass wire
    b. Elastic dumbbell
    c. Steel spring

20. Prior to bonding, the interior of the bracket is _____.

    a. coated with fluoride
    b. etched
    c. painted with adhesive
    d. a, b, and c

28 Periodontics

▼ LEARNING OBJECTIVES

The student will be able to:

1. Define these terms: coronal polish, dental prophylaxis, scaling, root planing, gingival curettage, gingivectomy, and gingivoplasty.

2. Identify these specialized instruments used in periodontics: periodontal probe, scalers, curettes, pocket marker, and periodontal knives.

3. State the use of the ultrasonic scaler, prophy angle, rubber cup, and brushes.

4. Describe the process of recording a periodontal examination.

5. Describe the manipulation and use of periodontal surgical dressings.

OVERVIEW OF PERIODONTICS

The goal of periodontal treatment is to free the tooth surfaces of calculus, plaque, debris, and diseased tissue so as to attain and maintain healthy periodontal tissues.

The following are the more commonly performed procedures related to attaining this goal.

Coronal polishing is only the polishing of the crowns of the teeth to remove plaque and extrinsic stains. It does *not* involve the removal of calculus.

Extrinsic stains are only on the exterior surfaces of the tooth and can be removed by polishing. **Intrinsic stains** are found within the enamel of the tooth and cannot be removed by polishing.

In some states, the extended function dental assistant (EFDA) is permitted to perform coronal polishing prior to procedures such as placement of the rubber dam.

A **dental prophylaxis** involves the removal of calculus, debris, plaque, and stains on the coronal surfaces of the teeth and into the gingival sulci. (**Supragingival calculus** is located *above*

the gingiva. **Subgingival calculus** is located *below* the gingiva in the gingival sulcus.)

The dentist and the registered dental hygienist (RDH) are the only members of the dental health team permitted by state law to perform this service.

Scaling is the removal of calculus from the tooth surfaces with periodontal instruments (Fig. 28–1).

Root planing is the removal of subgingival calculus that is embedded on cementum of the root. This results in a smooth surface, which encourages reattachment of the epithelial tissues.

Gingival curettage is the removal of the soft tissue lining and the diseased tissue of periodontal pockets. (When the depth of the gingival sulcus is greater than 3 mm, it is considered to be a periodontal pocket.)

A **gingivectomy** is the surgical removal of the diseased soft tissue wall of a periodontal pocket.

A **gingivoplasty** is the surgical procedure by which gingival deformities are reshaped to create normal and functional form.

477

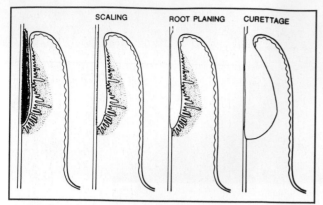

▼ **Figure 28-1**

Diagram comparing the tissues removed by periodontal procedures. On the left is diseased tissue. (Perry DA, Beemsterboer P, Carranza F: Techniques and Theory of Periodontal Instrumentation. WB Saunders, Philadelphia, 1990, p 4.)

INSTRUMENTATION FOR PERIODONTICS

Periodontal Probe

The periodontal probe is used to measure the depth of the gingival sulcus. This instrument is elongated and tapered, with a blunt point.

Millimeter gradations from 1 to 10 mm, in increments of 1 to 2 mm, are placed on the working end. The marks for 4 and 6 mm are omitted on the probe to facilitate reading (Fig. 28-2).

Scalers

A scaler is a periodontal instrument with cutting edges terminating in a sharp tip. Scalers are used primarily for the removal of supragingival calculus.

Scalers come in a wide variety of sizes and designs. They are usually provided as double-ended instruments. Bends in the shank, plus the size and shape of the blade, determine where the scaler is used (Figs. 28-3 and 28-4).

The **hoe scaler** is designed to remove easily accessible calculus. It has a single straight cutting edge with the blade turned at an angle of 99 to 100 degrees to the shank (Fig. 28-5A).

The **file scaler** is used to remove calculus on root surfaces in deep, narrow pockets. It has multiple cutting edges lined up as a series of miniature hoes (Fig. 28-5B).

Curettes

A curette is a periodontal instrument with sharp cutting edges and a rounded toe. Curettes are used for subgingival scaling and root planing.

The design of **universal curettes** allows them to be adapted to all surfaces of the teeth. They can be used for both supragingival and subgingival calculus removal.

Area specific curettes, such as the **Gracey curettes**, are scaling and root planing instruments designed to fit particular anatomic portions of the teeth (Fig. 28-6).

Pocket Marker

A pocket marker is similar in appearance to cotton pliers except that the tips are sharp and designed to pinch a small hole in the gingiva. A series of these markings may be used to outline the extent of surgery for a gingivectomy (Fig. 28-7).

Periodontal Knives

Periodontal knives are used to remove excessive and diseased gingival tissue during a gingivectomy and a gingivoplasty (Fig. 28-8).

Ultrasonic Scaler

The ultrasonic scaler is a power-driven device that is used to remove deposits of calculus and stains from the teeth. It may be used in conjunction with hand scaling.

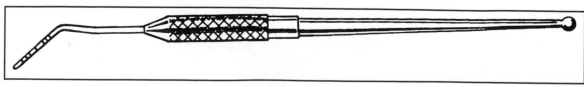

▼ **Figure 28-2**

Periodontal probe with gradations on the working end. (Torres HO, Ehrlich A: Modern Dental Assisting, 4th Ed. Philadelphia, WB Saunders, 1990, p 799.)

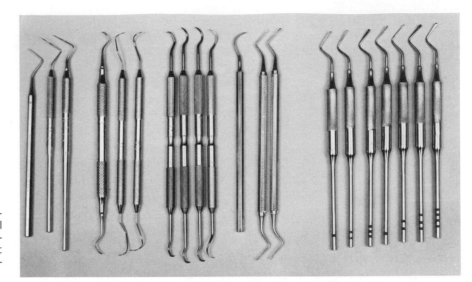

▼ Figure 28-3

Periodontal instruments. The three instruments on the left are periodontal probes. The remainder of the instruments are scalers. (Torres HO, Ehrlich A: Modern Dental Assisting, 4th Ed. Philadelphia, WB Saunders, 1990, p 798.)

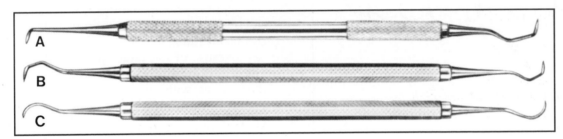

▼ Figure 28-4

Dental scalers. *A.* Goldman-Fox universal scaler. *B.* Jaquette scaler. *C.* Goldman sickle scaler. (Courtesy of Hu-Friedy, Chicago, IL.)

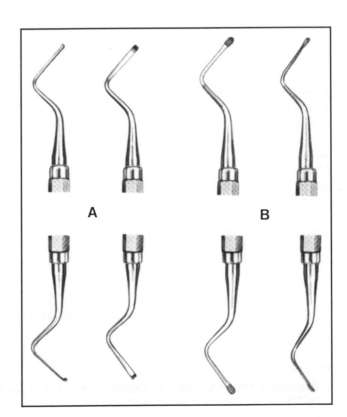

▼ Figure 28-5

Periodontal hoes and files. *A.* Hoes are used for the removal of easily accessible calculus. *B.* Files are used for calculus removal on root surfaces in deep, narrow pockets. (Courtesy of Hu-Friedy, Chicago, IL.)

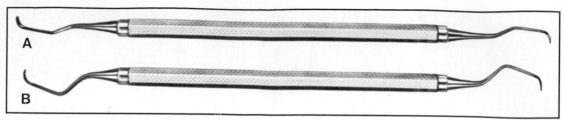

▼ **Figure 28–6**

Gracey curettes. *A.* Short, for incisors and cuspids. *B.* Medium contra-angle for premolars and molars and buccal and lingual surfaces. (Courtesy of Hu-Friedy, Chicago, IL.)

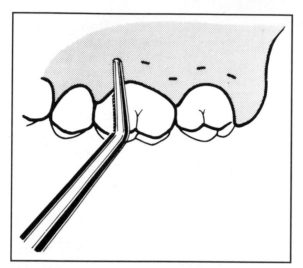

▼ **Figure 28–7**

Periodontal pocket marker. Makes pinpoint perforations that indicate pocket depth. (Carranza FA, Jr: Glickman's Clinical Periodontology, 7th Ed. Philadelphia, WB Saunders, 1990, p 800.)

The scaling action is caused by the rapid vibration of its removable tip. A sterile tip is placed just prior to treatment (Fig. 28–9).

Water, provided through a jet on the tip of the handpiece, cools the working tip and prevents overheating of the teeth being treated. The assistant may use the high volume evacuator (HVE) tip to remove water and debris from the oral cavity during the use of this instrument (Fig. 28–10).

Prophy-Jet

The prophy-jet is a specially designed handpiece that delivers a mixture of warm water and sodium bicarbonate. It is used to remove extrinsic stain and soft deposits.

The use of a lip lubricant helps to reduce any discomfort caused by the gritty debris generated by this instrument.

Because of the large quantity of aerosol spray given off, this is not the instrument of choice for the patient with infectious diseases such as acquired immunodeficiency syndrome (AIDS) or hepatitis.

Prophy Angle

The right-angle handpiece, which is specifically designed for use during a dental prophylaxis, is commonly referred to as a *prophy angle*. Review these handpieces in Chapter 12, "Rotary Dental Instruments."

Rubber Cups and Bristle Brushes

A rubber cup is used with the prophy angle to apply polishing paste and to polish the teeth (Fig. 28–11).

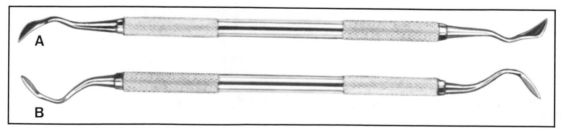

▼ **Figure 28–8**

Gingivectomy knives. *A.* Kirkland knife for the initial incision for gingivectomy. *B.* Orban knife with an angled blade and contra-angled shank particularly suitable for posterior applications. (Courtesy of Hu-Friedy, Chicago, IL.)

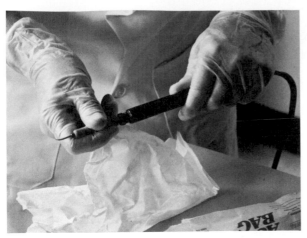

▼ **Figure 28 – 9**

Inserting the sterile scaling tip in the ultrasonic handpiece. (Torres HO, Ehrlich A: Modern Dental Assisting, 4th Ed. Philadelphia, WB Saunders, 1990, p 638.)

A rubber cup consists of a rubber shell with a web-shaped or rib-shaped configuration in the hollow interior. It is discarded after a single use.

Bristle brushes are also used for polishing. However, because the stiff bristles could damage delicate tissues or scratch restorations, use of the bristle brush is limited to the occlusal surfaces of the teeth.

THE PERIODONTAL EXAMINATION

The initial examination for the periodontal patient includes:

▼ A complete medical and dental history (see Chapter 14, "The Dental Examination").

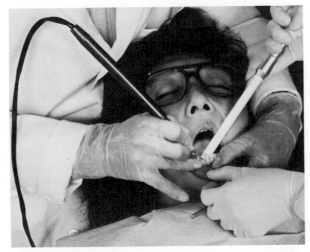

▼ **Figure 28 – 10**

The HVE is used with the ultrasonic scaler to remove excess water from the mouth. (Torres HO, Ehrlich A: Modern Dental Assisting, 4th Ed. Philadelphia, WB Saunders, 1990, p 639.)

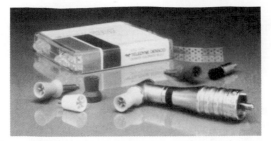

▼ **Figure 28 – 11**

Prophy angle, rubber prophy cups, and bristle brushes. (Courtesy of Teledyne Getz, Elk Grove Village, IL.)

▼ A thorough oral examination (see Chapter 14, "The Dental Examination").

▼ Radiographs.

▼ Occlusal analysis and tooth mobility.

▼ Evaluation of personal oral hygiene.

▼ Other diagnostic aids as needed (see Chapter 14, "The Dental Examination," and Chapter 17, "Alginate Impressions and Diagnostic Casts").

Radiographs

The diagnosis of periodontal conditions depends on an accurate radiographic survey. Each radiograph must represent a true periapical projection of the teeth and the alveolus.

Lack of accuracy in radiographic technique may cause distortion, which can result in a diagnostic error.

A current radiographic survey is produced so that the dentist may evaluate it and compare this with previous surveys and clinical findings.

Occlusal Analysis

The patient's occlusion is evaluated, and the dentist looks for indications of bruxism. These are likely to appear as abnormal abrasion and facets of wear on the tooth surfaces. (**Bruxism** is the involuntary grinding or clenching of the teeth.)

If bruxism is present, it may need to be corrected before the periodontal condition can be eliminated.

Tooth Mobility

The individual teeth are checked for mobility. (**Mobility** is the movement of the tooth within its socket.)

Mobility of the individual tooth is recorded using the numbers 0, 1, 2, and 3. (Some operators use the Roman numerals I, II, and III for recording mobility.)

The numbers stand for the following values:

0 — **normal**, that is, no mobility (some operators use N for normal, instead of 0).

1 — **slight mobility**, greater than normal.

2 — **moderate mobility** (total movement of 1 mm displacement).

3 — **extreme mobility** (the tooth moves more than 1 mm and in all directions).

Periodontal Indices

There are many indices used to describe various aspects of periodontal diseases. The dentist selects those indices to be included in the examination. (**Indices** is the plural of index. An index is an expression of clinical observations in numerical values.)

Dental Plaque Index

This index is used to describe the extent of plaque on the basis of the amount of tooth surface covered. There are several systems for scoring the plaque index. In one system this is scored from "0" (no plaque) to "3" (plaque covering more than one half of the tooth surface).

Bleeding Indices

Based on the principle that healthy tissue does not bleed, testing for bleeding may be a significant procedure for evaluation prior to treatment planning and after treatment. Several different systems of scoring bleeding are used.

Evaluation of Personal Oral Hygiene

The dentist or hygienist will evaluate the patient's home care program and provide additional instruction as necessary. (This is described in Chapter 5, "Preventive Dentistry and Nutrition.")

PERIODONTAL PROBING

During the periodontal examination, the periodontal probe is used to measure the depth of the

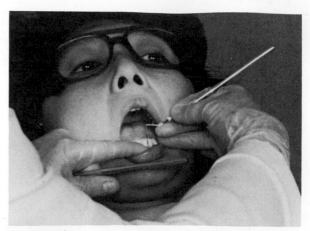

▼ **Figure 28–12**

Using the periodontal probe during a patient examination. (Torres HO, Ehrlich A: Modern Dental Assisting, 4th Ed. Philadelphia, WB Saunders, 1990, p 803.)

gingival sulcus at six points as it surrounds each tooth (Fig. 28–12).

These findings are charted on the patient's clinical record. The dentist may prefer to use a special periodontal chart that may be used for this purpose (Fig. 28–13).

There are six "readings" of pocket depth for each tooth:

▼ Mesiofacial.

▼ Facial.

▼ Distofacial.

▼ Mesiolingual.

▼ Lingual.

▼ Distolingual.

Instrumentation

▼ Basic setup.

▼ Periodontal probe.

▼ Cotton pellets.

▼ Sterile gauze squares, 2 × 2 inch.

▼ Mouth rinse (optional).

▼ Dental floss.

▼ HVE tip.

▼ Periodontal chart.

▼ Pencils (red, blue, and black).

Procedure

CHARTING A PERIODONTAL EXAMINATION

1 The patient is asked to rinse his mouth. The HVE tip is used to evacuate the oral cavity.

2 Gauze squares are handed to the operator. The operator dries the area to be examined.

3 The operator inserts the periodontal probe into the depth of the sulcus for the three measurements on the facial surface of each tooth in the arch: *distofacial, facial,* and *mesiofacial.*

The operator repeats this probing procedure for the three measurements on the lingual surfaces of each tooth in the arch: *distolingual, lingual,* and *mesiolingual.*

The operator repeats this process for the facial and lingual surfaces of the teeth in the opposite arch.

4 The assistant records the number of each

reading as it is dictated by the operator.

These findings are written as numbers (just under the tooth number) on the patient's clinical record (see Fig. 28–13).

5 The assistant may be asked to place corresponding dots on the line nearest the tooth surface to represent the depth of the pocket. (Each gradation line on the periodontal chart equals 2 mm.)

The dots are marked with a blue pencil.

Later the assistant may be asked to use a red pencil to make a line connecting these dots.

This line is a visual representation of the depth of the sulcus around the neck of each tooth.

6 The operator determines the mobility of each tooth by finger pressure. This information is also recorded by the assistant.

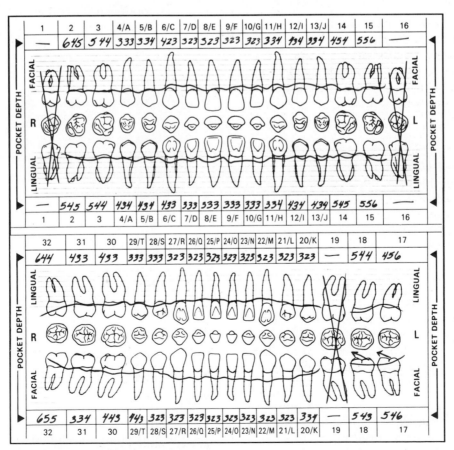

▼ **Figure 28–13**

Periodontal charting for a 40-year-old patient. (Courtesy of Colwell Systems, Inc, Champaign, IL.)

THE DENTAL PROPHYLAXIS

The assistant may be asked to aid the dentist or hygienist during the dental prophylaxis.

Instrumentation

▼ Basic setup.

▼ Disclosing tablets or solution.

▼ HVE tip.

▼ Scalers (assorted).

▼ Right-angle (prophy angle) handpiece.

▼ Prophy cup and brushes.

▼ Dental floss and tape.

▼ Mouthwash and paper cup.

Procedure

PERFORMING DENTAL PROPHYLAXIS

1. The patient is seated, draped, and given protective glasses to wear.

   The patient may be given a disclosing tablet to chew. If so, he is instructed to rub his tongue on all tooth surfaces to disclose the plaque and debris on the teeth.

2. If the ultrasonic scaler is used, the assistant may be asked to use the HVE tip to remove excess water from the patient's mouth.

   If the operator uses scalers and other hand instruments to remove plaque and calculus from all surfaces of the teeth, the assistant may be asked to use the air-water syringe and HVE tip to remove debris and excess water.

3. The operator polishes the teeth using prophy paste on a rubber cup and/or a bristle brush.

   The assistant may be asked to use the air-water syringe and HVE tip to remove debris and excess water.

4. The operator gently guides dental floss or dental tape between the contacts of the teeth. This polishes the interproximal surfaces of the teeth and detects any rough areas.

   The assistant should note any contact areas that "fray" the floss.

5. If the hygienist has performed the prophylaxis, the dentist examines the teeth and rechecks the questionable areas that were noted by the hygienist.

6. The dentist advises the patient on the necessity for additional treatment.

7. The hygienist or assistant instructs the patient on oral hygiene procedures for home care.

8. If no further treatment is indicated at this time, the patient is advised when to return to be checked for progress on his oral hygiene program.

PERIODONTAL DRESSING

Following periodontal surgery, such as a gingivectomy or a gingivoplasty, a periodontal surgical dressing is placed over a surgical site to reduce bleeding, protect the tissues, and minimize postoperative discomfort.

The dentist will state a preference for a eugenol type or a noneugenol type of periodontal dressing, and the assistant is responsible for mixing and preparing it.

The procedure described here is for mixing noneugenol type surgical dressing, which is less irritating to the tissues.

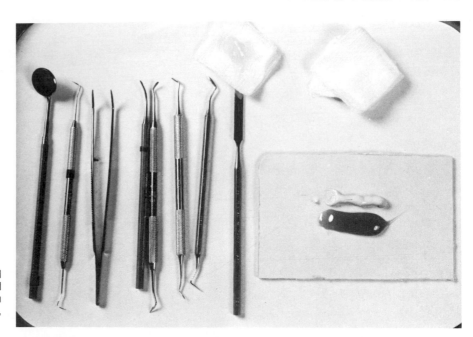

▼ **Figure 28-14**

Instrumentation for preparation and placement of periodontal surgical dressing. (Torres HO, Ehrlich A: Modern Dental Assisting, 4th Ed. Philadelphia, WB Saunders, 1990, p 813.)

Noneugenol Type Periodontal Dressing

Instrumentation (Fig. 28-14)

▼ Basic setup.

▼ Mixing pad (waxed).

▼ Spatula (medium, stiff blade).

▼ Noneugenol paste, base, and catalyst.

▼ Petroleum jelly.

▼ Oil of orange (to clean instruments).

▼ Sterile plastic gloves (to wear while mixing the material).

Procedure

MIXING NONEUGENOL TYPE PERIODONTAL DRESSING

1 Wearing sterile plastic gloves, extrude equal lengths of catalyst and base from the tubes onto a paper pad (approximately 2 inches for each quadrant).

2 Use the spatula to fold and mix materials on the pad quickly until the colors are evenly blended (Fig. 28-15).

Work quickly because the working time is limited.

Wipe the spatula clean immediately before the dressing hardens on it.

3 Test the material for tackiness (Fig. 28-16).

Tackiness leaves the material after 3 to 4 minutes.

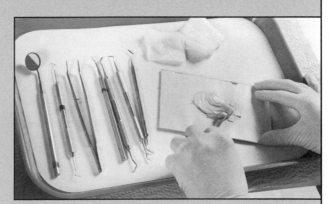

Figure 28-15 Mixing periodontal surgical dressing. (Torres HO, Ehrlich A: Modern Dental Assisting, 4th Ed. Philadelphia, WB Saunders, 1990, p 814.)

Continued on following page

The dressing mix retains its plastic quality for placement for approximately 10 to 15 minutes.

4. Coat gloved fingers with petroleum jelly and form ropes of the dressing mix (Fig. 28–17).

5. The material is now ready to be placed on the surgical site.

6. Use oil of orange to remove any material that has hardened on the spatula.

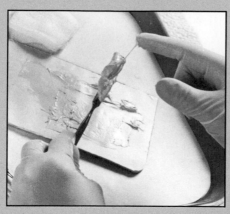

Figure 28–16 Testing for tackiness of periodontal surgical dressing mix prior to placement. (Torres HO, Ehrlich A: Modern Dental Assisting, 4th Ed. Philadelphia, WB Saunders, 1990, p 814.)

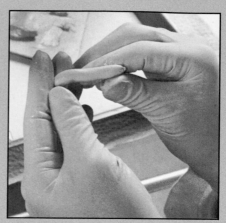

Figure 28–17 Forming a roll of periodontal surgical dressing prior to placement. (Torres HO, Ehrlich A: Modern Dental Assisting, 4th Ed. Philadelphia, WB Saunders, 1990, p 814.)

PREVENTIVE CARE FOR THE PERIODONTAL PATIENT

Establishing and maintaining a good home care program are essential for the periodontic patient. If oral hygiene is not adequately maintained, there is every likelihood that the periodontal disease will recur or become worse.

In addition to carrying out his home care program faithfully, it is important that the periodontic patient return frequently for professional prophylaxis and re-evaluation of his condition.

The patient is placed on a recall program so that he is seen regularly every few months. The dentist will determine the desired length of time between visits.

While the patient is under the ongoing care of the periodontist, he also returns to his regular dentist for routine checkups and any restorative care that may be necessary.

▼ EXERCISES

1. _____ calculus is located below the gingiva in the gingival sulcus.

   a. Subgingival
   b. Supragingival

2. A/An _____ is used to measure the depth of the gingival sulcus.

   a. explorer
   b. periodontal probe
   c. pocket marker
   d. scaler

3. _____ is the movement of the tooth within its socket.

   a. Bruxism
   b. Mobility
   c. Periodontal index

4. Periodontal knives are used to remove excessive and diseased gingival tissue during a gingivectomy and a gingivoplasty.

   a. true
   b. false

5. A bristle brush is used on the _____ surfaces of the teeth.

   a. facial
   b. interproximal
   c. occlusal
   d. a, b, and c

6. A/An _____ is a specially designed handpiece that delivers a mixture of warm water and sodium bicarbonate.

   a. prophy angle
   b. prophy-jet
   c. ultrasonic scaler

7. After the tackiness leaves the freshly mixed periodontal dressing, it will retain its plastic quality for placement for approximately _____ minutes.

   a. 2 to 5
   b. 5 to 10
   c. 10 to 15
   d. 15 to 20

8. When the depth of the gingival sulcus is greater than _____ mm, it is considered to be a periodontal pocket.

   a. 3
   b. 4
   c. 5
   d. 6

9. A dental plaque index of 3 indicates _____.

   a. minimal plaque
   b. no plaque
   c. plaque covering less than one half of the tooth surface
   d. plaque covering more than one half of the tooth surface

10. A _____ is the removal of the soft tissue lining and diseased tissue of periodontal pockets.

    a. gingival curettage
    b. gingivectomy
    c. prophylaxis
    d. root planing

11. Tooth mobility recorded as a 2 (or II) indicates _____ mobility.

    a. extreme
    b. moderate
    c. normal
    d. slight

12. A _____ has sharp cutting edges and a rounded toe.

    a. chisel
    b. file scaler
    c. hoe scaler
    d. surgical hoe

13. _____ involves the mechanical removal of calculus, debris, plaque, and stains on the coronal surfaces of the teeth and in the gingival sulci.

    a. Coronal polishing
    b. Curettage
    c. Prophylaxis
    d. Root planing

14. Coronal polishing _____ involve the removal of calculus.

    a. does
    b. does not

15. _____ type periodontal dressings are used to protect a surgical site.

    a. Calcium hydroxide
    b. Eugenol
    c. Noneugenol
    d. b and c

16. A _____ is the surgical removal of the diseased soft tissue wall of a periodontal pocket.

    a. curettage
    b. gingivectomy
    c. gingivoplasty
    d. prophylaxis

17. A _____ has cutting edges terminating in a sharp tip.

    a. curette
    b. Gracey curette
    c. periodontal knife
    d. scaler

18. If the hands are coated with petroleum jelly, it is not necessary to wear gloves while mixing periodontal dressing.

    a. true
    b. false

19. The freshly mixed periodontal dressing is shaped into _____ _____ of dressing mix.

    a. flat patties
    b. ropes
    c. small triangles

20. After use, the rubber cup used in the prophylaxis is _____ _____ .

    a. autoclaved
    b. disinfected
    c. discarded
    d. sterilized with dry heat

29 Endodontics

LEARNING OBJECTIVES

The student will be able to:

1. Describe the specialty of endodontics.
2. Identify the specialized instruments used in endodontics.
3. Describe the specialized diagnostic tests used in an endodontic examination.
4. State the need for a sterile field in endodontic treatment.
5. Describe assisting during endodontic treatment.

OVERVIEW OF ENDODONTICS

Endodontics, which is also known as *root canal therapy* (RCT), deals with diagnosis and treatment of diseases of the tooth pulp and the periapical tissues. Often this treatment makes it possible to save a tooth that otherwise would require extraction.

The patient in need of endodontic treatment is usually in severe pain because the nerve of the tooth is inflamed, dying, or infected. These patients should be scheduled and seen as quickly as possible for the relief of pain.

The general dentist may provide endodontic treatment or may refer the patient to an endodontist, who is a specialist in this type of treatment. If the patient is treated by an endodontist, he is referred back to the general dentist for placement of a permanent restoration.

Endodontic therapy consists of removing all remnants of the pulp and cleaning and enlarging the root canals. The final step is filling the canals so that they are sealed securely without having the filling material extend beyond the apex of the tooth.

Frequently endodontic therapy can be com-pleted in a single visit. However, there are situations in which two or more visits are necessary. A major concern throughout endodontic treatment is the control of infection in the tooth and the surrounding tissues.

INSTRUMENTATION FOR ENDODONTIC TREATMENT

Gates-Glidden Drills

Gates-Glidden drills are small, flame-shaped rotary cutting endodontic instruments with long shanks that are used with slow-speed handpieces (Fig. 29–1).

These drills are used to open and enlarge the root canal; however, the refinement of the canal preparation may be accomplished with hand-operated instruments.

Broaches

Barbed broaches are hand-operated instruments used primarily for removing pulp tissue, cotton

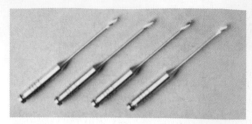

▼ **Figure 29–1**

Gates-Glidden drills. (Courtesy of Kerr Manufacturing Co, Romulus, MI.)

pellets, paper points, or other soft materials from the root canal (Fig. 29–2*A*).

Smooth broaches, which do not have barbs, are used as probes or pathfinders. Broaches are available in coarse, medium, fine, X-fine, XX-fine, and XXX-fine sizes.

Endodontic Files

Standard endodontic files are hand-operated instruments that come in a wide range of sizes (Figs. 29–2*B* and 29–3*A*).

Hedstrom files are hand-operated instruments that are designed with a cutting edge that runs in a continuous spiral (Fig. 29–2*C*).

When working with files to enlarge, shape, and smooth the root canal, the operator must use them in strict sequential order; that is, moving progressively from the smaller to larger size.

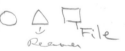

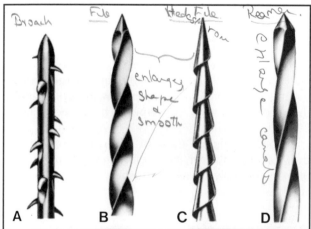

▼ **Figure 29–2**

Details of hand-operated endodontic instruments. *A.* Barbed broach. *B.* Standard file. *C.* Hedstrom file. *D.* Reamer. (Courtesy of Charles B. Schwed Co, Inc, Kew Gardens, NY.)

Reamers

Reamers are hand-operated instruments with a cutting edge. They are used to enlarge the canal during the process of endodontic treatment (Figs. 29–2*D* and 29–3*B*).

Handles, Sizes, and Color Coding

These instruments are supplied with a fixed plastic handle, which is known as a **style B** handle.

An alternative is a removable handle. The removable handle is used to adjust the working length of the instrument.

Files and reamers come in 20 different sizes ranging from the smallest (size 08) to the largest (size 140). The smaller the size of the instrument, the more delicate it is and the more easily it will break.

Six colors are used to color code the size of the instrument. In order to accommodate the complete range of sizes, the colors are reused. The following are examples of these color codes:

▼ White—size 15.

▼ Yellow—size 20.

▼ Red—size 25.

▼ Blue—size 30.

▼ Green—size 35.

▼ Black—size 40.

The assistant should become familiar with the color coding on the sizes most frequently used by the dentist.

Working Length

The working length of the tooth is the distance from the reference point to the apex of the root (but not beyond). The dentist may use an electronic "apex finder" to determine the working length.

The working length may also be determined by using a millimeter endodontic ruler to measure a radiograph with a "test file" in place. This film must accurately show the total length of all roots of the involved tooth, plus 1 to 2 mm around the apices (Fig. 29–4).

The working length is recorded on the patient's chart. Once the length has been determined, the endodontic instruments are measured and marked accordingly with the placement of stops.

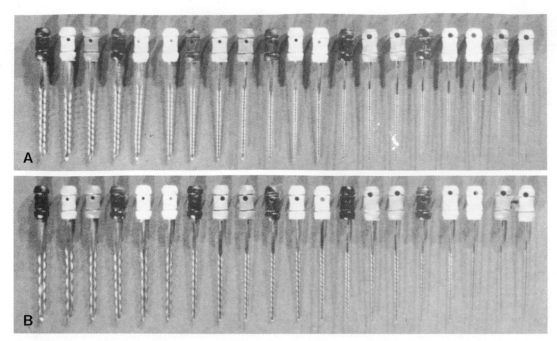

▼ **Figure 29-3**

Endodontic files and reamers. *A.* Standardized files with plastic handles. *B.* Standardized reamers with plastic handles. (Courtesy of Kerr Manufacturing Co, Romulus, MI.)

Stops are small, round sterile pieces of rubber or plastic that are placed on the broaches, reamers, or files to mark the working length.

Stops are used to prevent placing the instrument too far into the canal and perforating the apex. To provide an accurate measurement of the canal, the stop must be placed precisely at a right angle to the instrument.

The endodontic instruments with the stops in place are arranged in order of use (from smallest to largest).

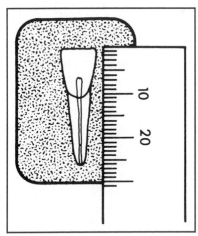

▼ **Figure 29-4**

Estimated working length determination using a millimeter ruler. (Walton RE, Torabinejad M: Principles and Practice of Endodontics. Philadelphia, WB Saunders, 1989, p 189.)

Glass Bead Sterilizer

A glass bead sterilizer is a small electrical unit with a recessed well that is filled with glass beads. The thermostat maintains the temperature of these beads at 450°F (232°C) (Fig. 29-5).

The glass bead sterilizer is used at chairside to sterilize files, reamers, and broaches. The instruments are placed, point down, in the sterilizer for 10 to 12 seconds immediately prior to their insertion into the canal. The instrument cools instantly before it is placed in the canal.

Irrigating Syringes

A sterile **Luer-Lok syringe** is used to irrigate and lubricate the root canal during treatment. The syringe has a chamber and plunger so that the solution may be drawn directly into the syringe.

A Luer-Lok syringe is made of plastic and is disposable. It is available in sizes 2 ml to 5 ml with a blunt 20- to 23-gage needle. The needle may be bent at an angle to facilitate access to the canal.

Irrigating Solutions

Sodium hypochlorite (common household bleach) is the solution most frequently used for

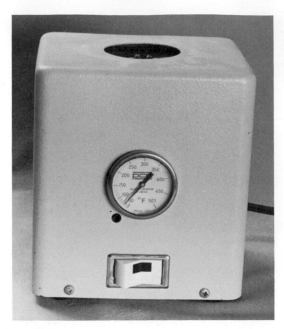

▼ **Figure 29-5**

A glass bead sterilizer suitable for chairside sterilization of endo-dontic hand-operated instruments. (Walton RE, Torabinejad M: Principles and Practice of Endodontics. Philadelphia, WB Saunders, 1989, p 155.)

irrigation of the root canal. It may be used as it comes from the bottle, or it may be diluted with 1 to 2 parts water.

At the beginning of the procedure, the irrigating solution is placed in a sterile dappen dish. The syringe is filled by immersing the syringe hub in the solution while withdrawing the plunger. This draws the solution up into the chamber of the syringe. The needle is then placed on the threaded hub and the syringe is ready for use.

During treatment, any excess irrigating solution is caught with a gauze square or by using the high volume evacuator (HVE) tip. Caution must be taken not to get the solution on the patient's clothing or skin.

Paper Points

Paper points, which are made of rolled absorbent sterile paper, are also referred to as *absorbent points.*

They are long and narrow and tapered to fit into the root canal. Paper points are used to place medicaments or dry the canal.

Paper points are available in assorted sizes (from coarse to fine) to adapt to the length and shape of the canals that are being treated.

Gutta-Percha Points

Gutta-percha points are slender, tapered, and pointed to fit the contours of the root canal. They are available in various sizes (fine, fine-medium, medium, medium-large, and large). These points are used to seal the treated root canal permanently.

Gutta-percha points may be disinfected by placing them in a cold chemical solution such as sodium hypochlorite. Gutta-percha points *cannot* be autoclaved because the high temperature would melt them, making them useless.

Lentulo Spiral — cement carrier.

Lentulo spirals, also known as *paste fillers*, are small, flexible instruments that are used to carry cement into the prepared root canal. These spirals are available for use as hand-operated instruments or for use in the low-speed handpiece.

Spreaders

A root canal spreader is a hand-operated, smooth, pointed, and tapered metal instrument. When heated, the spreader is used to pack the gutta-percha points (filling material) into the prepared canal space (Fig. 29-6A).

Condensers

Endodontic condensers, also known as *pluggers*, are stainless steel instruments with an elongated and pointed tip. They are used to aid in compressing the filling material when the root canal is being filled (Fig. 29-6B).

Special Care of Endodontic Instruments

Endodontic instruments are flexible and extremely delicate. Should an instrument break within the root canal, apical surgery or the extraction of the tooth may be necessary.

As the instruments are prepared for sterilization, they must be individually checked for any sign of wear, weakness, or fracture. If weakened or fractured, they are discarded.

Although a glass bead sterilizer is used at chairside, this does not replace regular cleaning and sterilization of these instruments after use.

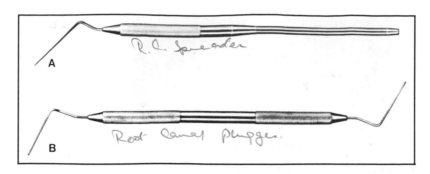

▼ **Figure 29–6**

Root canal spreader and plugger. *A.* Root canal spreader. *B.* Root canal plugger. (Courtesy of Hu-Friedy, Chicago, IL.)

THE ENDODONTIC EXAMINATION

The endodontic examination includes a complete medical and dental history, with emphasis on the current symptoms. Since it may be necessary to use or prescribe antibiotics during treatment, it is particularly important to identify any antibiotic sensitivities the patient may have.

The dentist also performs a visual examination and other specialized diagnostic procedures as indicated.

Radiographs

Periapical radiographs of the tooth in question are important. These radiographs are used for diagnostic purposes and in establishing the "working length" for the tooth.

Each radiograph must be accurate so as not to distort the tooth and must include the surrounding alveolus and periapical tissues.

Percussion

The dentist gently taps the tooth or teeth with a firm object (such as the blunt end of an instrument handle) to determine the extent of sensitivity. (This process is called **percussion**.)

The patient should be warned that if the tissues are inflamed, the tapping of a specific tooth will cause momentary discomfort.

Thermal Sensitivity Testing

To test the reaction of the tooth to cold, a cylinder of ice is placed in a gauze square and is brought into contact with the tooth (Fig. 29–7).

To test the reaction of the tooth to heat, it is touched with a heated instrument, with a mass of heated gutta-percha, or with a stick of heated impression compound (Fig. 29–8).

If the tooth responds painfully to the hot/cold stimulus, an acute abscess may be present.

Transillumination

The anterior teeth may be further examined by placing a fiberoptic light on their lingual surfaces. This light is reflected through the enamel and the dentin.

The dentist will notice if the translucency of the tooth varies from that of the other teeth in the arch, or the light may reveal a fracture of the tooth.

Pulp Vitality Testing

The pulp tester (vitalometer) is a high-frequency electronic instrument that is used to evaluate the vitality and response of the tooth in question (Figs. 29–9 and 29–10).

Because the patient's fear and apprehension could result in inaccurate readings, the use of the

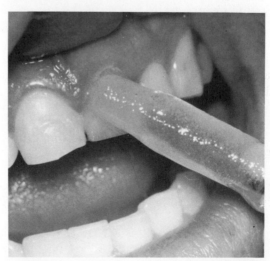

▼ **Figure 29–7**

The reaction of the tooth to cold is tested by the application of an ice stick to the labial surface. (Walton RE, Torabinejad M: Principles and Practice of Endodontics. Philadelphia, WB Saunders, 1989, p 61.)

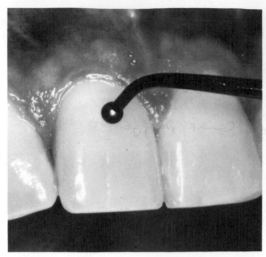

▼ **Figure 29-8**

The reaction of the tooth to heat is tested by the application of a heated ball burnisher to the labial surface. (Walton RE, Torabinejad M: Principles and Practice of Endodontics. Philadelphia, WB Saunders, 1989, p 62.)

test is explained to the patient before it is performed.

A control tooth is tested first to aid the patient in understanding that he will feel only a slight sensation on the tooth being tested. (A **control tooth** is a normal tooth. Preferably, the control tooth should be the same type of tooth in the same arch in the quadrant opposite the one that is affected.)

A tooth that is very sensitive will react more readily than a normal tooth. A tooth with a pulp that is dead or dying will not register at all.

Instrumentation

▼ Cotton rolls.

▼ Warm air syringe.

▼ Vitalometer (pulp tester).

▼ Toothpaste.

Procedure

TESTING PULP VITALITY

1 Assemble the tip into the pulp tester and turn it on.
  The indicator will show that the apparatus is functioning.
  Adjust the indicator to zero (0).

2 Inform the patient that he will feel a slight tingling or a warm feeling as the test progresses.
  Instruct the patient to raise his finger when he feels any sensation and assure him that the test will cease immediately.

3 Isolate the involved teeth with cotton rolls and dry them with warm air. Maintaining a dry field helps to prevent the current from leaking from the tooth to gingival tissues or metallic restorations. If this happens, it may cause an unnecessary and unpleasant sensation for the patient.

4 Apply a small amount of toothpaste to the recessed area on the tip of the pulp tester. The toothpaste serves as a conductor to complete the contact between the tip and the tooth. This complete contact is necessary to produce an accurate reading.

5 Place the tip of the pulp tester in the proper position on the control tooth. The tip must be firm against the tooth enamel at all times.
  Caution: Do not place the tip on a metallic restoration. To do so will cause the patient undue discomfort and result in an incorrect reading.

6 Slowly move the indicator from 0 upward.
  When the patient signals, stop moving the control and record the reading.
  Return the control to 0, and take a second reading on the control tooth. Record this reading.

7 Isolate the tooth suspected of causing the patient discomfort.
  Moisten the tip of the pulp tester with toothpaste, and place it on the enamel of that tooth. Do not place it on a metallic restoration.
  Slowly adjust the control until the patient indicates that he feels sensation.
  Record the reading number of the tooth and return the control to 0.
  After a few seconds, repeat this process to obtain and record a second reading.

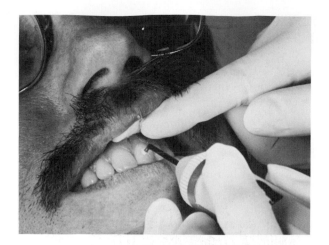

▼ Figure 29–9

Pulp vitality test. Vitalometer tip is placed on the facial surface of a maxillary central incisor. (Torres HO, Ehrlich A: Modern Dental Assisting, 4th Ed. Philadelphia, WB Saunders, 1990, p 666.)

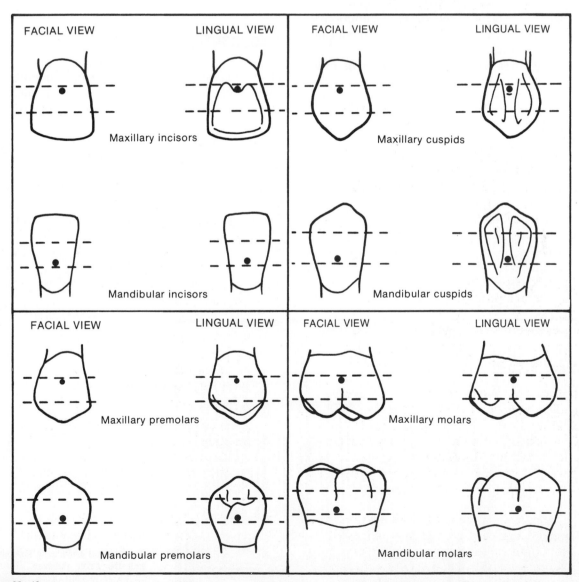

▼ Figure 29–10

Electric pulp testing of teeth. Dot represents approximate spot for placement of the electrode tip on the tooth surface. (The electrode is not placed if there is a metallic restoration present at the site.) (Torres HO, Ehrlich A: Modern Dental Assisting, 4th Ed. Philadelphia, WB Saunders, 1990, p 667.)

STERILE TECHNIQUE IN ENDODONTIC TREATMENT

The use of sterile technique is absolutely essential in endodontic treatment, and the principles of infection control must be followed precisely at all times.

Endodontic Kits and Packs

Endodontic instruments and accessories are frequently prepared in sterile packs or kits. Kits are metal boxes compartmentalized to retain the small endodontic instruments in an orderly fashion (Fig. 29–11).

Sterile Field

A sterile field may be established by draping with a sterile towel on the assistant's cart or endodontic instrument tray. Sterile endodontic instruments are placed on the sterile field.

If the pack was wrapped in a towel, when the pack is opened the *inside* of that towel forms the sterile field for the instruments.

Rubber Dam

The use of a rubber dam is mandatory in endodontic treatment. After it has been placed, the dam and the crown of tooth being treated are disinfected with a solution such as hydrogen peroxide, glutaraldehyde, or an iodophor.

PAIN CONTROL DURING ENDODONTIC TREATMENT

If there is any vitality remaining in the tooth to be treated, the dentist will administer a local anesthetic solution prior to endodontic therapy.

If the tooth is extremely sensitive, it may be necessary to inject additional anesthetic solution directly into the pulp.

If the tooth is nonvital (the pulp is already dead), the use of local anesthetic solution is not indicated. At subsequent visits, after the pulp has been removed, local anesthesia is not usually necessary.

The patient may be given a prescription for medication to control any anticipated postoperative discomfort. This prescription is noted on the patient's chart.

ENDODONTIC TREATMENT

The following are the basic steps in endodontic treatment. Frequently these steps are completed at a single visit. If these are *not* completed at the visit, it is necessary to place "temporary stopping" between visits.

Calcium hydroxide, gutta-percha, zinc oxide–eugenol cement, or a special cement (such as Cavit) may be used for this purpose. The temporary filling is removed when the tooth is reopened for additional treatment at a subsequent visit.

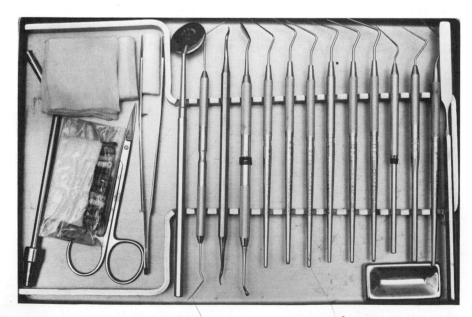

▼ Figure 29–11

Sterile metal endodontic instrument kit with the cover removed. (Torres HO, Ehrlich A: Modern Dental Assisting, 4th Ed. Philadelphia, WB Saunders, 1990, p 673.)

Instrumentation

- ▼ Basic setup.

- ▼ Local anesthetic setup (optional).

- ▼ Rubber dam setup.

- ▼ Disinfecting solution for rubber dam.

- ▼ Handpieces (high and low speed).

- ▼ Tapered fissure or round burs.

- ▼ Gates-Glidden drills *or* broaches (in sizes specified by the dentist).

- ▼ Reamers (sizes specified by dentist).

- ▼ Files (sizes specified by dentist).

- ▼ Millimeter measure.

- ▼ Stops.

- ▼ Luer-Lok syringe.

- ▼ Glass dappen dish.

- ▼ Irrigating solution (sodium hypochlorite diluted with equal parts of water).
- ▼ HVE tip.

- ▼ Paper points (fine, medium, coarse).

Procedure

PREPARING THE CANAL

1. If necessary, local anesthetic solution is administered.

2. The rubber dam is placed so that only the tooth to be treated is exposed. The crown of the tooth and the surface of the rubber dam are swabbed with disinfecting solution.

3. A bur may be used to obtain access to the pulp chamber.

4. The Gates-Glidden drill or barbed broaches (sequentially from the smallest to the largest) are used to open and clean the canals of pulp debris. (This process is called **debridement**.)

5. The working length of the canal is established and the stops are placed on the reamers and files.

6. Reamers and files are used to shape and clean the canals.
    These are used alternately with irrigation of the canals.
    The overflow of the irrigating fluid is caught with a gauze sponge or with the HVE tip.

7. A periapical radiograph is exposed with an instrument in place to verify the measurement of the length of the tooth.

8. When the dentist is satisfied with the canal preparation, the canals are dried by placing sterile paper points carefully into the opening of the tooth. The tooth is now ready to be filled.

Filling the Root Canal(s)

Instrumentation

- ▼ Gutta-percha points (assorted sizes).

- ▼ Isopropyl alcohol.

- ▼ Gauze squares.

- ▼ Cement setup (zinc phosphate cement may be used).

- ▼ Spreaders.

- ▼ Condensers.

- ▼ Lentulo spiral.

- ▼ Paper points.

- ▼ Cotton rolls.

- ▼ Bunsen burner and matches.

Procedure

FILLING THE ROOT CANAL

1. A gutta-percha **trial point** is placed and radiographed. (This is also known as the *master cone*.) The trial point is usually 1 to 1.5 mm short of the apex of the root canal.

2. While preparations are being made to cement the gutta-percha point, a paper point may be placed in the canal(s) to absorb moisture that might accumulate.

3. If zinc phosphate cement is to be used:
   Just prior to use, sterilize the slab and spatula by wiping them with a gauze square moistened with isopropyl alcohol.
   Mix the cement to a consistency similar to that used for the cementation of a cast restoration (see Chapter 20, ''Dental Cements'').
   Pass the lentulo spiral to the operator and hold the slab with the prepared mix close to the patient's chin.

4. The operator dips the lentulo spiral into the cement mix and rotates it to distribute the cement onto the dry walls of the canal.

5. Using the cotton pliers, hold the master cone at a right angle to the pliers.

   Coat the apical third of the cone with cement and pass this to the operator.

6. The operator places the master cone in the canal. Next, additional gutta-percha points may be placed alongside the master cone.

7. The operator uses condensers and spreaders, beginning with the widest and using progressively smaller sizes, to compact the gutta-percha points in the canal until full. The Bunsen burner is used to heat these instruments as necessary.
   By using a heated condenser, the excess gutta-percha material extending from the orifice of the canal is removed flush with the tooth surface.

8. *Optional:* Amalgam or composite restorative material may be used to fill the recessed area at the opening of the canal.

9. The successfully treated tooth will require a permanent restoration such as an onlay, inlay, or a full or veneer crown. The patient is referred back to his regular dentist for the preparation and placement of this permanent restoration.

▼ EXERCISES

1. To provide an accurate measurement of the canal, a stop is placed _____ to the long axis of the instrument.

   a. at an oblique angle
   b. at a right angle
   c. distal
   d. parallel

2. A _____ is used primarily for removing pulp tissue or other soft materials from the root canal.

   a. barbed broach
   b. smooth broach
   c. Hedstrom file
   d. reamer

3. During endodontic treatment, _____ is used to flush out the root canal.

   a. dilute sodium hypochlorite
   b. glutaraldehyde
   c. hydrogen peroxide
   d. iodine

4. During endodontic treatment, the canals are dried with _____ .

   a. cotton points
   b. gentle puffs of warm air
   c. gutta-percha points
   d. a and b

5. _____ is a diagnostic test that involves gently tapping the tooth to determine the extent of sensitivity.

   a. Mobility
   b. Palpation
   c. Percussion
   d. Transillumination

6. A size 10 file is _____ than a size 90 file.

   a. larger
   b. smaller

7. If the tooth responds painfully to hot/cold stimulus, a/an _____ may be present.

   a. acute abscess
   b. deep cavity
   c. irritated pulp
   d. periodontal pocket

8. Local anesthesia _____ indicated during the endodontic treatment of a nonvital tooth.

   a. is
   b. is not

9. When positioning the tip of the pulp tester, it _____ be placed on a metal restoration.

   a. should
   b. should not

10. After being placed, the rubber dam may be disinfected with _____ _____ .

    a. glutaraldehyde
    b. hydrogen peroxide
    c. sodium hypochlorite
    d. a or b

11. _____ are hand-operated instruments with a cutting edge that are used to enlarge the canal during the process of endodontic treatment.

    a. Broaches
    b. Endodontic files
    c. Gates-Glidden drills
    d. Reamers

12. A/An _____ is used at chairside to sterilize files, reamers, and broaches.

    a. dry heat sterilizer
    b. endodontic kit
    c. glass bead sterilizer
    d. hot oil sterilizer

13. When testing pulp vitality, a tooth with a pulp that is dead or dying will _____ .

    a. not respond at all
    b. respond more readily than the control tooth
    c. react more weakly than the control tooth

14. _____ points, also referred to as absorbent points, are available in assorted sizes to adapt to the length and shape of the canals being treated.

    a. Cotton
    b. Gutta-percha
    c. Paper
    d. Silver

15. When creating a sterile field for endodontic treatment, the instruments are placed on the _____ surface of the sterile towel.

    a. inside
    b. outside

16. At the _____ endodontic visit, a bur may be used to gain access to the pulp chamber.

    a. first
    b. second
    c. third

17. The gutta-percha trial point is also known as the master cone.

   a. true
   b. false

18. A glass bead sterilizer may be filled with glass beads or with _____
   _____.

   a. alcohol
   b. glutaraldehyde
   c. sand
   d. table salt

19. The _____d_____ of the tooth is the distance from the reference point to the tip of the root.

   a. apex
   b. master file
   c. test file
   d. working length

20. The slab and spatula used to mix the cement for the final filling of the root
   canal must be sterile.

   a. true
   b. false

30 Oral Surgery

▼ LEARNING OBJECTIVES

The student will be able to:

1. Describe the specialty of oral and maxillofacial surgery.
2. Identify the specialized instruments used in oral surgery.
3. Describe the assistant's role in oral surgery.
4. Describe the steps in a forceps extraction.
5. Provide presurgery and postsurgery instructions to the patient.

OVERVIEW OF ORAL SURGERY

Oral and maxillofacial surgery is the specialty of dentistry that includes the diagnosis and surgical adjunctive treatment of diseases, injuries, and defects involving both the function and esthetic aspects of the hard and soft tissues of the oral and maxillofacial regions.

The most commonly performed oral surgery procedure is the extraction of teeth. Generally, a tooth is extracted only when there are no alternatives (such as endodontic treatment or restorative procedures) by which the tooth can be restored to function in the arch.

SPECIALIZED INSTRUMENTATION FOR ORAL SURGERY

Each of the following specially designed instruments has a place in oral surgery (Figs. 30–1 through 30–5).

Elevators

Periosteal Elevator

The periosteal elevator, also known as a **periosteotome**, is used *prior* to the placement of the surgery forceps to detach the gingival tissues around the cervix (neck) of the tooth and to make a slight separation of the alveolus from the tooth.

The periosteal elevator is designed with a semi-spoon shape to fit under the free gingiva. However, to avoid unnecessary injury to the tissues, the working edges are sharp but slightly rounded, similar to a large spoon excavator (see Fig. 30–1; Figs. 30–4 and 30–5).

Root Elevator

The root elevator is designed to provide access to a fractured root. The handle of the instrument is bulbous and fits firmly in the hand with a palm-grasp.

The elevator nibs may be designed in pairs (right and left) and as *single, straight,* or *mitered*

505

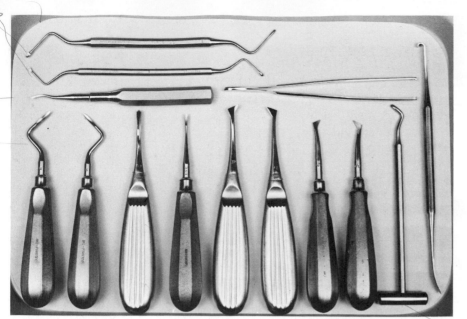

(Handwritten annotations: curette, root pick, rt pick, Root elevator)

▼ **Figure 30–1**

Surgical instruments. Top (*left*): two curettes and a root pick. Top (*right*): tissue forceps. *Left to right:* root picks (left and right pair), large straight elevator, small straight elevator, root elevators (left and right pair), small root elevators (left and right pair), T handle root elevator, a double-ended surgical instrument (the top is a tissue retractor; the bottom is a periosteal elevator). (Torres HO, Ehrlich A: Modern Dental Assisting, 4th Ed. Philadelphia, WB Saunders, 1990, p 821.)

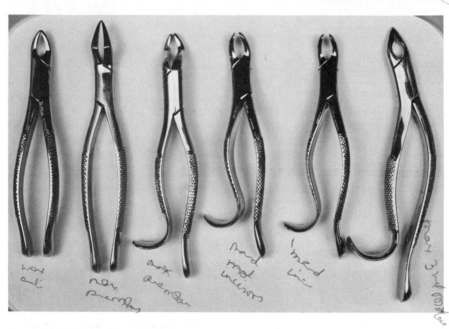

(Handwritten annotations: max ant, max premolar, max premolar, mand root incisors, 1 mand inc, mand 3rd molar)

▼ **Figure 30–2**

Surgical forceps. *Left to right*: maxillary anterior forceps, maxillary premolar forceps, maxillary premolar forceps, mandibular anterior forceps, mandibular molar forceps, maxillary third molar forceps. Note the little finger rest on the four instruments at the right. (Torres HO, Ehrlich A: Modern Dental Assisting, 4th Ed. Philadelphia, WB Saunders, 1990, p 821.)

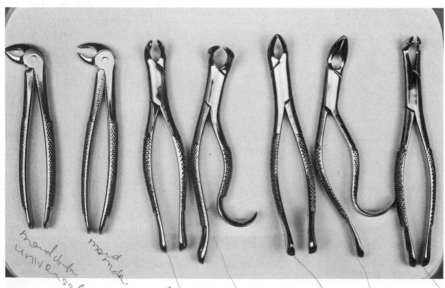

(Handwritten annotations: mand both universal, mand molar, mandibular molar universal, cowhorn mand mo, mand pg, mand molar, mand 3rd)

▼ **Figure 30–3**

Surgical forceps. *Left to right*: bird beak mandibular universal forceps (premolar and molar) (2), mandibular molar universal forceps, cowhorn mandibular molar forceps, mandibular posterior forceps, mandibular molar forceps, mandibular third molar forceps. (Torres HO, Ehrlich A: Modern Dental Assisting, 4th Ed. Philadelphia, WB Saunders, 1990, p 822.)

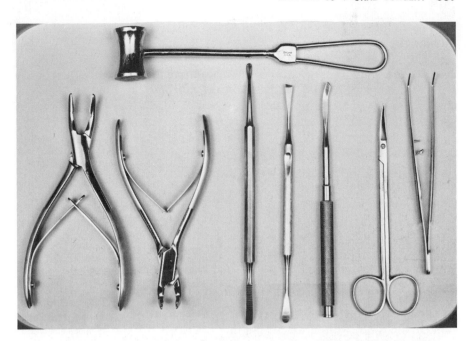

▼ **Figure 30–4**

Assorted surgical instruments. *Top*: surgical mallet. *Left to right*: straight rongeur, curved rongeur, bone file, periosteal elevator, bone chisel, tissue scissors, tissue pliers. (Torres HO, Ehrlich A: Modern Dental Assisting, 4th Ed. Philadelphia, WB Saunders, 1990, p 822.)

nibs. The design of the nib indicates the use of the instrument (see Fig. 30–1). (The **nib** is the working tip of the instrument.)

Tooth Elevator

The tip of the tooth elevator, also known as an **exolever,** is designed to be placed at the crown of an impacted tooth or fractured crown.

The instrument provides leverage to elevate the tooth from its socket and to avoid undue trauma to the tissues. The handle of the tooth elevator may be **T** shaped or rounded to provide the necessary leverage.

The dentist carefully places the rotational force to remove the tooth by literally easing it out of its socket. The action is similar to unscrewing an object from its socket (see Fig. 30–1).

Apical Elevator

An apical elevator, also known as a **root pick,** is designed to remove fractured root tips retained in the apical area of the tooth socket. The shank of the instrument has a slight angle to provide access within the socket (see Fig. 30–1).

An apical elevator may have an added barb on

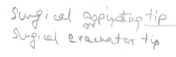

Surgical aspirating tip
or
Surgical evacuator tip

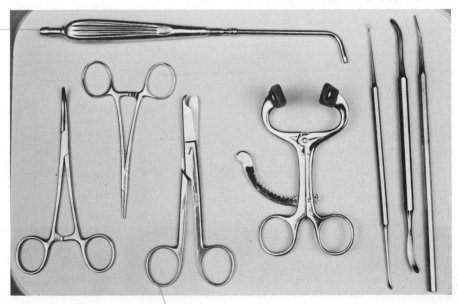

▼ **Figure 30–5**

Surgical instruments and accessories. *Top*: surgical aspirating tip. *Left to right*: curved hemostat, straight hemostat, suture scissors, bite block (mouth prop), double-ended curette and periosteal elevator, double-ended periosteal elevator, bone chisel. (Torres HO, Ehrlich A: Modern Dental Assisting, 4th Ed. Philadelphia, WB Saunders, 1990, p 823.)

Suture scissors

the tip to provide retention in grasping and removing the root tip.

The apical elevator is laid in the socket adjacent to the fractured root tip. The instrument is gently teased and brought slowly toward the oral cavity, not toward the apex of the socket. This action will loosen the root tip and remove it.

If pressure were applied downward in the socket, toward the apex, this might force the root tip out of the socket and into the surrounding alveolus or sinus.

Forceps

Forceps are used for the actual removal of the tooth from its socket after it has been slightly loosened with the elevators. The objective is to remove the tooth without fracturing the root tips.

The handles of forceps are designed for a palm-grasp position and may have a hook on one handle to provide additional leverage by providing placement for the little finger (see Figs. 30–2 and 30–3).

The beaks of the forceps are designed to fit the convexity (curve) of the crown with the nibs of the beaks placed onto the cementum of the tooth just below the cementoenamel junction.

The term **universal** means that the forceps may be used either on the left or right side of one dental arch or in some instances that it may be used on the maxillary or mandibular arch.

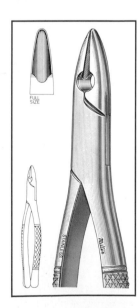

▼ Figure 30–6

Forceps for the extraction of maxillary anterior teeth. (Courtesy of Miltex Instrument Co, Lake Success, NY.)

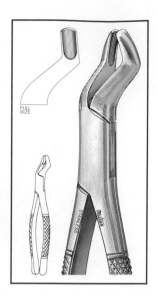

▼ Figure 30–7

Universal forceps for the extraction of maxillary molars. (Courtesy of Miltex Instrument Co, Lake Success, NY.)

Maxillary Anteriors

Several types of forceps used for the extraction of maxillary incisors and cuspids are shown in Figures 30–2 and 30–6.

Maxillary Premolars and Molars

Several types of forceps used for the extraction of maxillary premolars and molars are shown in Figures 30–2 and 30–7. These may be universal (left or right) or provided in pairs (specific to the left and right quadrants).

Mandibular Anteriors

Several types of forceps used for the extraction of mandibular incisors and cuspids are shown in Figures 30–2 and 30–8. Notice that the curve of the beaks is slightly downward when the handles of the forceps are grasped in the palm of the hand.

Mandibular Premolars and Molars

Several types of forceps used for the extraction of mandibular premolars and molars are shown in Figures 30–3 and 30–9. These may be universal (left or right) or provided in pairs (specific to the left and right quadrants).

Children's Teeth

To avoid trauma to the mandible or maxilla, dental forceps are more delicate in design for the extraction of children's smaller teeth (Fig. 30–10).

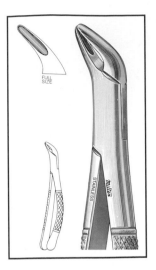

▼ Figure 30-8

Universal forceps for the extraction of mandibular anterior teeth, premolars and roots. (Courtesy of Miltex Instrument Co, Lake Success, NY.)

Curette

A curette has a small spoon-shaped blade, sharpened around the entire margin. The curette is used to remove debris and infectious material (abscess) from the apex of the socket after the tooth has been extracted.

Curettes come in varying sizes, and the shanks are straight or angled to enable the oral surgeon to reach different areas of the mouth. Curettes are often supplied as double-ended instruments (see Figs. 30-1 and 30-5).

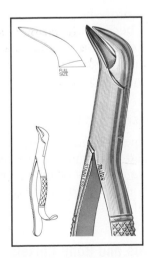

▼ Figure 30-9

Universal forceps for the extraction of mandibular molars. This instrument is commonly referred to as a cowhorn forceps. (Courtesy of Miltex Instrument Co, Lake Success, NY.)

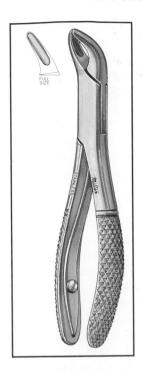

▼ Figure 30-10

Universal forceps for the extraction of primary incisors. Notice the spring handle on this instrument. (Courtesy of Miltex Instrument Co, Lake Success, NY.)

Rongeur

The rongeur is a bone cutting instrument that is similar in design to a forceps. The primary differences are that the rongeur has a spring between the handles and sharpened edges on the blades.

The blade of the rongeur may be end-cutting or side-cutting, depending on the design, and must be kept sharp (see Fig. 30-4).

The rongeur is used only to remove bone such as the sharp edges of the alveolar crest following extraction of the tooth. It is not used during the extraction of the tooth.

After each application of the rongeur, the dentist holds the instrument toward the assistant with the beaks open. To remove any bone fragments on the cutting edge, the assistant wipes the beaks clean with a sterile gauze square.

Bone File

A bone file is a sharp instrument used with a push-pull action (see Fig. 30-4). It is used to remove sharp bone fragments and to file down the rough margins of the alveolus following an extraction and the use of the rongeur.

To prevent pulverized bone or chips from

being left in the wound, careful cleansing of the instrument is necessary after each stroke. To do this, after each stroke, the dentist holds the instrument toward the assistant, who wipes the grooved end with a sterile gauze square.

Scalpel

The scalpel is a surgical knife with a sharp blade. It is designed to make an incision in the soft tissues of the oral cavity. The size and shape of the blade selected depends on the procedure being performed and on the dentist's preference.

Disposable scalpels, which are constructed with a plastic handle and a metal blade, are used once and discarded.

Reusable scalpel handles, which are metal, have blades that fit securely into a handle (see Fig. 30–13). The blade is discarded after a single use. The handle is sterilized prior to use.

Used scalpel blades are "sharps" and must be discarded appropriately (see Chapter 8, "Hazards Management in the Dental Office").

Hemostat and Needle Holder

A **hemostat** is a scissors-like surgical instrument. The blades of the hemostat are not sharp but have serrations, or grooves, to help hold an object or tissue. A mechanical lock on the handle keeps the blades closed so that the object is held securely.

Hemostats may be straight or curved, providing easy access for surgical procedures in various positions in the oral cavity (see Fig. 30–5).

A **needle holder** is a modified hemostat with a distinct groove in the beaks to provide space for placement and retention of the suture needle.

The handles of the hemostat and needle holder are held in place by a ratchet action. To position the hemostat, the beaks are placed on the object and the handles are gently forced together and manually locked.

To reposition the hemostat, one handle of the instrument is forced downward and sideways to release the ratchet and unlock the beaks.

Scissors

Tissue Scissors

Tissue scissors are delicately designed with curved or straight, tapered blades for severing the oral tissue in surgical procedures (see Fig. 30–4).

Suture Scissors

Suture scissors are similar in design but with stronger blades and are designed to cut only sutures (see Fig. 30–5).

Retractors

Tissue Retractors

Many different types of tissue retractors, or tissue pliers, are available. Retractors are used to hold and retract (hold back) tissue firmly during surgical procedures (see Fig. 30–1).

Retractors are always used very carefully to avoid undue trauma or damage to the delicate tissues.

Cheek and Tongue Retractors

These retractors may be large, curved, angled instruments made of metal or a plastic that can withstand sterilization procedures.

Retractors are designed to hold and retract the cheeks, the tongue, or a section of the mucosa during the surgical procedures.

Mouth Props

Mouth props are large angled or lock-type forceps with a rubber-covered extension to be used to prop the patient's mouth open mechanically. The rubber cover provides protection against injury to the enamel of the teeth during placement and removal (see Fig. 30–5).

The mouth prop is of particular importance during surgical procedures performed under general anesthesia because the patient does not have control of muscular action and will involuntarily close his mouth and/or swallow his tongue.

Surgical Burs

Specially designed surgical burs, with extra-long shanks, are used to remove bone and to cut or split the crowns or roots of teeth. These burs are made for both low-speed and high-speed handpieces.

Surgical Mallets and Bone Chisels

Bone chisels are used to remove bone or to split teeth. They must be sharp to be effective (see Figs. 30–4 and 30–5).

Some chisels are designed for use with a hand mallet (see Fig. 30–4). Another type is driven by a special handpiece described as an engine-driven oral surgical mallet.

Surgical Aspirating Unit

The objective of surgical aspiration is to maintain a clear field of operation for the oral surgeon, to increase patient comfort, and to prevent the patient from aspirating debris or fluids into the lungs.

The surgical aspirating unit provides high-power aspiration using a very fine tip, which is used to remove blood from the socket during the surgical procedure. The system may be portable, or it may attach to the central vacuum system.

Because the surgical aspirating tip is so fine and is often slightly curved, it may clog easily (see Fig 30–5). A metal stylet (fine wire) may be needed to keep it open during use and to clean it prior to sterilization.

The high volume oral evacuation system may be used both for oral evacuation and as an aid in retraction of the cheek or tongue as needed throughout the procedure. Aspirating and high volume evacuator (HVE) tips are sterilized prior to use and are included in the surgical pack.

Immediately following the surgery, the vacuum system should be flushed with copious amounts of water or a cleansing solution.

The portable surgical vacuum system has a glass tank to receive surgical fluids. Prior to surgery, the exterior of this tank is covered with a clean towel so that the contents will not be visible. Immediately following surgery, this container must be emptied and cleaned.

Operating Light

The assistant is responsible for adjusting the light to keep the surgical field properly lighted throughout the procedure. As usual, a clean "barrier" is placed on the light handle during operatory preparation.

However, during the procedure, as a further precaution, the assistant may hold a disinfecting wipe when she touches the handle of the light. This wipe is discarded after a single use.

PAIN CONTROL IN ORAL SURGERY

Sedation and Premedication

The trauma of extended surgical procedures may be avoided with the surgeon's cautious application of sedative preparations prior to or during the surgical process.

Sedation may be administered in conjunction with injections of local anesthetic solutions or by inhalation of nitrous oxide–oxygen prior to the initial injection.

Specialized Local Anesthesia Needs

A more profound (deeper) level of local anesthesia may be required in oral surgery than is required for most restorative procedures.

For this reason, additional injections may be made to block peripheral nerves in the surrounding tissues. Also, the surgeon may select a local anesthetic solution formula that has a longer duration.

General Anesthesia

General anesthesia may be indicated for some oral surgery patients. Although general anesthesia may be administered in the dental office, it presents a serious risk to the patient.

To ensure the patient's safety, a second professional (such as an anesthetist or anesthesiologist) who is specially trained in this field may be present to supervise the administration of general anesthesia.

THE CHAIN OF ASEPSIS

Asepsis means sterility, that is, the freedom from pathogenic microorganisms. Establishing and maintaining the chain of asepsis (sterility) means that the instruments, surgical drapes, and gloved hands of the surgical team must be sterile. Once established, the chain of asepsis must *not* be broken.

Contact with anything that is *not sterile* will break the chain of asepsis and will contaminate the surgical area. Therefore, the surgical team should remain in place until the procedure is complete.

Care and Sterilization of Surgical Instruments

The importance of sterility for surgical instruments cannot be overemphasized. Surgery disrupts the natural protective barriers of the soft and hard tissues of the oral cavity. Instruments that are not sterile may cause the surgical site to be contaminated with infectious microorganisms.

▼ If they cannot be cleaned immediately, surgical instruments should be placed in a holding solution so that blood will not dry on the instrument. (Dried blood is difficult to remove.)

▼ Hinged surgical instruments, such as forceps, should be placed in the ultrasonic cleaner in an open position.

▼ The hinge of a surgical instrument should be lubricated *before* the instrument is autoclaved. (Use only a lubricant recommended by the instrument manufacturer.)

▼ Never lock a hinged instrument during autoclaving. (Locking would prevent adequate sterilization and may damage the instrument.)

Surgical Pre-Set Trays

The oral surgeon informs the assistant of the procedure to be performed and any preference for specific instruments.

When selecting the instruments for the surgical tray, it is helpful if the assistant is able to visualize the position of the instruments during use. This helps to ensure that the correct instruments are chosen.

The assistant must be able to select, sterilize, and arrange the materials and instruments in sequence of use on a tray for each oral surgical procedure.

Not having the correct instrument or supplies can create a crisis. If in doubt as to whether an instrument should be included, it is better to include too many rather than to discover that a key instrument is missing.

To prepare a sterile surgical tray, all instruments for the procedure (even those that have already been sterilized) are wrapped and sterilized together.

The pack is opened at the time of surgery, with the instruments left lying on the inside of the wrap, which forms a sterile field.

When the tray is complete, it is covered with the *inside* surface of another sterile towel, which protects it until the time of use.

After surgery all instruments are sterilized again whether or not they were used.

Staff Preparation

Surgical Garb

The surgical team may wear sterile, disposable gowns over their regular office uniforms. They may also wear disposable surgical caps to confine their hair so that it does not contaminate the surgical site.

Hand Preparation and Surgical Gloves

The surgeon and assistant prepare their hands and arms with an intensive surgical scrub. The hands are then dried with a sterile, disposable towel and powdered lightly. Sterile latex gloves are placed over the hands.

The gloves worn during surgical procedures must be *sterile* latex gloves. (The latex gloves worn for routine procedures are clean, but not sterile.)

Once the team members have scrubbed and donned their gloves, it is essential that they not touch anything that is not sterile.

For this reason, the assistant does not scrub until she has completed all preparatory duties such as seating the patient and assembling necessary equipment, instruments, and materials.

FORCEPS EXTRACTION

A forceps extraction is sometimes described as a "simple extraction"; however, this name is misleading. All extractions are surgical procedures. There are no simple extractions—only extractions of increasing difficulty. A forceps extraction is usually performed on a tooth that:

1. Is at least partially erupted.
2. Has a solid, intact crown.

These two factors are important in making it possible for the surgeon to grasp the tooth with the forceps beyond the cementoenamel junction.

Presurgery Instructions to the Patient

Prior to surgery, the patient is seen by the oral surgeon for a presurgery diagnosis and planning visit. At this time, the following presurgery instructions are reviewed with the patient.

1. Get adequate rest prior to oral surgery.
2. If premedication has been prescribed, take it as directed by the dentist.
3. If general anesthesia is indicated, follow directions for not eating or drinking prior to the surgery.
4. Have someone accompany you to the office to drive you home following the surgery.
5. Plan your activities so that you will be able to

rest the remainder of the day following the surgery.

If necessary, the surgeon will request medical records from the patient's physician. The patient must sign a "release of information" form before this request can be made. These records must be received so that the surgeon can review them prior to the scheduled surgery.

The Assistant's Role

Day Before Surgery

1. Check that all patient records and radiographs are complete and in good order.
2. Verify that information has been received from the patient's physician as requested.
3. If a prosthesis is to be placed, check that it has been returned by the laboratory and is placed in a container with sterilizing solution.
4. Determine that the appropriate surgical packs have been prepared and sterilized.

Just Prior to Surgery

1. Establish and maintain the chain of asepsis while preparing the operatory.
2. Determine that the surgical aspirating equipment, nitrous oxide–oxygen unit, and accessories are all in readiness in the operatory.
3. Place an emergency kit in the operatory. If nitrous oxide–oxygen is not available, also place the emergency supply of oxygen.
4. Prepare the equipment, handpieces, surgical tray, and medicaments.
5. Once the surgical pack has been opened, the inner surface of a sterile towel is draped over the instrument tray to maintain sterility until the surgeon is ready to begin the procedure.

Patient Preparation

1. Check with the patient to determine that prescribed premedication was taken as directed. If not, the surgeon should be alerted immediately.
2. Seat and drape the patient. To protect the pa-

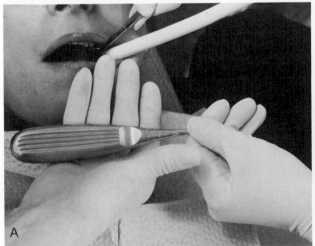
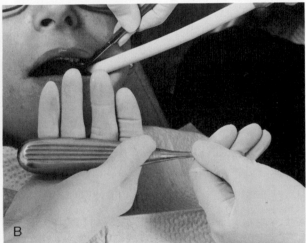
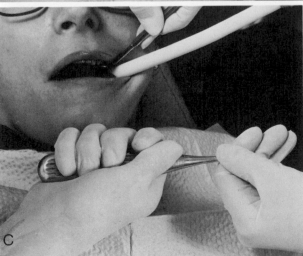

▼ **Figure 30–11**

Instrument exchange in oral surgery. *A.* The assistant grasps the elevator by the "working end" forward in the position of use (palm-thumb grasp). *B.* The assistant firmly places the elevator in the palm of the operator's hand. *C.* The assistant releases the instrument as the operator grasps it securely. (Torres HO, Ehrlich A: Modern Dental Assisting, 4th Ed. Philadelphia, WB Saunders, 1990, p 836.)

tient's clothing, a large plastic drape is commonly used in addition to a patient towel.

3. Adjust the chair into a comfortable reclining position.
4. Allay patient apprehension until the surgeon enters the operatory by staying and conversing with the patient. This is essential if premedication has been administered.

During Surgery

1. Maintain the chain of asepsis.
2. Pass and receive instruments (Figs. 30–11 and 30–12).
3. Aspirate and retract.
4. Maintain a clear operating field with adequate light.

5. Steady the patient's head and mandible if necessary.
6. Observe the patient's condition and anticipate the surgeon's needs.

Instrumentation

▼ Local anesthetic setup.

▼ Basic setup.

▼ Cotton-tipped swabs.

▼ Disinfecting solution (usually an iodine solution, such as Betadine).

▼ Periosteal elevator.

▼ Elevator (of operator's choice).

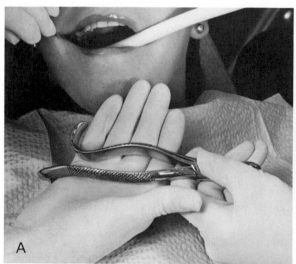
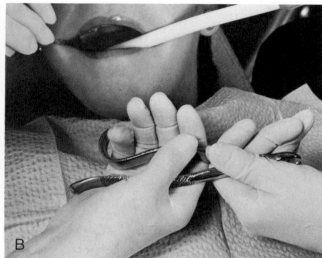
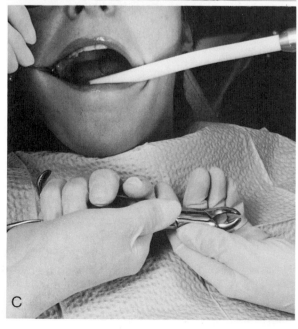

▼ **Figure 30–12**

Forceps exchange in oral surgery. *A.* The assistant grasps the forceps near the "working end" and places it firmly in the operator's hand toward the position of use. *B.* The hook on the handle is placed around the operator's little finger. This provides additional leverage during the tooth extraction. *C.* The assistant releases the forceps as the operator grasps it securely. (Torres HO, Ehrlich A: Modern Dental Assisting, 4th Ed. Philadelphia, WB Saunders, 1990, p 837.)

Procedure

A FORCEPS EXTRACTION

1. Using a pointed instrument, such as an explorer, the surgeon checks to be certain that there is adequate anesthesia of the gingival tissues and periodontium.

2. The patient is warned that he may feel some pressure during the extraction.

   The patient is also warned that he may hear grating or cracking sounds during the procedure.

3. The immediate area of the extraction is swabbed with disinfecting solution.

4. Using a periosteal elevator, the surgeon gently loosens the gingival tissue and compresses the alveolar bone surrounding the tooth cervix of the tooth.

   Optional: If indicated, the surgeon may use a scalpel to make an incision to prevent tearing the tissues.

5. If indicated, the surgeon may use a tooth elevator to loosen the tooth prior to placement of the forceps.

6. Extraction forceps are selected to provide good access and a firm grip on the tooth at the upper third of the root below the cementoenamel junction.

   The beaks of the forceps are placed parallel to the long axis of the tooth so that they firmly grip the crown at the cementoenamel junction.

7. The tooth is luxated in the socket to compress the bone and enlarge the socket. When this is complete, the tooth can be freely lifted, not pulled, from the socket (*Luxate* means to rock back and forth.)

8. The extracted tooth is examined to be certain that the root has not been fractured and left in the socket.

9. If the root tip has fractured, the surgeon uses root picks and root elevators to remove the fragments.

   The assistant vacuums the socket frequently to keep the root tip visible. If the suction loosens the root tip, it is removed from the aspirating tip and reassembled with the extracted tooth root to be certain that all fragments have been removed.

10. If indicated, sutures are placed to close the surgical site.

11. Several sterile gauze squares are folded into a tight pad to form a pressure pack.

    The cheek is retracted and the folded gauze is placed over the extraction site and out toward the lips or cheek (not over the tongue).

12. The patient is instructed to bite on the pack for at least 30 minutes to control the bleeding and to aid in clot formation. The patient is discouraged from talking while these packs are in place.

▼ Forceps (of operator's choice).

▼ Sterile gauze squares for pressure pack.

▼ Surgical scalpel (optional).

▼ Sutures (optional).

▼ Rongeur (optional).

▼ Bone file (optional).

▼ Surgical aspirator tips for HVE.

▼ Suture scissors.

IMMEDIATE POSTOPERATIVE CARE

Instructions to and Dismissal of the Patient

Following the directions of the dentist, the assistant will provide the postsurgical instructions to the patient. Instructions for home care should be provided both in verbal and in written form.

The individual accompanying the patient is also given the home care instructions. If the patient is given a prescription, the purpose and administration of the medication are also reviewed.

The patient may be given a written appointment card showing the day, date, and time that he is to return for a postoperative surgical checkup or for suture removal.

Control of Bleeding

The patient is given the following instructions regarding the control of bleeding:

▼ A pressure pack made of folded sterile gauze squares has been placed over the socket to control bleeding and to encourage clot formation and healing.

▼ Keep the pack in place for at least another 30 minutes. If the compress is removed too soon, this will disturb clot formation and may increase bleeding.

▼ If bleeding has not stopped when the original pack is removed, use the extra sterile gauze squares you were given to create and place an additional pressure pack.

▼ If bleeding continues, moisten a tea bag (which contains tannic acid), place it in a sterile gauze square, and place it over the surgical site. Bite firmly for about 20 minutes to apply pressure.

▼ If bleeding increases or does not stop, call the dental office.

▼ It is recommended that you limit your activities for a few days to avoid strenuous work or exercise. This recommended rest is to avoid hemorrhage at the site of surgery.

Control of Swelling

The patient is given the following instructions regarding the control of swelling:

▼ During the first 24 hours, a cold pack (an ice bag covered with a towel) is usually placed in a cycle of 20 minutes on and 20 minutes off. Cold slows the circulation in these tissues and helps to control swelling.

▼ After the first 24 hours, external heat may be applied to the surgical area. Heat increases the circulation in these tissues and promotes healing.

▼ After the first 24 hours, gently rinse the oral cavity with warm saline solution every 2 hours. (The percentage of salt in the solution should be approximately 1 teaspoon of salt to 8 ounces

of warm water. A stronger solution will irritate the tissue.)

Control of Pain

Analgesics, most commonly in the form of aspirin, are used to control minor discomfort following oral surgery.

If the patient is in extreme discomfort, stronger analgesics may be prescribed by the dentist. A record of this prescription is placed in the patient's chart.

Control of Infection

Antibiotics are administered to control any infection following surgery. Before prescribing, the dentist must study the patient's medical history to determine any sensitivity to antibiotics that the patient may have.

A form of **penicillin** is frequently used for gram-positive infections of the oral cavity. However, penicillin causes a severe allergic reaction in some patients.

Erythromycin is effective against gram-positive organisms; however, gastrointestinal disturbances may occur in patients who are given erythromycin.

A copy of the antibiotic prescription is placed in the patient's chart and noted on the treatment record.

Postoperative Visit

A postoperative visit may be scheduled so that the dentist can check on healing and, if necessary, remove the sutures.

After extensive surgery, the oral surgeon may request postsurgical radiographs to ascertain the removal of the pathologic condition and the extent of wound healing.

Within 6 to 8 weeks following surgery, the formation of regenerative bone may be detected on the radiograph.

SUTURES

As a rule, if a scalpel has been used, sutures will be needed. Sutures are placed using a suture needle and suture material (Fig. 30–13).

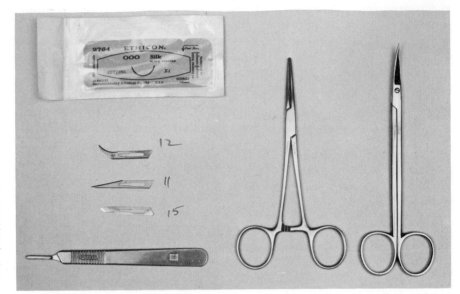

▼ **Figure 30–13**

Pre-set tray for scalpel use and suture placement. *Left* (top to bottom): sterile sutures, assorted scalpel blades, reusable scalpel handle. *Right (side of tray):* straight hemostat (for holding the suture needle) and curved scissors (for cutting tissues or sutures). (Torres HO, Ehrlich A: Modern Dental Assisting, 4th Ed. Philadelphia, WB Saunders, 1990, p 843.)

Suture Placement

Suture needles are curved, with sharp points and edges, and come in various sizes. The curvature of the needle makes it possible for the point of the needle to enter and leave the tissue in a small area.

Gut (organic) suture material is absorbed by the body and does not require removal. It may be used if suture placement is needed in a deeper area that is inaccessible for suture removal.

Nylon or silk sutures, the type commonly used in dentistry, are not absorbed by the body and must be removed once initial healing has occurred.

Prethreaded disposable suture needles are available in sterile packages and are ready for use.

A needle holder or hemostat may be used to hold the needle during suture placement.

Instrumentation

▼ Basic setup.

▼ Sterile prethreaded sutures and needle.

▼ Needle holder.

▼ Suture scissors.

▼ Sterile gauze squares, 2 × 2 inch.

Procedure

SUTURE PLACEMENT

1. The assistant locks the threaded suture needle in the needle holder and passes it to the surgeon. For access to the tissue, the needle is usually placed at a right angle to the hemostat.

2. The assistant retracts the tongue or cheeks to provide a clear line of vision as the surgeon places the sutures.

3. Following the tying of each suture, the as-sistant may be directed to use the suture scissors to cut the sutures, leaving approximately 2 to 3 mm of suture material beyond the knot.

4. The used suturing supplies are received from the surgeon and replaced on the surgical tray.

5. The assistant notes on the patient's chart the number and type of sutures placed.

Suture Removal

The nylon or silk suture is removed approximately 3 to 5 days after surgery, provided that adequate healing has taken place.

Instrumentation

▼ Basic setup.

▼ Cotton-tipped applicators.

▼ Surgical gauze squares, 2 × 2 inches.

▼ Antiseptic solution for irrigation (optional).

▼ Solution for disinfecting surgical site.

▼ Suture scissors.

▼ Cotton pliers.

Procedure

SUTURE REMOVAL

1 Examine the surgical site to evaluate healing. If healing is satisfactory, the sutures may be removed.

2 Swab the wound with an antiseptic solution to remove any debris. (An alternative is to irrigate the site.)

3 Use cotton pliers to hold the suture gently away from the tissue to expose the attachment of the knot.

4 Gently slip one blade of the suture scissors (which are held in the other hand) under the suture. Cut the suture near the tissue.

5 Use the cotton pliers to grasp the knot and gently slide the suture out of the tissue. Take care not to pull the knot through the tissue because this will cause unnecessary discomfort to the patient.

6 Count the sutures that have been removed and compare this with the number indicated on the patient's treatment record.

7 If there is bleeding, the surgical area may be irrigated again with the antiseptic solution. An alternative is to place a compress on the surgical site to encourage clotting.

▼ EXERCISES

1. A/An _____ is used to detach the gingival tissues around the neck of the tooth.

   a. curette
   b. elevator
   c. periosteal elevator
   d. rongeur

2. The handle of a root elevator is _____ .

   a. bulbous
   b. hinged
   c. serrated

3. The beaks of the forceps are designed to fit the ___Convexity___ of the tooth crown.

   a. apex
   b. cervix
   c. concavity
   d. convexity

4. The term universal means that the forceps may be used ___(d)___ _____ .

   a. in pairs
   b. on the left side of the dental arch
   c. on the right side of the dental arch
   d. b and c

5. The forceps used to extract _____ anterior teeth have a slight downward curve of the beaks.

   a. mandibular
   b. maxillary

6. The hook on the handle of some forceps provides ___a___ _____ .

   a. additional leverage
   b. an improved palm grasp
   c. an improved palm-thumb grasp

7. Nylon and silk sutures ___b___ _____ absorbed by the body.

   a. are
   b. are not

8. The working end of a rongeur is ___Sharp___ _____ .

   a. serrated
   b. sharp
   c. smooth

9. If a scalpel is used, ___d___ _____ will be needed.

   a. a bone file
   b. a curette
   c. antibiotics
   d. sutures

10. To lock a hemostat, the handles are _____ a _____.

    a. forced downward and sideways
    b. gently forced together
    c. twisted clockwise
    d. twisted counterclockwise

11. Used scalpel blades are _____ a _____.

    a. discarded as sharps
    b. disinfected
    c. sterilized
    d. b or c

12. A _____ a d t _____ has a ratchet type lock handle but does not have a sharp edge.

    a. hemostat
    b. needle holder
    c. rongeur
    d. a and b

13. During surgery, _____ c _____ are worn.

    a. latex gloves
    b. overgloves
    c. sterile latex gloves
    d. a and b

14. _____ b) _____ means sterility, that is, the freedom from pathogenic microorganisms.

    a. Asepis
    b. Sepsis

15. The surgical aspirating tip may be unclogged by _____.

    a. rinsing it with solution of sodium hypochlorite
    b. rotating the tip against the tissues
    c. turning the unit off
    d. using a metal stylet

16. To control immediate postoperative bleeding, a/an _____ may be used.

    a. heating pad
    b. ice pack
    c. pressure pack
    d. a and c

17. Before use, the glass tank of the portable surgical vacuum system is _____.

    a. autoclaved
    b. covered with a towel
    c. lined with plastic

18. After the surgical pre-set tray has been opened prior to use, the surface is covered with ———————————.

    a. a clean patient towel
    b. a fresh plastic barrier
    c. the inside surface of a sterile towel
    d. the outside surface of a sterile towel

19. The assistant scrubs and dons gloves ——————————.

    a. after the instruments and operatory are ready
    b. after the patient has been seated
    c. prior to seating the patient
    d. a and b

20. To control swelling in the first 24 hours, the patient should use ——————————.

    a. a moistened tea bag
    b. cold
    c. heat
    d. mouth rinses

Abrasion—Wearing, grinding, or rubbing away by friction.

Abscess—A localized collection of pus in a limited area.

Abscess, periapical—A localized area of pus formed at the apex of the root tip.

Abscess, periodontal—A localized area of pus, found in the periodontal tissues.

Abutment—A tooth, root, or implant used for the retention of a fixed or removable prosthesis. Also known as a *retainer*.

Acid etch—Treating tooth structure with an etching solution to provide retention for sealants, cements, restorative materials, or orthodontic brackets.

Acrylic—An organic resin from which various types of dental appliances, retainers, and devices are constructed.

Acute—Having a short and relatively severe course, as opposed to chronic.

Acute necrotizing ulcerative gingivitis (ANUG)—A painful, progressive bacterial infection of the gingiva.

Adhesion—The state in which two surfaces are secured together by chemical forces, mechanical interlocking forces, or both.

Aerobes—A variety of bacteria that must have oxygen in order to grow.

AIDS—Acquired immunodeficiency syndrome.

Alginate—The impression material most commonly used to create diagnostic casts.

Alloy—A substance consisting of two or more metals.

Alveolar bone—That part of the alveolar process that lines the sockets into which the roots of the teeth are affixed.

Alveolar mucosa—The mucous membrane covering the basal part of the alveolar process and continuing to form the lining of the cheeks and the floor of the mouth.

Alveolar process—The extension of the maxilla and mandible that surrounds and supports the teeth and forms the dental arches.

Alveolar socket—The cavity within the alveolar process in which the root of the tooth is held in position.

Alveolectomy—Excision of a part of the alveolar bone to achieve normal ridge contour preparatory to construction of a denture prosthesis.

Alveolitis—Inflammation and infection associated with a disturbance of the blood clot following tooth extraction. Also known as a *dry socket*.

Amalgam—An alloy in which mercury is one of the metals.

Amalgam carrier—A dental hand instrument used to carry and place freshly mixed amalgam in a cavity preparation.

Amalgamation—The process of forming an alloy by mixing mercury with another alloy.

Amalgamator—A device used to mix mercury and the amalgam alloy.

Anaerobes—A variety of bacteria that grow in the absence of oxygen and are destroyed by the presence of oxygen.

Anaerobes, facultative—Organisms that can grow in either the presence or the absence of oxygen.

Analgesics—Drugs that dull the perception of pain without producing unconsciousness. See also *Relative analgesia.*

Anaphylaxis—An allergic reaction that may be immediate, severe, and fatal.

Anatomy—The study of the structure of the body and its parts.

Anesthesia—The loss of feeling or sensation.

Anesthetic—A drug that produces the loss of feeling or sensation.

Angina pectoris—Severe substernal pain that is the result of narrowing of the coronary artery and decreased blood to the heart.

Angle former—A dental hand instrument used to accentuate line and point angles in the internal outline and retention form of a cavity preparation.

Angle, line—The junction of two walls (tooth surfaces) of a cavity preparation.

Angle, point—The junction of three walls (tooth surfaces) of a cavity preparation.

Anode—The electrically positive terminal in an x-ray tube.

Antagonists—Teeth in opposing arches that contact each other.

Anterior—Toward the front.

Anterior teeth—The maxillary and mandibular incisors and cuspids.

Antibiotic—A chemical substance that is able to inhibit the growth of, or to destroy, bacteria and other microorganisms.

Antihistamine—Drugs that counteract the release of histamine in allergic reactions.

Antiseptic—A substance that inhibits or kills microbes.

Apex—The anatomic area at the end of the tooth root.

Aphthous ulcer—A viral infection that causes recurring outbreaks of blister-like sores inside the mouth and on the lips.

Apical—Pertaining to the apex.

Apical curettage—Surgical removal of infectious material surrounding the apex of a tooth root.

Apicoectomy—The surgical removal of the apical portion of the tooth through a surgical opening made in the overlying bone and gingival tissues.

Appliance—A device used to provide function or therapeutic effect.

Arch—See *Mandibular arch* and *Maxillary arch.*

Articular disc—A cushion of tough specialized connective tissue within the temporomandibular joint. Also known as the meniscus.

Articulation—The contact relationship of upper and lower teeth as they move against each other.

Articulator—A mechanical device that represents the temporomandibular joints to which upper and lower casts of the dental arches may be attached to simulate mouth functions.

Artifact—A structure or appearance that is not normally present in the radiograph. Artifacts are produced by artificial means.

Asepsis—Absence of pathogenic microorganisms.

Attrition—Loss of tooth structure due to wear.

Atypical gingivitis—See *Gingivitis, HIV.*

Autoclave—A sterilizing device employing steam under pressure.

Avulsed—Torn away. Extraction by force. Also referred to as *evulsed.*

Bacteria—One-celled microorganisms with certain characteristics. Some, but not all, are pathogens.

Base—The layer of cement that acts as an insulator and protective barrier under a restoration.

Bevel—A slanting of the enamel margins of a tooth preparation. A cut with an angle of more than 90 degrees with a cavity wall.

Bicuspid—See *Premolar.*

Bifurcation—The anatomic area where roots divide in a two-rooted tooth.

Bilateral—Pertaining to both sides.

Binangle—An instrument having two off-setting angles in its shank.

Bite—An occlusal record of the relationship between the upper and lower teeth.

Blade—The sharpened working end of a dental hand instrument.

Bonding—The force by which a substance is secured in intimate contact with another substance. Bonding may be mechanical, chemical, or physical.

Bracket—A small attachment used to fasten the arch wire to the teeth or to the orthodontic bands.

Bridge—A prosthetic device consisting of artificial teeth (pontics) that is supported by cementing it to abutment teeth.

Broach—An instrument with barbs protruding from a metal shaft. Used in endodontic treatment.

Bruxism—The involuntary grinding or clenching of the teeth that damages both tooth surface and periodontal tissues.

Buccal—Pertaining to or adjacent to the cheek.

Bur—A rotary cutting instrument made of steel or tungsten carbide manufactured with cutting heads of various shapes and sizes.

Bur, friction-grip—A bur with a smooth shank that is held in place in the chuck of a handpiece.

Bur, latch-type—A bur with a notched shank that fits into a latch-type contra-angle handpiece.

Burnish—The process of smoothing a metal surface by rubbing.

Burnisher—A dental hand instrument used to smooth the edges at the margin of a metal restoration and the tooth surface.

Calculus—A hard mineralized deposit attached to the teeth.

Canal—The pulp chamber of a root.

Canine—See *Cuspid.*

Canker sore—See *Aphthous ulcer.*

Capsule—A fibrous sac that encloses a joint and limits its action. Also a gelatinous structure that surrounds some bacteria.

Caries—Dental decay. An infectious disease that progressively destroys tooth substance.

Cartilage—A flexible, white tissue around the ends of bones and joints.

Carver—An instrument used to shape a plastic material such as amalgam or wax.

Cassette—A light-proof container with intensifying screens in which extraoral x-ray films are placed for exposure to x-ray radiation.

Cast—Replica of the teeth or dental arch that is used as a working model.

Casting—The result of filling a mold with molten metal.

Cavity—A decay lesion or hole in a tooth.

Cavosurface, angle—An angle in a cavity preparation formed by the junction of the wall of the cavity with the exterior tooth surface.

CDA—Certified dental assistant. One who has

passed the Dental Assisting National Board (DANB) examination in chairside assisting.

Cementoenamel junction (CEJ) — The junction of the enamel of the crown and the cementum of the root at the cervix of the tooth.

Cementum — The substance covering the root surface of the tooth.

Centric occlusion — When the jaws are closed in a position that produces maximal stable contact between the occluding surfaces of the maxillary and mandibular teeth.

Ceramics — The art of making dental restorations from fused porcelain.

Cervical erosion — The wearing away of cementum that has been exposed as a result of gingival recession.

Cervix — Neck. The neck of a tooth at the cementoenamel junction.

Chisel — An instrument for cutting or cleaving tooth structure in the preparation of cavities.

Cingulum — A bulge or prominence of enamel found on the cervical third of the lingual surface of an anterior tooth.

Clasps — The attachments of a partial denture that grasp the natural teeth.

Cleoid — A carving instrument with a blade shaped like a pointed spade. Claw-like.

Coagulant — An agent that promotes the clotting of blood.

Cocci — Spherical or bead-shaped bacteria.

College pliers — See *Cotton pliers.*

Collimation — The elimination of peripheral radiation.

Composite — Resins used for tooth-colored dental restorations.

Concave — Inward curvature.

Condensation — The insertion and compression of a dental material into a prepared cavity.

Condenser — A dental hand instrument used to pack plastic-type restorative material into a cavity preparation.

Contour — The shape, form, or surface configuration of an object.

Contra-angle — An instrument having two or more off-setting angles. See also *Handpiece.*

Convex — Outward curvature.

Core — The central part. In a post and core restoration, the core is the portion that extends above the gingiva.

Cotton pliers — Pliers designed with plain or serrated points that are used as part of the basic dental setup. Also known as *college pliers.*

Crown, anatomic — The portion of the tooth that is covered with enamel.

Crown, cast — A cast restoration that covers the entire portion of a tooth that is normally covered with enamel.

Crown, clinical — The portion of the tooth that is visible in the mouth.

Curettage — Scraping or cleaning with a curette.

Curette — A hand instrument with a sharpened curved blade that is used with a scraping motion.

Curing — The act of polymerization of a chemical compound.

Cusp — A pointed or rounded eminence on the surface of a tooth.

Cusp of Carabelli — The "fifth" cusp located on the lingual surface of many maxillary first molars.

Cuspid — An anterior tooth with long thick root.

Dappen dish — A small clear glass mixing vessel.

Decay — See *Caries.*

Dentin — The material forming the main inner portion of the tooth structure, the crown, and the root.

Dentinocemental junction — The line of union of the cementum and dentin of the tooth.

Dentition — Natural teeth in the dental arch.

Denture — A substitute for missing teeth. May be complete (full) or partial.

Denture, duplicate — A second denture intended to be a copy of the original.

Dew point — The temperature at which condensation occurs.

Diagnosis — Recognizing a departure from normal, and distinguishing one disease or condition from another.

Diastema — An abnormal space between two adjacent teeth in the same arch, usually found between the maxillary central incisors.

Die — A replica of a single tooth or several teeth on which a restoration is fabricated.

Diplococci — Pair-forming cocci.

Direct technique — See *Technique, direct.*

Disc — Rotary instruments made of various abrasive materials, commonly using a metal or paper backing.

Disclosing solution — A coloring agent applied to the teeth to reveal dental plaque.

Discoid — A spoon-shaped instrument with a cutting edge around the total periphery.

Disinfectant — An agent used to kill pathogenic microorganisms without necessarily sterilizing the material.

Disinfection — The process of killing pathogenic agents by chemical or physical means. It does not include the destruction of spores and resistant viruses.

Distal — Away from the midline.

Dorsum — The upper surface of the tongue.

Droplet infection — See *Infection, droplet.*

Dry socket — See *Alveolitis.*

Edentulous — Without teeth. Usually meaning having lost all natural teeth.

EFDA — Extended function dental auxiliary. Also known as an *expanded function dental auxiliary.*

Embrasure — A V-shaped space in a gingival direction between the proximal surfaces of two adjoining teeth in contact.

Emesis basin — A kidney-shaped receptacle for fluids.

Enamel — The hard tissue that covers the anatomic crown of the tooth.

Epinephrine — A vasoconstrictor.

Equilibration — The act of putting the mandible in a state of balance with the maxilla.

Erosion — The superficial wearing away of tooth substance not involving bacteria.

Eruption — The migration of a tooth into functional position in the oral cavity.

Etchant — The acid solution or gel used to etch tooth structure.

Eugenol — A pale-colored liquid obtained from clove oil and other natural sources.

Evulsed — See *Avulsed.*

Excavator, spoon — A dental hand instrument with a sharp, bowl-shaped edge that is used to remove carious dentin.

Excursion — Movement of the mandible from the centric position to a lateral or protrusive position.

Exodontics — The science and practice of removing teeth.

Exothermic — The heat given off during a chemical reaction.

Explorer — A dental hand instrument with a fine tip that is used to detect caries and rough areas on the tooth surface.

Exposure — Uncovering, as in exposing a pulp via the opening in the wall of the pulp chamber. Also, when producing a radiograph, exposing the dental film and tissues to ionizing radiation.

Extrude — The migration of a tooth out of its normal occlusal position as a result of absence of opposing occlusal force, as when the contacting tooth in the opposite arch has been lost. Also, to force out, that is, dispensing impression material from an extruder gun.

Fabrication — Constructing or making a restoration.

Face bow — A caliper-like device that is used to record the relationship of the maxilla and mandible to the temporomandibular joints and to orient the models of both in this same relationship on an articulator.

Facial — Refers collectively to both the labial and the buccal surfaces of the teeth.

Facultative anaerobes — See *Anaerobes, facultative.*

Fauces — See *Pillars of fauces.*

Festooning — The carving of the base material of a denture to simulate the contours of the natural tissues being replaced.

File — A metal instrument with ridges or teeth on its cutting surfaces.

Finish line — The point at which the cavity preparation meets the external surface of the tooth.

Fissure — A deep groove or cleft, commonly the result of the imperfect fusion of the enamel.

Flange — The parts of the denture base that extend from the cervical areas of the teeth to the border of the denture.

Flash — Excess material that is squeezed out of a mold.

Fluorosis — Mottled enamel caused by excessive fluoride intake.

Foramen — A natural opening in bone or other structure.

Forceps — An instrument used for grasping or applying force to teeth, tissues, or other instruments.

Form, convenience — The methods used to gain access to the cavity preparation for the insertion and finishing of the restorative material.

Form, outline — The curved shape and border of the restoration and of the tooth.

Form, resistance — The form and thickness given to the tooth enamel, dentin, and restoration to prevent displacement or fracture of either structure.

Form, retention — The shape given to the tooth surfaces (cavity walls) to prevent the dislodgment of the restoration.

Fossa — A hollow, grooved, or depressed area in a bone or tooth. (Plural, *fossae.*)

Fracture — To break apart or rupture.

Framework — The metal skeleton that provides a basic support for the saddle and the connectors of the removable partial denture.

Frenum — A fold of mucous membrane attaching the cheeks and lips to the upper and lower arches, in some instances limiting the motions of the lips and cheeks. (Plural, *frena* or *frenula.*)

Fulcrum — The point or support on which a lever turns.

Gag reflex — Protective mechanism located in the posterior of the mouth. Contact with this area causes gagging, retching, or vomiting.

Gagging—The retching action caused by touching the posterior area (soft palate) of the mouth.

Gauges—Instruments used to measure dimensions.

Generic—Those drug (product) names that any business firm may use.

Germicide—A solution capable of killing all microorganisms except spores.

Gingiva—The mucous membrane tissue that immediately surrounds a tooth. (Plural, *gingivae*.)

Gingiva, attached—The portion of the gingiva extending from the gingival margin to the alveolar mucosa.

Gingiva, free—That part of the gingivae that surrounds the tooth and is not directly attached to the tooth surface.

Gingival curettage—The removal of soft tissue constituting the pocket wall by scraping with periodontal instruments.

Gingival margin—The most coronal portion of the gingiva surrounding the tooth.

Gingival margin trimmer—A dental hand instrument designed to bevel the cervical cavosurface walls of the cavity preparation.

Gingival sulcus—The shallow furrow formed where the gingival tip meets the tooth enamel.

Gingivectomy—The excision of the soft tissue wall of the periodontal pocket when the pocket is not complicated by extension into the underlying bone.

Gingivitis—Inflammation of the gingiva characterized clinically by changes in color, gingival form, position, surface appearance, and the presence of bleeding and/or exudate. Also known as *Type I periodontal disease.*

Gingivitis, HIV—Inflammation of the gingiva characterized by a bright red linear border along the free gingival margin. Also known as *atypical gingivitis.*

Gingivoplasty—The procedure by which gingival deformities (particularly enlargements) are reshaped and reduced to create normal and functional form.

Glutaraldehyde—A high-level disinfectant.

Gram-negative bacteria—Bacteria that are not stained by Gram stain.

Gram-positive bacteria—Bacteria that are stained by Gram stain.

Handpiece, contra-angle—An extension attached to a low-speed handpiece to form an offset angle.

Handpiece, high-speed—A dental handpiece that rotates at a speed between 100,000 and 800,000 rpm.

Handpiece, low-speed—A dental handpiece that rotates at a speed between 6000 and 10,000 rpm.

Handpiece, right-angle—An extension attached to a low-speed handpiece to form a right angle.

Handpiece, straight—A low-speed handpiece that may be used to hold rotary instruments that is most commonly used in the dental laboratory.

Hatchet—An angled hand-cutting instrument used to develop internal cavity form.

Hemorrhage—An abnormal loss of large quantities of blood.

Hemostat—A scissors-like surgical instrument with a static-type lock used to help hold an object or tissue.

Hepatitis A—An inflammation of the liver transmitted through contact with contaminated food or water. Also known as *infectious hepatitis.*

Hepatitis B—A viral infection of the liver. Also known as *serum hepatitis.*

Hepatitis C—A viral infection that is similar to hepatitis B as to mode of transmission and the presence of a carrier state.

Herpes simplex—A viral infection that causes recurrent sores.

Hoe—A dental hand instrument, used with a pull motion, that has the working blade at a right angle to the long axis of the handle.

Homogeneous—A mix with a uniform quality throughout.

HVE—High volume evacuator. Used to remove excess fluids and debris from the oral cavity.

Hypnotic—A drug that produces sleep.

Impaction—Any tooth that remains unerupted in the jaws beyond the time at which it should normally be erupted.

Impaction, bony—A tooth that is blocked by both bone (alveolus) and tissue (mucosa).

Impaction, soft tissue—A tooth that is blocked from eruption only by gingival tissue.

Impression compound—Thermoplastic impression material that is rigid at mouth temperature.

Incisal—Biting edge of an anterior tooth.

Incise—To cut or tear.

Incisive papilla—See *Papilla, incisive.*

Incisor—Anterior teeth with thin and sharp cutting edge.

Index—A core or mold used to record the relative position of a tooth or teeth to one another and/or to a cast.

Indirect technique—See *Technique, indirect.*

Infection, droplet—The type of infection transmitted by the droplets of water such as from sneezing or from handpiece spray.

Infection, self—Infective microorganisms present in the patient's mouth cause infection when they get into the blood stream during dental surgery. The patient infects himself.

Infectious hepatitis—See *Hepatitis A.*

Infiltration—Technique of applying anesthetic solution in the area immediately surrounding the tooth or teeth.

Inlay—A cast restoration prepared outside the mouth and cemented in a cavity preparation that is designed to restore one, two, or three surfaces of the tooth.

Interdental—See *Interproximal.*

Interproximal—Between the proximal surfaces of adjacent teeth.

Invaginate—To fold inward.

Iodophors—Disinfectants that are used in differing strengths as a surgical scrub and as a surface disinfectant.

Ion—An atom or group of atoms that carry a positive or negative electrical charge.

Irreversible—Incapable of returning to the original state.

Kilovolt—Unit of electrical potential equal to 1000 volts.

Labial—Of, or pertaining to, the lip.

Lamina dura—Thin, compact bone lining the alveolar socket.

Lateral—Toward the side.

Lateral excursion—A sliding position of the mandible to the left or right of the centric position, as related to the maxilla.

Leakage—Penetration of fluids between a dental restoration and the surrounding tooth.

Lentulo spiral—A fine, flexible, needle-like instrument capable of being inserted into a small hole.

Ligature—Cord, thread, or stainless steel wire used to bind teeth together or to hold structures in place.

Lingual—Of, or pertaining to, the tongue.

Lobe—A developmental segment of a tooth.

Local anesthesia—Deadening of sensation of a specific area through the administration of a drug that blocks nerve conduction.

Lumen—The space within a tube, such as a blood vessel or needle.

Luting—Bonding or cementing two unlike substances together.

Luxate—To dislocate, bend, or put out of joint.

Malocclusion—When the teeth in the upper and lower jaws do not come together correctly.

Mamelon—A rounded eminence on the incisal edge of a newly erupted incisor.

Mandibular arch—The teeth in position in the alveolar process of the mandible. Also known as the *lower jaw.*

Mandrel—A mounting device with a screw and a threaded end or a snap-on attachment to hold the disc in a dental handpiece.

Margin—In cavity preparations, the outside limit of the preparation.

Matrix—A metal or plastic band used to replace the missing wall of a tooth during placement of the restorative material.

Maxillary arch—The teeth in position in the alveolar process of the maxillae. Also known as the *upper jaw.*

Meniscus—The bottom of the elliptical curve where the water touches the dry side of the container. See also *Articular disc.*

Mesial—Toward the midline.

Microorganism—A living organism so small that it is visible only with a microscope.

Mobility—Movement of the tooth within its socket.

Model—Replica typically made of a gypsum product (a cast).

Molar—A posterior tooth with a broad occlusal surface for chewing.

Monococcus—A single coccus.

Mucosa—A mucous membrane consisting of an outer epithelial layer and a connective tissue layer.

Mucus—Secretions of the mucous membranes.

Nib—The working end or face of a dental hand instrument with a smooth or serrated surface.

Noble metals—Metals that are highly resistant to oxidation, tarnish, and corrosion. The noble metals used in dentistry are **gold** (Au), **palladium** (Pd), and **platinum** (Pt).

Occlusal—The chewing surfaces of the posterior teeth.

Occlusion—The contact between the maxillary and mandibular teeth in all mandibular positions and movements.

Occlusion, centric—See *Centric occlusion.*

Onlay—A cast restoration designed to restore the occlusal surface, the mesial-distal or lingual-facial margins, and frequently two or more cusps of the occlusal surface of a posterior tooth.

Opaque—The ability to block light.

Overbite—Vertical projection of upper teeth over the lowers.

Overhang—Excess restorative material projecting over the cavity margin.

Overjet—Horizontal projection of upper teeth over the lowers.

Over-the-counter drug—Sold or purchased without a prescription.

Palatal—Area involving the palate, or roof of the mouth.

Palate, hard—The bony anterior portion of the roof of the mouth.

Palate, soft—The posterior tissue portion of the roof of the mouth.

Palatine raphe—A narrow whitish streak in the midline of the palate.

Palpation—An examination technique of the soft tissues with the examiner's hand or finger tip.

Papilla—Gingiva filling the interproximal spaces between adjacent teeth. Projections located on the dorsum of the tongue that contain receptors for the sense of taste. (Plural, *papillae*.)

Papilla, incisive—A rounded projection at the anterior end of the palatine raphe.

Partial denture—Prosthetic device containing artificial teeth supported on a framework and attached to natural teeth by means of clasps.

Path of insertion—The lines or grooves parallel to the long axis that permit the rigid metal casting to be seated in the tooth. Also, the direction or path of a removable partial denture that permits the insertion and removal of the prosthesis.

Pathogen—A microorganism capable of causing disease.

Pathology—The study of disease.

Percussion—An examination technique that uses sharp, short blows to the involved tooth with a finger or instrument.

Periapical abscess—See *Abscess, periapical.*

Pericoronitis—An inflammatory process occurring over a partially erupted tooth.

Periodontal ligament—The tissues that support and anchor the tooth in its socket.

Periodontal scaling and root planing—The procedure designed to remove the microbial flora and bacterial toxins on the root surface or in the pocket, calculus, and diseased cementum and dentin.

Periodontitis—Inflammatory and destructive disease involving the soft tissue and bony support of the teeth.

Periodontitis, HIV—Periodontal lesions associated with AIDS. Also known as *AIDS virus–associated periodontitis.*

Periradicular—Around the root.

Pharmacology—The study of drugs, especially as they relate to medicinal uses.

Philtrum—The soft vertical groove running from under the nose to the middle of the upper lip.

Physiology—The study of the functions of the body systems.

PID—Position indicator device, used to direct and restrict the central beam in dental radiographic technique.

Pillars of fauces—The two arches at the back and sides of the mouth.

Pit and fissure—Faults that are the result of noncoalescence of enamel during tooth formation.

Plaque—A soft deposit on the teeth consisting of bacteria and bacteria products.

Post—A post or pin, usually made of metal, fitted into a prepared root canal of a natural tooth to improve retention of a restoration. Also known as a *dowel.*

Post dam—A seal at the posterior of a denture.

Posterior—Toward the back.

Posterior teeth—The maxillary and mandibular premolars and molars.

Premolar—A posterior tooth with points and cusps for grasping, tearing, and chewing.

Process—A prominence or projection of a bone.

Prophy angle—See *Handpiece, right-angle.*

Prophylaxis, oral—A scaling and polishing procedure performed to remove coronal plaque, calculus, and stains to prevent caries and periodontal disease.

Prosthesis—A replacement for a missing body part.

Protrusion—A position of the mandible placed as far forward as possible from the centric position as related to the maxilla.

Proximal—Nearest or adjacent to.

Proximal walls—The tooth surface, mesial or distal, that is nearest to the adjacent tooth.

Psychosedation—See *Relative analgesia.*

Pulp—The vital tissues of the tooth consisting of nerves, blood vessels, and connective tissue.

Pulpal floor—The floor of the cavity preparation, horizontal to the pulpal area of the tooth.

Pulpitis—Inflammation of the dental pulp.

Pumice—Ground volcanic ash that is used for polishing.

Quadrant—One of the four sections, or quarters, of the mouth.

Reamer—An instrument with a tapered metal shaft, more loosely spiraled than a file, used to clean and enlarge a root canal.

Recession—Loss of part or all of the gingiva over the root of a tooth.

Registered dental hygienist (RDH)—A licensed preventive oral health professional who provides educational, clinical, and therapeutic services.

Registration—The record of desirable jaw relations. Also, a form used to gather patient financial information.

Reimplant—Replacing a lost or extracted tooth into the alveolar process (socket).

Relative analgesia—The use of nitrous oxide and oxygen gases to achieve a state of patient sedation.

Retarder—A chemical that decreases the rate of a chemical reaction to allow a longer working time.

Retention—The result of adhesion, mechanical locking, or both.

Retrusion—A position of the mandible as far posterior as possible from the centric position, as related to the maxilla.

Ridge—A linear elevation on the surface of a tooth. Also, the remaining bone of the alveolar process in an edentulous arch.

Ruga—A fold in the mucosal tissue found on the roof of the mouth and in the stomach. (Plural, *rugae.*)

Saddle—The portion of the removable appliance that rests on the oral mucosa covering the alveolar ridge. It also retains the artificial teeth.

Scaling—A treatment procedure necessary to remove hard and soft deposits from the tooth's surface.

Sealant—Resin material used to seal pits and fissures to protect against caries.

Sedatives—Drugs that reduce excitability, create calmness, and allow sleep to occur as a secondary effect.

Self-infection—See *Infection, self.*

Sepsis—The presence of disease-producing microorganisms.

Serum hepatitis—See *Hepatitis B.*

Shaft—The elongated stem of an instrument that is designed for grip and to give leverage.

Shank—The tapered portion of the dental hand instrument between the handle and blade. The portion of a bur that fits into the dental handpiece.

Sinus—An air-filled cavity within a bone.

Slurry—A watery mixture or suspension of insoluble material.

Smear layer—The very thin organic film that is created when dentin and enamel are cut with rotary instruments. The layer of debris that adheres to dentin as a result of cavity preparation.

Spirochetes—Unicellular bacteria that have flexible cell walls, are capable of movement, and have a wave-like or spiral shape.

Spores—Protective form taken by some bacteria in order to withstand adverse conditions.

Staphylococci—Cocci that form irregular groups or clusters.

State Board of Dental Examiners—The administrative board designated to interpret and implement regulations under the State Dental Practice Act.

State Dental Practice Act—The law that contains the legal restrictions and controls on the dentist, dental auxiliaries, and the practice of dentistry within each state.

Sterilization—The process by which all forms of life are completely destroyed within a circumscribed area.

Stippling—A textured effect that is done to simulate the normal gingiva tissue.

Stones—Mounted rotary instruments used for polishing and refining restorations.

Streptococci—Chain-forming cocci.

Sulcus—A groove or depression. (Plural, *sulci.*) See also *Gingival sulcus.*

Supine—Positioned lying on the back with the face up.

Suture—The line where two bones are closely joined. Material used to close a surgical wound or injury with stitches.

Syncope—A temporary loss of consciousness caused by an insufficient blood supply to the brain. Also known as *fainting.*

Technique, direct—Shaping of a wax pattern in the mouth on the prepared tooth itself.

Technique, indirect—Shaping of a wax pattern on a model (die) of a prepared tooth.

Temporary filling—Material used to fill a tooth until cavity preparation or placement of a final restoration.

Temporomandibular joint—The articulation of the mandible with the temporal bone.

Tofflemire—A matrix retainer and band system used to replace the missing wall of a tooth while the restoration is being placed.

Trabecular bone—Bone spicules in cancellous bone that form a network of intercommunicating spaces that are filled with bone marrow.

Tragus—The cartilaginous projection anterior to the external opening of the ear.

Translucency—The relative amount of light transmitted through an object.

Trituration—Process of mixing mercury with amalgam alloy.

Tuberculosis—A disease caused by the tubercle bacillus.

Tuberosity—An elevation or protuberance on a bone.

Ultrasonic scaling—The use of an ultrasonic scaler to remove mineralized deposits from the tooth surfaces.

Undercut—The portion of a tooth that lies between the height of contour and the gingivae.

Universal numbering system—Identification of the teeth by numbering the permanent teeth from 1 to 32. Primary teeth are lettered from A to T.

Vasoconstrictor—Shrinks blood vessels.

Veneer—A layer of tooth-colored material (composite or porcelain) that is bonded or cemented to the prepared tooth surface.

Ventral—Refers to the front or belly side of the body.

Vermilion border—The exposed red portion of the upper or lower lip.

Virulence—The relative capacity of a pathogen to overcome body defenses.

Virus—Submicroscopic infectious agents.

Viscosity—The property of a liquid that causes it not to flow.

Wall, axial—A portion of a prepared tooth near the pulpal area and parallel with the long axis of the tooth.

Wedelstaedt chisel—A dental chisel with a modified curved shank.

Young's frame—A U-shaped metal or plastic frame used to hold rubber dam in place.

REFERENCES

Accepted Dental Therapeutics, 40th ed. Chicago, American Dental Association, 1984.

ADA Council on Dental Materials, Instruments and Equipment: Recommendations in radiographic practices: An update. JADA 119:115–117, 1989.

ADAA Principles of Ethics and Code of Professional Conduct. Chicago, American Dental Assistants Association, 1980.

AIDS: The disease and its implications for dentistry. JADA 15:395–403, 1987.

Air-water spray caution urged. CDA Journal 18(6):13, 1990.

American Dental Association principles of ethics and code of professional conduct. JADA 117:657–661, 1988.

American Medical Association Drug Evaluations, 6th ed. Philadelphia, WB Saunders, 1986.

Amsterdam M: The diagnosis and prognosis of the advanced periodontally involved dentition. CDA Journal 17(9):13–24, 1989.

Angle EH: Treatment of Malocclusion of the Teeth. Philadelphia, The SS White Dental Manufacturing Co., 1907.

Ash MM: Wheeler's Dental Anatomy, Physiology, and Occlusion, 6th ed. Philadelphia, WB Saunders, 1984.

Ash MM: Kerr and Ash's Oral Pathology, 5th ed. Philadelphia, Lea & Febiger, 1986.

Barr CE, Marder MZ: AIDS: A Guide for Dental Practice. Chicago, Quintessence Publishing, 1987.

Barton RE, Matteson SR, Richardson RE: The Dental Assistant, 6th ed. Philadelphia, Lea & Febiger, 1988.

Baum L, Phillips RW, Lund ML: Textbook of Operative Dentistry, 2nd ed. Philadelphia, WB Saunders, 1985.

Begg PR, Kesling PC: Begg Orthodontic Theory and Technique, 3rd ed. Philadelphia, WB Saunders, 1977.

Bell WH, Proffitt RP, Whits RP Jr: Surgical Corrections of Dentofacial Deformities, vols. 1 and 2. Philadelphia, WB Saunders, 1985.

Bohay R, Wood RE: Basic Concepts in Extraoral Radiography. ADAA, Chicago, 1990.

Bonewit K: Clinical Procedures For Medical Assistants, 3rd ed. Philadelphia, WB Saunders, 1990.

Boswell S: What do you say before you say hello? CDA Journal 18(9):25–28, 1990.

Buckalew AT: Care of the oral surgery patient. The Dental Assistant 59(5):14–16, 1990.

Carranza FA Jr: Glickman's Clinical Periodontology, 7th ed. Philadelphia, WB Saunders, 1990.

Carranza FA, Perry DA: Clinical Periodontology for the Dental Hygienist. Philadelphia, WB Saunders, 1986.

Chernega AB: Emergency Guide For Dental Auxiliaries. Albany, NY, Delmar Publishers, 1987.

Christensen GJ: Glass ionomer as a luting material. JADA 120(1):59–62, 1990.

Clemons GP, Reynolds MA, Agarwal S, et al: Current concepts in the diagnosis and classification of periodontitis. CDA Journal 18(5):33–38, 1990.

Cottone JA: Recent developments in hepatitis: New virus, vaccine, and dosage recommendations. JADA 120(5):501–508, 1990.

Crawford JJ: Clinical Asepsis in Dentistry. Mesquite, TX, Oral Med Press, 1987.

Current Procedural Terminology for Periodontics, 5th ed. Chicago, American Academy of Periodontology, 1987.

Davis WL: Oral Histology: Cell Structure and Function. Philadelphia, WB Saunders, 1986.

deLyre W, Johnson AN: Essentials of Dental Radiography for Dental Assistants and Dental Hygienists, 3rd ed. Englewood Cliffs, NJ, Prentice-Hall, 1985.

Dentist's Desk Reference: Materials, Instruments and Equipment, 2nd ed. Chicago, American Dental Association, 1983.

Dietz ER: Pit and fissure sealants. The Dental Assistant 57:11–17, 1988.

Dietz E: Update: Dental office waste management. Dental Economics 80(9):62–67, 1990.

Dorland's Illustrated Medical Dictionary, 27th ed. Philadelphia, WB Saunders, 1988.

Edwards C, Statkiewicz-Sherer MA, Ritenour ER: Radiation Protection for Dental Radiographers. Denver, Multi-Media Publishing, 1984.

Ehrlich A: Nutrition and Dental Health. Albany, NY, Delmar Publishers, 1987.

Exposure and Processing for Dental Radiography. Dental Radiography Series, Health Sciences Publication No. N-413. Rochester, NY, Eastman Kodak Co, 1990.

Facts About AIDS for the Dental Team. Chicago, American Dental Association, 1988.

Farman AG: Normal Radiographic Anatomy of the Teeth and Jaws. Chicago, ADAA, 1990.

Farman AG: Radiographic Pitfalls and Errors. Chicago, ADAA, 1990.

Farman AG: Concepts of radiation safety and protection. The Dental Assistant 60(1):11–14, 1991.

Farman AG, Curran AE: Biologic Effects of Radiation and Radiation Safety and Protection. Chicago, ADAA, 1990.

Farman AG, Curran AE: Film, Darkroom and Processing. Chicago, ADAA, 1990.

Farman AG, Fraunhofer JA: Radiation Physics, the Dental X-ray Machine and Diagnostic Imaging Theory. Chicago, ADAA, 1990.

Fletcher GGT: The Begg Appliance and Technique. London, Wright-PSG, 1981.

Fonseca RJ, Davis WN: Reconstructive Preprosthetic Oral and Maxillofacial Surgery. Philadelphia, WB Saunders, 1986.

Gerstein H (ed): Techniques in Clinical Endodontics. Philadelphia, WB Saunders, 1983.

Gould AR, Farman AG: Diseases of the Teeth and Jaws. Chicago, ADAA, 1990.

Graber LW: Orthodontics: State of the Art, Essence of the Science. St. Louis, CV Mosby, 1986.

Grant DA, Stern IB, Everett FG: Periodontics in the Tradition of Gottlieb and Orban, 6th ed. St. Louis, CV Mosby, 1988.

Grossman LI, Oliet S, Del Rio CE: Endodontic Practice, 11th ed. Philadelphia, Lea & Febiger, 1988.

Handwashing. Dental Product Report 25(2):85–95, 1991.

Holyroyd SV, Wynn RL, Requa-Clark B: Clinical Pharmacology in Dental Practice, 4th ed. St. Louis, CV Mosby, 1988.

Infection control: Fact and reality, a training program for dental offices. ADA News 19(4), 1988.

Infection Control in the Dental Office. Dental Radiography Series, Health Sciences Publication No. N-415. Rochester, NY, Eastman Kodak Co, 1990.

Ionizing Radiation Policy. University of California School of Dentistry, UCSF Medical Center, San Francisco, 1991.

Jablonski S: Illustrated Dictionary of Dentistry. Philadephia, WB Saunders, 1982.

Jacob SW, Francone CA, Lossow WJ: Structure and Function in Man, 5th ed. Philadelphia, WB Saunders, 1982.

Kerr DA, Ash MM, Millard HD: Oral Diagnosis and Treatment Planning, 7th ed. St. Louis, CV Mosby, 1987.

Kratochvil FJ: Partial Removable Prosthodontics. Philadelphia, WB Saunders, 1988.

Landesman HM, Wright WE: A technique for making impressions on patients requiring removable partial dentures. CDA Journal 14(6), 1986.

Langlais RP, Bricker SL, Cottone JA, et al: Oral Diagnosis, Oral Medicine and Treatment Planning. Philadelphia, WB Saunders, 1984.

Laskin DM: Oral and Maxillofacial Surgery, vol. 2. St. Louis, CV Mosby, 1985.

Levine N: Current treatment in dental practice. Philadelphia, WB Saunders, 1986.

Lovelace SE: Prosthodontics. CDA Journal 18(11):31–35, 1990.

Lovelace SE: Oral and maxillofacial surgery. CDA Journal 19(1):43–48, 1991.

Macdonald G: Chemical hazards: Regulations, identification and resources. CDA Journal 17(12):32–34, 1989.

Malamed SF: Handbook of Medical Emergencies in the Dental Office, 3rd ed. St. Louis, CV Mosby, 1987.

Management of Photographic Wastes in the Dental Office. Rochester, NY, Eastman Kodak Co, 1990.

Massler M, Schour I: Atlas of the Mouth, in Health and Disease, 2nd ed. Chicago, American Dental Association, 1982.

McCarthy FM: Medical Emergencies in Dentistry, 3rd ed. Philadelphia, WB Saunders, 1982.

McCarthy FM: Essentials of Safe Dentistry for the Medically Compromised Patient. Philadelphia, WB Saunders, 1989.

McLean JW: Cermet cements. JADA 120(1):43–47, 1990.

Miles DA, Williamson FF: Modified Radiographic Techniques and Special Patient Radiography. Chicago, ADAA, 1990.

Miles DA, VanDis ML, Jensen CW, et al: Radiographic Imaging for Dental Auxiliaries. Philadelphia, WB Saunders, 1989.

Miller CH: Implementing an office infection control program. The Dental Assistant 59(6):11–15, 1990.

Miller LM: Maintaining Esthetic Restorations. Houston, Reality Publishing, 1989.

Morris AC, Bohannan HM, Casullo DP: The Dental Specialties in General Practice. Philadelphia, WB Saunders, 1983.

Mount GJ: Restorations of eroded areas. JADA 120(1):31–40, 1990.

Moyers RE: Handbook of Orthodontics, 4th ed. Chicago, Year Book, 1988.

National Council Radiation Protection Report No. 35. Bethesda, MD, Health and Human Services Publications, Federal Drug Administration 84-8225, 1984.

National Research Council: Health Effects of Exposure to Low Levels of Ionizing Radiation. Washington, DC, National Academy Press, 1990.

Nester EW, Roberts CE, Lindstrom ME, et al: Microbiology, 3rd ed. Philadelphia, WB Saunders, 1983.

Nizel AE: Nutrition in Preventive Dentistry, 2nd ed. Philadelphia, WB Saunders, 1981.

Nortje CJ, Ferreira R, Parker EM: Intraoral Radiographic Technique. Chicago, ADAA, 1990.

OSHA: Hepatitis vaccine should be free to employees. ADA News 21(12):1, 1990.

Pedersen GW: Oral Surgery. Philadelphia, WB Saunders, 1988.

Perry DA, Beemsterboer P, Carranza FA: Techniques and Theory of Periodontal Instrumentation. Philadelphia, WB Saunders, 1990.

Peterson LJ, Ellis EE III, Hupp JR, et al: Contemporary Oral and Maxillofacial Surgery. St. Louis, CV Mosby, 1988.

Phillips RW: Skinner's Science of Dental Materials, 8th ed. Philadelphia, WB Saunders, 1982.

Phillips RW: Elements of Dental Materials for Dental Hygienists and Assistants, 4th ed. Philadelphia, WB Saunders, 1984.

Pincock JL: Orthognathic surgery. CDA Journal 19(2):31–39, 1991.

Pinkham JR, Casamassimo PS, Fields HW Jr, et al: Pediatric Dentistry: Infancy Through Adolescence. Philadelphia, WB Saunders, 1988.

Pontecorvo DA: Expanded duties: Results of ADAA's nationwide survey. The Dental Assistant 57:9–13, 1988.

Radiation Safety in Dental Radiography. Dental Radiography Series, Health Sciences Publication No. N-414. Rochester, NY, Eastman Kodak Co, 1990.

Reis-Schmidt T: Periodontal diagnosis and assessment. Dental Product Report 24(4):26–96, 1990.

Reis-Schmidt T: Periodontal therapy: Plaque control. Dental Product Report 25(3):28–94, 1991.

Reiter C: Assisting in periodontics: An overview. Dental Assisting July/August, 1983.

Reitz CD, Clark NP: The setting of vinyl polysiloxane and condensation silicone putties when mixed with gloved hands. JADA 116:371–374, 1988.

Roguszewski DH: Disinfecting impressions. Dental Product Report 25(3):62–70, 1991.

Rosenstiel SF, Land MF, Fujimoto J: Contemporary Fixed Prosthodontics. St. Louis, CV Mosby, 1988.

Runnells RR: Infection Control and Hazards Management. Fruit Heights, UT, IC Publications, 1989.

Schaefer ME: Infection control, OSHA and a hazards communication program. CDA Journal 18(8):53–58, 1990.

Stassler HE: Following manufacturer's directions ensures accurate impressions. Dental Office 10(5):5–6, 1991.

Sturdevant CM, Barton RE, Sockwell CL, et al: The Art and Science of Operative Dentistry, 2nd ed. St. Louis, CV Mosby, 1985.

The American Dental Association Regulatory Compliance Manual. Chicago, IL, The American Dental Association, 1990.

The glass ionomer cement. JADA 120(1):19–29, 1990.

Torres HO, Ehrlich A: Modern Dental Assisting, 4th ed. Philadelphia, WB Saunders, 1990.

Walton RE, Torabinejad M: Principles and Practice of Endodontics. Philadelphia, WB Saunders, 1989.

Waste handling and processing standards developing for dentistry. Dental Products Report 23:46–63, 1989.

Wei SHY: Pediatric Dentistry: Total Patient Care. Philadelphia, Lea & Febiger, 1988.

Index

Note: Page numbers in *italics* refer to illustrations.

A

Abbreviations, charting, 235
  for combinations of surfaces, 235
  for single surfaces, 235
  treatment, 235
Abscess, definition of, 99
  periapical, 99, *99*
  periodontal, 99, *99*
Abutment, definition of, 425
Acid attack, definition of, 83
Acid etch solution and gels, handling precautions for, 125
Acidosis, diabetic, as medical emergency, 138–139
Acquired immunodeficiency syndrome (AIDS), 96–97
  dental implications of, 97, *97*
  transmission of, 96
Acrylic resin, for custom trays, 401, 403–404
Activator light, for sealant curing, 458, *458*
Active life, of disinfectant solution, alteration of, 109–110
  definition of, 109
Acute dose, of radiation, 243
Acute necrotizing ulcerative gingivitis, 97. See also *Gingivitis.*
Aerobes, definition of, 92
AIDS. See *Acquired immunodeficiency syndrome (AIDS).*
Air compressor, central, 154
Air-water syringe, 153–154
  care of, 154
  in oral evacuation, 201
  uses of, 153
Ala, of nose, 42, *42*, 251
ALARA principle, radiography and, 244
Ala-tragus line, definition of, 251
Alcohol abuse, 314
Alginate impression(s), 283–293
  care of, *292*, 292–293
  diagnostic cast and, separation of, 300, *300*
  disinfection of, 114–115, *115*
  gypsum products and, 294–296
  instrumentation for, 284, *284*, 285
  laboratory plaster for, 294
  mandibular, 287–289

Alginate impression(s) *(Continued)*
  completion of, 292
  materials for, 283–284
    measuring of, 284, *284*
    mixing of, 287
    storing of, 284
    types of, 284
  maxillary, 290–291
  patient preparation for, 286
  preliminary, for crowns, 430
  taking of, qualified personnel for, 285
  tray selection and preparation for, 286
  wax-bite registration in, 293–294
Allergic reaction, as medical emergency, 138
Alloy(s), definition of, 375
  high noble, 423
  high-copper, 375
  mercury ratio to, 375, *376*
Alveolar canal, inferior, radiographic density of, 275
Alveolar crest, definition of, 46, *46*
Alveolar foramen, inferior, radiographic density of, 275
Alveolar mucosa, anatomic location of, 48
Alveolar nerve, anterior superior, anatomic distribution of, 40, *41*
  inferior, subdivision of, 42
  middle superior, anatomic distribution of, 40, *41*
  posterior superior, anatomic distribution of, 40, *41*
Alveolar process, 45–46, *46*
  alveolar socket of, 46
  cortical plate of, 46
  crest of, 46, *46*
  lamina dura of, 47
  trabeculae of, 46
Alveolar socket, definition of, 46
Alveolus, definition of, 46
Amalgam. See also *Alloy(s); Amalgam restoration(s).*
  advantages of, 373
  condensation of, 376–377
  definition of, 375
  disadvantages of, 373
  mixing of, procedure for, 382
  placement and condensing of, 382, *382*
  structure of, 375–377

Amalgam carrier, 170
  double-ended, 170, *171*
Amalgam carver, 171, *171*
Amalgam condenser, *171*
Amalgam file, *170*, 171
Amalgam knife, 171, *171*
Amalgam preparation bur, 182, *183*
Amalgam restoration(s), 373–384, *374*
  amalgam condensation in, 376–377
  capsule for, 376, *376*
  finishing and polishing of, 384, *384*
  preparation and placement of, 379–384
    amalgam mixing in, 382
    amalgam placement and condensing in, 382, *382*
    carving in, 383
    cavity preparation in, *380*, 380–381
    final steps of, 384
    instrumentation for, 379
    matrix and wedge placement in, 381
    occlusion adjustment in, 383, *383*
    sedative base and cavity liner placement in, 381, *381*
    Tofflemire retainer assembly in, 379–380
  pre-set tray for, 376, *376*
  terminology related to, 373–374
  trituration and, 375–376, *376*
Amalgamator, definition of, *127*, 376
American Dental Assistants Association, 15–16
  principles of ethics of, 16
Ampere, definition of, 246
Amphetamine abuse, 314
Anaerobes, definition of, 92
  facultative, 92
Analgesia, planes of, 316, 318
  relative (nitrous oxide–oxygen), 316–318
    administration of, 316, *317*
    advantages of, 316
    contraindications for, 316
    equipment care and, 318
    induction of, 317
    instrumentation for, 316
    recovery from, 318
Analgesics, definition of, 315
Anaphylactic shock, as medical emergency, 138